The Travel and Tropical Medicine Manual

THIRD EDITION

The Travel and Tropical Medicine Manual

ELAINE C. JONG, MD
Clinical Professor of Medicine
Founding Director, Travel and Tropical Medicine Service
Director, Student and Campus Health Service
University of Washington School of Medicine
Co-Director, Hall Health Travel Clinic
Hall Health Primary Care Center
Seattle, Washington

RUSSELL McMULLEN, MD
Associate Professor of Medicine
Co-Director, Travel and Tropical Medicine Service
University of Washington School of Medicine
Seattle, Washington

SAUNDERS
An Imprint of Elsevier

SAUNDERS
An Imprint of Elsevier

The Curtis Center
Independence Square West
Philadelphia, Pennsylvania 19106

THE TRAVEL AND TROPICAL MEDICINE MANUAL ISBN 0-7216-7678-2

NOTICE

Infectious disease is an ever-changing field. Standard safety precautions must be followed, but as new research and clinical experience broaden our knowledge, changes in treatment and drug therapy may become necessary or appropriate. Readers are advised to check the most current product information provided by the manufacturer of each drug to be administered to verify the recommended dose, the method and duration of administration, and contraindications. It is the responsibility of the licensed prescriber, relying on experience and knowledge of the patient, to determine dosages and the best treatment for each individual patient. Neither the publisher nor the author assumes any liability for any injury and/or damage to persons or property arising from this publication.

Previous editions copyrighted 1995, 1987

International Standard Book Number 0-7216-7678-2

Acquisitions Editor: Kimberly Murphy
Publishing Services Manager: Patricia Tannian
Project Manager: Melissa Mraz Lastarria
Book Design Manager: Gail Morey Hudson
Cover Design: Teresa Breckwoldt

GW/QWF
Printed in the United States of America.

Last digit is the print number: 9 8 7 6 5 4 3 2

Dedicated to

The Traveler—may there always be new frontiers

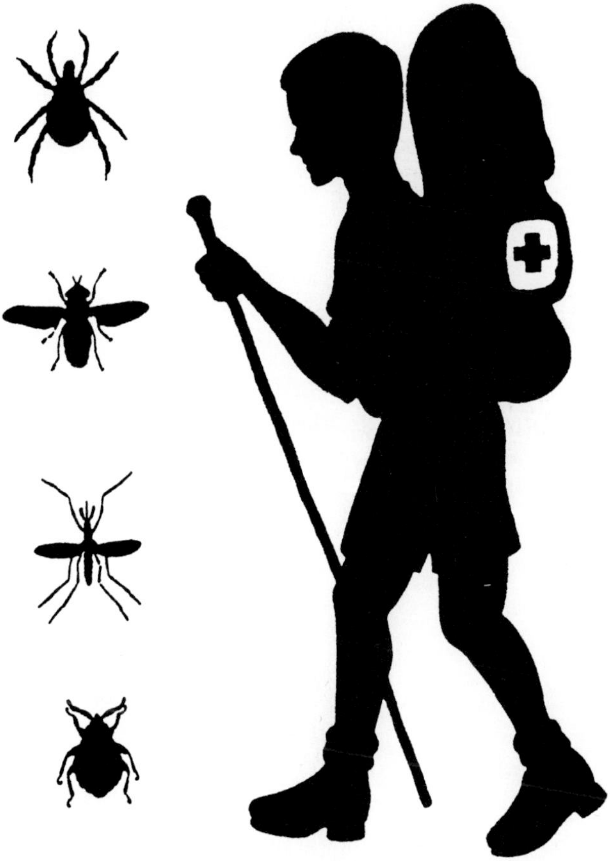

Contributors

SUSAN ANDERSON, MD
Travel, Tropical, and Wilderness Medicine Consultant
Clinical Assistant Professor of Medicine
Division of Infectious Disease and Geographic Medicine
Stanford University School of Medicine
Stanford, California

VERNON E. ANSDELL, MD, FRCP
Associate Clinical Professor
Department of Public Health Sciences and Epidemiology
University of Hawaii
Director, Tropical and Travel Medicine
Kaiser Permanente Hawaii
Honolulu, Hawaii

HOWARD D. BACKER, MD, MHP
Medical Consultant and Epidemiologist
Immunization Branch, Division of Communicable Disease Control
California Department of Health Services
Berkeley, California

AMY J. BEHRMAN, MD
Associate Professor, Emergency Medicine
Director, Occupational Medicine
University of Pennsylvania Health System
Philadelphia, Pennsylvania

THOMAS N. BETTES, MD, MPH
Director Clinical Services
American Airlines Medical Department
Fort Worth, Texas

STEPHEN A. BEZRUCHKA, MD, MPH
Senior Lecturer, Department of Health Sciences
University of Washington
Emergency Physician, Virginia Mason Hospital
Seattle, Washington

CONNIE CELUM, MD, MPH
Associate Professor, Medicine, University of Washington
Director, HIV Prevention Trials Unit, Harborview Medical Center
Seattle, Washington

MARTIN S. CETRON, MD
Adjunct Associate Professor, Medicine, Infectious Diseases
Emory University School of Medicine
Deputy Director and Chief Surveillance and Epidemiology
Division of Global Migration and Quarantine
Centers for Disease Control and Prevention
Atlanta, Georgia

ROY COLVEN, MD
Assistant Professor, Medicine (Dermatology), University of Washington
Section Head, Dermatology, Harborview Medical Center
Seattle, Washington

H. HUNTER HANDSFIELD, MD
Professor of Medicine, University of Washington
Director, Sexually Transmitted Disease Control Program
Public Health—Seattle & King County
Seattle, Washington

THOMAS R. HAWN, MD, PHD
Acting Instructor, Medicine, University of Washington Medical Center
Senior Research Scientist, Institute for Systems Biology
Seattle, Washington

CARTER D. HILL, MD, FACEP
Clinical Associate Professor, Medicine, University of Washington
Emergency Physician, Highline Community Hospital
Seattle, Washington

VITO R. IACOVIELLO, MD
Instructor, Medicine, Harvard Medical School
Boston, Massachusetts
Director, AIDS Related Services
Division of Infectious Diseases, Mount Auburn Hospital
Cambridge, Massachusetts

ELAINE C. JONG, MD
Clinical Professor of Medicine
Founding Director, Travel and Tropical Medicine Service
Director, Student and Campus Health Service
University of Washington, School of Medicine
Co-Director, Hall Health Travel Clinic, Hall Health Primary Care Center
Seattle, Washington

M. PATRICIA JOYCE, MD, FACP
Director, Medical Services, Infectious Disease
National Hansen's Disease Programs
Baton Rouge, Louisiana

KEVIN C. KAIN, MD, FRCPC
Director, Tropical Disease Unit
Professor of Medicine, University of Toronto
Toronto, Ontario, Canada

W. CONRAD LILES, MD, PhD
Associate Professor
Medicine, Division of Allergy and Infectious Diseases
University of Washington
Seattle, Washington

SHEILA M. MACKELL, MD
Staff Pediatrician, Flagstaff Medical Center
Flagstaff, Arizona
Pediatric Travel Medicine Consultant, Kaiser Permanente
Oakland, California

JEANNE M. MARRAZZO, MD, MPH
Assistant Professor, Medicine, University of Washington
Infectious Diseases, Harborview Medical Center
Medical Director, Seattle STD/HIV Prevention Training Center
Seattle, Washington

JONATHAN D. MAYER, PHD
Professor
Geography, Medicine, Family Medicine, Health Services
University of Washington
Seattle, Washington

RUSSELL MCMULLEN, MD
Associate Professor of Medicine
Co-Director, Travel and Tropical Medicine Service
University of Washington, School of Medicine
Seattle, Washington

ANNE C. MOORE, MD, PhD
Medical Epidemiologist, Division of Parasitic Diseases
Centers for Disease Control and Prevention
Atlanta, Georgia

CHARLES M. NOLAN, MD
Clinical Professor of Medicine, Department of Medicine
University of Washington
Director, Tuberculosis Control Program
Public Health—Seattle & King County
Seattle, Washington

THOMAS B. NUTMAN, MD
Head, Helminth Immunology Section
Head, Clinical Parasitology Unit
Laboratory of Parasitic Diseases, NIAID
National Institutes of Health
Bethesda, Maryland

CHRISTOPHER SANFORD, MD, DTM&H
Clinical Instructor
Department of Family Medicine
University of Washington, School of Medicine
Co-Director, Hall Health Travel Clinic, Hall Health Primary Care Center
Seattle, Washington

SUZANNE M. SHEPHERD, MD, DTM&H
Associate Professor, Emergency Medicine
Director of Education and Research
PENN Travel Medicine, University of Pennsylvania Health System
Philadelphia, Pennsylvania

WILLIAM H. SHOFF, MD, DTM&H
Associate Professor, Emergency Medicine
Director, PENN Travel Medicine
University of Pennsylvania Health System
Philadelphia, Pennsylvania

DAVID H. SPACH, MD
Associate Professor
Medicine, Division of Allergy and Infectious Diseases
University of Washington
Seattle, Washington

ALAN SPIRA, MD, DTM&H, FRSTM
Medical Director
The Travel Medicine Center
Beverly Hills, California

M. SEAN STROTHER, MD
Clinical Instructor
Department of Medicine, Division of Dermatology
University of Washington Medical Center
Seattle, Washington

MARI C. SULLIVAN, MSN, ARNP
American Embassy, Medical Unit
Bucharest, Romania
Medical Officer, Foreign Service
United States of America Department of State
Washington, DC

LARRY G. THIRSTRUP, MD
American Airlines Medical Department (Formerly)
Fort Worth, Texas

MATTHEW J. THOMPSON, MBChB, MPH, DTM&H
Assistant Professor, Department of Family Medicine
University of Washington
Seattle, Washington

WESLEY C. VAN VOORHIS, MD, PhD
Professor of Medicine
Department of Medicine, Division of Allergy and Infectious Diseases
University of Washington
Seattle, Washington

ABINASH VIRK, MD, DTMH
Assistant Professor, Division of Infectious Diseases
Mayo Graduate School of Medicine
Director, Travel and Geographic Medicine Clinic, Mayo Clinic
Rochester, Minnesota

NICHOLAS J. WHITE, OBE, DSc, MD, FRCP
Professor of Tropical Medicine
University of Oxford, United Kingdom
Mahidol University
Bangkok, Thailand

MARY E. WILSON, MD, FACP
Associate Professor, Medicine, Harvard Medical School
Boston, Massachusetts
Chief of Infectious Diseases, Mount Auburn Hospital
Cambridge, Massachusetts

Preface

Health care providers all over the world have experienced a dramatic increase in the quality and quantity of information available to them in real time brought about by modern communication technologies. The ability to rapidly share information and communicate with expert colleagues about challenging clinical scenarios has had a great impact on the practice of travel medicine. With the focus of travel and clinical tropical medicine on mobile populations and their exposures to ever-changing landscapes of communicable diseases and environmental hazards as they go from one place to another, one may ask how the printed publication of a basic manual on travel and tropical medicine will be relevant to the needs of today's clinicians, who have at their disposal a wealth of timely and frequently updated electronic information.

Based on the comments and helpful suggestions from readers of the first and second editions of the *Travel and Tropical Medicine Manual* (TTMM), it does appear that there is a continued and unique need for a practical, informed, and updated approach to travel and tropical medicine, written from a clinician's perspective and in the concise format offered by the TTMM. While the viewpoints expressed by the contributing authors are based on scientific medicine as currently practiced in developed countries, there is a common sensitivity to the practical aspects of health care delivery and decision-making in the field. The chapter authors have contributed their best efforts to introduce, summarize, and prioritize the medical approach to the clinical topics covered in each chapter in a succinct form, thus providing a framework for dealing with the abundance of information that streams in from electronic medical information systems.

While many clinicians new to travel and tropical medicine expressed how helpful it was to read the earlier editions of this manual from cover to cover for orientation, other experienced colleagues have commented how this manual has provided a comprehensive and convenient review of the field when studying for examinations or putting together educational presentations. Health care workers in the field have valued the portability of the manual and its emphasis on information for clinical application. So, while acknowledging the many excellent textbooks, references, and monographs currently available that go beyond the scope and depth possible in a manual, I hope that readers of this third edition of *The Travel and Tropical Medicine Manual* will continue to enjoy a familiar companion.

In closing, the inspiration and mentorship provided by the late Dr. Abraham Braude and by Drs. Seymour Klebanoff, Mickey Eisenberg, and Martin S. Wolfe over the past two decades are gratefully acknowledged.

In addition, the current edition of the TTMM would not have been possible without the dedicated assistance of John Martines and the enthusiasm of University of Washington colleagues, Drs. Christopher Sanford and Matthew J. Thompson.

Elaine C. Jong, MD
Seattle, Washington

Contents

SECTION III
FEVER

SECTION IV
DIARRHEA

SECTION V
SKIN LESIONS

SECTION VI
SEXUALLY TRANSMITTED DISEASES

SECTION VII
WORMS

The Travel and Tropical Medicine Manual

SECTION I

PRE-TRAVEL ADVICE

CHAPTER 1

Health Concerns of International Travelers

Elaine C. Jong

A new medical specialty, travel medicine, emerged in the 1980s in response to increasing geographic movements of people, going from relatively sanitary and industrialized environments of North America to destinations with the challenges of health standards and living conditions characteristic of developing economies and tropical environments. As Americans continue to pursue their exploration of the world for recreational, educational, business, religious, and humanitarian purposes, American physicians and other health care providers need to know how to counsel their traveling patients with regard to immunizations, malaria, diarrhea, and a wide variety of health issues.

The Centers for Disease Control and Prevention (CDC) in Atlanta, Georgia, the World Health Organization (WHO), other health agencies, and public and private information services issue periodic guidelines and health information for international travel. However, given that approximately 40 million Americans work or travel abroad each year, the guidelines are by necessity very general and may not be directly applicable to the individual traveler. In fact, a recent CDC guide for malaria prevention was issued with the statement, "These revised recommendations place increased emphasis on *individualized recommendations* for travelers, and increased responsibility on individual travelers and their physicians." International travelers should seek medical advice 4 to 6 weeks in advance of their departure date. *This allows adequate time for immunizations to be scheduled, for advice and prescriptions to be given, and for special information to be obtained when needed.*

The medical approach to travel becomes even more complex when the itinerary encompasses several countries at different stages of development, when the traveler has drug allergies or underlying chronic medical conditions, or when the traveler plans a long-term trip lasting months to years. Such travelers may need to start 3 or more months in advance of anticipated trip departure to complete vaccine series and other health documentation needed for issuance of visas, and for appropriate travel arrangements. Table 1-1 summarizes the steps for pretravel medical preparation.

All travelers should be advised to assemble the information listed in Table 1-2 in a concise and clearly written form to carry with them. In addition, travelers should carry a supply of medications adequate to last the duration of the trip and an extra pair of eyeglasses with a copy of the prescription for the corrective lenses.

Table 1-1
Pretravel Medical Recommendations

1. Consult personal physician, local Public Health Department, or travel clinic about recommendations for immunizations and malaria chemoprophylaxis after selection of the travel itinerary, but preferably 4 to 6 weeks in advance of departure.
2. Prepare a Traveler's Health History (Table 1-2) and the Traveler's Medical Kit (Table 1-6).
3. Carry a telephone credit card that can be used for international telephone calls, or make sure that the friends or relatives listed in the health history would accept an international collect call in case of an emergency.
4. Make sure to have the telephone number of your personal physician, including office and after-hours numbers, and a fax number if available. A business card attached to the Traveler's Health History is a handy way to carry this information.
5. Check medical insurance policy or health plan for coverage for illness or accidents occurring outside the United States.
6. Specifically inquire if the regular insurance policy or health plan will cover emergency medical evacuation by an air ambulance.
7. Arrange for additional medical insurance coverage or for a line of credit as necessary for a medical emergency situation.

Table 1-2
Traveler's Health History

International travelers should assemble the following information in a concise and clearly written form to carry with them:

1. An up-to-date immunization record (preferably the *International Certificates of Vaccination*).
2. A list of current medications by both trade name and generic name, as well as the actual dose.
3. A list of all medical problems, such as hypertension, diabetes, asthma, and heart disease (cardiac patients should carry a copy of the most recent electrocardiogram).
4. A list of known drug allergies.
5. ABO blood type and Rh factor type.
6. Name and telephone number (and telefax number, if available) of his or her regular doctor.
7. Name and telephone number of the closest relative or friend in the United States who might assist if the traveler incurs serious illness while out of the country.

IMMUNIZATIONS FOR TRAVEL

International travel exposes people to infectious diseases that are infrequently seen in the United States because of a generally high standard of sanitation and mandatory immunization practices. For example, adult travelers have acquired measles and chickenpox on trips abroad. Paralytic polio is transmitted outside the Western Hemisphere in developing countries where conditions favor oral-fecal transmission, and in other countries where routine immunizations do not reach a high level of coverage among susceptible populations. Thus all travelers should be questioned about their status with regard to the routine immunizations of childhood—tetanus, diphtheria, measles, mumps, rubella, and polio—and a primary series or booster doses of the vaccines should be given as appropriate. Vaccines against *Haemophilus influenzae* b, hepatitis B, varicella, and pneumococcal disease were added to the recommended childhood immunizations in the 1990s. The vaccines against *H. influenzae* b and measles are especially important for young infants going abroad, and the hepatitis B vaccine is important for children on prolonged visits to countries where the disease is endemic. The medical concerns for traveling children are addressed in Chapter 11.

All vaccinations administered to travelers should be recorded in a copy of the yellow booklet *International Certificates of Vaccination,* which is recognized by the World Health Organization (WHO). This record should be kept in a safe place with the passport, since it becomes a lifelong immunization record. There is a special page for validation of the yellow fever vaccine, which must be done in an official vaccination center, as well as additional pages to record the other vaccines.

Up-to-date information on areas where cholera and yellow fever are reported is best obtained from the CDC (www.cdc.gov/travel) or the WHO (www.who.org) web sites. The smallpox and cholera vaccines are no longer required for international travel according to WHO recommendations. Owing to relatively limited supplies and the fact that it must be given within 1 hour after reconstitution of the vaccine, the yellow fever vaccine is available only from official vaccination centers registered by the Department of Public Health in each state.

Some confusion exists over the difference between *required* vaccinations and *recommended* vaccinations. The CDC issues annual guidelines in its manual *Health Information for International Travel,* in which there is a listing, country by country, of vaccines required for entry. This document can be obtained in printed form for a fee from the Public Health Foundation (www.publichealthfoundation.org), or can be consulted through the CDC web site. Someone calling a travel clinic to ask which shots are required for a trip to Kenya or Venezuela, for instance, will be told by a person consulting the manual that yellow fever vaccine is not required for a traveler arriving from North America. Yet, if one refers to maps showing where yellow fever is endemic, one can see that Kenya and Venezuela both lie within the endemic zones. Thus yellow fever vaccine might be *recommended* to a traveler to those countries even though the vaccine is not a requirement for entry.

Other vaccines may be recommended to travelers, depending on their destinations, degree of rural exposure during travel, eating habits, purpose of the trip, and state of health. In this group are the typhoid fever vaccine, meningococcal vaccine, rabies vaccine, plague vaccine, and immune serum globulin (gamma globulin) or vaccine for hepatitis A protection. Certain travelers, such as health care workers, missionaries, Peace Corps volunteers, students, and any person likely to have household or sexual contact with residents in tropical or developing countries should consider being vaccinated for hepatitis B. Other travelers who are going to live or work in the People's Republic of China and other Asian countries need to consider Japanese encephalitis B vaccine. Details of travel immunizations are given in Chapter 4.

MALARIA

In addition to travel immunizations, a major consideration for international travelers is whether their travel will take them to an area where malaria is transmitted. Malaria has a worldwide distribution in tropical

Table 1-3
Recommendations to Avoid Mosquito Bites

1. Remain in well-screened areas, especially during the hours between dusk and dawn.
2. Sleep under mosquito netting if the room is unscreened.
3. Wear clothing that adequately covers the arms and legs when outdoors.
4. Apply mosquito repellent to exposed areas of skin when outdoors, and wear permethrin-treated outer clothing. The most effective mosquito repellents for application to skin surfaces contain *N,N*-diethyl-3-methylbenzamide or *N,N*-diethyl-m-tolazamide (DEET), which is also effective against biting flies, chiggers, fleas, and ticks. Clothing, as well as mosquito netting, can be sprayed with products containing permethrin. Permethrin does not repel insects but works as a contact insecticide that leads to the death of the insect. (See Table 1-4.)

and subtropical areas. It is reemerging in areas once considered to be free from risk. Data derived from CDC statistics show that during the 1980s, the greatest number of Americans with malaria acquired the infection in Africa; while fewer contracted malaria in Asia, South America, Central America, and Mexico, the risk in these other areas remained significant. In the 1990s, malaria transmission in all these regions continued to be a serious problem for the traveler, especially because of the emergence of new drug-resistant strains in areas where the use of chloroquine phosphate was once highly effective in malaria prevention against all malaria species.

Malaria is a protozoan parasite transmitted to humans by biting female anopheline mosquitoes. Chemoprophylaxis, or the taking of drugs to prevent clinical attacks of malaria, is recommended to most travelers going to malarious areas. The standard chemoprophylactic regimens are discussed in Chapter 5. In some areas of Africa, South America, Asia, and the South Pacific, infections with chloroquine-resistant *Plasmodium falciparum* malaria (CRPF) are a risk to travelers. Updated information on the risk of CRPF is published periodically in the CDC publication *Morbidity and Mortality Weekly Report*. Drugs useful in the prevention of chloroquine-resistant malaria include mefloquine (Larium), Doxycycline (Doryx, Vibramycin), and atovaquone/proguanil (Malarone). These and other antimalarial drugs are discussed in Chapters 5 and 17.

Since the risk of infection is related to the number of bites sustained, and since current malaria chemoprophylaxis regimens are not completely protective, all travelers should follow certain simple precautions when visiting or staying in malarious areas (Tables 1-3 and 1-4). In addition to preventing bites from mosquitoes spreading malaria, these precautions help the traveler avoid bites from other mosquito species and insects that spread a variety of diseases in tropical and subtropical areas, for which there are no prophylactic drugs or vaccines (e.g., dengue fever, hemorrhagic fever, several forms of encephalitis, leishmaniasis, trypanosomiasis, filariasis).

DIARRHEA

Between 30% and 60% of travelers to tropical countries are affected by "traveler's diarrhea." This illness is characterized by sudden onset of four to five bowel movements of watery diarrhea per day, sometimes accompa-

Table 1-4
Insect Repellents and Insecticides*

Examples of Insect Repellents Containing DEET for Skin Application

Ultrathon Insect Repellent: 35% DEET in polymer formulation, up to 12 hr protection against mosquitoes; also effective against ticks, biting flies, chiggers, fleas, gnats (distributed by Amway and Travel Medicine Inc, Northampton, MA).

DEET Plus Insect Repellent: 17.5% DEET with 2.5% R-326, apply every 4 hr for mosquitoes, every 8 hr for biting flies (Sawyer Products, Safety Harbor, FL 34695-0188).

Controlled Release DEET Formula: 20% DEET in "submicron encapsulation" protein formulation that provides sustained release while limiting the skin's exposure to DEET (Sawyer Products, Safety Harbor, FL.)

Examples of Permethrin-Containing Insecticides for Application to External Clothing and Mosquito Nets (see Fig. 1-1)

Permethrin for Clothing Tick Repellent: Contains permethrin in a non-aerosol pump spray can; repels ticks, chiggers, mosquitoes, and other bugs (Sawyer Products, Safety Harbor, FL 34695-0188). One application lasts 4 weeks or more.

PermaKill Solution: 13.3% permethrin liquid concentrate supplied in 8-oz bottle, can be diluted (⅓ oz permethrin concentrate in 16 oz water) to be used with a manual pump spray bottle; or diluted 2 oz in 1½ cups of water to be used to impregnate outer clothing, mosquito nets, and curtains (Sawyer Products, Safety Harbor, FL 34695-0188). Permethrin impregnation of garments or mosquito netting will achieve protection for up to 1 year or good for 30 launderings.

*Brand names are given for identification purposes only and do not constitute an endorsement.

nied by abdominal cramps, malaise, nausea, and vomiting. An attack typically lasts 3 to 6 days.

The pathogens causing gastrointestinal disease are acquired mostly through fecal-oral contamination, and preventive strategies to avoid illness include careful selection of food and water. Adequate means for purification of water vary depending on the water source. Bringing water to a boil is probably the most reliable way to kill pathogens up to 20,000 feet above sea level. Water purification tablets are convenient and commercially available, and are almost as effective as boiling when the water is at 20° C (68° F); the water-tablet mixture is shaken or stirred every 5 minutes for a total duration of 30 minutes. For a summary of commonly used chemical methods for water purification, see Table 1-5. Small water purification filters have become a popular and reasonably priced alternative used by many travelers; the devices using iodine-resin technology have proved to be effective against the broadest range of pathogens. Water purification is discussed in detail in Chapter 7.

Owing to widespread publicity in the lay press, many travelers want to know more about the use of antibiotic capsules or tablets to prevent diarrhea while traveling. A "Traveler's Diarrhea Consensus Development Panel," convened by the National Institutes of Health in January 1985, advised against using drugs as a preventive measure for traveler's diarrhea; the chief objections cited were the occurrence of undesirable side effects and the potential for allergic reactions. The panel acknowledged

How to Apply Permethrin to your Clothing

Use permethrin (Permanone®) to treat clothing, mosquito netting, or tent fabric.
Do not apply permethrin on your skin.

Spraying–Lay out the clothing to be sprayed. For shirts and trousers, spray the front of each garment for 60-90 seconds. Use a slow sweeping motion, holding the can about 12 inches from the fabric. Spray inside cuffs. Turn the garment(s) over and repeat. For socks and bandanas, spray for 30 seconds per side. The fabric should be slightly damp. Hang up to dry. You'll need 1/2 to 2/3 of a can to treat a shirt and trousers. The sprayed garments, even after multiple launderings, will kill mosquitoes and ticks for about six weeks. This is because permethrin binds tightly to the fabric.

All fabrics, even your best silk shirt, can be treated without leaving an odor or a stain. Permethrin is also safe to humans. Very little is absorbed through the skin and even these small amounts are rapidly neutralized by the body. Minor rashes only have been reported from skin contact.

Impregnating–Soaking protective clothing or mosquito netting in a permethrin solution is a method used to achieve longer protection. Follow the directions below using the 4 Week Tick Killer 13.3% solution. Treated fabric will kill insects for several months.

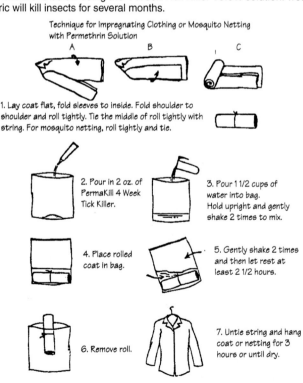

Technique for Impregnating Clothing or Mosquito Netting with Permethrin Solution

1. Lay coat flat, fold sleeves to inside. Fold shoulder to shoulder and roll tightly. Tie the middle of roll tightly with string. For mosquito netting, roll tightly and tie.
2. Pour in 2 oz. of PermaKill 4 Week Tick Killer.
3. Pour 1 1/2 cups of water into bag. Hold upright and gently shake 2 times to mix.
4. Place rolled coat in bag.
5. Gently shake 2 times and then let rest at least 2 1/2 hours.
6. Remove roll.
7. Untie string and hang coat or netting for 3 hours or until dry.

Fig. 1-1 How to apply permethrin to your clothing. (Courtesy of Rose SR: *International Travel Health Guide,* Northampton, MA, 1993, Travel Medicine.)

Table 1-5
Methods for Purification of Water*

Method	Brand name	Quantity to be added to 1 quart or 1 liter of water
Iodine compound tablets†	Potable Aqua, Coughlins	Two tablets are added to water at 20° C, and the mixture is agitated every 5 minutes for a total of 30 minutes.
Chlorine solution, 2%-4%	(Common laundry bleach)	Two to four drops are added to water at 20° C, and after mixing, the solution is kept for 30 minutes before drinking.
Iodine solution†	(2% tincture of iodine)	Five to ten drops of iodine are added to water at 20° C, and after mixing, the solution is kept for 30 minutes before drinking.
Heat		Water is heated to above 65° C for at least 3 minutes. (At 20,000 ft altitude or 6000 m, water boils at 70° C.)

*The methods presented here are sufficient to kill *Giardia* cysts in most situations. Heat is the best method when tested in a laboratory situation. (See Chapter 7 for more detailed information.)
†Iodine-containing compounds should be used with caution during pregnancy.

that for the short-term traveler, the risk of traveler's diarrhea might be decreased by daily prophylactic doses of bismuth subsalycylate (Pepto-Bismol), or even daily doses of antibiotics. This subject is discussed in detail in Chapter 6.

Medical Emergencies During Travel

Emergency medical care abroad is not a subject likely to be broached by the average travel agent, for fear of alarming the potential traveler. Yet American travelers, especially those planning long-term travel (trips of 3 weeks or longer), the very young and the very old, and those with special medical conditions (cardiac, pulmonary, gastrointestinal, or hematologic problems; pregnancy; human immunodeficiency virus [HIV] infection; organ transplant) need to have a plan in case the need for emergency medical care arises. Even the young traveler in perfect health can break a leg, be involved in a motor vehicle accident, or be bitten by a rabid dog.

People planning trips to exotic places, but who will stay in urban, first-class hotels, may have relatively easy access to English-speaking physicians with Western-style biomedical training. However, many places where modern tourists go are far from English-speaking medical practitioners and Western-style hospitals. Medications for treatment of certain infections and special medical conditions may not be available under any circumstances. Thus, for such travelers, pretravel counseling, preparation of the traveler's medical kit, and a medical emergency evacuation plan are of great importance.

Finding a Physician in a Foreign Country

For travelers with specific medical conditions, referral to friends or colleagues in foreign countries can often be obtained before the trip from the regular U.S. physician.

American embassies often have lists of English-speaking physicians. The U.S. State Department has a 24-hour emergency number (see Appendix) for overseas citizens. University or other teaching hospitals can be relied on to provide good-quality care and are likely to have staff members who speak English.

Travelers can join the International Association for Medical Assistance to Travelers (IAMAT) before departure. Among its many services, this nonprofit organization provides lists of English-speaking physicians in most countries (see Appendix).

Emergency Information Needed

The Traveler's Health History (Table 1-2) and the *International Certificates of Vaccination* should be carried with the passport at all times. Although a medical-alert bracelet or necklace (available from pharmacies or by mail; see Appendix) is recommended to travelers, people offering assistance in some countries may not recognize the significance of, or even look for, such identification.

Payment for Services

Coverage for emergency medical services abroad should be verified with the regular insurance company or health care plan before the trip. Medicare will not cover services provided in foreign countries, with the exception of an urgent problem arising en route from the United States to Alaska that requires medical treatment in Canada. Several companies specializing in medical insurance for travelers are listed in the Appendix.

Payment for medical services abroad is customarily due when care is given, but travelers will need to save the receipts for reimbursement by their health coverage plan. Insurance companies are unlikely to pay for procedures or treatments that are experimental or not available in the United States.

Emergency Medical Care En Route

At the time of writing, most commercial airplanes carry a minimum of first-aid supplies. Generally, oxygen is available only in the event of cabin decompression, although some airlines carry small portable tanks for medical emergencies. Patients with chronic pulmonary conditions requiring supplemental oxygen must make arrangements at the time of reservation for supplies of in-flight portable oxygen tanks. Advanced life-support equipment and drugs may not be available for passengers with acute cardiac or pulmonary emergencies, although some aircraft do carry portable cardiac defibrillators. In the event of a serious medical emergency that occurs during flight, most commercial aircraft will reroute and land at the closest commercial airport. Chapter 2 presents further details of air carrier health issues.

Commercial international cruise ship lines carrying fee-paying passengers are required by maritime law to have a physician on board at sea. The qualifications of the ship's physicians and the availability of advanced life-support equipment and drugs may vary from line to line, so specific inquiries should be made.

Emergency Evacuation Home

Some commercial airlines will allow passage of a seriously ill person back to the United States only when that person is accompanied by a licensed physician. Payment of the physician and purchase of his or her round-trip airfare must be provided in such cases.

In other cases, emergency evacuation home must proceed by way of specially equipped aircraft (helicopters and fixed-wing aircraft), which usually carry their own teams of medical personnel, including physicians and nurses. Costs for such evacuations can run to tens of thousands of dollars, depending on geographic conditions and medical needs.

Emergency evacuation insurance is available; however, prospective subscribers need to read the terms carefully, since some plans provide only for evacuation to the nearest regional medical center, not for transport back to a medical facility in the traveler's home country. Given that very ill people would prefer to receive a customary standard of care, evacuation of a patient to a foreign medical center, where English may be spoken as a second language and where medical protocols are different, may not be as satisfactory as evacuation back to the United States. Names and addresses of organizations arranging international emergency transport services for their members are given in the Appendix.

Emergency Blood Transfusion

The traveler's blood type, if known, should be listed in the Traveler's Health History and/or in the space provided in the *International Certificates of Vaccination* booklet. If an urgent blood transfusion becomes necessary, however, and the blood type is unknown, the traveler's blood can be quickly typed and then tested against the donor's blood. However, in certain parts of the world, certain blood types may not be easily obtainable. For instance, in the People's Republic of China, the predominant blood type is A-positive among the resident population.

Travelers with bleeding problems or tendencies (e.g., those on anticoagulation therapy or those with a history of bleeding peptic ulcers) should probably get information from their local blood bank before they leave about resources in the countries to be visited.

WILDERNESS AND ADVENTURE TRAVEL

The more remote from access to established medical care facilities, the more the traveler has to anticipate self-care or peer-care for medical problems that might occur. Many of the medical concerns arising during adventure travel are covered throughout this book. However, the treatment of serious injuries and trauma in the wilderness and the approach to survival skills are beyond the scope of this book. Specific preparation and equipment may be needed for survival in wilderness settings or extreme environments.

The adventure or expedition traveler planning a remote and/or challenging route is advised to obtain accurate information regarding the physical difficulty and inherent environmental risks associated with the trip itinerary, to carefully review the qualifications and personalities of the trip leader(s) and fellow adventurers, to query the dietary arrangements for the trip, and to verify the possibilities for emergency evacuation. In addition, adventure travelers should acquire advanced first aid skills and prepare themselves to be in optimal physical condition before departure. Further information may be obtained from consulting some of the references listed at the end of the chapter, as well as by contacting The Wilderness Medical Society (see Appendix).

THE TRAVELER'S MEDICAL KIT

Table 1-6 presents recommendations for a traveler's medical kit for an average international trip. Depending on geographic locations, types of activities planned, and underlying health, the traveler may augment the kit with regular prescription medications, medication for high-altitude sickness, antifungal preparations, pesticide preparations for ectoparasites, and additional antiparasitic drugs. Pulmonary patients may need to make arrangements for portable oxygen supplies and even oxygen concentrator machines, and peritoneal dialysis patients may travel with dialysate fluids and accessories, and need advance reservations for access to dialysis services at destination (see Chapter 14).

Prescription Medications

Travelers should not pack their entire supply of prescription medications into checked luggage, since the baggage could be lost in transit. At least a few days' supply of necessary medications should be taken in hand-held luggage. Preferably, the entire supply of usual prescription medications, enough to last the whole trip, should be taken in the hand-held luggage.

SUMMARY OF CONSIDERATIONS FOR HEALTH AND TRAVEL

Travelers need to be counseled about common medical problems of international travel that may be related to the mode of transportation, changes in altitude, changes in time zones, increased exposure to sun, taking of new drugs, insect bites, and changes in climate and humidity (Chapters 2, 8, 9, and 10). When the traveler has an underlying medical condition, travel arrangements and health recommendations become increasingly important (Chapter 14). Travelers with HIV infection need thoughtful pretravel counseling on vaccines, potential drug interactions, geographic infectious disease hazards, and access to medical care during travel (Chapter 13).

Contingency plans for a medical emergency should be discussed openly and the need for special travel insurance coverage considered with all travelers regardless of underlying health. Even a healthy young traveler is at risk for contracting a serious illness or accidental injury during travel.

It is important to know the female traveler's reproductive plans or whether she is pregnant. The physical demands and geographic factors of travel may influence the pregnancy. Additionally, certain required or recommended vaccines may be contraindicated, as may some drugs used for malaria chemoprophylaxis or for the relief of common traveler's ailments (Chapter 12).

If an extended stay outside the United States is anticipated (6 months or more), even generally healthy persons should have a routine physical examination, including an evaluation of tuberculosis status (skin test or screening chest x-ray study), routine screening laboratory tests, and blood typing. The long-term traveler should also have a complete dental examination. Sometimes the form and content of the pretravel medical evaluation will be dictated by the requirements of the sponsoring employer or agency, the insurance carrier, or even the application for foreign resident status or foreign work permits. Requests from foreign governments for pretravel syphilis serology, HIV serology, examination of a stool specimen for ova and parasites, and chest x-ray study are not uncommon when Americans apply for foreign residency (Chapter 15).

Table 1-6
The Traveler's Personal Medical Kit*[†]

Below are listed some of the suggested items for the traveler's personal medical kit. Not all of these items are necessary or appropriate for every traveler: items should be selected based on the style of travel and destination(s).

Prescription Items*

Antibiotics, General: Antibiotics may be useful for travelers at risk for skin infections, upper respiratory infections (URIs), and/or urinary tract infections (UTIs), as well as for treatment of traveler's diarrhea (TD).

Skin infections:

Cephalexin, (or cephradine) 500-mg capsule. One PO q6h × 7 days

Mupirocin 2% *(Bactroban)* topical antibiotic ointment. 15-g tube or 1-g foil packets. Apply to infected skin lesions three times a day.

Upper respiratory tract infections:

Trimethoprim 160-mg/sulfamethoxazole 800-mg double-strength tablet (TMP/SMX DS). One PO q12h × 7 days; or

Doxycycline, 100 mg capsule. One PO q12h × 7 days; or

Azithromycin, 250-mg tablet. Two PO first dose, followed by one POq 24 h × 4 additional days.

Urinary tract infections (uncomplicated):

TMP/SMX DS tablet: One PO q12h × 3 days; or

Norfloxacin, 400-mg tablet: One PO q12h × 3 days.

Multipurpose Antibiotics: These would provide empiric coverage for skin infections, URI, and UTI. (Note that ciprofloxacin and levofloxacin are commonly used for treatment of traveler's diarrhea as well):

Amoxicillin 875 mg plus clavulanate 125 mg tablet (*Augmentin* 875 mg). One PO q12h × 3-7 days; or

Ciprofloxacin *(Cipro)*, 500 mg tablet. One PO q12h × 3-7 days; or

Levofloxacin *(Levoquin)*, 500 mg tablet. One PO q24h × 3-7 days.

Allergic Reactions: (To bee, wasp, yellow jacket, or hornet stings; food, etc.)

EpiPen emergency injection of epinephrine:

Use according to package directions for severe reaction to bee sting or for other allergic reaction causing shortness of breath or wheezing; or swelling of the lips, eyes, throat, or severe hives. This will give short-acting relief. As soon as the afflicted person can swallow, give them *Benadryl* tablets as directed below.

Benadryl (diphenhydramine), 25-mg tablet:

Take two tablets by mouth immediately, then one to two tabs q6h × 2 days following an allergic reaction. Use *Benadryl* alone for mild to moderate allergic skin reactions and itching, and take Benadryl following the use of the *EpiPen.*

Medrol DosePack (methylprednisolone):

For use with severe and persistent allergic reactions or skin rashes. Follow the instructions for the tapering dose schedule in the packet. May be required in addition to Benadryl for severe allergic reactions.

Ventolin (albuterol) inhaler (MDI, multidose inhaler):

Use for asthma attacks or for allergic reactions that cause persistent wheezing. Two puffs 2 minutes apart, each inhaled as deeply as possible into the lungs. Do this four times a day.

Cough Suppressant: A small bottle of prescription cough syrup or a few tablets of codeine-containing medication (*Tylenol #3* tablets will serve this purpose, as well as that of medication for severe headache or pain).

*Dosage information applies to adults in good health without contraindications to the given drug.
[†]Trademark names are provided for identification only and do not constitute an endorsement.

Continued

Table 1-6—cont'd
The Traveler's Personal Medical Kit

Diarrhea Treatment: An antimotility drug such as loperamide *(Imodium)* plus an antibiotic (e.g., trimethoprim/sulfamethoxazole, ciprofloxacin, levofloxacin, azithromycin) may be prescribed for self-treatment (see Chapter 6).

High-Altitude Illness: Acetazolamide *(Diamox)* may be prescribed for prophylaxis of high-altitude illness for high-altitude destinations (see Chapter 9).

Jet Lag: In some cases, a short-acting sleeping medication is helpful in treating sleeping problems associated with jet lag (see Table 8-2).

Malaria Pills: As the malaria situation in many countries continues to change, malaria chemoprophylaxis changes as well. Updated information on the malaria situation for specific destination(s) needs to be carefully reviewed, and appropriate medications prescribed (see Tables 5-3 and 5-4).

Motion Sickness: Travelers who experience motion sickness may be prescribed a medication for this (see Table 8-4).

Nausea and Vomiting: *Compazine* (prochloperazine), 25-mg rectal suppository. This may be helpful when oral medications cannot be tolerated and an injectable antiemetic is not available.

Pain Relief: A modest supply of prescriptive pain medication may be needed for headache, toothache, or musculoskeletal injury.

Tylenol #3 (acetaminophen with 30 mg codeine) tablets: one to two tablets PO q4-6h prn severe headache or pain; or

Dilaudid (hydromorphone), 2-mg tablets: one to two tablets PO q4h for relief of severe pain (useful for people allergic or intolerant to codeine).

Nonprescription Items

Aspirin, acetaminophen *(Tylenol)*, ibuprofen *(Advil, Nuprin)*, or naproxen *(Aleve)*: For general relief of minor aches and pains or headache.

Antibiotic Ointment: (*Neosporin* or Bacitracin) for topical application on minor cuts and abrasions.

Antifungal Powder or Cream: For travelers prone to athletes' foot and/or other fungal skin problems.

Antifungal Vaginal Cream or Troches: For women prone to yeast vaginitis associated with changes in climate or after antibiotic use.

Decongestant Tablets *(Actifed, Sudafed, Contac, etc.)*: For nasal congestion due to colds, allergies, or water sports.

Diarrhea Prevention: Bismuth subsalicylate *(PeptoBismol)* tablets may be taken, two tablets qid every day of the trip to prevent traveler's diarrhea (see Table 6-3).

Hydrocortisone 1% Cream: For topical relief of itching due to insect bites or sunburn.

Laxative: For relief of "traveler's constipation" due to changes in diet and schedule. Patients with a history of this problem may need to take a fiber supplement and/or a stool softener.

Oral Rehydration Solution: *WHO-ORS* (Jianas Brothers, Kansas City, MO) or *CeraLyte* (Jessup, MD.): packets of balanced oral rehydration salts and sugar to be mixed in purified water safe for drinking for fluid replacement and rehydration during severe diarrhea (see Table 6-4).

Diseases spread by sexual and intimate contact should also be discussed with the international traveler, especially those going abroad for an extended stay. In addition to the sexually transmitted diseases (STDs) frequently seen in northern temperate climates (gonorrhea, syphilis, chlamydia, hepatitis B, and infection with herpes simplex virus and HIV), lymphogranuloma venereum, chancroid, and granuloma inguinale are a risk in many tropical and developing countries (Chapters 36 through 39).

Table 1-6—cont'd
The Traveler's Personal Medical Kit

Throat Lozenges: For relief of throat irritation due to air pollution or upper respiratory infection.
General Health and First Aid Supplies
Antiseptic Solution: Topical solution for cleansing of minor cuts and abrasions (*Hibiclens*).
Bandages: Adhesive bandage strips with sterile pad *(BandAids)*, 4 × 4-inch sterile gauze pads 2-inch roll gauze dressing.
Elastic Bandage: For minor sprains *(Ace wrap)*.
Eyeglasses: If corrective lenses are used, bring an extra pair of eyeglasses along.
Case (Waterproof): To hold medications and supplies.
Condoms (Latex): For prevention of sexually transmitted diseases.
Insect Repellent (with DEET): For topical application to exposed areas of skin (see Tables 1-3, 1-4).
Insecticide Spray (with Permethrin): For application to external clothing, mosquito nets, curtains, etc. (see Tables 1-3, 1-4).
Moleskin: For prevention of blisters on feet.
Safety Pins: The rustproof baby diaper pin types are useful for all kinds of emergency repairs, pinning room curtains shut, hanging laundry on wire hangers, etc.
Sanitary Supplies (Menstruating Women): Tampons, sanitary napkins (these may not be readily available in tropical and developing parts of the world).
Scissors: For general use, if not included in pocket knife.‡
Swiss Army Knife (or similar): An all-purpose gadget, especially useful if tweezers and scissors are included.‡
Sunglasses: With UV light protective lenses.
Sunscreen: Any brand with sun protective factor (SPF) sufficient to protect against UV-A and UV-B.
Tape, Adhesive: For first aid wound care.
Tape, Duct: For general repairs, creating splints, etc.
Tick Pliers: For participants in outdoor activities; to remove ticks safely and completely (see Fig. 1-2).
Toilet Paper: Often not available in public rest facilities when one is in desperate need (buy a compact roll, available in sporting supply stores).
Towelettes (Premoistened): For cleaning hands.
Thermometer, Oral: Very important for assessment of illness while traveling.
Venom Extractor Pump: To extract venom from venomous insect stings and snake bites (see Fig. 1-3).
Water Disinfection Chemicals: See Table 1-5.
Water Disinfection Device, Portable: See Table 7-6.

‡As a result of heightened airline security concerns, pocket knives, scissors with pointed tips, nail files with pointed ends, box cutters, and all sharp implements must be transported in the checked baggage; such implements in carry-on bags will be confiscated at airport security checkpoints for boarding passengers.

The prevalence of HIV infection is of course many times higher than the number of acquired immunodeficiency syndrome (AIDS) cases reported, and the infection is present in all countries. In Africa and Asia, heterosexual intercourse is a major mode of transmission of HIV. Recent reports suggest that sexual contact with residents of developing countries occurs with surprising frequency among tourists, business travelers, and expatriate workers. International travelers need to be warned of the risk of sexual contact with strangers, regardless of sexual orientation, and

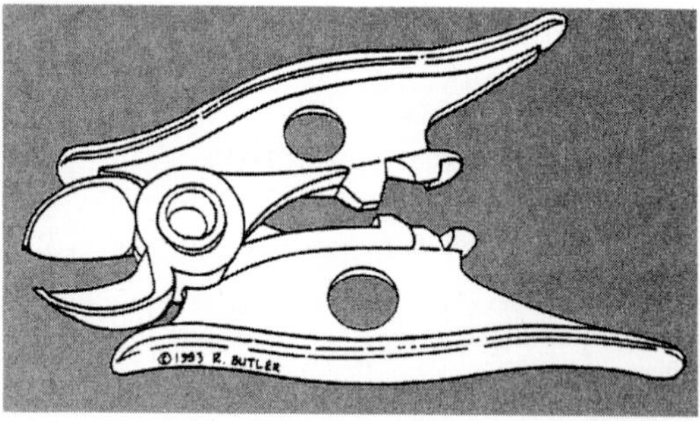

Fig. 1-2 The tick plier. A lightweight plastic device for safe and complete removal of ticks. (See the Appendix for mail-order suppliers.)

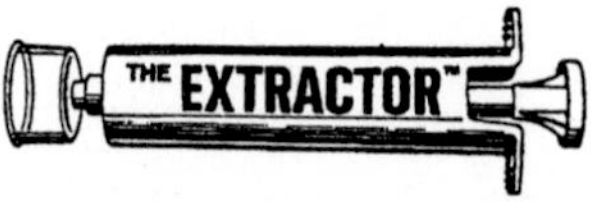

Fig. 1-3 The extractor. Venom extractor pump for first aid treatment of venomous insect stings and snake bites. (See Appendix for mail-order suppliers.)

particularly of contact with sex-industry workers, in whom HIV infection and other STDs are more prevalent.

Personal safety has emerged as another important issue in traveler's health. Recent studies have shown that motor vehicle accidents (25%) and other injuries and accidents (15%, including drownings and falls from height) accounted for more deaths in American travelers than infectious diseases and other illnesses (10%). Heart attacks and other cardiovascular problems in male travelers over 60 years old accounted for 50% of reported deaths, but probably do not represent a preventable consequence of travel. Recommendations for travel with chronic medical conditions are given in Chapter 14.

Finally, when the traveler returns home with a significant change in health, providers of medical care need to be acquainted with the signs and symptoms of serious tropical diseases. For example, misdiagnosis of a case of *Plasmodium falciparum* malaria as the "flu" can lead to tragic consequences for the patient, or an occult infection with *Strongyloides stercoralis* may threaten the health of a patient who has survived organ transplantation but must be maintained on immunosuppressive drugs. A patient passing a large intestinal worm, while usually not facing a life-threatening situation, may still present to an emergency room in a state of extreme anxiety and fright. An appreciation of the geographic distribution of tropical and exotic diseases and the risk factors contributing to the transmission of disease can help the health care provider to generate an appropriate differential diagnosis for illness occurring in the returned traveler.

REFERENCES

Auerbach PS, editor: *Management of wilderness and environmental emergencies,* ed 4, St Louis, 2000, Mosby.

Centers for Disease Control: *Health information for international travel,* Washington, DC, 2001-2002, Government Printing Office, HHS Publication No. (CDC) 2001-8280.

Fujimoto G, Robin M, Dessery B: *The travelers medical guide,* San Diego, KW Publications *(in press).*

Hargarten SW, Baker SP: Fatalities in the Peace Corps: a retrospective study: 1962-1983, *JAMA* 254:1326, 1985.

Hargarten SW, Baker T, Guptill K: Fatalities of American travelers: 1975-1984. In Steffen R et al, editors: *Travel medicine. Proceedings of the First Conference on International Travel Medicine,* Berlin, 1989, Springer-Verlag.

Hargarten SW, Baker T, Guptill K: Injury deaths and American travelers. In Steffen R et al, editors: *Travel medicine: Proceedings of the First Conference on International Travel Medicine,* Berlin, 1989, Springer-Verlag.

Holmes KK: The changing epidemiology of HIV transmission, *Hosp Pract* 26(11):153, 1991.

International Association for Medical Assistance to Travellers (IAMAT) Directory of English-Speaking Physicians. Guelph, Ontario, IAMAT. (revised periodically).

Jong EC: *The guide to healthy travel,* ed 2 Guelph, Ontario, 2002, IAMAT.

Jong EC: Advice to travelers. In Strickland GT, editor: *Hunter's tropical medicine,* ed 8, Philadelphia, 2000, WB Saunders.

Jong EC, McMullen R: General advice for the international traveler, *Infect Dis Clin North Am* 6:275, 1992.

Lackritz EM et al: Imported *Plasmodium falciparum* malaria in American travelers to Africa: implications for prevention strategies, *JAMA* 265:383, 1991.

National Institutes of Health Consensus Development Conference: Travelers' diarrhea, *JAMA* 253:2700, 1985.

Rose SR: *International travel health guide,* Northampton, MA, 2001, Travel Medicine, Inc, (updated annually).

Steffen R et al: Health problems after travel to developing countries, *J Infect Dis* 156:84, 1987.

Tainter S, Jong EC: The traveler's medical kit. In Jong EC, Keystone JS, McMullen R, editors: *The travel medicine advisor,* Atlanta, 1991, American Health Consultants.

United States Department of State, Bureau of Consular Affairs: *A safe trip abroad,* Superintendent of Documents, Government Printing Office, Washington, DC, 1990, DOS Publication 9493.

Weiss EA: *A comprehensive guide to wilderness and travel medicine,* Berkeley, CA, 1992, Adventure Medical Kits.

Wilson ME: *A world guide to infections: diseases, diagnosis, distribution,* New York, 1991, Oxford University Press.

Wilson ME, von Reyn DF, Fineberg HV: Infections in HIV-infected travelers: risks and Prevention, *Ann Intern Med* 114:582, 1991.

CHAPTER 2

Air Carrier Issues in Travel Medicine

Thomas N. Bettes and Larry Thirstrup

The issues facing aviation medicine today mirror the concerns of the global medical community. As the global community is concerned with the changing health of our biosphere, so too, is there similar interest in the quality and character of the cabin air in which the modern air traveler is surrounded. There is a mistaken perception that the poor quality of the cabin air actually facilitates the spread of disease. It might be supposed that in a world where modern air transport allows one to travel to another continent within hours, the threat of a plague might somehow ensue, but epidemiologic data clearly refute this notion. However, it is only through careful adherence to preexposure and postexposure guidelines that aircraft cabins are kept from becoming frequent vectors for infectious disease. Similarly, by adhering to the new standard of care applied to the prehospital arena, aviation medicine is saving countless lives in the cases of sudden death and other in flight emergencies through the use of automatic external defibrillators (AEDs) and enhanced emergency medical kits (EMKs). Despite this new technology, the best prevention for an inflight emergency is to keep it from occurring in the first place by establishing standard embarkation criteria. This chapter acquaints the general clinician with these somewhat esoteric issues while adding to the armamentarium of the well-seasoned travel physician.

CABIN AIR QUALITY

Both the traveling public and the aviation community have several misconceptions with regard to cabin air quality. It is generally thought that symptoms of fatigue, cephalgia, dysequilibrium, and upper respiratory symptoms are caused by recirculated air. Nonobjective terms such as "sick airplane syndrome," a variant of "sick building syndrome," have been used by the media and public. Several well-known myths explain how cabin air supposedly contributes to poor air quality. These myths are discussed in detail as the determinants of cabin air quality are reviewed (Table 2-1).

It is helpful for the physician and layperson alike to divide the issue of air quality into the five variables that contribute in some part to the overall milieu of the ambient air in the aircraft: pressurization, ventilation, contamination, humidity, and temperature (Table 2-2).

Pressurization

Almost without exception, the cabin environment is kept pressurized to 8000 ft. This level was chosen through research performed on pilots in

Table 2-1
Myths Regarding Cabin Air Quality

Aircraft ventilation systems cause a build up of contaminants.
Aircraft ventilation systems cause the spread of pathogens.
Decreased quantity of O_2 in cabin causes adverse symptoms.
Increased CO_2 in cabin causes adverse symptoms.

Table 2-2
Variables Contributing to Cabin Air Quality

Pressurization
Ventilation
Contamination
Humidity
Temperature

early NASA studies and is believed to be the altitude that most of the general public can tolerate without exhibiting signs or symptoms of altitude sickness. This altitude maintains the average individual on the upper flat part of the oxygen dissociation curve (Fig. 2-1). Most healthy individuals tolerate this altitude well. Although the percentage of O_2 remains the same at normal flight altitude as it does at sea level (21%), the partial pressure of O_2 decreases from 103 to 69 mm Hg at 8000 ft. This pressure ensures that about 90% of all hemoglobin will be saturated in the healthy individual. However, individuals with significant pathology, such as those with chronic obstructive pulmonary disease, recent myocardial infarction, or unstable angina, might suffer significant decompensation from even minor alterations in their O_2 dissociation curve. The clinician should be aware of this possibility when advising these patients who are considering air travel without supplemental oxygen. This topic is discussed further in the section on passenger acceptance and the Air Carrier Access Act (14 CFR Part 382).

Ventilation

The myth that aircraft ventilation contributes to poor quality of cabin air is unfounded. Depending on the type of aircraft, about half the cabin air is recirculated. The other half is outside air that is supplied by engine compressors, cooled by air-conditioning packs, and then blended with recirculated air. As a reference point, an office building may recirculate between 65% and 95% of its air. Older aircraft such as the Boeing 727 and McDonald-Douglas DC-9 do not recirculate air at all. It is only with the fuel crisis in the 1970s that modifications were made to newer aircraft to decrease the amount of outside air brought into the cabin by the engines, thereby decreasing fuel consumption. It is of note that the outside air brought into the cabin is virtually sterile.

Despite these modifications to newer aircraft, cabin air is exchanged in its entirety quite frequently. Consider the Boeing 767 used both in

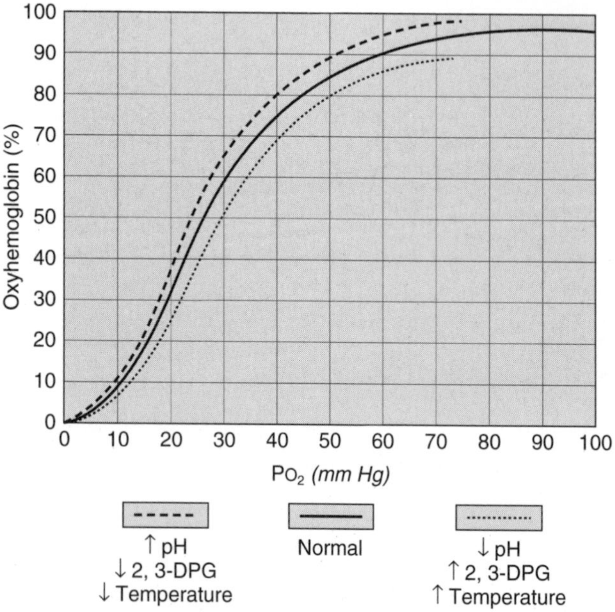

Fig. 2-1 The O_2 dissociation curve. (Brittenham GM: 5 Hematology: II red blood cell function and disorders of iron metabolism. In Dale DC, Federman DD: *WebMD Scientific American Medicine,* New York, 2002, WebMD.)

domestic and long-haul international travel. The cabin air is exchanged entirely every 2 to 3 minutes. Thus cabin air is exchanged approximately 20 to 30 times per hour. Compare that with the average household, which exchanges its volume only about 5 times per hour.

Clearly a large volume of air enters and exits the cabin in a short time. Without precise modifications, passengers would experience severe drafts. Engineering modifications have reduced this "wind tunnel effect" by using laminar flow. Cabin air enters from air ducts running the length of the cabin overhead. Air supplied then exits at approximately the same row, thereby reducing airflow in fore and aft directions, which effectively limits the spread of passenger-generated contaminants (Fig. 2-2).

Contamination

Although the laminar flow minimizes spread of passenger-generated contaminants, the major barrier to particulate matter on all modern aircraft is the HEPA (high efficiency particulate air) filter; this is the standard filter used in most intensive care units in hospitals, operating rooms, and industrial clean rooms. A rating is given on efficiency based on the ability of the filter to remove particles greater than 0.3 μm. For comparison, bacteria and fungi are usually larger than 1 μm. Viruses however, may range in size from 0.003 to 0.05 μm; clumping of the virus facilitates its removal via the HEPA filter.

Studies have been done in which air samples were collected from various locations and sampled for microorganisms. Locations included mu-

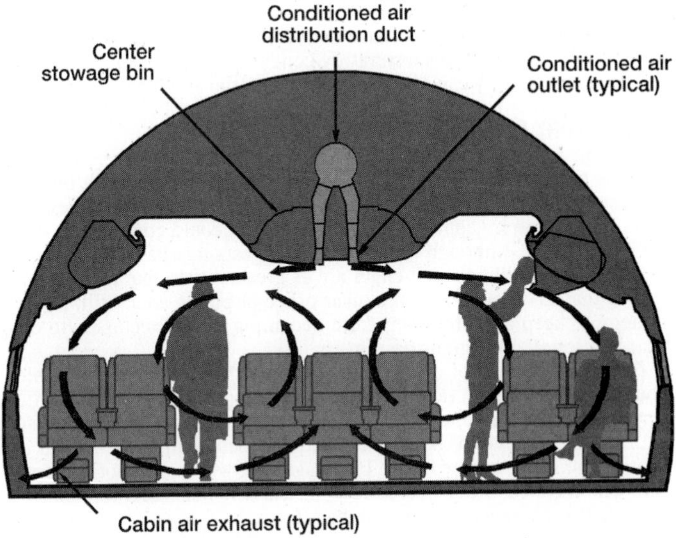

Fig. 2-2 Cabin picture demonstrating air flow. (Copyright The Boeing Company.)

nicipal buses, shopping malls, sidewalks, downtown streets, and airport departure lounges; microbial aerosol levels in the cabin were much lower than in other public locations. Results from these studies contradict the myth that aircraft are large-scale "mixing chambers" for microorganisms. Although there is a risk of disease transmission based on the number of passengers and the close proximity, the risk does not appear to be any greater than that associated with other public transportation.

In addition to pathogenic organisms, there is concern regarding other contaminants including carbon dioxide, carbon monoxide, and ozone. Carbon dioxide levels have been equated with poor air quality, and recommendations have been made with regard to safe levels by ASHRAC (American Society of Heating Refrigeration and Air Conditioning). However, these parameters are not appropriate for aircraft, since there are different sources of contamination and population densities. Nonetheless, data collected on 92 different U.S. flights found carbon dioxide, carbon monoxide, and ozone levels well below Federal Aviation Agency (FAA) and Occupational Safety and Health Administration standards. Thus symptoms of fatigue, headache, nausea, and upper respiratory tract are far more likely to stem from other factors including flight duration, noise levels, dehydration, and circadian dysrhythmia.

Humidity and Temperature

The cabin milieu is much like that of a desert environment (12% to 21%); relative humidity can be between 5% and 35% on most aircraft. The low humidity is caused by the frequent renewal of cabin air with outside air, which is well below 0° F and thus contributes little appreciable moisture or heat in the cabin. Air bled off the engines must be circulated and warmed to bring it to a comfortable range. Exposure to this environment for prolonged periods is known to cause dehydration as a result of insensible water loss and exacerbates respiratory conditions. Of interest, however, is that the low humidity can actually inhibit bacterial and fungal growth.

RESPIRATORY DISEASE TRANSMISSION ISSUES

Increasing awareness regarding multiple drug-resistant tuberculosis infections has led to concern by the traveling public. Along with the false perception that cabin air circulates poor quality air, many also believe that a passenger with mycobacterial or other illness could conceivably infect the entire cabin. Although the literature suggests that passengers in contiguous areas of the aircraft cabin are at greatest risk, that risk does not exceed that associated with any other office or public area. Still, the best strategy to keep aircraft cabins from becoming global vectors is to deny boarding for all contagious passengers.

Despite the policy of most major airlines to reduce exposure to infectious diseases through denial of boarding, exposure does occur. Certain tenets regarding the spread of infectious disease and the postexposure notification process are based on literature documenting the spread and natural history of source cases. In considering whether to notify passengers who traveled with a source case, air carriers must be aware that data indicate that passengers are not at the same risk.

It is important to document the level of infectiousness of the source passenger. In the case of *Mycobacterium tuberculosis,* factors such as anatomic involvement, positive acid-fast bacillus (AFB) smears, history of transmission, prior treatment of the source case, proximity to the source case, and duration of exposure must be considered. The literature shows that proximity to the source case is one of the most important variables in the transmission of infectious disease. Thus a passenger traveling in first class need not necessarily be notified of a source case seated in the rear of the aircraft in the coach section. Similarly, those whose exposure was limited to less than 8 hours are unlikely to need notification. Important exceptions to this rule should be noted. Consider the case of an airline delayed on the ground for 3 hours as a result of engine problems during which the ventilation system was inoperative; 54 passengers were on board the flight and 72% became infected with influenza. The attack rate varied linearly with time spent on board the aircraft. This scenario shows that any alteration from standard boarding, taxi, and takeoff protocols might be significant in determining infectivity of source case and need to notify.

The Centers for Disease Control and Prevention (CDC) recommendations published in March 1995 take all of these factors into consideration. Their position in general is that the risk of transmission is low, and the airline should consider "infectiousness" of passenger and prior treatment. Risk of transmission is also affected by length of flight and proximity to source case. Additionally, any extra variables such as ground delays or inoperative ventilation systems should be considered. Passengers should then be notified if all of the criteria are met.

Notification should be made by the airline in cooperation with public health departments. The preferred mode of notification is by a letter containing potential exposure and follow-up recommendations. The letter should explain the disease involved and contact information. Issues hampering this effort include the long delay between source travel and airline notification date, as well as inability to reliably contact passengers who traveled with the source passenger because of inaccurate/variable record keeping.

DENIAL OF BOARDING/PASSENGER ACCEPTANCE

Strict regulations must be followed in the case of a patient requiring oxygen to embark on a long flight. The FAA considers oxygen to be hazardous cargo. Oxygen, as well as any other oxidizing agents, can pose serious hazards to the safety of the aircraft and passengers. Consider the downing of an airliner that killed all on board because oxygen-generating cylinders were inappropriately stored in the cargo.

For the passenger who requires supplemental oxygen, it is imperative that the physician be acquainted with each carrier's policy regarding supplemental oxygen. Most carriers require a fixed interval of time to prepare the aircraft before embarking any passenger who requires oxygen. Further, the passenger must have a physician's statement attesting to the ability of the patient to be cleared to an altitude of 8000 ft with the use of supplemental oxygen. The statement must include flow rates, continuous or intermittent usage, and type of delivery system—mask versus nasal cannula. Additionally, the physician must consider the need for ground oxygen during layover or transfer. Typically, such service is not available from the airline and must be arranged in advance.

Although the airline may make certain regulations to ensure the safety of the traveling public, it may not limit the ability of those with disabilities to board the aircraft, with rare exception. The Air Carrier Access Act of 1986 was established to ensure that persons with disabilities, as per the Americans with Disabilities Act (ADA) definition, were treated without discrimination in any way, consistent with safe carriage of all passengers. This act, known as the FAA final rule, required the department of transportation to publish air carrier access guidelines adopted in March 1990 (14 CFR Part 382). The regulation, which applies only to U.S.-based carriers, states that a carrier may not refuse carriage of a passenger solely based on disability. Nor can it limit the number of disabled individuals on a flight. Further, a carrier may not limit transportation of an individual simply because his appearance or behavior is disturbing. Some take this to mean that any "sick" passenger must be accepted.

There are a few exceptions to the FAA final rule: A carrier may refuse to transport an individual if the carrier deems transportation of the passenger to be a risk to health or safety of the public, or a clear violation of FAA rules. For example, an air carrier might justifiably refuse boarding to a disabled individual who is unable to perform exit row functions and no other seat is availabile. Also, a carrier may refuse boarding to a passenger known to harbor communicable disease or a passenger who requires respiratory equipment not compatible with the aircraft.

The responsibility to accept all disabled or ill passengers who do not pose a risk to the traveling public resulted in the establishment of the complaint resolution official (CRO). This position is specifically mandated by Air Carrier Access Rules to resolve complaints or disagreements regarding the transportation of individuals with disabilities. This official or department is usually in a central location and may involve discussion with an in-house consultant or physician. The physician may request information regarding the clinical scenario before making a decision with regard to acceptance or denial of passenger boarding. The CRO may also be asked to make a decision regarding diversion of a flight during which the safety of a passenger or crew member might be jeopardized if it were to continue. Clearly, the issue of traveling with a disability or medical need can best be accomplished through early communication with the air carrier and its special assistance coordinator. Help for physicians who must advise passengers on travel or medical certifications is also available though the Aerospace Medical Association.

IN-FLIGHT MEDICAL EMERGENCIES

With the aging of the population and the increase in air travel, the number of in-flight medical emergencies has increased. Before the late 1980s, information about the frequency and type of in-flight emergencies was sparse because of inconsistent reporting or reporting of events by non-medical personnel. One study published in *JAMA* overreported the number of in-flight deaths because it included airline accidents during the years covered in the analysis. More than 63% of the nonaccidental deaths that occurred were caused by sudden cardiac arrest.

Further research into the types of emergencies and equipment needed led the FAA to pass the 1986 FAR requirement (121.309). This regulation mandated air carriers to adhere to a certain standard for medical kits. It has been subsequently amended to apply to commuter air carriers with 10 to 30 seats. A minimum of four basic medications are required: dextrose 50%, adrenaline, diphenhydramine, and nitroglycerin tablets. Some first aid items and basic instruments are also mandated.

Passage of the Aviation Medical Assistance Act of 1997 helped to further enhance the provisions of the on-board medical kit. It also called for the adoption of a Good Samaritan protection policy, which held faultless any rescuer who assisted a passenger in need. Before the adoption of this policy, there was the perceived notion that physicians or other medical personnel might have been reluctant to render aid for fear of legal repercussions.

Automatic External Defibrillators

The role of the AED is expanding. According to data published by the American Heart Association, sudden death occurs in about 1000 people every day in the United States. The chance of survival in such an event is less that 1 in 10. As is the teaching for all basic and advanced rescue personnel, the adage "shock first and shock fast" is of paramount importance. Because ventricular fibrillation is the most common and most treatable rhythm disturbance found at time of cardiac death, the importance of AEDs cannot be overestimated.

The AED is currently approved for use in air carriers in the United States, although not mandated until the year 2003. The small portable device fits safely and unobtrusively in any overhead bin or closet and can be operated by almost anyone with a minimum of training. Rescue personnel who are versed in Basic Life Support as taught by the American Heart Association should at least be familiar with such equipment, even if they are not proficient with a particular model. Most major air carriers carry this equipment on board and have trained their crew in its use. The importance of ready access to AED by first responders cannot be overstated, since the survivability of a sudden death event decreases by 7% to 10% with each passing minute. If air carriers are to continue to make a difference in the prevention of sudden cardiac deaths, the use and availability of such life saving devices must be encouraged.

Other issues regarding in-flight emergencies and EMKs are certain to be encountered. Debate continues with regard to who may have access to

AEDs and EMKs on board U.S. air carriers; for the moment, the decision is made by each individual carrier. It is hoped that standard criteria might soon be adopted to ensure ready access to all qualified personnel, thereby increasing the availability of these life-saving technologies.

REFERENCES

CDC: Exposure of passengers and flight crew to *Mycobacterium tuberculosis* on commercial aircraft, 1992-1995, *MMWR* 44:137, 1995.

Driver CR et al: Transmission of *M. tuberculosis* associated with air travel, *JAMA* 272:1031, 1994.

Kenyon TA et al: Transmission of multidrug-resistant *Mycobacterium tuberculosis* during a long airplane flight, *N Engl J Med* 334:933, 1996.

Klontz KC et al: An outbreak of influenza A. Taiwan/1/86 (H1N1) infections at a naval base and its association with airplane travel, *Am J Epidemiol* 129:341, 1989.

McFarland JW, Hickman C, Osterholm MR, MacDonald KL: Exposure to *Mycobacterium tuberculosis* associated with air travel, *JAMA* 272:1031, 1994.

Medical guidelines for airline travel, Alexandria, Virginia, 1997, Aerospace Medical Association.

Miller MA, Valway SE, Onorato IM: Tuberculosis risk after exposure on airplanes, *Tubercle Lung Dis* 77:414, 1996.

Moore M, Fleming KS, Sands L: A passenger with pulmonary/laryngeal tuberculosis: no evidence of transmission on two short flights, *Aviat Space Environ Med* 67:1097, 1996.

Moser MR et al: An outbreak of influenza aboard a commercial airliner, *Am J Epidemiol* 110:1, 1979.

Rayman R: Commentary on inflight medical kits, *Aviat Space Environ Med* 69:1007, 1998.

Wick RL Jr, Irvine LA: The microbiological composition of and airliner cabin air, *Aviat Space Environ Med* 66:220, 1995.

World Health Organization: *Tuberculosis and air travel: guidelines for prevention and control,* Geneva, 1998, WHO.

CHAPTER 3

Emerging Diseases and the International Traveler

Jonathan D. Mayer

In 1992, the Institute of Medicine released a landmark report entitled *Emerging Infections: Microbial Threats to Health in the United States.* The report was issued in response to a growing realization that minimizing the importance of infectious diseases in the United States and elsewhere constituted false complacency. The continuing impact of infectious diseases had been grossly underestimated, and the emergence of human immunodeficiency virus/acquired immunodeficiency syndrome (HIV/AIDS) and other infectious diseases was and still is alarming. Emerging infectious diseases have become a major topic of scholarly study in public health, infectious diseases, medical geography, and related disciplines. Emerging diseases must be an important consideration in travel medicine. Infectious diseases remain the top cause of mortality worldwide.

There is no universally accepted definition of emerging infectious diseases, and all attempts at definition have been understandably vague. Most definitions suggest that emerging infections are those with increasing incidence at local, regional, or international scales. Infectious diseases that are becoming more common, newly recognized, genuinely novel in humans, exhibiting resurgence, and spreading from epicenters are all included under the rubric of emerging infectious diseases. Also included in most discussions of disease emergence are those diseases that exhibit antimicrobial resistance, such as malaria and, in some populations, tuberculosis. There is widespread agreement that most emerging diseases do not appear de novo; rather, they are recently recognized. Some diseases, such as HIV/AIDS, and probably less common diseases such as Ebola hemorrhagic fever, probably appeared owing to species jumps. Many well-known infectious diseases, such as yellow fever and African trypanosomiasis have well-understood cycles that involve nonhuman animal reservoirs.

The examples of emerging diseases that are considered in this chapter are among those that constitute major threats to the traveler. Many "exotic" tropical hemorrhagic fevers such as those resulting from the Ebola virus are not included here. Although Ebola fever has a high case-fatality rate, it does not constitute a threat to the typical traveler, and less than 1000 cases have been identified in indigenous populations in Africa since its recognition more than two decades ago. The emerging and resurgent diseases are specifically discussed in other chapters of this book; this chapter provides a general framework for understanding the new global transmission modes for emergent and resurgent diseases.

There have been many attempts to compile lists of emerging diseases, and the lists are long including a 61 page list of emerging diseases and their symptoms, geographic distributions, and treatments in the Institute of Medicine's *Emerging Infections: Microbial Threats to Health in the United States* (pp 199-260). Numerous emerging infectious diseases, some of which constitute potential risks to international travelers, are discussed in the journal *Emerging Infectious Diseases,* published by the Centers for Diseases Control and Prevention (CDC) in the United States. This valuable journal is available on the worldwide web at: *http://www.cdc.gov/ncidod/EID/index.htm.* It is also available in hard copy. Several hundred emerging infections have been mentioned in the Federation of American Scientists' Program for Monitoring Emerging Diseases (ProMED), which is a simple bulletin board system that contains the most recent reports of disease outbreaks. The archives for ProMED are available on the web at: *http://www.healthnet.org/programs/promed.html.* Bulletins are sent out via electronic mail, and free subscriptions are available to individuals by registering one's e-mail address at the web site.

CAUSES AND RECOGNITION OF DISEASE EMERGENCE

Many factors are responsible for disease emergence. These include greater contact with previously isolated populations, contact with diseases that have sylvatic cycles owing to deforestation and travel into uninhabited areas, an increasingly interconnected world with air transportation that is highly accessible to relatively affluent populations, changes in land use and demographic patterns, and disruption of stable ecosystems. Antimicrobial resistance is largely due to genetic adaptation of microbes to prophylactic and treatment agents and to the overuse of broad-spectrum antibiotics. Recognition of new and emerging diseases has developed largely as a result of good surveillance systems, spatial clusters of disease occurrence, increasing incidence and prevalence, pathognomonic signs, and easily recognized signs and symptoms.

SPECIFIC DISEASES

Because so many Americans and citizens of other developed countries travel frequently for leisure and business, their travel itineraries and possible geographic exposures should be considered in any differential diagnosis where the etiology is not obvious. Clinicians must inquire about immediate and past travel itineraries, and the information should be as specific as possible in terms of the cities or areas of the countryside visited. If possible, the patient or other knowledgeable person should be asked about the specific types of geographic environments with which the patient has had contact. Their activities, such as swimming in stagnant water, walking through areas with exposed pools of water and puddles, or drinking tap water in developing countries, should also be subject to inquiry.

Airborne Diseases

With regard to viral and bacterial airborne pathogens, the greatest risks to other travelers and to casual contacts, both en route and at their successive destinations, are respiratory diseases whose incubation periods are longer than the actual travel time. Under certain conditions, it is possible that many people on an intercontinental airline trip could be infected with an airborne pathogen from an index case from a traveler on the same flight (see Chapter 2). Clinically apparent disease would not be detected until well after the end of the airline trip, and the spread of a new respiratory pathogen would therefore be both geographically dispersed and rapidly spreading. Of all emerging diseases, new strains of influenza and multiple drug-resistant tuberculosis constitute the two most serious threats to public health in the future. Travelers are especially subject to developing these diseases because of their exposure to many people.

Influenza

Although influenza is hardly a new disease, it is considered to be an emerging disease because of its demonstrated potential for genetic shift. It has been present in pandemic form, owing to major antigenic shifts, in many different outbreaks. The most notorious of these was the influenza pandemic of 1918-1919 in which more than 20 million people died worldwide. There is reasonable evidence to conclude that there was a major antigenic shift, and the population was immunologically naïve to the new strain. For reasons that are not completely clear, the pandemic was most fatal for younger adults between 20 and 40 years old.

The widely available trivalent influenza vaccine is recommended officially in the United States for those over 50 years old, or other categories of individuals, such as those with cardiorespiratory diseases, and health care workers. It is also prudent to recommend influenza vaccination for all international travelers because they are likely to travel by airplane, where conditions could facilitate rapid transmission of influenza. Needless to say, the trivalent vaccines, which are agreed on every February for the following flu season at an international consensus conference, provide no protection against major genetic shifts. These genetic shifts cannot be anticipated. The only effective prophylaxis is well known: isolation. Short of this extreme measure, frequent hand washing and, for influenza A outbreaks, the use of amantadine or rimantadine, or other anti-influenza drugs are the only effective prophylactic measures.

Tuberculosis

Tuberculosis is considered to be an emerging disease because it is becoming increasingly resistant to available antimicrobial agents, and because it accounts for the greatest number of deaths worldwide of any infectious disease. No effective vaccine is available for tuberculosis, and the potential is great for new drug resistant strains to spread rapidly. In the case of tuberculosis, there have been documented cases of transmission on commercial aircraft.

Plague

During a possible outbreak of plague in India in 1994, airports of entry in the United States were prepared to quarantine anyone who exhibited symptoms of pneumonic plague, since the threat of rapid spread of this contagious disease could have been serious. There is some dispute in the literature about whether the febrile disease in India in the areas surrounding Surat was, in fact, plague; but its containment, if it was plague, was a matter of luck. That pneumonic plague can arise again is indisputable, and its potential for rapid and fatal spread is great.

Vector-Borne Diseases

Many of the diseases that are considered to be emerging are vector-borne diseases. Lyme disease (Lyme borreliosis) is highly endemic in the upper Midwest of the United States, New England, and the Middle Atlantic States and is present in low intensity along the Pacific Coast west of the coastal mountain ranges, from north of San Francisco to Vancouver Island. It is present in Scandinavia, Europe, and Russia, where the disease is known as erythema chronicum migrans. Malaria is pantropic, and there is some evidence and much speculation that the ecologic changes associated with global warming may result in the reappearance and new appearance of malaria in more temperate zones. Dengue fever is also pantropic, and is experiencing epidemics in the Americas, the Pacific Basin, and the tropical areas of the Pacific Rim.

To a large extent, the vectored diseases may be considered together in terms of prevention, as simple preventive measures significantly decrease the risk of contracting the diseases. These measures include wearing long-sleeved shirts and pants, which can be quite comfortable if they are made of white or light-colored cotton, even in tropical areas. Additional measures are the application of insect repellent to clothing and exposed skin areas (see Chapter 1). Knowledge of which specific places within a given locality have endemic vector-borne disease is frequently useful, since it may be possible to avoid exposure to those areas. Most anopheline mosquito species take their blood meals close to dawn and dusk, and avoidance of areas where there is likely to be increased risk of mosquito bites at these times is wise. On the other hand, the *Aedes aegypti* and *Aedes albopictus* mosquitoes, which are the vectors for dengue fever, take their meals throughout the day.

Lyme Disease

Lyme disease is considered to be an emerging disease. Its incidence and prevalence rates in the midwestern United States and the Northeast have both increased markedly over the past two decades. Deer ticks *(Ixodes scapularis)* are the vectors for Lyme disease. Many small rodents, but particularly the white-footed mouse, *Peromyscus leucopus,* are highly competent animal reservoirs. The microgeography of the distribution of the East Coast and Midwestern varieties of Lyme disease parallels the distribution of white-tailed deer. These deer are not particularly competent reservoirs, but serve as the "transportation" for the ixodid ticks. Ticks have no powers of locomotion, and the white-footed mice do not move far; however, this is different in the daily paths of the deer, who travel miles at a time. Thus a typical environment for Lyme disease in the United States is a brushy or grassy area that is at the edges of more forested areas.

Deer are edge dwellers, and people tend to come into contact with nature precisely where the deer are most common—at the edges of forests. This is frequently quite literally in the backyards (or front) of suburban houses. Several studies have shown that Lyme disease is most commonly contracted within a few hundred feet of home. This is relevant for domestic and international travelers to endemic areas, since Lyme disease is so prevalent. Its prevalence in ecologically similar areas in much of northern Europe and Scandinavia is also high. Lyme disease is also found in Austria, and the prevalence of seropositivity of residents of cities such as Vienna is quite high. Travelers to all of these areas should be cautioned about the importance of wearing appropriate attire, using insect repellents, and checking their bodies for ticks.

The probability of contracting the disease is directly related to the length of time that the tick is attached, which can be for 2 days or more. Ticks should be gently removed from the skin with tweezers or forceps, grasping the ticks as close to the epidermis of the person as possible. Care must be taken not to detach the mouthparts from the rest of the tick, since this still allows the injection of the pathogen, a spirochete called *Borrelia burgdorferi.*

Dengue Fever

As previously mentioned, a number of regions in the world are experiencing major epidemics of dengue fever, and there is limited but suggestive evidence that global environmental changes may be resulting in the northward and southward movement of the mosquito vectors from tropical areas. There have been more than a dozen cases of dengue that have been indigenously acquired in the United States, mostly in Texas. Dengue is considered to be an emerging disease because it is present in epidemic proportions in many areas of the tropics and because it seems to be diffusing into areas that were previously dengue-free.

Dengue virus infection can present on a continuum from subclinical to a hemorrhagic state leading to shock syndrome and disseminated intravascular coagulation. Typically, an international traveler who contracts dengue will experience symptoms that range from nonspecific flu-like manifestations to debilitating symptoms that take months to resolve. Dengue is rarely fatal in the typical traveler. Fatalities occur mostly among young children who have previously been exposed to one of the four dengue serotypes and are then exposed to another serotype. There is no vaccine or specific treatment available for dengue; treatment is symptomatic, and conservative measures such as adequate hydration and rest are of tantamount importance (see Chapter 18).

The mainstay of prophylaxis are the same as for other insect vector-borne diseases: using insect repellents and wearing long-sleeved shirts and long pants outdoors, even in the hot tropical environments where dengue is most commonly found. Because there is no effective treatment or vaccine for dengue, travelers must realize that their risk of being exposed to dengue is a major risk of travel to certain tropical urban and rural locales, and the use of preventive measures cannot be overemphasized.

Malaria

Like dengue, malaria is considered to be an emerging disease; there is some evidence that it is undergoing northward and southward movement into more temperate areas because of possible global environmental change and because its incidence and prevalence rates are increasing in many areas. Whereas malaria appeared to have been almost eradicated in the 1960s, resistance to medications and insecticides has led the World Health Organization (WHO) to acknowledge that malaria eradication is no longer a reasonable goal. Rather, there is an initiative at WHO called the "Rollback Malaria Initiative"; as the name implies, reduction in malaria prevalence is the most that can be expected.

There have been several reports of "airport malaria" in the United States and Europe, where individuals who live within several kilometers of major international airports contract malaria, although they have not been in areas where malaria is endemic. Experimental studies show that anopheline mosquitoes can survive in the wheelwells of commercial aircraft, and the putative mode of transmission is that the anophelines fly several kilometers and infect individuals who live near airports. There are also some case reports of indigenously acquired malaria in the United States thought to be transmitted from undiagnosed immigrants with malaria infections. It is well to remember that many competent anopheline vectors are already present in the United States and that as recently as the 1930s, malaria was endemic in the Tennessee River Valley. In the nineteenth century, malaria was present as far north as upstate New York and Oregon in the summers.

The prevention and treatment of malaria are discussed elsewhere (Chapters 5 and 7). From the viewpoint of malaria as an emerging disease, it is crucial to realize that strains of *Plasmodium falciparum* and, to a lesser extent, *Plasmodium vivax* develop rapid resistance to new prophylactic drug agents. The resistance is most intense in Thailand and in sub-Saharan Africa, where 90% of the malaria cases occur. It appears likely that there will be an effective vaccine for malaria in the next decade, but in the meantime, prophylaxis with mefloquine, doxycycline, atovaquone/proguanil, or other agents that are more effective than chloroquine for prophylaxis will remain the mainstay of malaria prevention in the traveler.

Food-Borne Diseases

A number of food-borne diseases are usually included under the rubric of emerging diseases. These include *E. coli* 0157:H7 and variant Creutzfeldt-Jakob disease (CJD), secondary to bovine spongiform encephalopathy or "mad cow disease."

E. coli 0157:H7

The syndromes associated with contamination of the meat supply with this pathogen were first described in the early 1980s. The presentation of the associated symptoms can range from mild diarrhea to hemolytic-uremic syndrome (HUS), principally in children. When this disease progresses to HUS, it can lead to renal failure, multiorgan failure, and, occasionally, death. This disease was originally identified in the United States, but it is clear that it occurs in many countries outside the United States. The pathogen has been isolated from fecal samples and from the guts of bovines, sheep, and other food sources. In the slaughtering process, the intestinal contents may contaminate the butchered meat, either because of intestinal perforation, or because of the loss of bowel control that animals experience immediately before slaughter. The pathogen is particularly likely to present a hazard in inadequately cooked hamburgers, because the pathogen that is present on the surfaces of large cuts of meat is mixed throughout ground meat.

E. coli colitis is by no means restricted to the United States, and its initial recognition in the 1980s in the United States has led to better recognition and surveillance in other countries as well. This is not exclusively a disease of travelers, but travelers to the United States and from the United States to other countries must realize that they may be at risk of developing the disease. It is both a travel-associated and a non-travel-associated disease. In the major outbreak of this disease on the West Coast of the United States in the 1990s, most of those who were affected contracted the disease in their home communities.

There is no effective treatment for this form of colitis, nor is there a vaccine. Recent efforts and funding in the United States have been directed to improving the sophistication of the microbiologic techniques of testing meat samples. Meat inspectors have relied on the gross appearance of the inspected meat, rather than more sophisticated microbiologic analysis. Ensuring that hamburgers and other chopped meat products are "well-done" or cooked to a core temperature of about 155° F is an essential step in prevention. Hamburgers should not appear pink in their interiors. This simple measure can eliminate most cases of the hamburger meat-associated colitis. Many restaurants, including fast-food chains, now refuse to serve rare hamburgers to their customers.

Outbreaks of *E. coli* 0157:H7 disease have also involved fresh fruits and vegetables and unpasteurized juices. It is presumed that fecal contamination of the produce during harvesting and processing leads to the presence of the pathogen in the final vended products.

Variant Creutzfeldt-Jakob Disease (vCJD)

Reports of seemingly idiopathic encephalopathy emerged in the United Kingdom in the 1990s. The symptoms and both the gross appearance and histology of the brains of affected individuals at necropsy suggested a similarity to CJD, but there were symptomatic differences. Like HUS, vCJD constitutes a long and interesting story of disease associated with the meat processing industry. vCJD occurs because of the ingestion of meat contaminated by central nervous system (CNS) tissue from cattle with bovine spongioform encephalopathy. Supplementation of cattle feed with offal from the same species has been a common practice throughout many areas of the world. This is no longer the practice in the UK, owing to rapid recognition of the probable route of contagion. The European Union placed an embargo on the shipment of beef from the UK, but cases of vCJD are now appearing in other European countries. The possibility exists that this disease could also appear in the United States through indigenous transmission, but this has not yet occurred. It may be prudent for travelers to the UK and other European countries to avoid beef products, although the actual risk of contracting this fatal disease may be low. Slaughtering practices have been modified, but because of a long incubation period, it is not yet clear that the risk of contracting nvCJD has been eliminated. It has a long latency period, and although the epidemic curve is decreasing, new cases could occur.

Water-Borne Diseases

Just as there are a number of emerging food-borne diseases, there are also a number of travel and non-travel-associated waterborne diseases. These include cholera and cryptosporidiosis. Cholera is considered to be an emerging disease because of its geographic diffusion patterns and its reintroduction to the Americas, and because of its increasing prevalence. Cryptosporidiosis is a newly recognized diarrheal disease that is both indigenously acquired in the United States and can be contracted in many other countries as well.

Cholera

Cholera, like so other "emerging diseases," is not a new disease. It has been present historically in many countries of the world. The world is experiencing a new pandemic of cholera, however, and it has been introduced into the United States. Prevention and treatment of cholera is discussed elsewhere (Chapters 4, 6, and 25). It was introduced into the Americas when a ship arriving from Asia dumped its bilge water into the Pacific Ocean off the coast of Peru, introducing the disease into Peru. It spread rapidly throughout many areas of Latin America and has moved northward to the United States. Recent studies suggest that phytoplankton may serve as reservoirs for vibrio-associated diseases. As with other emerging diseases, the spread of cholera can be traced to patterns of migration and travel, as well as to the shipment of food that can have fecal contamination from cholera carriers.

Cryptosporidiosis

This disease is responsible for thousands of cases of moderate to severe diarrhea worldwide. It is caused by *Cryptosporidium parvum* and constitutes a risk for travelers, as well as local populations. The largest documented outbreak of cryptosporidiosis was in Milwaukee in the 1990s, where more than 400,000 people developed diarrhea, more than 1000 people were hospitalized, mostly for rehydration, and more than a dozen people died. All of these people were immunocompromised because of a variety of factors, including immunosuppression resulting from HIV/AIDS, cancer, chemotherapy, and other factors. The Milwaukee outbreak was due to a breakdown in the mechanism of the local water filtration plant and by fecal contamination of the rivers that drain in to Lake Michigan by runoff from agricultural land. *C. parvum* is impervious to chlorination and other chemical treatments.

C. parvum is ubiquitous, and cases have been described in returned travelers. For the traveler, heat and filtration of potentially contaminated water are the most reliable ways to prevent cryptosporidiosis (Chapter 7). There is no specific treatment for cryptosporidiosis, although some evidence suggests that paromomycin may be helpful in certain cases. Antimotility agents are contraindicated, and adequate hydration is the only active measure that is appropriate once an individual contracts the disease. This disease should be part of the differential diagnosis of diarrhea in the returning traveler, although traveler's diarrhea caused by toxigenic *E. coli* will usually be the most common illness (see Chapters 25 and 26).

THE DANGER OF EMERGING DISEASES

The world is highly interconnected through global commerce and jet travel and subject to the rapid spread of emerging and resurgent diseases. What happens in one area can rapidly affect other areas at great distances. This has enormous implications for travel medicine, because a disease that is endemic in one area can become epidemic in another area quite rapidly. Those providing pretravel counseling and posttravel treatment need to be aware of outbreaks in regions in which the traveler will be visiting, or from which the traveler is returning.

REFERENCES

Greenwood B, De Cock K, editors: *New and resurgent infections: prediction, detection, and management of tomorrow's epidemics,* Chichester UK, 1998, John Wiley and Sons.

Krause RM, editor: *Emerging infections: biomedical research reports,* New York, 1998, Academic Press.

Lederberg J, Shope RE, Oaks SC Jr, editors: *Emerging infections: microbial threats to health in the United States,* Washington DC, 1992, National Academy Press.

Morse SS, editor: *Emerging viruses,* New York, 1993, Oxford University Press.

Roizman B, editor: *Infectious diseases in an age of change: the impact of ecology and behavior on disease transmission,* Washington DC, 1995, National Academy Press.

Scheld WM, Craig WA, Hughes JM, editors: Emerging infections, ed 2, Washington DC, 1998, ASM Press.

Wilson ME, Levins R, Spielman A, editors: *Disease in evolution: global changes and emergence of infectious diseases,* New York, 1994, New York Academy of Sciences.

CHAPTER 4

Immunizations for Travelers

Elaine C. Jong

Recommendations for travel immunizations are based on a personalized risk-assessment of each traveler and trip itinerary, and knowledge of current health conditions at a given destination. Most travelers want protection against vaccine-preventable diseases, yet acceptance of recommended travel immunizations may depend largely on cost, number of doses, and route of administration (oral versus injection). Many first-time international travelers are surprised by the number of vaccines that may be considered for a given trip itinerary. On the other hand, experienced repeat travelers may be pleased by the availability of new vaccines that may be better tolerated and provide greater efficacy with a longer duration of protection compared with older products.

Travelers planning adventure or expedition travel, extended stays abroad, or whose work may necessitate multiple trips abroad with very short notice should be encouraged to seek advice for travel immunizations well in advance (up to 6 months) of anticipated departure. This allows time for optimal scheduling of vaccine doses and procurement of vaccines that may be in short supply or difficult to obtain. For travelers with little advance notice, accelerated schedules may be used for some travel vaccines, and multiple vaccine doses may be given at different sites on the same day, limited only by the recipient's tolerance for multiple injections and associated minor adverse side effects. Up to 6 live virus vaccines may be given on the same day without interfering with immune efficacy. Table 4-1 lists some conditions that may cause vaccine interactions or interfere with the expected immune protection. In general, attenuated live virus vaccines and bacterial vaccines are contraindicated during pregnancy and in persons with altered immune competence (see Chapters 12, 13, and 14). This chapter describes adult travel immunizations. Pediatric travel immunizations are covered in Chapter 11.

ROUTINE IMMUNIZATIONS

Immunizations may be organized into three categories called the "3 Rs": routine, required, and recommended. Routine immunizations are those usually given as part of standard childhood immunization programs, and may include vaccines for diphtheria/pertussis/tetanus, polio, hepatitis B, *Haemophilus influenzae* B, measles/mumps/rubella, varicella, and pneumococcal disease. When individuals seek travel immunizations, this is a

Table 4-1
Vaccine Interactions

Vaccine	Interaction	Precaution
Immune globulin	Measles/mumps/rubella (MMR) vaccine	Give these vaccines at least 2 weeks before immune globulin (IG) or 3-5 mo after IG, depending on IG dose received.
Oral typhoid vaccine	Antibiotic therapy	Do not administer oral typhoid vaccine (OTV) concurrently with antibiotics.
Oral typhoid vaccine	Malarone malaria chemoprophylaxis	Schedule an interval of at least 10 days between final dose of oral typhoid vaccine and proguanil (Malarone = atovaquone + proguanil)
Rabies vaccine (HDCV) intradermal series	Chloroquine malaria chemoprophylaxis	Complete rabies vaccine (intradermal series) at least 3 weeks before starting chloroquine malaria chemoprophylaxis; use rabies vaccine intramuscular series if 3-week interval is not possible.
Virus vaccines, live (MMR, OPV, varicella, yellow fever vaccine)	Other live virus vaccines	Give live virus vaccines on same day, or separate doses by at least 1 month.
Virus vaccines, live (MMR, OPV, varicella, yellow fever vaccine)	Tuberculin skin test (PPD)	Do skin test on same day as receipt of a live virus vaccine, or 3 weeks after, because live virus vaccines can impair the response to PPD skin test.
Yellow fever	Cholera vaccine (parenteral)	Give the two vaccines on same day or at least 3 weeks apart.

Updated from Jong EC: Immunizations for international travelers. In *The Travel Medicine Advisor,* Atlanta, 1993, American Health Consultants.

natural opportunity for them to catch up on any missed doses of the routine immunizations. Adult travelers may need boosters for tetanus/diphtheria, polio (for travel outside the Western Hemisphere), and measles (if a second dose after infancy was not received). Adults born before hepatitis B was incorporated into the routine childhood vaccine series may require the full hepatitis B vaccine primary series for protection. Those lacking a definite history of varicella (chickenpox) infection may benefit from immunization, since varicella is a disease of young adults rather than childhood in many tropical countries. In some communities and areas of the United States, where there are recurrent outbreaks or heightened levels of transmission of hepatitis A virus infections, the hepatitis A vaccine is included among the routine immunizations of childhood. The primary vaccine schedules and booster intervals for routine immunizations for adults are given in Table 4-2.

Table 4-2
Dosage Schedules for Adult Routine Immunizations

Vaccine	Primary series	Booster interval
Hepatitis B (Engerix B) (accelerated schedule)	3 doses* IM at 0, 1, and 2 mo	A fourth dose is recommended 12 mo after the first dose to ensure long-lasting immunity
Hepatitis B (Engerix B) (standard schedule)	3 doses* IM at 0, 1, and 6 mo	Need for booster not determined
Hepatitis B (Recombivax) (standard schedule)	3 doses* IM at 0, 1, and 6 mo	Need for booster not determined
Influenza virus	1 dose* IM or SC	Annual immunization with current vaccine
Measles/mumps/rubella (MMR)† (for children ≥15 mo and adults)	1 dose* SC	Boost measles vaccine at 12-18 yr old; if a second dose was not received after childhood, boost measles vaccine *once* in adult life before international travel for people born after 1957 and before 1980
Pneumococcus (Pneumovax) (23-valent)	1 dose* SC	1 booster 5 years after the first dose, if the primary dose was received at <65 years of age
Poliomyelitis, enhanced inactivated (E-IPV) (killed vaccine, safe for all ages)	Give doses* 1 and 2 SC or IM 4-8 wk apart; give dose 3 6-12 mo after dose 2	Give booster dose *once* to people before travel in areas at risk, if 5 or more years since the last dose of vaccine
Tetanus and diphtheria toxoids adsorbed (Td) (for children ≥7 yr old and for adults)	3 doses* SC or IM; give doses 1 and 2 4-8 wk apart, give dose 3 6-12 mo later	Routine booster dose every 10 yr
Varicella† (Varivax) (for children ≥13 yr old and for adults)	2 doses* SC given 4-8 weeks apart	None

Adapted from Jong EC: Immunizations for international travelers. In *The Travel Medicine Advisor,* Atlanta, 1993, American Health Consultants.
IM, Intramuscular; *SC,* subcutaneous.
*See manufacturer's package insert for recommendations on dosage.
†May be contraindicated in patients with any of the following conditions: pregnancy, leukemia, lymphoma, generalized malignancy, immunosuppression from HIV infection or treatment with corticosteroids, alkylating drugs, antimetabolites, or radiation therapy.

REQUIRED TRAVEL IMMUNIZATIONS

The immunizations for international travel identified as "required" usually refer to those regulated by the World Health Organization (WHO). In past years, yellow fever, cholera, and smallpox vaccines were subject to WHO regulations. However, the requirements for cholera and smallpox vaccines for international travel were dropped several decades ago. At the present time, yellow fever vaccine is the only one that may be required for entry into member countries according to current WHO regulations.

The international traveler should have all current immunizations recorded in *The International Certificates of Vaccination,* a document in booklet form printed on yellow paper and approved by the WHO. The booklet has a special page for official validation of the yellow fever vaccine, and is recognized as an official document all over the world. Recent copies of the booklet (after 1988) do not contain a separate page for cholera vaccine validation because the WHO officially removed cholera vaccination from the International Health Regulations in 1973. If given, the cholera vaccination can be recorded in the space provided for "Other Vaccinations" in the newer booklets. Copies of *The International Certificates of Vaccination* may be ordered from the U.S. Government Printing Office (see Appendix).

Yellow Fever Vaccine

Yellow fever is a viral infection transmitted by *Aedes aegypti* mosquitoes in equatorial South America and Africa. The endemic zones are shown in Fig. 4-1. The yellow fever (YF) vaccine is a live attenuated viral vaccine prepared from the 17D strain of YF virus (YF Vax, Aventis, formerly Pasteur Merieux Connaught). The WHO controls the production of YF vaccine, sets requirements, and approves certain laboratories for its manufacture. The vaccine leads to seroconversion rates of 95% or higher and a duration of immunity of at least 10 years, and possibly lifelong. The YF vaccine is given as a single dose for primary immunization; the recommended booster interval is 10 years (Table 4-3). The vaccine is contraindicated in infants less than 6 months old because of the age-related risk of encephalitis after immunization. If possible, YF immunization should be delayed until the infant is at least 9 months old. The vaccine is generally not recommended during pregnancy except when travel to a highly endemic area cannot be avoided or postponed by the pregnant traveler, and the risk of the actual disease is thought to be greater than the theoretical risk of adverse effects from the vaccine.

Additional contraindications to receiving the YF vaccine include immune suppression caused by underlying disease (e.g., malignancy, HIV infection, congenital immune deficiency) or by medical therapy (e.g., medication with daily corticosteroids, cancer chemotherapy, radiation therapy, organ transplant therapy). Most travel experts would consider administering yellow fever vaccine to travelers at risk if the CD4 cell count were ≥400 μl in an HIV-infected person, or if the corticosteroid dosage was ≤20 mg prednisone per day. The vaccine virus is cultured in eggs and is not recommended for persons with a history of severe allergy (anaphylaxis) to eggs. A review of reports submitted to the Vaccine Adverse Events Reporting System (VAERS) from 1990 though 1997 found a rate of 1/131,000 for anaphylaxis after immunization with YFV. The package insert contains instructions for skin-testing persons with an uncertain history of allergy to egg.

A recent report from the GeoSentinel Network clinical sites showed that the risk of rare, serious adverse effects associated with yellow fever vaccine increases with age in adult vaccine recipients (≥65 years old). Thus, careful review of the proposed itinerary with regard to risks and benefits of YF vaccine is particularly important for senior travelers.

If a person for whom the vaccine is contraindicated must travel to a country where yellow fever vaccine is required for entry, a signed statement on letterhead stationery that states that the yellow fever vaccine

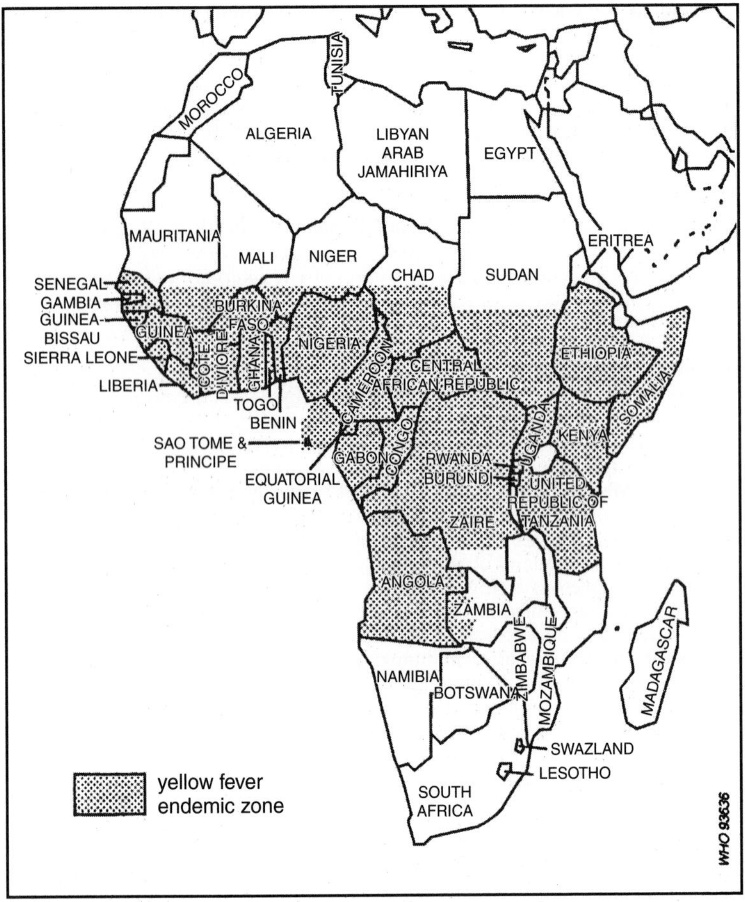

Fig. 4-1 Yellow fever endemic zones. (From W.H.O., in Centers for Disease Control and Prevention: *Health information for international travel, 2001-2002,* Washington, DC, 2001, US Government Printing Office.)

could not be given to the traveler because of medical contraindications will be accepted in lieu of the vaccination statement, according to WHO regulations.

Cholera Vaccine

The whole cell, inactivated parenteral cholera vaccine commonly used in the past was not highly efficacious, even when the primary series of two doses given a week or more apart was received. Therefore, as previously mentioned, the WHO dropped its endorsement of a requirement for this

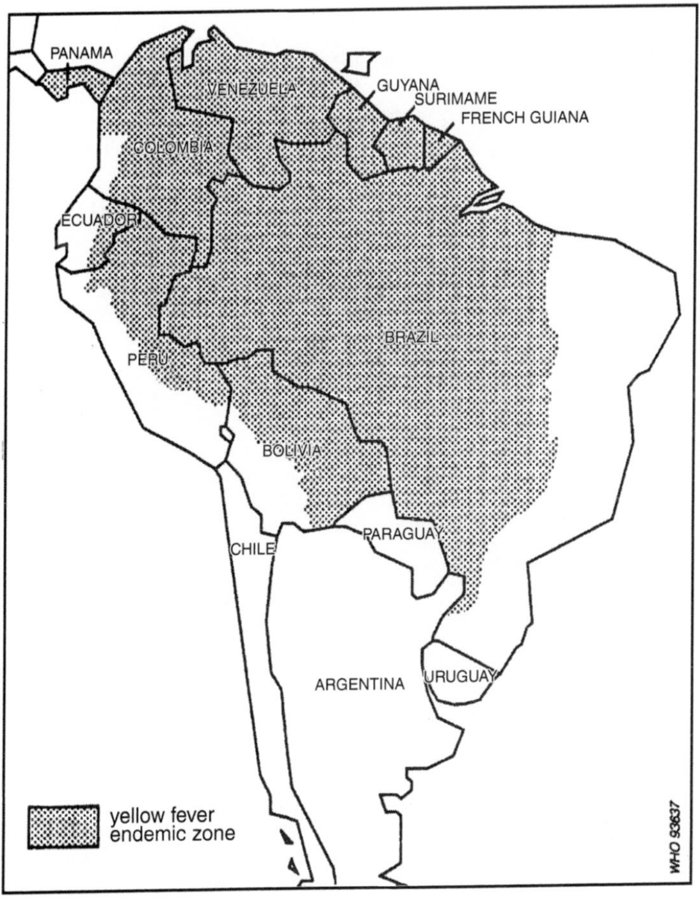

Fig. 4-1, cont'd For legend see opposite page.

vaccine for entry into any country. Nonetheless, some countries still could request (unofficially) a cholera vaccine for travelers arriving from cholera-endemic areas as a condition for entry. If this situation is anticipated, a single dose of one of the newer cholera vaccines should meet this requirement and should be recorded in the traveler's *International Certificates of Vaccination* (see earlier discussion). Alternatively, the traveler without cholera vaccine documentation in such a situation may be able to pay a penalty fee in lieu of actual immunization at the border.

New oral cholera vaccines have been developed that appear to offer improved protection compared with the traditional parenteral cholera vaccine. The live-attenuated oral cholera vaccine CVD-HgR (Orachol,

Table 4-3
Dosage Schedules for Adult Travel Immunizations

Vaccine	Primary series	Booster interval
Cholera, parenteral	2 doses* SC or IM 1 wk or more apart	6 mo
Cholera, oral (Orachol, Mutacol)	1 dose* PO according to package directions	Need for booster not determined
Hepatitis A+B (Twinrix)	3 doses* by IM injection at 1, 2, and 6 months	Need for booster not determined
Immune Globulin (hepatitis A protection)	1 dose* IM in gluteus muscle (2 ml dose for 3 mo protection; 5 ml divided dose for 5 mo protection)	Boost at 3- to 5-mo intervals depending on initial dose received for continued risk of exposure
Japanese Encephalitis (JE Vax)	3 doses* SC on days 0, 7, and 30	Booster dose may be given after 2 yr
Meningococcus (A/C/Y/W-135) (Menimmune)	1 dose* SC	None
Plague	1st dose (1 ml IM); 2nd dose (0.2 ml IM) 4 wk later; dose 3 (0.2 ml IM) 3-6 mo after dose 2	Boost if risk of exposure persists: give first 2 booster doses (0.1-0.2 ml) 6 mo apart, then give 1 booster dose at 1- to 2-yr intervals as needed
Rabies, human diploid cell vaccine (HDCV) (Imovax)	3 doses* (0.1 ml ID) on days 0, 7, and 21 or 28	Boost after 2 yr or test serum for antibody level (must not use chloroquine prophylaxis until 3 wk after completion of ID vaccine series)
Rabies (HDCV) or rabies vaccine absorbed (RVA) or Rabies (PCEC) (RabAvert)	3 doses* (1 ml IM in the deltoid area) on days 0, 7, and 21 or 28	Boost after 2 yrs or test serum for antibody level
Tick Borne Encephalitis (FSME-Immun)	3 doses* SC at months 0, 1-3, and 9-12 months after dose #2	Boost 3 years after the last dose
Tick Borne Encephalitis (Encepur), (Rapid Schedule)	3 doses* SC on 0, 7, 21 days	Boosters at 12-18 months, and 3-5 years.
Tuberculosis (BCG vaccine)‡	1 dose* percutaneously with multiple-puncture disk	Revaccination after 2-3 mo in those who remain tuberculin negative to 5 TB skin test
Typhoid, Vi capsular polysaccharide (Typhim Vi)	1 dose* SC	Boost after 2 yr for continued risk of exposure
Typhoid, oral (Vivotif) (for persons ≥6 years of age)	1 capsule* PO every 2 days for 4 doses	5 yr
Yellow fever† (YF Vax)	1 dose* SC	10 yr

Adapted from Jong EC: Immunizations for international travelers. In *The Travel Medicine Advisor,* Atlanta, 1993, American Health Consultants.

SC, Subcutaneous; *IM,* intramuscular; *PO,* orally; *ID,* intradermal.

*See manufacturer's package insert for recommendations on dosage.

†Caution, may be contraindicated in patients with any of the following conditions: pregnancy, leukemia, lymphoma, generalized malignancy, immunosuppression from HIV infection or treatment with corticosteroids, alkylating drugs, antimetabolites, or radiation therapy.

‡Withdrawn from market by manufacturer, March, 2002.

Swiss Serum Institute, or Mutachol, Berna) is available in Western Europe, Latin America, and Canada. United States release of the vaccine is pending Food and Drug Approval (FDA) approval. The vaccine is given as a single oral dose and appears to provide significant protection for 6 months or longer in field trials in endemic areas. Travelers going to cholera-endemic or cholera-epidemic areas are encouraged to follow food and water precautions as recommended for prevention of all forms of travel-associated diarrhea. Some practitioners recommend that people with underlying gastric conditions, such as achlorhydria or partial gastric resection, or on medications that block gastric acid production (H_2 blockers), which may increase susceptibility to cholera infection, be priority candidates for cholera immunization when the new vaccine becomes available.

Smallpox Vaccine

The smallpox vaccine (vaccinia virus vaccine) is no longer available commercially. Limited supplies are released on a case-by-case basis from the CDC based on individual review. Research scientists and health care workers who work with the smallpox virus and closely related viruses are candidates for immunization. The last case of smallpox acquired through natural transmission was reported in 1977, and the requirement for smallpox vaccine for international travel was removed from the WHO regulations in 1982.

RECOMMENDED TRAVEL VACCINES

Recommended travel vaccines are given to travelers based on the anticipated level of risk of exposure. Vaccines in this category may include hepatitis A, immune globulin (for hepatitis A), hepatitis B, typhoid fever, meningococcal meningitis, rabies, Japanese encephalitis, plague, and tick-borne encephalitis. Immunization against tuberculosis (bacillus Calmette-Guérin [BCG] vaccine) or a tuberculosis skin test (purified protein derivative [PPD]) may also be recommended for some travelers. Brief descriptions of each vaccine are given in the following discussion. Table 4-3 lists doses and schedules for primary immunizations and boosters.

Immune Globulin and Hepatitis A Vaccine

Hepatitis A is a serious viral infection with an oral-fecal transmission pattern similar to polio, cholera, typhoid, and traveler's diarrhea. Hepatitis A infections are reported to be the leading cause of vaccine-preventable illness occurring among nonimmune international travelers, where the incidence rate can be as high as 20 cases/1000 travelers/month among travelers doing rural or adventure travel in developing countries. A lower rate, 3 to 6 cases/1000 travelers/month, has been observed among travelers going to tourist areas or hotels and resorts in developing countries.

Hepatitis A infections are less serious when acquired in early childhood, when they may present as mild anicteric illnesses. Although the hepatitis A case fatality rate associated with acute infections is less than 0.1% in childhood from <1 to 14 years old, the rate is 0.4% from 15 to 39 years old, 1.1% in persons over 40 years old, and rises to 2.7% persons over 50 years old.

Although up to 60% of adults over 40 years old from industrialized countries may have immunity to hepatitis A through clinical or subclinical infection, most travelers less than 40 years old are susceptible. In nonimmune travelers going to hepatitis A endemic areas when there is less than 2 weeks remaining before departure, immune globulin (IG, purified human immune globulin) may be used to provide temporary protection against hepatitis A virus infection through the passive transfer of preformed antibodies against hepatitis A present in the IG (at least 100 IU/ml). Duration of protection is dependent on dose, with a dose of 0.06 ml/kg administered as a deep intramuscular injection into the gluteus maximus muscle providing up to 5 months of protection (Table 4-3).

If time allows, a serum test for hepatitis A antibody should be performed in people who are of foreign birth, resided overseas, travel frequently in nonindustrialized countries, give a history of a previous illness with jaundice, or were born before 1945; unnecessary immunization may be avoided if a person has protective antibodies from hepatitis A infection in the past.

The use of IG for protection against hepatitis A in travelers has been largely supplanted by use of the inactivated hepatitis A vaccines. Several safe and highly efficacious inactivated hepatitis A virus (HAV) vaccines have become available commercially since the 1994 release of Havrix (GlaxoSmithKline, formerly SmithKline Beecham, Philadelphia, PA). Havrix is an inactivated HAV vaccine, derived from the HM-175 viral strain, and given by injection. The others include VAQTA (Merck Vaccine Division, West Point, NJ), an inactivated parenteral HAV vaccine derived from the CR-326F strain; AVAXIM (Aventis, formerly Pasteur Merieux, Paris, France), an inactivated parenteral HAV vaccine derived from the GBM viral strain; and Epaxal Berna (Swiss Serum Research Institute, Berne, Switzerland), an inactivated parenteral virosomal HAV vaccine derived from the RG-SB viral strain. Havrix and VAQTA are available in the United States and Canada at the present time, as well as worldwide. The other vaccines are distributed mostly in Western Europe.

The immunization schedules for all the hepatitis A vaccines listed here consist of a single primary dose given by intramuscular injection into the deltoid muscle, resulting in protective antibody titers within 2 to 4 weeks (98% to 100% seropositivity rate). The first vaccine dose is followed by a booster dose 6 to 12 months later, producing levels of antibody predicted to give protection up to 10 years or more by mathematical modeling.

In some cases, travelers return for their booster dose of inactivated hepatitis A vaccine later than the recommended time of 6 to 12 months after the primary dose. Based on the results of clinical studies, delaying the booster dose up to 66 months after primary vaccination did not seem to influence the anamnestic immune response to the booster dose. However, significantly more late travelers (≥24 months) had lost detectable antibodies than control subjects (6 to 12 months) before administration of the booster dose. These findings suggest that a booster dose given later than the recommended 6 to 12 months will still be highly effective.

Vaccine interchangeability, that is, when one of the inactivated hepatitis A vaccines is used for the primary dose, and then a hepatitis A vaccine made by a different manufacturer is used for the booster dose, has been studied among several of the vaccines listed previously. It appears from the preliminary results of clinical studies that Havrix and VAQTA may be used interchangeably without significant loss of protective antibody levels elicited (data on file, Merck Vaccine Division, West Point, NJ), although this practice is not recommended or officially approved at this time.

Concurrent Administration of Hepatitis A Vaccine with Immune Globulin

When hepatitis A vaccine is given to at-risk travelers less than 2 weeks before trip departure, some experts have recommended that a dose of immune globulin (IG) be given concurrently to protect the traveler in the window of time before vaccine-induced antibodies reach protective levels. Although clinical studies showed that geometric mean titers of serum antibodies against hepatitis A were significantly lower for healthy adult subjects receiving both vaccine and IG, the antibody levels were nevertheless substantially higher than the cutoff of assay seropositivity (20 mIU/ml) and much higher than IG alone. These differences were clinically insignificant.

Hepatitis B Vaccine

Hepatitis B vaccine was added to the list of vaccines recommended for routine immunization of children in the United States in the early 1990s. However, many adult travelers at potential risk of infection would not have received hepatitis B vaccine as a routine immunization. In many parts of Asia and Africa, up to 15% of the general population may be asymptomatic carriers of hepatitis B virus. Travelers going to Asia and Africa who will live and work among the residents, such as missionaries, health care staff, volunteer relief workers, teachers, students, adventure travelers, and other travelers who might have intimate or sexual contact with the residents, should consider immunization against hepatitis B.

Two recombinant hepatitis B vaccines are available, Recombivax (Merck Vaccine Division, West Point, NJ) and Engerix B (GlaxoSmithKline, Philadelphia, PA). The standard dosage schedule for both vaccines consists of doses administered by injection at 0, 1, and 6 months. Engerix B vaccine has an FDA-approved accelerated dosage schedule of 0, 1, and 2 months. This may allow full immunization of a traveler with limited time before departure; however, a booster dose at 12 months is recommended to ensure long-lasting immunity.

Among travelers who are at high risk of hepatitis B exposure, such as health care workers, relief workers, missionaries, long-term travelers, and expatriates, the possibility of vaccine recipients who do not seroconvert with protective levels of antibody after immunization should be considered. Known risk factors are increasing age (>30 years old), chronic medical conditions, obesity, smoking, male gender, and vaccine administration into the buttock. Anti-HBs testing should be performed 1 to 6 months after the last dose of vaccine. If there is no seroconversion (≥10 mIU/ml), one dose of hepatitis B vaccine should be given, and the anti-HBs titer rechecked 4 to 12 weeks later. If there is still no measurable antibody response, the second series is completed with two additional doses given 1 and 6 months after.

Hepatitis A+B Vaccine

A hepatitis A+B combination vaccine (Twinrix) was released in 2001 by GlaxoSmithKline (GSK). This vaccine contains 720 Elisa units of hepatitis A antigen and 20 μg of hepatitis B antigen, and the primary immunization series consists of three doses given at 0, 1, and 6 months. The use of this combination vaccine will be convenient for travelers and other persons who need protection against both diseases, and decrease the total number of vaccine injections required (3 versus 5). A clinical research study has reported that an accelerated dosing schedule of 0, 7, and 21 days elicits a high level of protective antibody against hepatitis A and, to a lesser degree, against hepatitis B 1 month after the third dose. A fourth dose at 12 months is recommended to boost the longevity of the immune response to the accelerated schedule. This alternative schedule has not yet received FDA approval.

Typhoid Fever Vaccine

The incidence of typhoid fever among American travelers is relatively low (58 to 174 cases per 1 million travelers), but among reported cases in the United States, 62% were acquired during international travel. Transmission appears particularly high in Mexico, Peru, India, Pakistan, and Chile. Sub-Saharan Africa and Southeast Asia are also regarded as areas of increased risk for typhoid fever.

Avoidance of potentially contaminated food and drink during travel is important, even if the typhoid vaccine is received. Protection against typhoid fever afforded by immunization may be overwhelmed by ingestion of highly contaminated food: protection rates of 43% to 96% were reported in field trials with the oral live-attenuated typhoid vaccine among residents of endemic areas. However, limited data are available to predict actual protection rates in people who travel from nonendemic areas to endemic areas for typhoid. The risk of typhoid fever infections to the traveler is further heightened by the multidrug resistance patterns emerging in *Salmonella typhi* strains around the world to antibiotics commonly used in the treatment of gastrointestinal infections, including the widely used fluoroquinolone drugs.

The oral typhoid vaccine (Vivotif, Berna, Coral Gables, FL) contains a live attenuated strain of *Salmonella typhi* bacteria (Ty21A). The vaccine is in capsule form and is recommended for people 6 years of age and older. A primary (or booster) series consists of four capsules, one taken every other day over the course of a week. The booster interval is 5 years. A liquid suspension form of this vaccine is expected in the near future; this may facilitate administration of the vaccine to children and others who have difficulty swallowing capsules. Persons who were previously immunized with one of the typhoid vaccines given by injection, and who now desire immunization with the oral vaccine, should receive the full four-capsule series.

Safety of the live oral Ty21A typhoid vaccine in immune-compromised persons has not yet been demonstrated, and this vaccine should not be administered to these persons. The vaccine is not recommended for pregnant women because of lack of data (Category C). The live oral typhoid vaccine should not be administered during an acute gastrointestinal illness, or if the individual is receiving treatment with sulfonamides or other antibiotics.

Conditions interfering with multiplication of the vaccine strain bacteria in vivo may result in an insufficient bacterial antigen stimulus to induce a protective response. The antimalarial drugs chloroquine and mefloquine may be administered concomitantly with the oral typhoid vaccine without decreasing the immune response rate. However, proguanil, one component of the atovaquone/proguanil (Malarone) fixed-dose combination drug used for prevention and treatment of chloroquine-resistant malaria, does significantly decrease the immune response to oral typhoid vaccine. Therefore proguanil and atovaquone/proguanil should be administered 10 or more days after the final dose of the vaccine. Concomitant administration of the oral polio vaccine or the yellow fever vaccine does not appear to suppress the immune response of the oral typhoid vaccine.

A highly purified Vi capsular polysaccharide vaccine (Typhim Vi, Aventis, formerly Pasteur Merieux) elicits immunity 10 days after receipt of a single primary dose by intramuscular injection. In contrast to the older inactivated whole-cell vaccine, also given by injection, the Vi polysaccharide typhoid vaccine is usually very well tolerated, has a low rate of adverse effects, and is safe for use in children >2 years old, pregnant women, and travelers with a compromised immune system. The booster interval for the Vi polysaccharide typhoid vaccine is 2 years.

The use of the injectable heat-phenol-inactivated whole-cell typhoid vaccine has been largely supplanted by the more modern vaccines, the oral typhoid vaccine and the Vi polysaccharide typhoid vaccine. The old inactivated whole-cell typhoid vaccine consisted of two doses given 4 weeks apart for primary immunization, and a booster dose after 3 or more years. The inactivated whole-cell vaccine was associated with troublesome side effects consisting of significant soreness at the injection site, headache, low-grade fever, and general malaise for 1 or 2 days after immunization.

Typhoid Fever Vaccine Combined with Hepatitis A Vaccine

Typhoid fever and hepatitis A viral infections are both transmitted through oral-fecal contamination of food and beverages; thus protection against both diseases is indicated in many international travelers. Several studies have shown that simultaneous administration of the Vi polysaccharide typhoid vaccine (Typhim Vi) and hepatitis A vaccine (Havrix or VAQTA) at different injection sites results in no significant increase in adverse side effects nor in impaired efficacy of either vaccine. One limited study showed that combining both vaccine preparations in the same syringe was also feasible, so a combined formulated vaccine against both typhoid fever and hepatitis A might offer more convenience to the traveler and be a product consideration at some time in the future.

Meningococcal Vaccine

The meningococcal vaccine is required for entry by Saudi Arabia for travelers to that country during the time of the annual religious pilgrimage (the Hajj) to Mecca in late spring. The vaccine is also recommended for people going to live and work in certain areas of Africa (sub-Saharan) and South America (Brazil) where outbreaks of the disease are frequent among the residents. The meningococcal vaccine is currently recommended by the CDC and the American College Health Association for incoming freshmen who will live in dormitories on the campuses of American colleges and universities, because of a recently recognized increased risk of meningococcal transmission in such populations.

The meningococcal polysaccharide vaccine (Menimmune, Aventis, Swiftwater, PA) is a quadrivalent vaccine inducing immunity against serogroups A, C, Y, and W-135. A single dose appears to provide immunity for at least 3 years. Vaccine efficacy is variable in young children, and a second dose of vaccine after 2 or 3 years is recommended for children living in high-risk areas who received the first vaccine dose at less than 4 years of age. In some countries, the bivalent meningococcal polysaccharide vaccine containing serogroups A and C is commonly available, and does not protect travelers in outbreaks involving serogroup Y or W-135 disease.

Rabies Vaccine

Animal bites, especially dog bites, present a potential rabies hazard to international travelers who travel to rural areas in Central and South

America, the Middle East, Africa, and Asia. Preexposure rabies immunization is recommended for rural travelers, especially adventure travelers who go to remote areas, and for expatriate workers, missionaries, and their families living in countries where rabies is a recognized risk. Preexposure rabies immunization simplifies the postbite medical care of a person following an animal bite in a high-risk area. Without preexposure immunization, the bitten person needs double treatment with both rabies immune globulin (RIG) and a series of five doses of a modern tissue culture-derived vaccine administered as soon as possible after the incident. Both RIG and high-quality rabies vaccine doses may be difficult for the international traveler to access in the areas of greatest rabies risk. More detailed recommendations for postbite treatment are discussed later.

The rabies vaccine is an inactivated virus vaccine, and three products are commonly available: human diploid cell vaccine (HDCV, Imovax, Aventis, Swiftwater, PA), rabies vaccine absorbed (RVA, GlaxoSmithKline, Philadelphia, PA), and purified chick embryo cell (PCEC, Rabavert, Chiron, Emeryville, CA) vaccine. These vaccine products may be used interchangeably in the preexposure rabies immunization: a total of three doses (1.0 ml each) of rabies vaccine are administered by intramuscular injection on days 0, 7, and 21, or 28.

An HDCV rabies vaccine (Imovax) product is marketed for administration by intradermal injection. A smaller vaccine dose (0.1 ml each) is used for the intradermal primary series on 0, 7, and 21 or 28 days, a schedule similar to that for the intramuscular series. The intradermal doses are less expensive than the intramuscular doses, but require advance planning: efficacy of the intradermal vaccine series is compromised if chloroquine prophylaxis against malaria is started within 3 weeks after the third dose of intradermal vaccine. If there is not sufficient time before departure, an intramuscular rabies vaccine series should be given. The usual booster interval for rabies vaccine is 2 years. However, if time permits, serologic testing may show persistence of protective antibody levels, so the booster dose may be delayed to 3 or even 4 years after the last dose on the basis of annual testing. This sparing of vaccine doses received could be beneficial to recipients who have a long-term need for protection (veterinarians, field biologists, laboratory workers, and expatriates living in high-risk areas).

Mild local reactions to rabies vaccine are common and consist of erythema, pain, and swelling at the injection site. Mild systemic symptoms including headache, dizziness, nausea, abdominal pain, and myalgias may develop in some recipients. In approximately 5% of people receiving booster doses of HDCV for preexposure prophylaxis and in a few receiving postexposure immunization, a serum sickness-like illness characterized by urticaria, fever, malaise, arthralgias, arthritis, nausea, and vomiting may develop 2 to 21 days after a vaccine dose is received.

Rabies vaccine adsorbed (RVA) vaccine was originally produced by the Michigan Department of Public Health, and is now distributed by GlaxoSmithKline. This inactivated virus vaccine is derived from virus grown in tissue culture cells in medium free of human albumin. The RVA vaccine may be used for intramuscular administration only. Data are accumulating on the incidence of reactions after immunization with this preparation. The PCEC rabies vaccine is also grown in tissue culture cells in medium free of human albumin, may be used for intramuscular administration only, and also appears to have a low adverse effects profile associated with revaccination doses, although data are still accumulating.

Rabies Exposure After-Bite Care

Receipt of preexposure rabies immunization simplifies the care of a person if a high-risk bite is sustained; in addition to immediate wound care (vigorous cleansing, debridement, loose approximation of skin edges, and antibiotics to prevent wound infection), two additional 1-ml intramuscular doses of rabies vaccine on days 0 and 3 are recommended for optimal protection.

If a person who has not received preexposure rabies vaccine is bitten while in a rabies-endemic area, postexposure care for the bite includes a dose (20 IU/kg) of rabies immune globulin (RIG), with one-half the dose infiltrated at the wound site if possible and the remainder given by intramuscular injection. In addition, five doses (1 ml) of rabies vaccine should be given by intramuscular injection on days 0, 3, 7, 14, and 28.

Safe supplies of rabies immune globulin and rabies vaccine are difficult to obtain in many rabies-endemic areas. The supply of RIG in developing countries is likely to be derived from horse serum (in contrast to the human-derived RIG product available in industrialized countries). Administration of horse-derived RIG is accompanied by a significant risk of serum sickness. The rabies vaccines available in developing countries are often Semple-type vaccines, derived from infected brain tissue of laboratory animals. Such preparations have a potential for adverse side effects and decreased protective efficacy compared with the modern tissue culture-derived rabies vaccines.

Japanese Encephalitis Virus Vaccine

Japanese encephalitis (JE) is a viral infection transmitted by *Culex* mosquitoes in Asia and Southeast Asia. Transmission is year round in the tropical and subtropical areas and during the late spring, summer, and early fall in temperate climates. Pigs and some species of birds are natural reservoirs of the virus, while the mosquito vectors breed extensively in flooded rice fields and irrigation projects.

JE virus is not considered a risk for short-term travelers visiting the usual tourist destinations in urban areas and developed resort areas. For visitors to rural areas during the transmission season, the estimated risk for JE during a 1-month period is 1:5000 or 1:20,000 per week. The risk of infection can be greatly decreased by personal protective measures to prevent mosquito bites: wearing protective clothing, using insect repellents, and sleeping under permethrin-treated bed nets. Nonetheless, because JE has been acquired by short-term travelers to endemic rural areas, and because agricultural projects bordering on urban areas can bring infected mosquitoes into the proximity of susceptible urban dwellers, the vaccine should be offered to travelers going on trips of any length to rural areas (especially areas of pig farming), and to expatriate workers, missionaries, and students who plan to live, work, or travel in urban, suburban, or farming communities in endemic areas.

An inactivated viral vaccine (JE Vax, Biken, distributed by Aventis, Swiftwater, PA) consisting of three doses given by injection over the course of a month is available for administration to travelers determined to be at significant risk. A schedule consisting of doses at 0, 7, and 30 days appears to result in a higher seroconversion rate and geometric mean titer of antibody among recipients than does a 2-week accelerated schedule consisting of doses at 0, 7, and 14 days. A booster dose of vaccine may be given 2 to 3 years after the primary immunization for continued risk of exposure.

Adverse reactions to Japanese encephalitis vaccine (JEV) include local pain and swelling at the site of injection in about 20% of recipients, systemic symptoms (fever, headache, malaise, rash) in about 10% of recipients, and hypersensitivity reactions (mainly urticaria, angioedema, or both) in 15 to 62 per 10,000 vaccinees. Hypersensitivity reactions reported occurred after the first, second, or third dose of vaccine, either almost immediately afterward or with delays of up to 2 weeks after receipt of the vaccine dose. Limited data suggest that persons who have had urticarial reactions to *Hymenoptera* envenomation and to other stimuli might be at greater risk than others of JEV-induced hypersensitivity reactions. The CDC recommends that vaccinees be directly observed for 30 minutes after receipt of JEV and that they not depart on their travel until 10 days after the last JEV dose to ensure access to familiar medical care systems should such a delayed adverse reaction occur.

Plague Vaccine

Plague, a bacterial disease caused by *Yersinia pestis,* is enzootic among wild rodents in countries of Africa, Asia, and the Americas. Plague is transmitted to humans by fleas or direct contact with infected animals. Person-to-person spread is common through respiratory secretions. International travelers going on standard tourist itineraries to countries where plague is reported are unlikely to be at risk. Persons who are at high risk of exposure include field biologists and those who will reside or work in rural mountainous or upland areas, where avoidance of rodents and fleas is difficult.

Plague vaccine is a killed bacterial vaccine with poorly documented protective efficacy. Availability of the vaccine for ordinary travelers is limited. Primary immunization consists of three doses of vaccine given by intramuscular injection over 10 months. Side effects include pain, redness, and induration at the site of injection. Systemic symptoms consisting of fever, headache, and malaise may occur after repeated doses.

Some medical consultants suggest the use of prophylactic tetracycline (500 mg by mouth four times a day for 7 days) immediately after exposure to plague-infected animals or humans as an alternative to plague vaccine. The efficacy of using tetracycline prophylaxis has not been studied in a controlled clinical trial, but is derived from use of the drug in the treatment of plague.

Tick-Borne Encephalitis Vaccine

Tick-borne encephalitis (TBE) is caused by infection with either of two closely related viruses: Central European encephalitis virus (CEEV) in Europe (Austria, Czechoslovakia, Germany, Hungary, Poland, Switzerland, northern Yugoslavia) and Russian Spring Summer encephalitis virus (RSSEV) in the Commonwealth of Independent States (the former Soviet Union) during the months of April through August. There is overlap of the areas of transmission in Eastern Europe. TBE is transmitted to humans by bites from infected *Ixodes ricinus* ticks usually found in forested areas of endemic regions. However, systemic infection after ingestion of unpasteurized dairy products from infected cows, goats, or sheep can also occur.

Vaccination against TBE is not available in the United States. A vaccine named FSME-Immun TBE Vaccine is manufactured by Immuno (Vienna, Austria) and is available in Canada and Europe. The vaccine is produced in chick embryo cell cultures; primary immunization consists of three doses given by subcutaneous injection over the course of a year. The limited availability of the vaccine and the relatively long immunization schedule mean that most travelers from North America who anticipate a need for protection against TBE will not be able to obtain the vaccine. Another TBE vaccine called Encepur TBE Vaccine is manufactured by Chiron, Behring, Germany, and has a rapid schedule option of 0, 7, and 21 days with booster doses scheduled at 12 to 18 months and at 3 to 5 years; however, this vaccine is not currently available in North America.

Travelers planning outdoor activities (hiking, biking, camping) in areas where TBE is a risk need to rely on personal protection measures to prevent tick bites. They should wear protective clothing when outdoors, use insect repellents containing *N,N*-diethyl-meta-toluamide (DEET) on exposed areas of skin, and treat their outer clothing with a permethrin-containing insecticide. All travelers to such areas should be advised to avoid ingestion of unpasteurized dairy products.

Tuberculosis (BCG Vaccine)

Travelers who will live among foreign residents or who will work in foreign orphanages, schools, hospitals, or other facilities may be at significant risk of exposure to infection with tuberculosis (TB), which is commonly spread from person to person by inhalation of infected respiratory droplets in closed environments. Such travelers should be skin tested with tuberculin (PPD) and control antigens (such as *Candida* and *Trichophyton*) before and after the trip. Persons who convert to a skin test positive status after international travel need further evaluation and are candidates for consideration of prophylactic treatment with isoniazid or other drugs to prevent TB disease. However, people going on short trips for tourism or business to countries where tuberculosis is much more common among the general population than in the United States are not considered to be at great risk of contracting TB.

The BCG (Bacillus Calmette-Guérin) vaccines are used widely all over the world for childhood immunization against tuberculosis, although this has never been a public health policy in the United States. There is no consensus on the protective efficacy of BCG vaccines, and estimates of protection have varied from study to study. Epidemiologic data suggest that the vaccine may be more useful in protecting children from disseminated extrapulmonary complications of tuberculosis than in protecting adults from primary pulmonary infection. Persons immunized with BCG vaccine become PPD skin test positive for many years afterward, regardless of the degree of protection conferred by the vaccine. As a result, the PPD skin test cannot be used as a reliable indicator of infection in recipients, and this situation can contribute to a delay in diagnosis in people who have contracted tuberculosis infection despite BCG vaccination.

Occasionally, children in families going abroad for extended residence are requested by the receiving country to provide proof of BCG vaccination to qualify for a visa. A BCG vaccine is commercially available in the United States and is approved by the American Academy of Pediatrics Committee on the Control of Infectious Diseases for use in children going to live in areas where tuberculosis is prevalent or where there is a likelihood of exposure to adults with active or recently arrested tuberculosis. The BCG vaccine also might be considered appropriate in the case of uninfected (PPD skin test-negative) health care workers who are going to work in areas where there is a high endemic prevalence of tuberculosis in the population, and who will have limited access to medical diagnosis and treatment.

Like other live attenuated vaccines, BCG vaccine is contraindicated in people with immunosuppression caused by congenital conditions, chemotherapy, radiation therapy, HIV infection, or another condition resulting in impaired immune responses. Pregnancy also is considered a relative contraindication.

Lyme Disease Vaccine

A vaccine against Lyme disease caused by infection with U.S. strains of *Borrelia burgdorferi* became available in 1999. Immunization with the Lymerix vaccine manufactured by GlaxoSmithKline (Philadelphia, PA) showed 80% to 90% protective efficacy among adult populations studied. The vaccine is directed against the OSP A (outer surface protein A) of *B. burgdorferi,* and is approved for use in persons 15 to 70 years old who live or work in known Lyme disease transmission risk areas and are exposed to ticks frequently or for long periods. The original vaccine schedule called for two primary doses given 1 month apart, with a booster dose at 12 months after the first. An alternative vaccine schedule was then been approved, where the three doses of vaccine are given on a schedule of 0, 1, and 6 months. The Lymerix vaccine was withdrawn from the market by the manufacturer in March, 2002. For persons who were unable to receive the vaccine, one study showed that among subjects 12 years of age and older, a single 200-mg dose of doxycycline given within 72 hours after an *Ixodes scapularis* tick bite could prevent the development of Lyme disease.

Influenza Vaccine and Pneumococcal Vaccine

Annual immunization against viral influenza is recommended for all people over 50 years old. Influenza vaccine is also recommended for special groups of patients at increased risk from complications of viral influenza. These patients include those with chronic respiratory disease (emphysema, asthma), ischemic heart disease, transplanted organs, renal failure, and impaired immune response from congenital conditions, acquired illness, or immunosuppressive therapy. The 23-valent polysaccharide vaccine against pneumococcal pneumonia is a one-time-only injection and is recommended for the same groups mentioned.

In addition to the elderly and the ill, "flu" vaccine is also recommended for all health care workers and for international travelers because prolonged air travel, fatigue, and exposure to crowds in various closed environments predispose them to respiratory infections. In recent years, the CDC has identified a particular risk for viral influenza infections among travelers during the summer sailing season of Alaska cruise ship tours. The risk is thought to be associated with exposure of susceptible travelers to influenza-infected persons among the other travelers and tourist industry staff, particularly those from the Southern Hemisphere where the seasonal climate patterns are opposite those in the Northern Hemisphere. If flu vaccine is unavailable for travelers during the summer months, the use of one of the antiviral drugs active against influenza virus, either for chemoprophylaxis or early treatment, should be discussed with travelers who will be at risk.

CONCLUSION

Despite the availability of safe, highly efficacious vaccines against many of the diseases that are health risks to international travelers, there are several factors that influence travelers' acceptance of immunization recommendations. Practical concerns include the time available before trip departure, past history of allergies to or intolerance of specific vaccines, avoidance of multiple vaccine doses administered by injection, and the traveler's overall budget for pretravel health preparations. Other factors influencing the traveler's choice of travel immunizations include his or her cultural perceptions of the health risks presented by a given itinerary, whether or not adventure travel away from normal tourist routes is planned, and anticipated access to organized medical care in case of medical illness while traveling abroad.

REFERENCES

Bock HL et al: Does the concurrent administration of an inactivated hepatitis A vaccine influence the immune response to other travelers vaccines? *J Travel Med* 7:74, 2000.

Centers for Disease Control and Prevention: *Health information for international travel,* Atlanta, 2001-2002, DHHS.

Centers for Disease Control and Prevention: Prevention and control of meningococcal disease and meningococcal disease and college students: recommendations of the Advisory Committee on Immunization Practices (ACIP), *MMWR* 49 (No.RR-7):1, 2000.

Centers for Disease Control and Prevention: Immunization of health-care workers: recommendations of the Advisory Committee on Immunization Practices (ACIP), *MMWR* 46:No.RR-18, 1997.

Centers for Disease Control and Prevention: Prevention of varicella: recommendations of the Advisory Committee on Immunization Practices (ACIP), *MMWR* 45 (No. RR-11):1, 1996.

Jong EC: Immunizations for international travel, *Infect Dis Clin North Am* 12:249, 1998.

Jong EC et al. An open randomized study of inactivated hepatitis A vaccine administered concomitantly with typhoid fever and yellow fever vaccines, *J Travel Med* 9:66, 2002.

Kollaritsch H et al: Safety and immunogenicity of live oral cholera and typhoid vaccines administered alone or in combination with anti-malarial drugs, oral polio vaccine or yellow fever vaccine, *J Infect Dis* (in press).

Landry P et al: Inactivated hepatitis A vaccine booster given ≥24 months after the primary dose, *Vaccine* 19:399, 2000.

Poland GA: Hepatitis B immunization in health care workers. Dealing with vaccine nonresponse, *Am J Prev Med* 15:73, 1998.

Ryan ET, Kain KC: Health advice and immunizations for travelers, *N Engl J Med* 342:1716, 2000.

Thompson RF: *Travel & routine immunizations,* 2001 edition. Milwaukee, 2001, Shoreland.

Walter EB et al: Concurrent administration of inactivated hepatitis A vaccine with immune globulin in healthy adults, *Vaccine* 17:1468, 1999.

CHAPTER 5

Malaria Prevention

Kevin C. Kain and Elaine C. Jong

Malaria is the most important parasitic disease in the world. Human malaria is a blood-borne protozoal infection caused by four species of the genus *Plasmodium: P. falciparum, P. vivax, P. ovale,* and *P. malariae.* The infection is transmitted through the bite of infected female *Anopheles* mosquitoes. Less commonly, malaria may be transmitted by blood transfusion, with shared needle use, and congenitally from mother to fetus. Ecologic change, economic and political instability, combined with escalating malaria drug resistance, has led to a worldwide resurgence of this parasitic disease. In 1998 the World Health Organization estimated there were 273 million cases and more than 1 million deaths resulting from malaria.

Malaria is not just a problem in the developing world, however. The combination of increases in international travel and increasing drug resistance has resulted in a growing number of travelers at risk of contracting malaria. It is now estimated that as many as 30,000 travelers from industrialized countries contract malaria each year, with record numbers of cases being documented in Europe and North America over the last 5 years. However, this incidence is likely to be an underestimate because of the failure to take into account those that are diagnosed and treated abroad and the prevalence of underreporting. In North America and Europe, there has been an increase in imported *P. falciparum* cases, with the majority acquired in Africa (80% to 95%) despite the fact that travel to Africa represents a minority of all travel from either continent.

The overall case fatality rate of imported *P. falciparum* malaria varies from 0.6% to 3.8% but may be much higher in the elderly. The fatality rate of severe malaria may be 20% or greater even when managed in modern intensive care units; however, cases of imported malaria and associated fatalities remain largely preventable, provided high-risk travelers use appropriate chemoprophylaxis and measures to reduce insect bites, and physicians promptly recognize infections and initiate appropriate treatment.

APPROACH TO MALARIA PREVENTION

All travelers to malarious areas:

- Must be aware of the risk of malaria and understand that it is a serious infection.
- Know how to help prevent it.
- Seek medical attention urgently if they develop a fever during or after travel.

This chapter highlights the important principles of malaria prevention. The interested reader is referred to Table 5-1 and references for additional sources of information and country-specific malaria risk.

Protection against malaria can be summarized into the following four principles:

1. **Assessing individual risk.** Estimating a traveler's risk is based on a detailed travel itinerary and specific risk behaviors of the traveler. The risk of acquiring malaria varies according to the geographic area visited (e.g., Africa versus Southeast Asia), the travel destination within different geographic areas (e.g., urban versus rural travel), type of accommodations (camping versus well-screened or air conditioned), duration of stay (1 week business travel versus 3-month overland trek), time of travel (high or low malaria transmission season), elevation of destination (malaria transmission is rare above 2000 meters), and efficacy of and compliance with preventive measures used (e.g., treated bed nets, chemoprophylactic drugs). Additional information can be obtained from studies that estimate risk of malaria in travelers using malaria surveillance data and the numbers of travelers to specific destinations. These studies show a higher risk of infection, particularly with *P. falciparum,* in Africa and New Guinea compared with Asia or Latin America. Risk of infection if no chemoprophylaxis is used varies from >20% per month in regions of Papua (formerly Irian Jaya), to 1.7% to 2.4% per month in West Africa, to 0.01% per month to Central America. Of note, the estimated risk of malaria for travelers to Thailand in one study was 1:12,254, which may be less than the risk of a serious adverse event secondary to malaria chemoprophylaxis. Such data can help provide an estimate of the cost/benefit ratio for the use of various chemoprophylactic drugs in different geographic areas. Good sources of updated malaria information and country-specific risk are available on line from the Centers for Disease Control and Prevention (CDC), the World Health Organization (WHO), and Health Canada (Table 5-1).

Table 5-1
Health Resources for Travel

Web Site Recommendations for Country Specific Malaria Risk:

http://www.cdc.gov
U.S. Centers for Disease Control and Prevention. See Travelers' Health section.

On-line references include full text *Health Information for International Travel, 2001-2002* with full adult and pediatric recommendations, including malaria risks and recommendations. Information also available at telephone 888-232-3228.

http://www.who.org
World Health Organization. See *International Travel and Health Information* resource page for travelers. Includes updates on country specific malaria risk.

http://www.hc-sc.gc.ca
Health Canada Online Resource Page. Search "travel" information. See Canadian Laboratory Centre for Disease Control recommendations and updates for preventing and treating malaria in travelers.

Table 5-2
Checklist for Travelers to Malarious Areas

The following is a checklist of key issues to be considered in advising travelers.

1. Risk of malaria
   Travelers should be informed about their individual risk of malaria infection and the presence of drug-resistant *P. falciparum* malaria in their areas of destination. Pregnant women and adults taking young children should question the necessity of the trip.
2. Antimosquito measures
   Travelers should be instructed how to protect themselves against mosquito bites.
3. Chemoprophylaxis (when appropriate)
   Travelers should be:
   a. Advised to start chemoprophylaxis before travel, to use prophylaxis continuously while in malaria endemic areas and for 1 or 4 weeks after leaving such areas (depending on drug used).
   b. Questioned about drug allergies and other contraindications for drug use.
   c. Informed that antimalarial drugs can cause side effects; if these side effects are serious, medical help should be sought promptly and use of the drug discontinued. Mild nausea, occasional vomiting, or loose stools should not prompt discontinuation of chemoprophylaxis; but medical advice should be sought if symptoms persist.
   d. Warned that they may acquire malaria even if they use malaria chemoprophylaxis.
   e. Warned that they may receive conflicting information regarding antimalarial drugs overseas, but that they should continue their prescribed medication unless they are experiencing moderate to severe adverse effects.
4. In case of illness travelers should be:
   a. Informed that symptoms of malaria may be mild, and that they should suspect malaria if they experience *a fever or flulike illness* (unexplained fever).
   b. Informed that malaria may be fatal if treatment is delayed. Medical help should be sought promptly if malaria is suspected, and a blood sample should be taken and examined for malaria parasites on one or more occasions (if possible, blood smears should be brought home for review).
   c. Reminded that self-treatment (if prescribed) should be taken only if prompt medical care is not available and that medical advice should still be sought as soon as possible after self-treatment.
   d. Reminded to continue to take chemoprophylaxis in cases of suspect or proven malaria.
5. Special categories:
   a. Pregnant women and young children require special attention because of the potential effects of malaria illness and inability to use some drugs (e.g., doxycycline).

Adapted from International Travel and Health, Geneva, 2000, World Health Organization.

2. **Preventing mosquito bites (personal protection measures).** All travelers to malaria-endemic areas need to be instructed in how best to avoid bites from *Anopheles* mosquitoes that transmit malaria. Any measure that reduces exposure to the evening and night-time feeding female *Anopheles* mosquito will reduce the risk of acquiring malaria. Insecticide-impregnated bed nets (permethrin or similarly treated) are safe for children and pregnant women and are an effective prevention strategy that is underused by travelers. Additional details are provided in Chapter 1.

3. **Use of chemoprophylactic drugs where appropriate.** The use of antimalarial drugs and their potential adverse effects must be weighed

against the risk of acquiring malaria (as described previously). The following questions should be addressed before prescribing any antimalarial.

a. Will the traveler be exposed to malaria?
b. Will the traveler be in a drug-resistant *P. falciparum* zone?
c. Will the traveler have prompt access to medical care (including blood smears prepared with sterile equipment and then properly interpreted) if symptoms of malaria were to occur?
d. Are there any contraindications to the use of a particular antimalarial drug?

▼ An overview of antimalarial drug regimens based on drug-resistance zones is provided in Fig. 5-1 and Table 5-3. It is important to note that a number of travelers to low-risk areas, such as urban areas and tourist resorts of Southeast Asia, continue to be inappropriately prescribed antimalarial drugs that result in unnecessary adverse events but little protection. Improved traveler adherence with antimalarial drugs will likely result when travel medicine practitioners make a concerted effort to identify and carefully council the high-risk traveler and avoid unnecessary drugs in the low-risk individual.

4. **Seeking early diagnosis and treatment if fever develops during or after travel.** Travelers should be informed that although personal protection measures and antimalarials can markedly decrease the risk of contracting malaria, *these interventions do not guarantee complete protection.* Symptoms resulting from malaria may occur as early as 1 week after first exposure and as late as several years after leaving a malaria zone whether or not chemoprophylaxis has been used. Most travelers who acquire falciparum malaria will develop symptoms within 3 months of exposure. Falciparum malaria can be effectively treated early in its course, but delays in therapy may result in a serious and even fatal outcome. The most important factors that determine outcome are early diagnosis and appropriate therapy. Travelers and health care providers alike must consider and urgently rule out malaria in any febrile illness that occurs during or after travel to a malaria-endemic area (see Chapters 17 and 18).

CURRENT CHEMOPROPHYLACTIC DRUG REGIMENS

Antimalarial drugs are selected based on individual risk assessment (as discussed previously) and drug-resistance patterns (Figs. 5-1 and 5-2 and Tables 5-1, 5-3, and 5-4). Chloroquine-resistant *P. falciparum* (CRPF) is now widespread in all malaria-endemic areas of the world, except for Mexico, the Caribbean, Central America, Argentina, and parts of the Middle East and China. *P. falciparum* malaria resistant to chloroquine and mefloquine is still rare except on the borders of Thailand with Cambodia and Myanmar (Burma). Resistance to sulfadoxine-pyrimethamine is now common in the Amazon basin and Southeast Asia and is emerging in various regions of Africa. Chloroquine-resistant *P. vivax* is also becoming an important problem, particularly in Papua New Guinea, Papua, Vanuatu, Myanmar, and Guyana.

Chloroquine-Sensitive Zones

Chloroquine is the drug of choice for travel to areas where chloroquine resistance has *not* been described; it is suitable for people of all ages and for pregnant women. Because insufficient drug is excreted in breast milk, nursing infants should be given chloroquine. Except for its bitter taste, chloroquine is usually well tolerated. Dark-skinned persons may experience

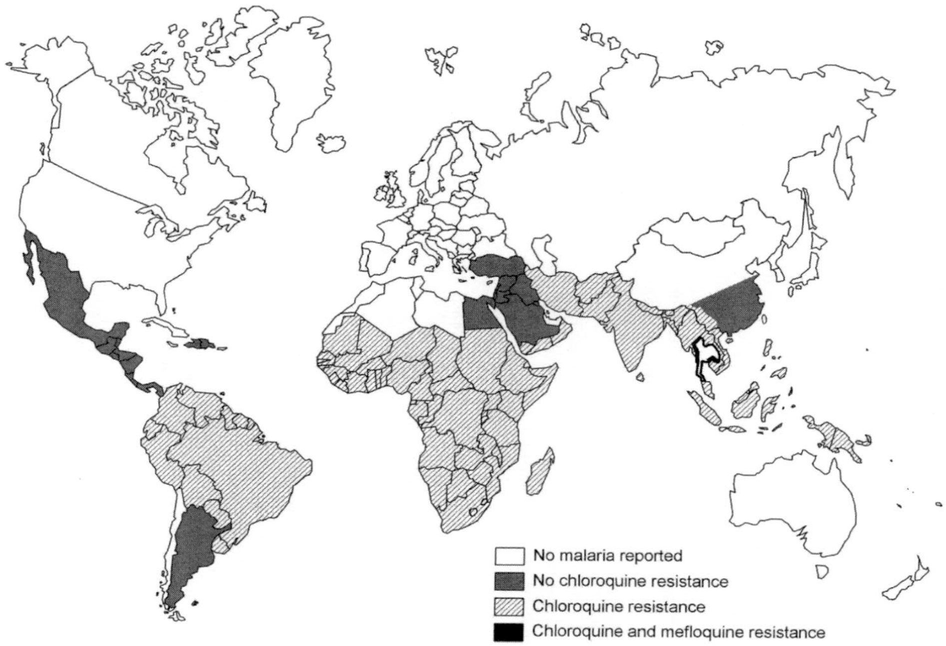

Fig. 5-1 Map of malaria-endemic areas and zones of drug-resistance. NOTE: This is meant as a visual aid *only.* The reader is referred to additional important details of malaria drugs and country-specific malaria risk available on-line (see Table 5-1) or references. (From Health Canada. Recommendations for the prevention and treatment of malaria among international travelers, *CCDR* 26S2, 2000.)

Table 5-3*
Malaria Chemoprophylactic Regimens for At-Risk Individuals According to Zones of Drug-Resistance

Zone	Drug(s) of choice†	Alternatives
No chloroquine resistance	Chloroquine	Doxycycline
Chloroquine resistance	Mefloquine or atovaquone/proguanil or doxycycline	1st choice: primaquine‡ 2nd choice: chloroquine plus proguanil§
Chloroquine and mefloquine resistance	Doxycycline	

Adult Doses

Chloroquine phosphate:	300 mg (base) weekly
Mefloquine:	250 mg (salt in United States; base elsewhere) weekly
atovaquone/proguanil	One tablet daily
Doxycycline:	100 mg daily
Primaquine:	30 mg (base) daily‡
Proguanil:	200 mg daily

Note: Protection from mosquito bites (insecticide-treated bed nets, DEET-based insect repellents, etc) is the first line of defense against malaria for *all* travellers. In the Americas and Southeast Asia, chemoprophylaxis is recommended *only* for travellers who will be exposed outdoors during evening or night time in rural areas.

*See detailed information in Table 5-4.

†Chloroquine and mefloquine are to be taken one week before entering malarial areas, continuing during the stay in malarial areas, and for 4 weeks after leaving malarial areas. Doxycycline and proguanil may be started 1 day before entering malarial areas, but must be continued for 4 weeks after departure, atovaquone/proguanil, and primaquine are started 1 day before entering the malarial area and may be discontinued 7 days after leaving the malaria-endemic area.

‡Contraindicated in G6PD (glucose-6-phosphate dehydrogenase) deficiency and during pregnancy. *not* presently licensed for this use. Must perform a G6PD level before prescribing.

§Chloroquine plus proguanil is less efficacious than mefloquine or doxycycline in these areas.

generalized pruritis that is not indicative of drug allergy. Retinal toxicity that may occur with long-term high doses of chloroquine used in the treatment of other diseases is extremely unlikely with chloroquine given as a weekly malaria chemosuppressive agent. Concurrent use of chloroquine interferes with antibody response to intradermal human diploid rabies vaccine.

Chloroquine-Resistant Zones

For many travelers to these areas, a choice between mefloquine (Larium), atovaquone-proguanil (Malarone), or doxycycline (Vibramycin) will have to be made. Less commonly primaquine or chloroquine plus proguanil is used. Deciding which agent is best requires an individual assessment of risk of malaria and the specific advantages and disadvantages of each regimen (see Table 5-5). For drugs such as mefloquine, doxycycline, and chloroquine/proguanil to be optimally effective, they need to be taken for

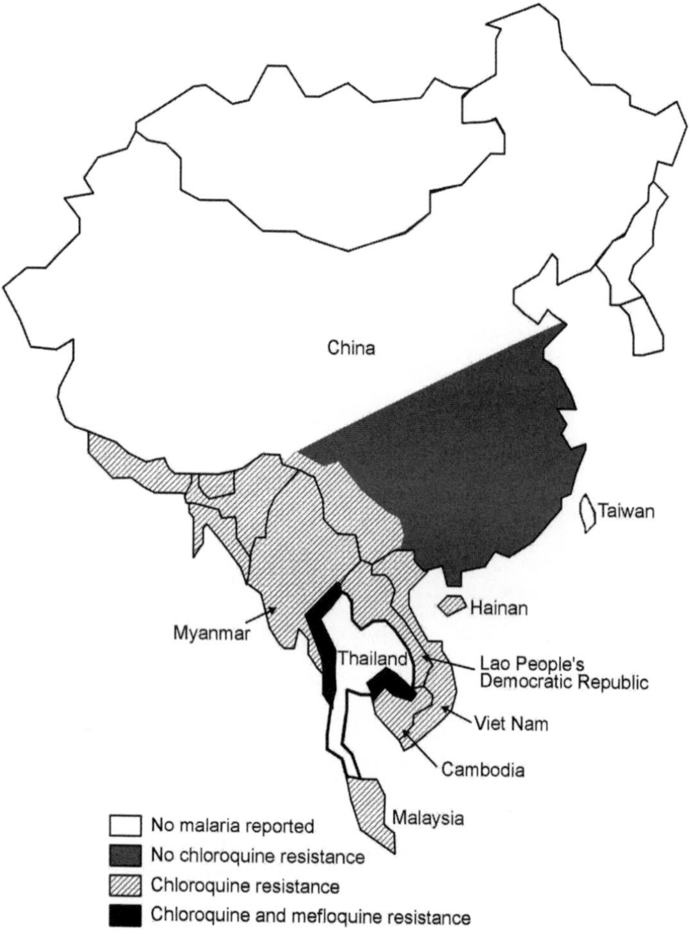

Fig. 5-2 Close-up map of malaria-endemic areas and zones of drug resistance in Southeast Asia. NOTE: This is meant as a visual aid *only.* The reader is referred to additional important details of malaria drugs and country specific malaria risk available on-line (see Table 5-1) or in references. (From Health Canada. Recommendations for the prevention and treatment of malaria among international travelers, *CCDR* 26S2, 2000.)

4 weeks after leaving a malaria-endemic area, although traveler adherence with this component has traditionally been poor. Agents such as atovaquone/proguanil and primaquine are called *causal* prophylactics because they kill malaria early in its life cycle in the liver, and therefore may be discontinued 1 week after leaving an endemic area (Fig. 5-3).

Text continued on p. 64

Table 5-4
Antimalarial Drugs, Doses,* and Adverse Effects (listed alphabetically)

Generic name	Trade name	Packaging	Adult dose	Pediatric dose	Adverse effects
Atovaquone/proguanil	Malarone	250 mg atovaquone and 100 mg proguanil (adult tablet)	Prevention: 1 tablet daily Treatment: 1000 mg atovaquone and 400 mg proguanil (4 tablets) once daily × 3 days	Prevention: 11-20 kg ¼ tablet 21-30 kg ½ tablet 31-40 kg ¾ tablet 40 kg 1 tablet Treatment: 20 mg/kg atovaquone and 8 mg/kg proguanil once daily × 3 days	Frequent: nausea, vomiting, abdominal pain, diarrhea, increased transaminases Rare: seizures, rash
Chloroquine[†] phosphate	Aralen	150 mg base	Prevention: 300 mg base once weekly Treatment: 1.5 g base × 3 days[‡]	Prevention: 5 mg base once weekly 5-6 kg or <4 mo: 25 mg base 7-10 kg or 4-11 mo: 50 mg base 11-14 kg or 1-2 yr: 75 mg base 15-18 kg or 3-4 yr: 100 mg base 19-24 kg or 5-7 yr: 125 mg base 25-35 kg or 8-10 yr: 200 mg base 36-50 kg or 11-13 yr: 250 mg base	Frequent: pruritis in black-skinned individuals, nausea, headache Occasional: skin eruptions, reversible corneal opacity Rare: nail and mucous membrane discoloration, nerve deafness, photophobia, myopathy, retinopathy with daily use, blood dyscrasias, psychosis and seizures, alopecia

Continued

Table 5-4
Antimalarial Drugs, Doses,* and Adverse Effects (listed alphabetically)—cont'd

Generic name	Trade name	Packaging	Adult dose	Pediatric dose	Adverse effects
				50 kg or 14 yr: 300 mg base Treatment: 25 mg salt/kg total over 3 days	
Doxycycline	Vibramycin Vibra-Tabs, Doryx	100 mg	Prevention: 100 mg once daily Treatment: 1 tablet twice daily for 7 days (plus Quinine) (See Chapter 17)	Prevention: 1.5 mg salt/kg once daily (max 100 mg daily) $<$25 kg or $<$8 yr: contraindicated 25-35 kg or 8-10 yr: 50 mg 36-50 kg or 11-13 yr: 75 mg $\geq$50 kg or $\geq$14 yr: 100 mg Treatment: 1.5 mg salt/kg twice daily (max 200 mg daily) $<$25 kg or $<$ 8 yr: contraindicated 25-35 kg or 8-10 yr: 50 mg twice daily 36-50 kg or 11-13 yr: 75 mg twice daily 50 kg or $\geq$ 14 yr: 100 mg twice daily (plus Quinine) (see Chapter 17)	Frequent: GI upset, vaginal candidiasis, Photosensitivity Occasional: Rare: allergic reactions, blood dyscrasias, azotemia in renal diseases, hepatitis

Mefloquine	Lariam	250 mg base	Prevention: 250 mg base once weekly Treatment: see text	Prevention: <5 kg: no data 5-9 kg: 1/8 tablet 10-19 kg: 1/4 tablet 20-30 kg: 1/2 tablet 30-45 kg: 3/4 tablet 45 kg: 1 tablet once weekly Treatment: see text	Common: transient dizziness diarrhea, nausea, vivid dreams, nightmares, irritability, mood alterations, headache, insomnia Rare: seizures, psychosis, prolonged dizziness
Quinine		330 mg salt	Prevention: Not indicated Treatment: See text	Prevention: Not indicated Treatment: See text	Common: Cinchonism
Primaquine		15 mg base	Prevention: Prophylaxis: 30 mg base daily (see text) Terminal prophylaxis or radical cure: 15 mg base/day for 14 days[§]	Prevention: 0.5 mg base/kg daily Terminal prophylaxis or radical cure: 0.3 mg base/kg/day × 14 days[¶]	Occasional: GI upset, hemolysis in G6P deficiency, methemoglobinemia
Proguanil	Paludrine	100 mg	Prevention: 200 mg daily NOTE: Not recommended as a single agent for prophylaxis	Prevention: 5-8 kg or <8 mo: 25 mg (1/4 tablet) 9-16 kg or 8 mo-3 yr: 50 mg (1/2 tablet) 17-24 kg or 4-7 yr: 75 mg (3/4 tablet)	Occasional: anorexia, nausea mouth ulcers Rare: hematuria

Continued

Table 5-4
Antimalarial Drugs, Doses,* and Adverse Effects (listed alphabetically)—cont'd

Generic name	Trade name	Packaging	Adult dose	Pediatric dose	Adverse effects
			Treatment: see text	25-35 kg or 8-10 yr: 100 mg (1 tablet) 36-50 kg or 11-13 yr: 150 mg (1½ tablets) ≥50 kg or ≥ 14 yr: 200 mg (2 tablets) Treatment: see text	
Pyrimethamine-sulfadoxine	Fansidar	25 mg pyrimethamine and 500 mg sulfadoxine	Prevention: no indication Treatment: 3 tablets (75 mg pyrimethamine—1500 mg sulfadoxine)	Prevention: no indication Treatment: 2-3 mo: ¼ tablet 4-11 mo: ½ tablet 1-2 yr: ¾ tablet 3-4 yr: 1 tablet 5-9 yr: 1.5 tablets 10-11 yr: 2 tablets 12-13 yr: 2.5 tablets ≥4 yr: 3 tablets	Occasional: headache, nausea folate deficiency Rare: Stevens-Johnson syndrome, erythema multiforme, toxic epidermal necrolysis

G6PD, Glucose 6-phosphate dehydrogenase.
*Dose for chemoprophylaxis, unless specified for "Treatment."
†Chloroquine sulfate (Nivaquine) is not available in the United States and Canada, but is available in most malaria-endemic countries in both tablet and syrup form.
‡Generally, 2 tablets twice per day on days 1 and 2, then 2 tablets on day 3 (total of 10 tablets).
§Doses are increased to 30-mg base/day for primaquine-resistant *P. vivax*.
¶Doses are increased to 0.5-mg base/kg/day for primaquine-resistant *P. vivax*.

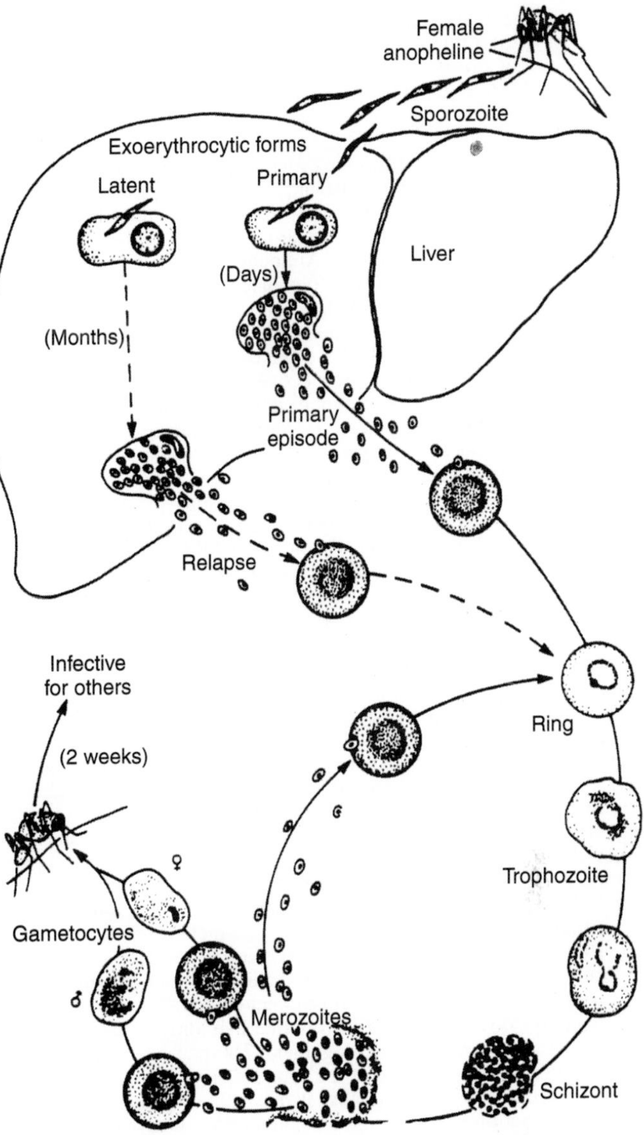

Fig. 5-3 Life cycle of the malaria parasite in humans. (From Wyler DJ: Plasmodium and Babesia. In Gorbach SI et al, editors: *Infectious diseases,* Philadelphia, 1992, WB Saunders.)

This advantage makes these drugs attractive for high-risk but short-duration travel. It is important to note that none of these agents is ideal, and all carry a risk of adverse events that are distressing enough to travelers that 1% to 7% will discontinue their prescribed chemoprophylactic regimen.

Mefloquine

Mefloquine (MFQ) is an efficacious chemoprophylactic agent (protective efficacy >90%) against drug-resistant *P. falciparum* and *P. vivax* malaria. It is currently listed as one of the drugs of choice by the CDC and WHO for most high-risk travelers to chloroquine-resistant regions such as sub-Saharan Africa and New Guinea. Although there is general agreement about MFQ's efficacy, it is MFQ's tolerance that has recently been called into question. However, based on data from well-designed trials (prospective, randomized trials), mefloquine would appear to be better tolerated than the popular media would have travelers believe. Six randomized, double-blind trials and seven prospective comparative studies failed to show significant differences in overall adverse events or discontinuation rates between MFQ and other chemoprophylactic drug regimens. Overall MFQ withdrawal rates in comparative trials were estimated to be 1%, indicating high acceptance rates compared with other chemoprophylactic regimens and suggesting that only a small number of individuals would need to switch to an alternative drug regimen. In placebo-controlled trials, significantly more participants discontinued MFQ (overall 3.3%; most commonly for gastrointestinal upset and dizziness) than placebo. In a recent randomized trial comparing mefloquine to Malarone in nonimmune travelers, both agents were effective and well tolerated, but Malarone was better tolerated than mefloquine.

Approximately 25% to 50% of MFQ users report side effects, the majority of which are mild and self-limited. The most frequent adverse events reported by MFQ users are nausea, strange dreams, dizziness, mood changes, insomnia, headache, and diarrhea. Severe neuropsychiatric reactions (psychosis, convulsions) are infrequent with prophylactic doses and are reported to occur in approximately 1/6,000 to 1/13,000 individuals. Less severe but nonetheless troublesome neuropsychologic adverse events (e.g., anxiety, depression, nightmares) disabling enough to result in drug discontinuation are reported in 0.2% to 3.9% of users. There is no evidence that the long-term use of mefloquine (>1 year) is associated with additional adverse effects and side effects may decrease with longer-term use.

Contraindications to the use of mefloquine include a history of psychiatric illness or seizure disorder or a past severe reaction to mefloquine. Precautions include use in pregnancy, especially the first trimester; children weighing less than 5 kg; cardiac conduction disturbances or arrhythmia; and the concurrent use of quinine-like drugs (halofantrine and mefloquine should not be used together). The package insert for mefloquine also cautions about use of the drug by drivers, pilots, and machine operators because of concerns that it may affect spatial orientation and motor coordination. There are no data on mefloquine use by scuba divers; caution is advised because of the risk of neurologic symptoms developing at depth and because signs and symptoms of decompression illness (dizziness, headache, nausea, fatigue) may be attributed to the drug, thus potentially delaying recognition and appropriate treatment for the decompression problem.

For a traveler to a CRPF destination who plans to engage in special physical activities such as those mentioned previously and who cannot take atovaquone/proguanil or doxycycline (see later discussion), a practical approach would be to start the traveler on mefloquine approximately 3 weeks before departure and monitor for adverse events. It has been suggested by many travelers that if the drug is taken in the evening, side effects are mostly relegated to the hours of sleep and effects on physical performance the next day are potentially lessened.

Mefloquine is metabolized through the liver and can cause an asymptomatic increase in the liver function tests during therapy. The drug should be avoided in travelers with chronic hepatic dysfunction. Travelers on drugs such as warfarin or cyclosporin A should start mefloquine 3 to 4 weeks in advance of departure, so that prothrombin times or cyclosporin A levels can be monitored and adjusted as needed.

For travelers who will be at immediate high risk of drug-resistant falciparum malaria, consideration may be given to the use of a loading dose of mefloquine. Data from several trials indicate that mefloquine taken once a day for 3 days before travel followed by standard weekly doses is an effective way to rapidly achieve therapeutic blood levels (in 4 days compared with 7 to 9 weeks with standard weekly dosing of mefloquine). Approximately 2% to 3% of loading-dose recipients discontinued mefloquine (most commonly for gastrointestinal upset and dizziness) and most of these did so during the first week. Alternatively, mefloquine can be initiated 2 to 3 weeks before travel to achieve higher blood levels before entering malaria-endemic areas. Either strategy permits an assessment of drug tolerance before travel and allows a change to a suitable alternative if required.

Atovaquone Plus Proquanil (Malarone)

Malarone is a fixed-dose combination of atovaquone and proguanil hydrochloride. Atovaquone acts by inhibition of parasite mitochondrial electron transport at the level of the cytochrome bc_1 complex and collapses mitochondrial membrane potential. The plasmodial electron transport system is a thousand-fold more sensitive to atovaquone than the mammalian electron transport system, which likely explains the selective action and limited side effects of this drug. Proguanil is metabolized to cycloguanil, which acts by inhibiting dihydrofolate reductase (DHFR). The inhibition of DHFR impedes the synthesis of folate cofactors required for parasite DNA synthesis; however, it appears that the mechanism of synergy of proguanil with atovaquone is not mediated through its cycloguanil metabolite. In studies, proguanil alone had no effect on mitochondrial membrane potential or electron transport, but significantly enhanced the ability of atovaquone to collapse mitochondrial membrane potential when used in combination. This might explain why proguanil displays synergistic activity with atovaquone even in the presence of documented cycloproguanil resistance or in patient populations who are deficient in cytochrome P-450 enzymes required for the conversion of proguanil to cycloguanil.

The combination of atovaquone and proguanil is effective against *P. falciparum* malaria strains that are resistant to a variety of other antimalarial drugs. Drug resistance to atovaquone appears to be associated with mutations in the cytochrome *b* gene.

Volunteer challenge studies have established that atovaquone and proguanil have causal prophylactic activity (i.e., activity against the liver stage parasite). As a causal chemoprophylactic agent, travelers would be required to take it only during periods of exposure and for 1 week after departure from malaria-endemic areas. This would avoid the requirement to complete 4 weeks of prophylaxis after exposure (a common reason for nonadherence with standard regimens) and may be particularly useful for travelers with short exposures in high-risk areas.

Three double-blind, randomized, placebo-controlled chemoprophylaxis trials have been conducted in long-term residents in Kenya, Zambia, and Gabon. The overall efficacy for preventing malaria in these semi-immune participants was 98% (95% CI, 91.9% to 99.9%). The most common reported adverse events attributed to treatment with study drug were headache, abdominal pain, dyspepsia, gastritis, and diarrhea. However, of note, all adverse events occurred with similar frequency in subjects treated with placebo or atovaquone/proguanil, and no serious adverse events were attributed to atovaquone/proguanil.

Studies among nonimmune travelers have recently been completed. In randomized, double-blind studies, approximately 2000 nonimmune subjects traveling to a malaria-endemic area received either atovaquone/proguanil, daily for 1 to 2 days before travel until 7 days after travel, mefloquine or chloroquine/proguanil, from 1 to 3 weeks before travel until 4 weeks after travel. No confirmed diagnosis of malaria occurred with either atovaquone/proguanil or mefloquine, but three documented cases of falciparum malaria occurred in travelers using chloroquine/proguanil. All drugs were well tolerated, but Malarone was significantly better tolerated than either mefloquine or chloroquine/proguanil in these studies.

Taken together, the studies to date indicate that atovaquone-proguanil is a well-tolerated and efficacious chemoprophylactic regimen for *P. falciparum.* The most common adverse effects are gastrointestinal, which can be reduced by taking Malarone with food. Additional data are required to establish efficacy against non-falciparum malaria but pivotal trials are underway.

Doxycycline

Another alternative for individuals unable to take mefloquine or atovaquone/proguanil is doxycycline. In comparative trials, doxycycline has been shown to have equivalent efficacy to mefloquine, with reported protective efficacy of >90% (95% CI, 80% to 98%). Doxycycline is also efficacious against mefloquine-resistant falciparum malaria but must be taken *every day* to work. Noncompliance with this daily regimen is the major reason for doxycycline failures. Doxycycline is contraindicated during pregnancy, in breastfeeding women and in children less than 8 years old. Long-term safety (>3 months) of daily doxycycline has not been established among travelers, but chronic use for months to years by young healthy adults in acne treatment protocols is a common clinical practice. Doxycycline may cause gastrointestinal upset and rarely esophageal ulceration, which is less likely to occur if the drug is taken with food and copious amounts of fluid. It should not be taken simultaneously with Pepto-Bismol or antacids. Doxycycline may be photosensitizing in some individuals; using a sunscreen (UV A&B) may reduce this problem. Doxycycline may also increase the risk of vaginal candidiasis; therefore women at risk of yeast vaginitis should carry antifungal vaginal suppositories or cream.

Primaquine

Primaquine is an 8-aminoquinoline that has activity against both blood and tissue (liver) stages of malaria and therefore can eliminate infections that are developing in the liver (causal prophylaxis). Randomized controlled trials of primaquine as a prophylactic agent (0.5 mg base/kg/day; adult dose 30 mg base/day) have shown a protective efficacy of 85% to 95% against both *P. falciparum* and *P. vivax* infections. Primaquine was as well or better tolerated than other standard regimens but may cause nausea and abdominal pain that can be decreased by taking the drug with food. Of importance, primaquine may cause oxidant-induced hemolytic anemia with methemoglobinemia, particularly in individuals with a deficiency of glucose 6-phosphate dehydrogenase (G6PD). It is contraindicated in patients with G6PD deficiency and also during pregnancy. If not already documented, a traveler's G6PD status should be determined with a G6PD blood test before primaquine is prescribed. In the absence of contraindications, primaquine may be a useful alternative prophylactic agent and because of its causal activity may be discontinued 1 week after leaving an endemic area. It is currently under review by the Food and Drug Administration for licensure for this indication.

If the risk of *P. vivax* infection is thought to be particularly high (e.g., long term expatriates, soldiers) consideration may be given to the use of primaquine phosphate ("radical" or "terminal" prophylaxis) to eliminate latent hepatic parasites; this is given at the conclusion of the standard posttravel chemoprophylaxis regimen.

Chloroquine Plus Proguanil

Another alternative for travelers with contraindications or intolerance to mefloquine, atovaquone/proguanil, or doxycycline is the combination of weekly chloroquine plus daily proguanil. This dosing schedule can be confusing to travelers, and, to avoid potential toxicity (e.g., taking daily chloroquine), it needs to be carefully explained. Proguanil is not available in the United States but is available in Canada, Europe, and many endemic countries. The combination of proguanil and chloroquine is considered safe during pregnancy. Reported side effects of proguanil include mouth ulcerations, gastrointestinal upset, and hair loss. The gastrointestinal side effects may be lessened by taking the drugs with meals. Chloroquine plus proguanil is more efficacious in sub-Saharan Africa than chloroquine alone, but it is considerably less efficacious than doxycycline, mefloquine, or atovaquone/proguanil providing only approximately 50% to 70% protective efficacy. There is little recent data on the efficacy of this combination outside of Africa (e.g., Indian subcontinent). A number of failures have been reported in travelers taking this combination, and users must be informed that they are taking a less efficacious regimen.

Chloroquine and Mefloquine-Resistant Zones

In these regions along the Thai-Myanmar and Thai-Cambodian border, doxycycline is the chemoprophylactic drug of choice. Atovaquone/proguanil may also be effective in these areas.

In summary, the use of mefloquine and other drug regimens should be carefully directed at high-risk travelers where their benefit most clearly outweighs the risk of adverse events. None of the available regimens are ideal for all travelers and the travel medicine practitioner should attempt to match the individual's risk of exposure to malaria to the appropriate regimen based on drug efficacy, tolerance, and safety. As a guide to facilitate decision making, we have generated a Clinical Utility Score, in which different attributes of each drug regimen, such as efficacy, tolerance, convenience, and cost, are weighted based on clinical trials and experience with these drugs (Table 5-5). The scores assigned are arbitrary and other groups and users may weight each variable somewhat differently depending on the specific needs and risk of drug-resistant malaria. For example, a traveler to rural Papua may weight efficacy more heavily than cost or convenience.

Table 5-5
Clinical Utility Score for Current Malaria Chemoprophylactic Regimens

Drug	Efficacy*	Tolerance†	Convenience‡	Causal§	Cost¶	Total
Mefloquine	3	1	3	0	2	9
Doxycycline	3	2	2	0	3	10
chloroquine/ proguanil	1	2	1	0	2	6
Azithromycin	2	2	2	0	1	7
Primaquine	2	2	1**	2	3	10
atovaquone/ proguanil	3	3	2	2	11	1

*Efficacy: 1 = <75%; 2 = 75-89%; 3 = ≥90%.
†Tolerance: 1 = occasional disabling side effects; 2 = rare disabling side effects; 3 = rare minor side effects.
‡Convenience: 1 = daily and weekly dosing required; 2 = daily dosing required; 3 = weekly dosing required.
§Causal: 0 = no causal activity; 2 = causal prophylactic (may be discontinued within a few days of leaving risk area)
¶Cost: 1 = > US$100/month; 2 = US$ 50-100/month; 3 = <US$ 50/month.
**Requires a pretravel G6PD level resulting in a lower convenience score.
NOTE: Scores and weighting are arbitrary and can be modified/individualized to specific travelers and itineraries.

Dosing regimens may affect the traveler's acceptance of and compliance with the regimen prescribed. Chloroquine and mefloquine are taken once weekly beginning 1 to 3 weeks before travel, during travel, and for 4 weeks after leaving the endemic area. Doxycycline and proguanil are taken once a day beginning 1 to 2 days before travel, during travel, and for 4 weeks after leaving an endemic area. Atovaquone/proguanil and primaquine are taken once a day beginning 1 to 2 days before travel and during travel; because they are active against liver stages of malaria, they can be discontinued 1 week after leaving an endemic area.

Other Drugs

Tafenoquine (WR 238605)

Tafenoquine is a 8-aminoquinoline related to primaquine, which has activity against both asexual (blood and liver) and sexual (gametocyte) stages of the parasite. This drug has a long half-life permitting a weekly or even longer dosing regimen. Like primaquine, tafenoquine is contraindicated in G6PD deficiency and pregnancy but otherwise is more active and appears to be better tolerated than primaquine. Randomized controlled trials with tefanoquine have shown that it is effective given both weekly or as a loading dose before travel. However additional studies are required before this drug can be licensed for malaria prevention.

Azithromycin

Azithromycin is an azalide antimicrobial agent that has been evaluated as a chemosuppressive agent in a number of studies. Although protective against *P. vivax* (>90%), protective efficacy against *P. falciparum* (70% to 83%) is generally considered to be too low to rely on azithromycin as a single agent to prevent falciparum malaria.

Pyrimethamine Plus Sulfadoxine (Fansidar)

This drug combination interferes with folic acid metabolism in the parasite: pyrimethamine inhibits dihydrofolate reductase, and sulfadoxine inhibits dihydropteroate synthetase. Fansidar was used as a weekly chemoprophylactic regimen against CRPF in the 1980s, but an unacceptable rate of serious and sometimes fatal hypersensitivity reactions that developed during therapy with the weekly dose resulted in withdrawal of the recommendation for its use in prophylaxis. At present, Fansidar is reserved for therapy.

Pyrimethamine Plus Dapsone

This drug combination is marketed as Maloprim in many malaria-endemic areas outside the United States and, like Fansidar, interferes with folic acid metabolism in the parasite. This drug combination is not as efficacious as mefloquine, atovaquone/proguanil, or doxycycline in preventing malaria. However, the tablets containing the fixed-dose combination are relatively inexpensive and often sold over the counter in foreign countries; thus travelers have been known to start taking this drug during travel in lieu of more efficacious antimalarial drugs, at the advice of other travelers or local pharmacies. Travelers should be told to avoid Maloprim and educated about the possible and potentially serious dose-related toxicity (bone marrow suppression) of this drug combination.

Standby Malaria Therapy

Most travelers will be able to obtain prompt medical attention when malaria is suspected and therefore *will not require a self-treatment regimen.* Under unusual circumstances individuals at risk of malaria may be unable to seek medical care within 24 hours and may require self-treatment for presumptive malaria. However, because of the nonspecific symptoms of malaria, the potentially serious risk of incorrectly treating another disease and the potential toxicity of malaria therapy, self-treatment should never be undertaken lightly; consultation with a tropical medicine expert is recommended before individuals are placed on self-treatment protocols. Travelers should be advised that the clinical presentation of malaria is variable and may mimic other diseases. An alternate diagnosis that requires treatment may be present, particularly in travelers who have been compliant with chemoprophylaxis. The most frequent symptoms of malaria are fever, headache, and generalized aches and pains. Fever, which may or may not be cyclical, is almost always present. Malaria can be misdiagnosed as "influenza" or another febrile illness, so that an early and accurate diagnosis is essential. Travelers for whom self-treatment has been recommended should be told that self-treatment is *not* considered definitive treatment but is a temporary lifesaving measure until they can receive medical attention. Self-treat for malaria should be used only if travelers develop fever *and* professional medical care is not available within 24 hours. After self-treatment medical attention should still be sought as soon as possible.

Halofantrine is *not* recommended for self-treatment of malaria (see later). Mefloquine is *not* an ideal self-treatment regimen because of an increase in neuropsychiatric adverse events observed when treatment doses of mefloquine are used. In some countries, a combination of mefloquine and Fansidar is marketed under the name Fansimef, which should not be confused with mefloquine. Fansimef is not recommended for the prevention or treatment of malaria. Individuals who are on chemosuppression should never attempt treatment with the same drug, as there is the potential for additive toxicity and reduced efficacy.

Rapid detection of malaria using dipsticks may be available to some travelers. The sensitivity and specificity of these tests in research labs appears promising (>90%). However the accuracy of these tests is not known in the hands of nonexperienced operators and with unrefrigerated conditions in the tropics. A summary of self-treatment regimens is presented in Table 5-6.

Malarone (Atovaquone Plus Proguanil)

Malarone (see the previous discussion) is an attractive agent for emergency self-treatment, provided the traveler is not taking this agent for prophylaxis. Apart from occasional gastrointestinal intolerance (reduced by taking the drug with food), treatment doses of Malarone are well tolerated (adult dose, 4 tablets per day times 3 days). It is safe for children (>11 kgs), but its safety in pregnancy and during breast feeding are unknown, and until additional data are available it should be avoided in these situations (see Chapter 12).

Fansidar

Fansidar is a fixed-dose combination of pyrimethamine and sulfadoxine. Fansidar has been recommended for use as a single 3-tablet oral dose (adult dose; for travelers not allergic to sulfa drugs) for emergency self-treatment of suspected CRPF when the traveler is remote from regular

Table 5-6
Self-Treatment Regimens* (to be used only if fever develops and medical care is not available within 24 hours):

A. For individuals in chloroquine-sensitive regions and not on chloroquine prophylaxis: Self-treatment with chloroquine should be taken (see Table 5-4). *Seek medical help as soon as possible.* Chloroquine prophylaxis should be started.

B. For individuals in chloroquine-sensitive regions and already on chloroquine prophylaxis: Self-treatment with Malarone should be taken (see Table 5-4). *Seek medical help as soon as possible.* Chloroquine prophylaxis should be resumed.

C. In chloroquine or chloroquine- and mefloquine-resistant *P. falciparum* regions, treatment recommendations for uncomplicated *P. falciparum* include the following (see Table 5-4): Begin oral Malarone (see Table 5-4). *Seek medical help as soon as possible.* Mefloquine or other appropriate prophylaxis should be resumed.
OR
Begin oral quinine and doxycycline (see Table 5-4). *Seek medical help as soon as possible.* Mefloquine or other appropriate prophylaxis should be resumed.
OR
Begin oral quinine plus Fansidar (see Table 5-4) (Sub-Saharan Africa/Indian subcontinent only). *Seek medical help as soon as possible.* Mefloquine or other appropriate prophylaxis should be resumed.

*If vomiting occurs within 30 to 60 minutes of dose, repeat full dose. If vomiting occurs 1 to 2 hours after dose, repeat one half dose.

medical care (see Table 5-4). Recent studies have shown increasing resistance to Fansidar among CRPF strains in Southeast Asia, the Amazon River Basin, and east Africa, which now limit the utility of Fansidar for standby treatment in high-risk travelers in these areas.

Mefloquine

Mefloquine may serve as an emergency self-treatment drug, if the traveler is not already taking mefloquine for prophylaxis, or is not being treated with closely related drugs such as quinidine or halofantrine. However, mefloquine-associated neuropsychiatric reactions have been reported to be 60 to 100 times more frequent at treatment doses (approximately 1 in 100 to 1 in 1700 treatment courses) than as a prophylactic agent. High-grade resistance to mefloquine has been reported in Southeast Asia, along the Burmese and Cambodian borders of Thailand: quinine plus tetracycline, or one of the artemisinin derivatives plus mefloquine is recommended for treatment of malaria acquired in this region. Elsewhere resistance to mefloquine remains uncommon.

Quinine Sulfate Plus Tetracycline

Quinine is not usually recommended in the category of emergency self-treatment of malaria, although it is one of the cornerstones of drug treatment for CRPF (see Chapter 17). However, field biologists and other travelers going on prolonged remote trips in CRPF areas may wish to prescribe the regimen of oral quinine plus tetracycline for standby emergency treatment of suspected malaria. Most patients taking quinine at the doses recommended for treatment of malaria develop symptoms of cinchonism: mild to severe nausea, vomiting, headache, and ringing in the ears, which makes adherence with this regimen challenging, especially in cases of self-treatment.

Halofantrine

Halofantrine is a phenanthrene methanol compound related to mefloquine, but with a different profile of pharmacokinetics, toxicity, and antimalarial activity. Recent published reports have documented a dose-related prolongation of the QT_c interval on electrocardiograms (ECG) in more than 60% of patients being treated with halofantrine at standard doses. Numerous ventricular tachyarrhythmias, sometimes leading to death, have been attributed to halofantrine and the WHO and other experts no longer recommend the use of this drug for self-treatment.

SPECIAL THERAPEUTIC CONSIDERATIONS

The Pregnant Traveler

Travel by pregnant women or women who might become pregnant to destinations where CRPF malaria is transmitted should be avoided or deferred when possible. This advice is based on the fact that the most effective antimalarial regimens against CRPF are neither recommended nor adequately studied during pregnancy, especially in the first trimester. On the other hand, malaria during pregnancy is associated with low-birth-weight infants and significant maternal mortality.

If a pregnant woman must travel to a CRPF malarial endemic area, the use of insect repellents and treated bed nets (see Chapter 1) should be strongly encouraged. If the travel is to an area where there is intense transmission of CRPF with high-grade chloroquine resistance and travel cannot be deferred, mefloquine may be considered for chemoprophylaxis after the first trimester of pregnancy. For areas with less intense transmission, chloroquine and proguanil chemoprophylaxis can be considered. Even though the combination of chloroquine and proguanil is not ideal, it may provide partial protection.

The Infant Traveler

Malaria chemoprophylaxis in the very young infant is difficult to achieve. Although most antimalarial drugs taken by the mother will be present in breast milk, drug concentrations are not considered high enough to provide an adequate protective dose to the nursing infant. Thus malaria prevention in the nursing infant must be addressed separately from what is recommended to the mother.

For pediatric travelers to malarious areas where chloroquine is still effective, the chloroquine dose can be adjusted based on weight (see Table 5-4). Chloroquine phosphate pediatric suspension is available in some destination countries, but not in the United States or Canada. If the suspension is not available, chloroquine phosphate tablets (250 mg salt = 150 mg chloroquine base) can be ground up by the pharmacist, and the weight-adjusted dose plus a filler can be put into capsules. Once a week, the capsule can be opened and the chloroquine powder mixed into a syrup to be given to a child. Chocolate syrup is recommended over fruit syrups and jams, as chocolate can effectively mask the extremely bitter taste of the chloroquine and make the mixture palatable to a child.

The dosage of proguanil can also be adjusted based on weight. Malarone (available in a one-quarter strength pediatric tablet) and mefloquine dosage for children can be adjusted based on weight for those weighing more than 11 kg and 5 kg, respectively. Doxycycline is contraindicated in children less than 8 years old. In addition to chemoprophylaxis, the use of insect repellents formulated for pediatric use and insecticide-impregnated bed nets are recommended (Chapters 1 and 11).

The HIV-Infected Traveler

P. falciparum malaria has been shown to increase HIV-1 replication and increase proviral loads and may cause faster progression of HIV-1 disease. HIV-1 infection also appears to make malaria worse and is associated with higher parasitemia infections and an increase in clinical malaria.

Furthermore, as in other travelers, a CRPF malaria infection could result in a serious and life-threatening illness, so insect precautions and malaria chemoprophylaxis appropriate to the itinerary should be strongly encouraged. Potential problems related to malaria chemoprophylaxis are these: Will the antimalarial drugs recommended for a particular itinerary interact with drugs the traveler is already taking, or result in toxic drug reactions? Travel advice for the HIV-infected traveler is discussed more fully in Chapter 13.

The Traveler Without a Spleen

Overwhelming infection from encapsulated bacteria such as *Haemophilus influenzae, Streptococcus pneumoniae,* and *Neisseria meningitidis* (meningococcus) is a recognized risk in persons who have undergone splenectomy. Medical advisors have postulated that malaria also would be more difficult to control in the splenectomized host, since the spleen serves as a major site for removal of parasitized red cells from the circulation. A review of the clinical course and treatment of malaria in a group of splenectomized patients, although based on a limited number of observations, suggested that splenectomized patients with malaria fare no better or worse than other patients with comparable malaria infections.

PRIMAQUINE FOR TERMINAL PROPHYLAXIS

Terminal chemoprophylaxis or "the radical cure" refers to treatment with primaquine phosphate, an antimalarial compound that can eradicate latent malaria (*P. vivax* or *P. ovale*) incubating in the liver. The standard adult regimen consists of primaquine phosphate at a dose of 26.3 mg (salt) (15 mg base) daily for 2 weeks. An alternative regimen consists of three 26.3 mg (salt) tablets (45 mg base) once a week for 8 weeks (see Table 5-4). Common side effects are nausea and malaise.

The risk of latent hepatic malaria infections causing attacks of malaria beyond the standard 4-week period of posttravel malaria chemoprophylaxis increases with the degree of exposure to mosquito bites in the malarious area. Although posttravel primaquine therapy is not routinely advised, travelers who spent prolonged periods in rural areas of malarious countries or who report an inordinate number of mosquito bites may be candidates for primaquine therapy.

Treatment with primaquine is usually initiated at the time of the last dose of posttravel chemoprophylaxis, or of the last dose of treatment for a malaria attack caused by *P. vivax* or *P. ovale.* Primaquine can cause severe hemolytic anemia in persons with red cells low in G6PD, which is more common in persons of African, Asian, or Mediterranean origin. G6PD testing should be used before initiation of primaquine therapy. Primaquine is also contraindicated during pregnancy.

Primaquine-Resistant or Tolerant *P. vivax*

P. vivax strains that do not respond to standard dose of primaquine (adults, 15 mg base/day) used for terminal prophylaxis have been reported from Papua, Papua New Guinea, India, South America, and Somalia. After treatment for a malaria attack caused by *P. vivax* from these areas, or in individuals who have suffered a relapse despite standard dose primaquine, primaquine should be given at two times the standard daily dose (adults, 30 mg base/day). Primaquine in higher than standard doses can be associated with nausea and vomiting, which can be reduced by giving the drug with food. Primaquine is contraindicated in G6PD deficiency and during pregnancy, and G6PD levels should always be checked before using this agent.

REFERENCES

Centers for Disease Control and Prevention: *Health information for international travel,* Washington DC, 2001-2002, Government Printing Office.

Hogh B et al: Atovaquone/proguanil versus chloroquine/proguanil for malaria prophylaxis in non-immune travelers: Results from a randomised, double-blind study, *Lancet* 2000.

International Association of Medical Assistance to Travelers (IAMAT): World Malaria Risk Chart. Guelph, Ontario, February, 1992.

Kain KC: Prophylactic drugs for malaria: why do we need another one? *J Trav Med* 6:S2, 1999.

Kain KC et al: Malaria deaths in visitors to Canada and in Canadian travelers: a case series, *CMAJ* 164:654, 2001.

Karwacki JJ et al: Proguanil-sulphonamide for malaria chemoprophylaxis, *Trans R Soc Trop Med Hyg* 84:55, 1990.

Lell B et al: Randomised placebo-controlled study of atovaquone plus proguanil for malaria prophylaxis in children, *Lancet* 351:709, 1998.

Lell B et al: Malaria chemoprophylaxis with tafenoquine: a randomised study, *Lancet* 355:2041, 2000.
Lobel HO et al: Long-term malaria prophylaxis with weekly mefloquine, Lancet 341:848, 1993.
Luzzi GA et al: Treatment of primaquine-resistant *Plasmodium vivax* malaria, *Lancet* 340:310, 1992.
Nosten F, van Vugt M: Neuropsychiatric adverse effects of mefloquine. What do we know and what should we do? *CNS Drugs* 11:1, 1999.
Ryan ET, Kain KC: Health advice and immunizations for travelers, *N Engl J Med* 342:1716, 2000.
Shanks GD et al: Efficacy and safety of atovaquone/proguanil for suppressive prophylaxis against *Plasmodium falciparum* malaria, *Clin Infect Dis* 27:494, 1998.
Steffen R, Fuchs E, Schildknecht J: Mefloquine compared with other malaria chemoprophylactic regimens in tourists visiting East Africa, *Lancet* 341:1299, 1993.
Weinke T et al: Neuropsychiatric side effects after the use of mefloquine, *Am J Trop Med Hyg* 45:86, 1991.
White NJ: Antimalarial drug resistance: the pace quickens, *J Antimicrob Chemother* 30:571, 1992.
Whitworth J et al: Effect of HIV-1 and increasing immunosuppression on malaria parasitemia and clinical episodes in adults in rural Uganda: a cohort study, *Lancet* 356:1051, 2000.
World Health Organization: Drug alert: halofantrine. Change in recommendations for use, *Wkly Epidemiol Rec* 68:269, 1993.
World Health Organization: *International travel and health: vaccination requirements and health advice 2002,* Geneva, Switzerland, 2002, World Health Organization.

CHAPTER 6

Traveler's Diarrhea: Prevention and Self-Treatment

Matthew J. Thompson and Elaine C. Jong

Traveler's diarrhea is a common concern of international travelers and is usually a self-limited illness consisting of 4 to 6 days of watery diarrhea, sometimes accompanied by low-grade fever, nausea, abdominal cramping, headache, and general malaise. It can affect up to 60% of travelers during a 2-week trip, depending on their destination. Highest attack rates are seen with travel to Africa, Asia, Latin America, and the Middle East; intermediate rates are found in the newly independent states of the former Soviet Union, southern Europe, Israel, South Africa, and the Caribbean; lowest attack rates are seen in most of Europe, North America, Japan, Australia, and New Zealand (Table 6-1).

Although traveler's diarrhea is commonly thought to be a problem when travelers from northern temperate climates go to tropical developing areas, it is increasingly recognized that acute gastroenteritis can occur among travelers going in the other direction. Indeed, traveler's diarrhea may be considered as an acute illness occurring when the normal ecology of a person's gastrointestinal tract is upset by exposures to new foods, spices, and microorganisms.

There are many pathogens known to be associated with traveler's diarrhea; they include bacteria, viruses, and parasites. Pretravel vaccinations can provide varying degrees of protection against certain enteric infections, although typhoid and hepatitis A may not present with diarrhea.

Common-sense food and water precautions during travel can help guard against the other specific infectious agents, but even if travelers attempt to select safe food and water, what is served to them may have been contaminated in the process of storage, preparation, and handling. The immune protection afforded by vaccination and natural immune mechanisms of the gastrointestinal tract (mainly gastric acidity) can be overwhelmed by the ingestion of heavily contaminated food and water. Finally, some pathogens can cause disease after ingestion of a relatively low infectious inoculum. Thus, despite pretravel use of the available vaccines, and careful selection of food and water during travel, the risk of contracting diarrhea remains high.

Most travelers, especially short-term business or pleasure travelers, are unwilling to be ill for 4 to 6 days; a rational plan for prevention and presumptive self-treatment of diarrhea based on epidemiologic considerations and safety of available medications is thus important.

Table 6-1
Risk Factors for Traveler's Diarrhea

Travel destination	Highest risk in Africa, parts of Asia, Latin America, and the Middle East
Age	Highest in infants and young adults
Source of food and water	Quality may depend on type of travel, adherence to dietary precautions.
Type of travel	Adventurous travelers, prolonged stays
Decreased gastric acidity	Acid-reducing medications, achlorhydria, hypochlorhydria, gastrectomy
Immune deficiency	Human immunodeficiency virus infection with low CD4 count Immunoglobulin A deficiency
Blood group O	Increased risk of severe disease with *Vibrio cholorae* El Tor

ETIOLOGY

Data on the etiology of traveler's diarrhea have been limited because most illness occurs during travel, and the duration of illness is relatively short. Travelers are usually well enough by the time they return home that medical attention is not required. The common infectious etiologies of traveler's diarrhea are listed in Table 25-1. In general, bacteria are responsible for the majority of cases of traveler's diarrhea, with viruses and parasites accounting for significantly lower numbers. However these depend heavily on the geographic region, time of year, and presence of local outbreaks. In up to half the cases of traveler's diarrhea, no etiologic agent can be identified. Occasionally, bloody or mucoid stools and a higher fever signal that the diarrheal illness is caused by one of the more serious invasive pathogens.

Published studies have implicated enterotoxigenic strains of *Escherichia coli* (ETEC) bacteria as the most common identifiable cause of acute diarrhea in travelers visiting developing and tropical countries. The ETEC are similar to the *E. coli* bacteria that are part of the normal enteric flora, but the strains associated with watery diarrhea have acquired plasmids coding for the production of powerful enterotoxins. Both a heat-stable and a heat-labile toxin have been identified. The heat-labile toxin of ETEC is similar to cholera toxin; it causes prolonged secretion of isotonic fluid containing high amounts of bicarbonate and potassium throughout all segments of the small bowel via stimulation of adenylate cyclase. The heat-stable toxin alters fluid transport via stimulation of guanylate cyclase in the jejunum and ileum only. A diarrhea-producing strain of ETEC may produce one or both of the toxins.

In the last decade, *Campylobacter* species, mostly *C. jejuni,* have also become recognized as common etiologic agents of traveler's diarrhea. *C. jejuni* was implicated in up to 17% of cases of traveler's diarrhea in Thailand in one study, but other causes of diarrhea were selected against because the patients were taking doxycycline as prophylaxis against malaria. There also appears to be seasonal variance in rates of *Campylobacter* infections: the peak incidence of infection in the United States is in the summer, whereas in North Africa it is during the drier winter months.

Table 6-2
Ten Tips for Selection of Safe Food and Water

1. Drink purified water or bottled carbonated water.
2. Eat foods that are thoroughly cooked and served piping hot.
3. Eat fruits that have thick skins (they should be peeled at the table by the traveler).
4. Avoid salads made with raw vegetables, especially leafy green vegetables.
5. Do not use ice cubes in any beverages, even beverages containing alcohol.
6. Only eat and drink dairy products made from pasteurized milk.
7. Avoid shellfish and raw or undercooked seafood, even if "preserved" or pickled with lemon or lime juice or vinegar.
8. Do not buy and eat food sold by street vendors.
9. If canned beverages are cooled by submersion of the can in a bucket of ice water or in a stream, be sure to dry off the outside of the container before drinking the contents.
10. Use purified water for brushing teeth and for taking medications.

Other bacterial enteric pathogens less frequently isolated in cases of traveler's diarrhea include species of *Salmonella, Shigella, Aeromonas, Plesiomonas shigelloides, Vibrio cholerae, V. parahaemolyticus, V. vulnificus, and Yersinia enterocolitica* (see Table 25-1).

Norwalk virus, implicated in outbreaks of food-borne gastroenteritis, is a common cause of diarrhea in adults and accounts for 10% to 15% of the cases of traveler's diarrhea. Rotavirus is less common in adults and accounts for only 5% to 14% of traveler's diarrhea. Infections with hepatitis A virus or hepatitis E (enterically transmitted non-A, non-B) virus also should be considered among etiologies of traveler's diarrhea.

The parasites causing acute diarrhea in travelers are usually protozoans, including *Giardia lamblia, Cryptosporidium sp., Cyclospora cayetanensis, Entamoeba histolytica, Isospora belli,* and *Dientamoeba fragilis.* Although less common, cases of helminthic infections have also caused diarrhea in travelers.

Food, fish, and shellfish poisoning also should be considered in cases of acute diarrhea in travelers (Chapters 27 and 28).

PREVENTION OF TRAVELER'S DIARRHEA

Preventive strategies for traveler's diarrhea include dietary protective measures, appropriate immunizations, and chemoprophylactic agents and should be tempered by the purpose, duration, and style of the trip.

Dietary Protective Measures

Advice on food and water precautions that can help to reduce the risk from all forms of traveler's diarrhea are given in Table 6-2. Details on techniques for water purification are given in Chapter 7. In general adherence to such protective measures are more difficult to sustain in longer term or adventurous travelers. Families with small infants may also consider keeping young infants off the ground and maintaining breastfeeding during the trip (see Chapter 11).

Immunization

Few vaccines are currently available to prevent the most common causes of traveler's diarrhea. The vaccines against typhoid are quite effective, whereas the oral cholera vaccines appear moderately effective against non-O139 strains. In contrast the parenteral cholera vaccine is of little benefit. The inactivated hepatitis A vaccines are extremely effective.

Chemoprophylaxis

Medications that can be used to prevent traveler's diarrhea are given in Table 6-3.

Bismuth Subsalicylate

A daily regimen of bismuth subsalicylate (Pepto-Bismol) taken at a dose of two tablets (or 60 ml of the 17.5 mg/ml suspension) four times a day, every day of the trip, for up to 3 weeks, has been reported to significantly decrease the incidence of traveler's diarrhea. Unfortunately, this regimen is rather costly and bulky and can no longer be recommended for routine prophylaxis.

The exact mechanism of action of bismuth subsalicylate has not been fully described, although the subsalicylate may reduce fluid secretion on the basis of antiprostaglandin effect. Adverse effects can include a black-colored tongue, constipation, and tinnitus. Bismuth subsalicylate is a pharmacologic agent of relatively low toxicity, yet it must be used with caution for prophylaxis in certain kinds of patients (those with salicylate

Table 6-3
Drug Regimens Used for Prevention of Traveler's Diarrhea*

Drug	Adult dosage	Comments
Bismuth subsalicylate (Pepto-Bismol)	2 tablets (262 mg) qid *or* 30 ml liquid (262 mg/15 ml) qid	Less effective than antibiotic prophylaxis; contraindicated in people allergic to aspirin, people on other salicylate-containing drugs, pregnancy. Not recommended for children.
Trimethoprim 160 mg/ sulfamethoxazole 800 mg (Bactrim, Septra)	1 tablet qd	Contraindicated in people allergic to sulfa; less effective than other antibiotics in many parts of the world.
Doxycycline 100 mg (Vibramycin, Doryx)	1 tablet qd	Contraindicated in pregnancy, age <8 years; highest efficacy shown in Africa.
Ciprofloxacin 500 mg (Cipro)	1 tablet qd	Contraindicated in pregnancy, age <18 years. Beware of drug interaction with theophylline.
Norfloxacin 400 mg (Noroxin)	1 tablet qd	Contraindicated in pregnancy, age <18 years. Beware of drug interaction with theophylline.
Ofloxacin 200 mg (Floxin)	1 tablet qd	Contraindicated in pregnancy, age <18 years. Less interaction with theophylline.

*The use of antimicrobials for the prophylaxis of travelers diarrhea is an unlabeled use.

sensitivity, bleeding disorders, impaired renal function, or peptic ulcer disease, or those who are already on salicylate therapy). The maximum recommended dose of 240 ml/day results in taking salicylate approximately equivalent to eight 325-mg aspirin tablets. Bismuth subsalicylate is not recommended for children, owing to the risk of Reye's syndrome.

Antibiotic Prophylaxis

Most prophylactic antibiotic regimens involve taking a single daily dose throughout the trip. Although not recommended for routine use, antibiotics for prevention of traveler's diarrhea may be appropriate in certain circumstances. Travelers such as business travelers, politicians, athletes, and honeymooners taking short (1 to 2 week) trips, where even a single day of illness could seriously ruin the purpose of the trip, might consider antibiotic prophylaxis. In addition, prophylaxis may be prudent in travelers with inflammatory bowel disease, brittle diabetes, acquired immunodeficiency syndrome or chronic renal impairment.

The effectiveness of antibiotic prophylaxis depends on the spectrum of activity of the antibiotic used relative to the antibiotic-resistance patterns among the local bacterial pathogens. Daily doses of doxycycline, trimethoprim-sulfamethoxazole (TMP/SMX), norfloxacin, ciprofloxacin, and ofloxacin have been shown to be successful in diarrhea prevention studies. TMP/SMX is the drug of choice for prevention of diarrhea in noncoastal western Mexico; however, in most of the developing world (South America, Africa, Asia) there is widespread resistance to TMP/SMX among the enteric pathogens. Although there are increasing reports of quinolone resistance, these antibiotics (norfloxacin, ciprofloxacin, and ofloxacin) are generally effective against a wide range of enteric bacterial pathogens including *E. coli, C. jejuni, Shigella, Salmonella, Vibrio, Aeromonas, Plesiomonas,* and *Yersinia.* Significant resistance among *Campylobacter sp.* and *Shigella sp.* in countries such as Thailand now limits their utility as preventive agents. Azithromycin is commonly recommended for empiric treatment in these areas, but is not usually used for prophylaxis. The doses of drugs used in prevention of diarrhea are shown in Table 6-3.

Antibiotic prophylaxis may lessen the risk of traveler's diarrhea, but susceptibility to infection with antibiotic-resistant bacteria and other pathogens may be increased as a result of the regimen's altering the normal enteric flora. In addition, the risk of severe sulfa allergic reactions (including erythema multiforme progressing to Stevens-Johnson syndrome or toxic epidermal necrolysis), adverse effects of the tetracyclines (gastrointestinal upset, phototoxic skin reactions, *Candida* vaginitis), and adverse effects of the quinolone antibiotics (gastrointestinal upset, headache, drug interactions) must be considered. For most travelers, it is preferable to carry antibiotics to be used for presumptive treatment of traveler's diarrhea rather than take antibiotics for prophylaxis.

EMPIRIC SELF-TREATMENT

The majority of travelers will do well if they are instructed to follow the guidelines for safe food and water selection, and if they carry a supply of appropriate medications for empiric self-treatment of traveler's diarrhea. Treatment of traveler's diarrhea consists of (1) oral rehydration, (2) symptomatic treatment, and (3) presumptive antibiotic treatment. Diagnosis and treatment of the traveler returning with diarrhea is discussed further in Chapter 25.

Oral Rehydration

Dehydration resulting from abnormal losses of body fluids through watery diarrhea can accentuate the general feeling of misery. Travelers having five or more watery bowel movements a day need to pay special attention to oral rehydration with safe liquids. In mild cases of traveler's diarrhea, a wide variety of liquids can be used, including water, canned juices, carbonated caffeine-free beverages, bouillon, and sports diuretics. In more severe diarrhea, and in the presence of dehydration, many of these liquids contain excess sugar and insufficient electrolytes for optimal replacement. In such cases commercially formulated preparations for fluid replacement can be purchased in powdered form convenient for mixing in 1-L volumes. The World Health Organization Oral Rehydration Formula is given for comparison (Table 6-4). A tablet form is manufactured overseas for mass oral rehydration programs in disaster areas.

Symptomatic Treatment

Regardless of specific etiology, most people will feel better with symptomatic relief from frequent stools and abdominal cramps.

Bismuth subsalicylate taken in treatment doses (Table 6-5) can rapidly reduce the number of stools (by approximately 50%) and is a reasonable choice for initial treatment of frequent watery stools in adults. Travelers must be warned, however, that they should not take doses of antibiotics and bismuth subsalicylate at the same time, because the *bismuth subsalicylate may significantly decrease absorption of the antibiotic.* The influence of bismuth subsalicylate on the absorption of doxycycline has been studied, but data are not presently available with regard to the specific interaction of bismuth subsalicylate and the quinolone antibiotics. Published studies show a clinically significant decrease in absorption of quinolones owing to concurrent therapy with antacids (containing aluminum and magnesium, or calcium), sucralfate, or nutritional supplements containing ferrous sulfate and zinc. If diarrhea develops while using bismuth subsalicylate prophylaxis, or if a treatment dose of bismuth subsalicylate was taken but is not giving adequate relief, it may be as long as 6 hours before an oral dose of antibiotic will be completely bioavailable and effective.

Table 6-4
World Health Organization Oral Rehydration Solution

Mix with 1 L of purified water:		Final solution will contain:	
Sodium chloride	3.5 g	Sodium	90 mEq/L
Potassium chloride	1.5 g	Potassium	20 mEq/L
		Chloride	80 mEq/L
Sodium bicarbonate	2.5 g	Base (bicarbonate, citrate, or lactate)	30 mEq/L
OR			
trisodium citrate	2.9 g		
Glucose	20 g	Glucose	20 g/L

*Commercially available as WHO-ORS from the manufacturer: Jianas Brothers, St Louis, Mo.

Loperamide (Imodium) and the combination of diphenoxylate HCl and atropine sulfate (Lomotil) are useful for obtaining rapid symptomatic relief from frequent bowel movements and abdominal cramps; these two drugs are synthetic opioids and work because of an antiperistaltic effect on the intestines, which slows intestinal transit and delays excretion. Although studies have been performed using loperamide and antibiotics in combination for traveler's diarrhea, Lomotil may promote invasiveness of pathogens in dysenteric diarrhea, causing prolongation of illness and increased risk of complications. Antimotility agents should therefore be avoided in patients with dysentery, as well as in young children because of the risk of side effects such as respiratory depression, drowsiness, and ileus. Clay-based products such as attapulgite or kaolin (Kaopectate) bind water in the colon and can increase the solid consistency of stools. Their efficacy in traveler's diarrhea has been fairly limited.

Finally, several studies have examined the use of probiotics such as lactobacillus or acidophilus in acute diarrhea. A genetically modified strain of human lactobacillus (Lactobacillus GG) has been used successfully to reduce the duration of symptoms in viral and antibiotic-associated acute diarrhea. Although experience in travelers is fairly limited at this time, it may provide a useful addition to the travel medicine kit.

Empiric Antibiotic Treatment

Several studies have shown that if *self-treatment with loperamide plus one of the antibiotics* is started right after the onset of nondysenteric traveler's diarrhea, relief can be obtained by many patients within 24 hours. Travelers may stop the antiperistaltic drug when symptomatic relief from cramps and frequent watery stools is obtained, but should continue taking the antibiotic according to the regimen selected, regardless of duration of symptoms (Table 6-5). Choice of antibiotic is dictated by several factors, particularly the resistance profile of the enteric pathogens likely to be encountered at the destination, age of the traveler, and any underlying medical illnesses.

In diarrheal illness with frequent watery stools, rapid transit times may rush an orally administered antibiotic through the bowel leading to suboptimal intraluminal concentrations and absorption of the drug. The use of an antiperistaltic drug concurrent with an antibiotic probably "traps" the antibiotic in the intestinal tract, leading to higher intraluminal concentrations of the antibiotic and more effective systemic absorption.

Quinolones are active against the majority of bacteria commonly implicated in travel-acquired diarrhea; they are also relatively free of major side effects; however, reduced doses may be advisable in elderly travelers or those with impaired renal function. Although they are generally accepted as the antibiotics of choice for empiric treatment in adults, growing quinolone resistance of *Campylobacter* sp. in certain developing countries such as Thailand now poses a significant threat to their utility there.

TMP/SMX had previously been considered a reasonable second choice for adults and the antibiotic of choice for children. However, it is not effective against *Campylobacter,* now recognized as a major cause of travel-acquired diarrhea. In addition, ETEC, *Shigella,* and other bacteria previously sensitive to TMP/SMX have demonstrated increasing resistance; the effectiveness of this combination outside of portions of Mexico and Central America is being called into question.

Azithromycin appears to offer several advantages over quinolones and TMP-SMX. It is more efficacious than ciprofloxacin for treating resistant strains of *Campylobacter* and multidrug-resistant *Shigella* sp., while main-

Table 6-5
Drugs for Empiric Self-Treatment of Traveler's Diarrhea

Drug	Adult dosage	Comments*
Symptomatic Medications		
Bismuth subsalicylate (Pepto-Bismol) tablets	2 tablets (262 mg) or 30 ml liquid (262 mg/15 ml) q30 minutes × 8 doses	The maximum recommended dose is 240 ml/day (16 tablets).
Diphenoxylate + Atropine (Lomotil)	2 tabs first dose, then 1 after each loose stool; do not exceed 8 tablets in 24 hr	Antiperistaltic drug; do not use in dysentery; available by prescription.
Loperamide (Imodium)	Take 2 caplets (2 mg each) for first dose then 1 after each loose stool; do not exceed 8 caplets (16 mg) in 24 hr	Antiperistaltic drug; do not use in dysentery; sold over the counter; liquid form available for pediatric dosing-use dose adjusted for weight on package insert.
Antibiotics		
Tetracycline	500 mg PO q6h *or* 2.5 g as a single oral dose	Do not use in pregnancy or in children <8 years old.
Doxycycline (Vibramycin, Doryx)	100 mg PO q12h × 6 doses	Do not use in pregnancy or in children <8 years old.
TMP/SMX (Bactrim, Septra)[§]	160-mg/800-mg tablet (one double-strength tablet) q12h × 6 doses Pediatric dose: 8 mg/kg trimethoprim daily in 2 divided doses	Do not use in sulfa-allergic patients. May be less effective in many areas of the world.
Azithromycin (Zithromax)	500 mg on day 1, then 250 mg day 2 onwards until diarrhea resolves. Pediatric dose 10 mg/kg on day 1, then 5 mg/kg on day 2 onwards.	Drug of choice for most children with traveler's diarrhea, and for adults in areas of high enteric bacterial resistance (e.g., Thailand)
Norfloxacin (Noroxin)	400-mg tablet q12h × 6 doses	Do not use in pregnancy or in children <18 years old.
Ciprofloxacin (Cipro)	500-mg tablet q12h × 6 doses; *or* 750-mg tablet once at start of diarrhea symptoms	Do not use in pregnancy or in children <18 years old.
Ofloxacin (Floxin)	200-mg or 300-mg tablet q12h × 6 doses[‡]	Do not use in pregnancy or in children <18 years old.
Levofloxacin (Levaquin)	500 mg q24h × 3 to 5 doses	Do not use in pregnancy or in children <18 years old.
Furazolidone[§]	100-mg tablet q6h × 7-10 days. Pediatric dose (16.7 mg/5 ml suspension): 1 mo-1 yr, 8-17 mg q6h; 1yr-4yr, 17-25 mg q6h; ≥5 yr 25-50 mg q6h	Consider second-line agent for children with traveler's diarrhea.[§] Avoid ≤1 month of age.

* See Chapter 11 for pediatric guidelines on treatment of diarrhea.
‡ This drug has been studied for this use at both doses.
† *Vibrio cholerae* O139 strain not susceptible.
§ Unlabeled use.

taining similar efficacy against most other enteric bacterial pathogens. Thus it should be considered as the drug of choice in children and a second choice for adults traveling to high diarrhea risk areas. For travelers to areas such as Thailand, however, where resistance to quinolones is widespread, it may be considered the drug of choice for all age groups.

Tetracycline or doxycycline may be useful for treatment of acute diarrhea in areas where resistance to the tetracycline drugs is not widespread among the bacterial enteric pathogens and may represent a less expensive antibiotic alternative to the quinolones for the budget-minded traveler. The vibrios (including *V. cholerae*) are usually sensitive, as are some isolates of *C. jejuni.* The single high-dose tetracycline regimen given in Table 6-5 was effective in treating even tetracycline-resistant shigellosis in Thailand, and a lower single dose (1 g tetracycline) was reported to be effective against cholera.

Rifaximin, a derivative of rifamycin, is a poorly absorbed antibiotic that is beginning to be studied for use in traveler's diarrhea. In early studies it appears to have equal efficacy to quinolones in treating traveler's diarrhea in adults. There is also limited experience with furazolidone, which may be an option for children.

Any illness that is characterized by high fever ($>102°$ F), severe abdominal pain, or the passage of grossly bloody stools (dysentery) is serious; and medical help should be sought as soon as possible. However, if self-treatment is the only option, then *the antibiotic selected should be used alone, without the antiperistaltic drug.*

Approximately 60% or more of cases of traveler's diarrhea are due to bacterial pathogens. If the diarrhea was caused by a viral infection, the course of antibiotic self-therapy is unlikely to influence the outcome; if the diarrhea was caused by a resistant bacterial agent or by a parasite, the illness will persist beyond the 3-day empiric treatment regimen, and the traveler needs to seek medical consultation.

SPECIAL CONSIDERATIONS

People stricken with diarrhea who are unable to tolerate oral rehydration owing to severe nausea and vomiting may require medical attention and intravenous fluids in a hospital. In particular, this may be the case in hot climates, where insensible water loss is greater and where dehydration may be a danger (Chapter 8).

Treatment of children with bloody diarrhea is complicated by the association between antibiotic treatment of the *E.coli* O157H7 strain and the subsequent development of hemolytic uremic syndrome. However, it is not thought that this strain of *E.coli* is highly prevalent in developing countries. It may be prudent to reserve antibiotics for children with bloody diarrhea that is severe or dysenteric in nature, pending further diagnostic evaluation and studies.

People taking diuretics need to be especially cautious in the face of severe watery diarrhea and probably should stop the diuretic during the acute diarrheal illness. Such people should seek medical attention for a blood pressure check, an examination of the heart and lungs, and a serum potassium check, in the event of severe diarrhea lasting more than 1 or 2 days.

In the case of many pathogens, the severity of diarrhea is inoculum dependent. People with decreased gastric acidity resulting from achlorhydria, gastric resection, frequent antacids, or medication with H_2 blocking agents or proton pump inhibitors may be more susceptible to illness and therefore may be in special need of pretravel medical counseling on preventive measures for traveler's diarrhea.

CHOLERA EPIDEMICS IN THE WESTERN HEMISPHERE, ASIA, AND AFRICA

The cholera epidemic in the Western Hemisphere, which was first recognized in Peru in January 1991, has now spread to almost all other countries in Latin America. The outbreak was an extension of the continuing seventh pandemic of *Vibrio cholerae* O1, biotype El Tor, which began in Indonesia in 1961. Approximately 400,000 cases of cholera were reported by the end of the first year, with the greatest number of cases being reported by Peru, Ecuador, Colombia, Bolivia, Brazil, Guatemala, Mexico, and El Salvador. Cholera transmission is associated with inadequately treated water supplies and poor sanitation that are present in many parts of the tropical and developing world.

Travelers may be overly concerned about the risk of cholera from news coverage of the epidemic in the popular media. Indeed, tourism to Peru dropped off markedly when the outbreak was first reported. However, the pandemic of cholera has continued for decades in many areas of Africa, Asia, and the South Pacific, and this has not deterred Americans from traveling to those regions. Many residents of cholera-endemic areas live in poor health under impoverished conditions; they often succumb rapidly to cholera because of dehydration, especially if oral rehydration cannot be started soon enough. In contrast, most tourists are in good overall health and are less likely to be exposed to contaminated water supplies.

Relatively few cases of cholera have been reported among American travelers to Latin America, mainly because they do not typically depend on the water and sanitation systems used by the local residents who have been most affected by the epidemic. Those Americans who have contracted cholera had eaten raw or contaminated seafood, or had eaten food sold from street vendors.

In 1992, a non-O1 cholera serogroup, *V. cholerae* O139 (Bengal) was identified as the causative organism in large outbreaks in India and has been subsequently isolated in several countries in Asia (Bangladesh, China, India, Malaysia, Nepal, Pakistan, and Sri Lanka) in 1993. The clinical disease produced by this strain appears to be the same as that caused by *V. cholerae* O1.

In 1994, outbreaks of cholera cause by *V. cholerae* O1, biotype El Tor, serotype Ogawa, were reported among Rwandan refugees in the Rwanda-Zaire border camps. Indeed the majority of all cases of cholera worldwide are found in Africa. Sporadic outbreaks continue in many countries; up to date information should be obtained from the Centers for Disease Control and Prevention (CDC) or one of the commercial travel medicine information sources. Although oral rehydration therapy remains the treatment of choice, intravenous fluids and appropriate antibiotics may need to be administered to severely dehydrated patients (Table 6-5). For cholera patients with severe illness and dehydration resulting from *V. cholerae* O1 strains, tetracycline (500 mg every 6 hours for 3 to 5 days) or doxycycline (300 mg daily for 3 to 5 days) are usually the antibiotics of choice. Single doses of doxycycline (300 mg) have been shown in some studies to be as effective as longer courses. However, fluctuating resistance to tetracyclines occurs in several parts of the world and is growing to TMP/SMX, chloramphenicol, and ampicillin. Alternative antibiotic choices may include 5-day courses of erythromycin (250 mg every 6 hours for adults, 40 mg/kg/day divided into four doses for children), furazolidone (100 mg every 6 hours for adults, 5 mg/kg/day divided into four doses for children), TMP/SMX, or ciprofloxacin. *V. cholerae* O139 strains are resistant to TMP/SMX and to furazolidone.

The parenteral cholera vaccine presently in use is not highly efficacious, and the World Health Organization (WHO) has dropped cholera as a recommended vaccine for the average traveler, even one going to cholera-endemic areas (Chapter 4). Travelers need to understand that the vaccine is not very effective and that it is *not* a significant mechanism for the prevention of cholera. Instead, travelers should be encouraged to follow the guidelines for safe food and water selection (Table 6-1).

An oral live vaccine against cholera (strain CVD103-HgR) is now available in Europe and other areas. The oral vaccine has a protection rate of 62% to 100%, with protection lasting at least 6 months, possibly years; however, the available injectable vaccines and oral vaccines that are directed against *V. cholerae* O1 do not provide protection against *V. cholerae* O139.

American travelers who go off normal tourist routes in areas of cholera transmission might be at risk of infection with cholera. If they are in good health, however, they would be expected to recover uneventfully, provided they start oral rehydration and self-treatment with antibiotics (tetracycline, doxycycline, quinolones, trimethoprim-sulfamethoxazole, or furazolidone) soon after symptoms are noted.

If a family with children is going to visit or work in an area of active cholera transmission, furazolidone or erythromycin might be used for treatment of cholera in children, as tetracyclines are contraindicated in children less than 8 years old, and quinolones are not approved for use in children less than 18 years old. Furazolidone in adult doses can also be used to treat cholera in adults unable to take tetracyclines or quinolones (Table 6-4), except in areas where resistant O139 strains are prevalent.

REFERENCES

Alam AN, Alam NH, Ahmed T, Sack DA: Randomised double blind trial of single dose doxycycline for treating cholera in adults, *Br Med J* 300:1619, 1990.

Black RE: Epidemiology of travelers' diarrhea and relative importance of various pathogens, *Rev Infect Dis* 12:S73, 1990.

Centers for Disease Control: Update: cholera—Western Hemisphere, *MMWR* 40:860, 1991.

DuPont HL et al: Five versus three days of ofloxacin therapy for traveler's diarrhea: a placebo-controlled study, *Antimicrob Agents Chemother* 36:87, 1992.

DuPont HL et al: Prevention of traveler's diarrhea (emporiatric enteritis). Prophylactic administration of subsalicylate bismuth, *JAMA* 243:237, 1980.

Ericsson CD, DuPont HL: Traveler's diarrhea: approaches to prevention and treatment, *Clin Infect Dis* 16:616, 1993.

Genta RM: Diarrhea in helminthic infections, *Clin Infect Dis* 16(suppl 2):S122, 1993.

Giannella RA, Broitman SA, Zamcheck N: Influence of gastric acidity on bacterial and parasitic enteric infections, *Ann Intern Med* 78:271, 1973.

Hoge CW et al: Trends in antibiotic resistance among diarrheal pathogens isolated in Thailand over 15 years, *Clin Infect Dis* 26:341, 1998.

Isolauri E et al: A human *Lactobacillus* strain (*Lactobacillus casei* sp strain GG) promotes recovery from acute diarrhea in children, *Pediatrics* 88:90, 1991.

Mattila L et al: Seasonal variation in etiology of traveler's diarrhea, *J Infect Dis* 165:385, 1992.

McAuley JB, Michelson MK, Schantz PM: Trichinella infection in travelers, *J Infect Dis* 164:1013, 1991.

Motala C, Hill ID, Mann MD, Bowie MD: Effect of loperamide on stool output and duration of acute infectious diarrhea in infants, *J Pediatr* 117:467, 1990.
Ortega YR et al: Cyclospora species: a new protozoan pathogen of humans, *N Engl J Med* 328:1308, 1993.
Petrucelli BP et al: Treatment of traveler's diarrhea with ciprofloxacin and loperamide, *J Infect Dis* 165:557, 1992.
Radandt JM, Marchbanks CR, Dudley MN: Interactions of fluoroquinolones with other drugs: mechanisms, variability, clinical significance, and management, *Clin Infect Dis* 14:272, 1992.
Sack RB, Rahman M, Yunus M, Khan EH: Antimicrobial resistance in organisms causing diarrheal disease, *Clin Infect Dis* 24(suppl 1):S102, 1997.
Steffen R: Worldwide efficacy of Bismuth subsalicylate in the treatment of traveler's diarrhea, *Rev Infect Dis* 12:S80, 1990.
Swerdlow DL, Ries AA: Cholera in the Americas: guidelines for the clinician, *JAMA* 267:1495, 1992.
Tauxe RV et al: Antimicrobial resistance of *Shigella* isolates in the USA: the importance of international travelers, *J Infect Dis* 162:1107, 1990.
Taylor DN et al: Etiology of diarrhea among travelers and foreign residents in Nepal, *JAMA* 260:1245, 1988.
Taylor DN et al: Treatment of traveler's diarrhea: ciprofloxacin plus loperamide compared with ciprofloxacin alone, *Ann Intern Med* 114:731, 1991.
Wong CS et al: The risk of hemolytic-uremic syndrome after antibiotic treatment of *Escherichia coli* O157:H7 infections, *N Engl J Med* 342:1930, 2000.
World Health Organization: Cholera in 1999, *Wkly Epidemiol Rec* 75:249, 2000.
World Health Organization: Cholera in 1998, *Wkly Epidemiol Rec* 74:257, 1999.
World Health Organization: Cholera outbreak among Rwandan refugees, *Wkly Epidemiol Rec* 69:221, 1994.

CHAPTER 7

Water Disinfection

Howard D. Backer

RISK OF WATER-BORNE INFECTION

Water disinfection is an essential component of the prevention strategy for enteric infections. In developing countries surface water may be highly contaminated with human waste. Urban tap water may be contaminated from aged, overwhelmed sanitation plants and deteriorating water distribution systems. Bottled water is a convenient solution, but in some places it may not be superior to the tap water. Moreover, the plastic bottles create a huge ecological problem since most countries where personal water treatment is necessary do not recycle. Even in developed countries with low rates of diarrhea illness, wilderness travelers who rely on surface water for drinking should take steps to ensure microbiologic quality. In the United States, there have been recent water-borne outbreaks of *Giardia, Shigella, E. coli* 0157:H7, and *Cryptosporidium,* all from surface water—but the latter two caused outbreaks from treated municipal water as well!

The list of potential water-borne pathogens is extensive and includes bacteria, viruses, protozoa, and parasitic helminths. More than 120 different enteric viruses alone can be transmitted by fecal contaminated water. Most of the organisms that can cause traveler's diarrhea can be water-borne; however, the majority of travelers' intestinal infections are probably transmitted by food. Cholera is well known to cause extensive water-borne outbreaks. Water is considered the main route of transmission for hepatitis E and one of the potential routes for hepatitis A and salmonellosis. Several organisms considered emerging pathogens are occasionally or commonly water-borne, including *E. coli* 0157:H7 and *Cryptosporidium.*

Risk of illness depends on the number of organisms ingested, which in turn depends on degree of water contamination from human and animal waste, immune status and individual susceptibility, virulence of the organism, and number of organisms ingested (Table 7-1). Microorganisms with small infectious dose can even cause illness through recreational water exposure such as swimming because of inadvertent water ingestion. Organisms that have been implicated recently in outbreaks resulting from recreational water exposure (including several in the United States) include *Giardia, Cryptosporidium, Shigella, E. coli* 0157:H7, gastroenteritis from unidentified enteric viruses, hepatitis A, and hepatitis E.

Persistence of microorganisms in water facilitates the potential for transmission; cold water greatly prolongs survival (Table 7-2). Some enteric bacteria can also survive and even multiply in organic-rich tropical

Table 7-1
Minimal Infectious Dose

Organism	Minimal infectious dose
Salmonella	10^5
Vibrio cholerae	10^3
Cryptosporidium	30
Giardia	10
Poliovirus	2-20
Rotavirus	1

Table 7-2
Survival of Microorganisms in Water

Organism	Survival
Vibrio cholerae	4-5 weeks in cold water
G. lamblia	2-3 months at 5° C-10° C 10-28 days at 15° C
Cryptosporidium	12 months in cold water
Enteric viruses	6-10 days at 15° C-25° C 30 days at 4° C
Hepatitis A	12 weeks in temperate water 6-12 months in cold water
Salmonella, Shigella	Half-life 16-24 hours in temperate stream

waters. There is a common misconception that streams "purify" themselves over a short distance. Natural die-off of organisms and the disinfection effects of ultraviolet light do decrease the number of viable microorganisms, but these are not reliable enough to ensure potable water in a stream. Microorganisms also clump to particles and settle to the bottom in still water, but are easily stirred up and redistributed. This does suggest that when taking surface water from a lake, one should try to obtain the water from underneath the surface, where particles float from surface tension, while still not disturbing bottom sediment.

Many organisms, such as *Giardia, Salmonella,* and *Cryptosporidium* can be zoonoses and have animal reservoirs; but most surface water contamination probably comes from human fecal contamination. It is important to properly dispose of personal waste. Bury feces 6 to 10 inches in the soil, at least 100 feet from any water source and any natural drainage.

Accurate information concerning water quality is difficult to obtain in any country. Where sanitation systems are lacking, which is still the case in most rural areas of developing countries, all surface water should be considered highly contaminated and tap water should be highly suspect. Any water that receives partially treated wastes is likely to contain pathogenic microorganisms, especially protozoa. *Giardia* and *Cryptosporidium* can be found in most surface waters, even in North America. Unfortunately, chemical and nuclear wastes from industrial dumping and agricultural and mining run-off may be unrecognized or unacknowledged pollutants of water supplies. The long-term traveler or expatriate to a given area should try to obtain information from his or her Consulate or other local expatriates about the safety of the local water supplies and available alternatives.

FIELD TECHNIQUES FOR WATER TREATMENT

Fortunately, there are reliable field methods for ensuring the microbiologic safety of drinking water. The three main methods to eliminate microorganisms from water are heat, chemicals, and filtration. Other techniques may be needed to improve the aesthetic quality of the water or to remove chemical contamination. Each technique is discussed along with its respective advantages and disadvantages. Understanding the principles of water disinfection helps in choosing a method appropriate for the risk, location, and size of the group.

Definitions

To understand discrepancies in recommendations, it is useful to define some terms. *Disinfection,* the desired result of field water treatment, means the removal or destruction of harmful microorganisms. Technically, it refers only to chemical means such as halogens, but the term can be applied to heat and filtration. *Pasteurization* is similar to disinfection but specifically refers to the use of heat, usually at temperatures below 100° C to kill most pathogenic organisms. Disinfection and pasteurization should not be confused with *sterilization,* which is the destruction or removal of all life forms. The goal of disinfection is to achieve *potable* water, indicating that a water source, on average over a period of time, contains a "minimal microbial hazard," so the statistical likelihood of illness is acceptable. *Purification* is the removal of organic or inorganic chemicals and particulate matter to remove offensive color, taste, and odor. It is frequently used interchangeably with disinfection, but purification may not remove or kill enough microorganisms to ensure microbiologic safety.

Heat

The advantages of heat for water disinfection are the following:

- ▼ It is widely available.
- ▼ It imparts no additional taste to the water.
- ▼ It is the only single-step process that inactivates all enteric pathogens.
- ▼ Efficacy of heat treatment is not compromised by contaminants or particles in the water as is halogenation and filtration.

The major disadvantages of heat are the following:

- ▼ Heat does not improve the taste, smell, or appearance of poor quality water.
- ▼ In many areas fuel is scarce or unavailable: 1 kg of wood is required to boil 1 L of water.
- ▼ Liquid fuels are expensive for developing countries and heavy to carry for wilderness traveler.

Heat inactivation of microorganisms is exponential and follows first-order kinetics. Thermal death point is reached in a shorter time at higher temperatures, whereas lower temperatures are effective with a longer contact time. Pasteurization uses this principle to kill food-borne enteric food pathogens and spoiling organisms at temperatures between 60° C and 70° C, well below boiling.

Table 7-3
Data on Heat Inactivation of Microorganisms

Organism	Lethal temperature/time
Giardia	55° C for 5 min 100° C immediately
E. histolytica	Similar to *Giardia*
Nematode cysts	50° C-55° C (Time not specified but should be similar to cryptosporidium)
Helminth eggs, larvae, cercariae	45° C-55° C for 20 min
Cryptosporidium	64.2° C for 2 min 72° C heated up over 1 min
E. coli	55° C for 30 min 60° C-62° C for 10 min
Salmonella and *Shigella*	65° C for <1 min
V. cholerae	100° C for 30 sec
Enteric Viruses	55° C-60° C for 20-40 min 70° C for <1 min
Hepatitis A	85° C for 1 min 60° C for 19 min (in shellfish)
Hepatitis E	60° C for 30 min
Bacterial spores	>100° C

Heat resistance varies with different microorganisms, but common enteric pathogens are readily inactivated by heat (Table 7-3). Bacterial spores (e.g., *Clostridium* spp.) are the most resistant; some can survive 100° C for long periods. *Clostridium* spores are wound pathogens that are ubiquitous in soil, lake sediment, tropical water sources, and the stool of animals and humans; but they are rarely water-borne enteric pathogens. Thus water sterilization is not necessary for drinking, since these most resistant organisms are not enteric human pathogens.

Protozoan cysts, including *Giardia, Entamoeba histolytica,* and *Cryptosporidium* are sensitive to heat, killed rapidly at 55° C to 60° C. Parasitic helminth eggs and larvae, and cercariae of schistosomiasis are equally susceptible to heat.

Vegetative bacteria and most enteric viruses are killed rapidly at temperatures above 60° C and within seconds by boiling water. Hepatitis A virus (HAV) should respond to heat similarly to other enteric viruses, but data suggest that it has increased thermal resistance compared with some other enteric viruses.

In recognition of the difference between pasteurizing water for drinking purposes and sterilizing for surgical purposes, most sources now agree that boiling for 10 minutes is not necessary. Because there is little data for HAV, the Centers for Disease Control and Prevention and the Environmental Protection Agency still recommend boiling for 1 minute to allow for an extra margin of safety. Although the boiling point decreases with increasing altitude, this is not significant with regard to the time and temperature required for thermal death (Table 7-4). Heating water on a stove or fire takes time, which counts toward disinfection while the temperature rises from 55° C to the boiling temperature. Therefore any water brought

Table 7-4
Boiling Temperature Altitude

Elevation	Boiling point
10,000 ft	90° C
14,000 ft	86° C
19,000 ft	81° C

to a boil should be adequately disinfected. For an extra margin of safety, the water should be brought to a boil, the stove turned off, and the pot covered for a few minutes before using the water.

Although attaining boiling temperature is not necessary, it is the only easily recognizable endpoint without using a thermometer. The use of hot tap water has been suggested to prevent traveler's diarrhea in developing countries; following the simple measure of "too-hot-to-touch" as a reliable indicator of adequate temperature for pasteurization of water. Testing shows considerable variation in the temperature of hot tap water (most between 55° C and 60 °C, but some lower) and in maximum tolerated temperature-to-touch (below 55° C for some people). If no other means of water treatment is available, using hot tap water that has been kept hot in a tank for some time is a reasonable alternative. Travelers staying in hotels or other accommodations with electricity can conveniently bring water to a boil with a small electric heating coil, or with a lightweight electric beverage warmer brought from home.

Temperatures adequate for pasteurization can be achieved by solar heating using a solar oven or simple reflectors in hot sunny climates.

Filtration

Filtration is appealing because the procedure is simple and adds no taste. Field devices that rely solely on mechanical filtration to remove microorganisms are usually adequate for cysts and bacteria, but may not reliably remove viruses, which are a major concern in water with high levels of fecal contamination (e.g., in developing countries). It is true that most viruses adhere to larger particles or clump together into aggregates that may be removed by the filter, or the viruses adhere to the filter media by electrochemical attraction. However, this is not adequate assurance, since the infectious dose of enteric viruses may be quite small. Some filters can remove viruses. Reverse osmosis filters that desalinate will also remove viruses; however, these are currently too expensive and slow for use in a hand pump for land travel. Iodine resin filters will kill bacteria and viruses. General Ecology has data that their First-Need mechanical filter will remove viruses, ostensibly by electrochemical means.

Filter pore size required for reliable removal of microorganisms is not straightforward because microorganisms can vary from expected size and have some elasticity, allowing them to deform under pressure, squeezing through filter pores (Table 7-5). Most field filters are not membranes, but rather depth filters, with mazelike passageways that trap particles and organisms smaller than the average passage diameter. The functional removal rate of various organisms is more important than the rated pore size of the filter. Good testing data are needed to back claims, but little

Table 7-5
Susceptibility of Microorganisms to Filtration

Organism	Approximate size	Maximum filter pore size
Nematode eggs	30 × 60 μm	20 μm
Giardia	6-10 × 8-15 μm	3-5 μm
Entamoeba histolytica	5-30 (average 10) μm	
Cyclospora	8-9 μm	3-5 μm
Cryptosporidium oocysts	2-6 μm	1 μm
Enteric bacteria	0.5 × 3-8 μm	0.2-0.4 μm
Viruses	0.03 μm	0.01 μm

objective, comparative testing is available. The Environmental Protection Agency (EPA) has proposed rigorous testing standards that are now used by most manufacturers to substantiate claims. Filters are expensive and their weight and bulk may be significant if carrying the gear oneself. A cracked filter element or a leaking seal that allows channeling of water around the filter will let contaminated water pass through the device.

Micropore filters clog quickly if the water is dirty or has a lot of suspended particles and eventually will clog from filtering apparently clear surface water. The user should know how to clean or replace the filter element to reestablish flow. Laboratory paper filters with a pore size of about 20 to 30 μm or even coffee filters can be used to prefilter the larger particulate debris from dirty water and can also retain parasitic eggs and larvae.

If the water supply is suspected of being heavily contaminated with biologic wastes, then heat or chemical treatment of the water after filtration is necessary to kill viruses. Prefiltration and microfiltration allow lower halogen doses to be used for the chemical inactivation step. Several iodine resin filters incorporate prefiltration, micropore filtration, and chemical inactivation steps into their design.

Filters for foreign and wilderness travelers are described in Table 7-6.

CLARIFICATION

The appearance of cloudy water can be improved by several other means. Large particles will settle out over a period of several hours by *sedimentation.* The supernatant can then be filtered and/or chemically treated. Smaller suspended particles can be removed by *coagulation-flocculation.* A pinch of alum (an aluminum salt) is added to a gallon of water, mixed well, and then stirred occasionally for 30 to 60 minutes. The small particles clump (flocculate) and then settle out over minutes to hours. The supernatant is then decanted, or the mixture is poured through a paper filter before proceeding with microfiltration and/or chemical treatment.

Granular Activated Charcoal

Granular activated charcoal (GAC) "purifies" by removing organic pollutants, chemicals, and radioactive particles by adsorption. This improves objectionable color, taste, and smell from water. Although some microorganisms will adhere to GAC or become trapped in charcoal filters, GAC does *not* remove all microorganisms; thus, it does not disinfect. In fact, charcoal beds become colonized rapidly with nonpathogenic bacteria.

Text continued on p. 102

Table 7-6
Field Water Treatment Devices

Product lines are continuously evolving, and prices change frequently and vary widely. Comments, corrections and additions are appreciated (HDBacker@aol.com).

For most of these products, claims are substantiated only by company sponsored and designed testing. Some results have been extrapolated to similar products. All new products must be tested using a standardized EPA protocol. Depending on claims, filters must demonstrate removal or inactivation of 10^3 cysts (99.9%), 10^4 viruses (99.99%), and 10^6 bacteria under varying water conditions of temperature and turbidity. These protocols are controversial and are being reviewed by a consensus panel. Objective, comparable test results for these products are not available.

Filter capacity is especially variable, depending on clarity of water. Numbers provided for capacity are usually maximal, using clean water. Comparative testing for filter capacity using slightly turbid river water and following manufacturer instructions for cleaning revealed markedly different valves for some filters. All field water has some sediment that clogs filters and reduces flow and capacity. For all filters, it is recommended to pump dilute bleach solution through the unit after each trip and before storage to decrease bacterial growth in the filter.

Katadyn — **www.katadyn.com** **http://www.katadyn.net/** **(800) 755-6701**

Product	Price	Structure/Function
		All filters contain a 0.2 micron ceramic candle filter; silver impregnated to decrease bacterial growth. Large units also contain silver quartz in center of filter.
Katadyn Pocket filter	$200	Hand-pump; 40″ intake hose and strainer, zipper case; Size: 10″ × 2″; Weight: 23 oz; Flow: 0.75-1 L/min; Capacity 13,000 L.
Mini ceramic filter	$90	Smaller, lighter hand-pump; 31″ intake hose and strainer, hard plastic enclosure and pump; Size: 7 × 2.75 × 1.75″; Weight: 9 oz; Flow: 0.5 L/min; Capacity: approx 7,000 L.
Katadyn Combi	$160	Small hand-pump with ceramic filter and activated charcoal stage; can brush ceramic to clean or separately replace elements; Size: 2.4 × 10.4″; Weight: 19 oz; Flow: 1.0 L/min; Capacity up to 50,000 L, 200 L for charcoal.
Expedition	$890	Large hand pump with steel stand; Size (packed in case): 23″ × 6″ × 8″; Weight: 12 lbs; Flow: 4 L/min; Capacity (per filter element) to 100,000 L.
Drip filter Ceradyn and Gravidyn	$160-$190	Gravity drip from one plastic bucket to another with 3 ceramic candle filter elements. Ceradyn filter candles are ceramic only, while Gravidyn filter candles combine ceramic and activated carbon elements; Size: 18" × 11" diameter (26" high when assembled); Weight: 9 lbs 4 oz; Flow: 1 pt/hr (10 gal/day); Capacity to 100,000 L.
Bottle	$45	Drink through bottle with three-stage water filter: cyst filter for protozoa, ViruStat Iodine resin, activated carbon; fits into standard cycle bottle holder; holds 0.6 L; Capacity 100 L.
Camp S Syphon filter	$100	Gravity siphon filter element available alone or with a 10 liter water bag: 12 × 2"; Weight: 2lb; Flow: 2 gal/hr; Capacity 5,000-20,000 L

Continued

Table 7-6
Field Water Treatment Devices—cont'd

Katadyn
Claims
Removes bacterial pathogens, protozoan cysts, parasites, nuclear debris. Clarifies cloudy water. If filter clogs, brushing the filter element (which can be done hundreds of times before needing to replace filter element) can restore flow. Claims for removal of viruses by ceramic filters not made in United States, although testimonials offered imply effectiveness in all polluted waters. Viral claims are made for Bottle. Pocket Filter has a lifetime warranty.

Comments
Well-designed, durable products that are effective for claims. However, high filter volume capacity is optimistic and not likeky to be achieved filtering average surface water. Backpacker Magazine field tests found the flow comparatively slow, requiring more energy to pump and frequent cleaning. Abrading the outer surface can effectively clean ceramic filters, but it is necessary to use the gauge to indicate when filter thickness becomes too thin.

Pocket Filter is the original, individual or small group filter design. Metal parts make it durable, but the heaviest for its size. Minifilter was designed to be lighter and more cost competitive. Expedition filter is popular for larger groups, especially river trips where weight is not a factor. Complete virus removal cannot be expected, although most viruses clump or adhere to larger particles and bacteria that can be filtered. Silver impregnation does not prevent bacterial growth in filters. Bottle filter with iodine resin allows no contact time and may not provide complete viral protection in all situations.

PUR Water Filters **http://www.katadyn.com**
Now owned by Katadyn, North America

Product	**Price**	**Structure/Function**
Guide	$80	Hand pump with 150 micron intake filter, 0.3 micron pleated filter with 143 square-inch surface area and carbon cartridge; Size: 9.5″ × 2.25″; Weight: 14 oz; max Flow: 1.0 L/min (36 stokes/L); Capacity: 100 gal/cartridge
Pioneer	$30	Hand pump filter (0.3 micron fiberglass disk) attaches to top of water bottle. Size: 2.5″ × 4.5″; Weight: 8 oz; Flow: 1 L/min; Capacity: 20 gal.
Hiker	$60	Hand pump with 0.3 micron pleated glass fiber with 107 square-inch surface; micro-filter and activated carbon core; Size: 6.5″ × 2.5″ × 3.5″; Weight: 11 oz; Flow: 1 L/min (48 stokes/L); Capacity: 200 gal

PUR Water Filters
Claims
Guide and Hiker are microfilters designed for high quality surface water. They will eliminate *Giardia, Cryptosporidium* and most bacteria; activated carbon core "reduces chemicals and pesticides, plus improves taste of water." Filters with large surface area are "guaranteed not to clog for 1 year."

Comments
PUR's popular Explorer with an iodine resin filter is not currently available.

Information on Purifiers from Katadyn-PUR web site:

Table 7-6
Field Water Treatment Devices—cont'd

Comments—cont'd

"Procter and Gamble (prior owners of PUR) stopped selling PUR purifiers in June 2000-they are currently not available. A quality control test indicated that the PUR Voyageur did not remove 99.99% of viruses in every condition when the StopTop carbon cartridge was used. The test did indicate full effectiveness against protozoa and bacteria.

Owners of PUR water purifiers may still use them. For full antivirus effectiveness, we advise consumers to pass water through the purifier twice and allow at least 30 minutes contact time for cold highly polluted water. PUR microfilter and purifier cartridges are interchangeable. If you already have a PUR water purifier and need a replacement cartridge, you can convert your unit to a microfilter by installing either a Hiker or Guide microfilter cartridge. Replacement cartridges are available at all outdoor stores. Until purifiers are available, use an EPA-registered disinfectant following microfiltration for complete virus protection."

Guide and Hiker were designed for the domestic backpacking market with higher water quality, where cysts and bacteria are a threat, but viruses are less of a problem. The Hiker received top ratings by Backpacker magazine for field tests evaluating user-friendliness. They may be used with a halogen disinfectant for international travel or conditions where high levels of contamination are possible.

PUR Marine Products **http://www.katadyn.com/**
Reverse Osmosis Filters

Product	Price	Structure/Function
Desalinator Survivor 06	$550	Hand operated pump, reverse osmosis membrane filter with prefilter on intake line; Size: 2.5″ × 5″ x 8″; Weight: 2.5 lb; Flow: 40 strokes/min yields 1 L/hr.
Survivor 35	$1425	Hand operated pump, reverse osmosis membrane filter with prefilter on intake line; Size: 3.5″ × 5.5″ × 22″; Weight: 7 lbs; Flow: 1.2 gal/hr (75 ml/min).

PUR Reverse Osmosis Filters

Claims

Reverse osmosis units desalinate, removing 98% salt from seawater by forcing water through a semi-permeable membrane at 800 PSI. In the process, microorganisms are filtered out. The manual operation of these units makes them unique and useful for survival at sea or for use in small craft without power source. Larger, power operated units also available.

Comments

Reverse osmosis units are included here for sea kayaking and small boat journeys in open water. Most large ocean-going boats use reverse osmosis filters. These units can obviate the need for relying solely on stored water or can be carried for emergency survival. The U.S. military uses truck mounted reverse osmosis filters on land for their ability to handle brackish water and remove all types of microorganisms. Reverse osmosis filters could be used for land-based travel, but are prohibitively expensive for most people and the flow rates are inadequate (1 liter per hour, not per minute). Desalination units will remove microorganisms, including viruses, which are larger than sodium molecules. Note that the company does not make claims for viral removal because they assume that the membrane is imperfect and some pores will be imprecise, perhaps allowing viral passage.

Continued

Table 7-6
Field Water Treatment Devices—cont'd

Exstream Water Technologies — **www.exstreamwater.com**
Now owned by Katadyn — **http://www.katadyn.com/**

Product	Price	Structure/Function
Orinoco Mackenzie Sungari	$40 $45 $60	Drink-through water bottles with four-stage cartridge containing prefilter for sediment, 1 micron cysts filter, penta-iodide resin then coconut-carbon scrubber. Orinoco wgt: 7.45 oz, capacity 26 oz (bike bottle style); Mackenzie wgt 7.95 oz, capacity 34 oz; Sungari similar to Orinoco with holster and torso pack

Exstream
Claims and Comments
Passed EPA tests to remove 3-log cysts, 4-log viruses, and 6-log bacteria. Patented ion-release technology and carbon scrubber dramatically reduce residual iodine. I5 is 1000 times more effective than I3 resin.

Similar design to WTC Sport Bottle (see comments below). Drink-through design limits to day use.

British Berkfeld — **(800) 350-4170**
U.S. distributor: James Filter — **http://www.jamesfilter.com/**

Product	Price	Structure/Function
Big Berkey Smaller versions available with variable numbers of filter elements.	$279	Stacked stainless steel containers with four 9" ceramic filters with activated carbon core; gravity flow; wgt: 6.0 lbs; assembled size 19.5" × 8.5"; flow:1.3 gallons/hr.; 2.4 gallon capacity of lower container.
LP-2	$145	Food grade high density polypropylene with 2 ceramic elements, gravity flow; wgt: 4 lbs; size: 24" × 10"; flow: ½ gal/hr; capacity of lower container: 2.4 gal.

British Berkfeld
Claims and Comments
Filter design is very similar to Katadyn Drip Filter. These filters are excellent for stationary base camps or expatriate homes. Ceramic filter is 0.9 micron absolute, but filters >99.99% of particles larger than 0.5 micron. Removes 100% cysts and 4 to 5-log bacteria. For complete protection, requires chlorine treatment as first step.

AquaRain Filter Systems — **(800) 572-2051**
www.aquarain.com

Product	Price	Structure/Function
AquaRain 400 AquaRain 200 Siphon Water filter	$239 $189 $32	Stainless steel containers (3 gallon each) with 2 or 4 silver impregnated ceramic filters with carbon core; gravity flow; wgt: 10 lbs; size 22" × 10.25"; flow: 32 gallons/day with 4 elements, 16 gal/day with 2; capacity 30,000-60,000 gallons.

Table 7-6
Field Water Treatment Devices—cont'd

AquaRain
Claims and Comments
Similar design as Berkfeld and Katadyn, although ceramic elements differ slightly (see previous comments). 0.2 micron absolute pore size, removes 100% cysts and 4-log reduction of bacteria. No claims for viruses. Clean ceramic elements 200 times before replacement.

General Ecology, Inc. **(610) 363-7900**
www.general-ecology.com

Product	Price	Structure/Function
First-Need Deluxe Water Filter	$85	All filters (except Microlite) contain 0.1 micron (0.4 micron absolute) "Structured matrix" filter in removable canister. Hand pump with intake strainer; outflow end connects directly to common water bottle; self-cleaning prefilter float; Size: 6″ × 6″, Weight: 15 oz; Flow: 1.6 L/min; Capacity: 100-400 liters.
Microlite	$35	Structured Matrix filter 0.5 microns (nominal) with activated carbon; hand pump, 24" intake hose and strainer; attaches directly to wide-mouth or bike bottle, soda bottle, or use outlet spout; Size: 5.5″ × 2.5″; Weight: 8 oz; Flow: 0.5 L/min; Capacity: 50 L/cartridge.
Trav-L-Pur	$144	Filter and hand pump in rectangular housing (1.5 pt Capacity); pour water into housing, then pump through prefilter and microfilter; Size: 4.5″ × 3.5 × 6.75″; Weight: 22 oz; Flow: 1-2 pt/min; Capacity: 100-400 L. (Carrying case included.)
Base Camp	$500	Stainless steel casing and hand pump connected with tubing; Capacity 1000 gal; canister Size 4.8 × 5.4″; pump 1.5″ × 10.5″; Weight: 3 lbs; Flow: 2 L/min. (Carrying case included.)

General Ecology Filters
Claims
First Need Filter is a proprietary blend of materials including activated charcoal. "Microfiltration" with 0.1 micron retention (0.4 absolute) "removes bacteria and larger pathogens" (cysts, parasites). "Adsorption and molecular sieving": carbon absorbers remove chemicals and organic pollutants that cause color and taste; cavities in surface of adsorption material draw particles in deeper. Does not remove all dissolved minerals or desalinate. Proprietary process also creates ionic surface charge that removes colloids and ultra-small particles through "electrokinetic attraction." Has passed laboratory tests as a purifier, which means reducing test virus by 10^4, as well as bacteria by 10^6 and Cryptosporidium by 10^3.

Microlite removes sediment, protozoan cysts, algae, chemicals (including iodine), and improves color and taste of water. Iodine tablets are included to kill bacteria and viruses when these organisms are a concern.

Continued

Table 7-6
Field Water Treatment Devices—cont'd

General Ecology
Comments
Reasonable design, cost, and effectiveness. All units (except Microlite) use the same basic filter design. Most testing with *E. coli* and *Giardia* cysts show excellent removal. Charcoal matrix will remove chemical pollutants. This is the only company that has met EPA standards for 4-log reduction of viruses through filtration without halogens. However, they do not claim to remove all viruses, since they have not been able to test with the hepatitis virus. Despite viral claims, recommend caution in highly polluted water; prior disinfection with halogen would guarantee disinfection, and carbon would remove halogen. The filter cannot be cleaned, although it can potentially be back flushed; so it must be replaced when clogged.

The Microlite is designed primarily for day-use or light backpacking. Used alone, it makes microbiologic claims for protozoan cysts *(Giardia* and *Cryptosporidium)* only. Iodine or chlorine should be used as pretreatment with this filter for all water except pristine alpine water in North America. This filter is compact, lightweight and designed for low volume use with inexpensive, easily changed filter cartridges.

Base Camp is for large groups. It also comes with an electric pump and can be hooked up in parallel to provide large quantities of water for disaster relief.

MSR and Marathon Ceramics **(206) 624-7948**
(Marathon Ceramics is a Division of MSR and subsidiary of REI) **www.msrcorp.com**

Product	Price	Structure/Function
MSR Waterworks II Total Filtration System (All filter elements replaceable)	$130	Four filter elements of decreasing pore size: porous foam intake filter, 10 micron stainless steel wire mesh screen, cylindrical ceramic filter with block carbon core, then 0.2 micron pharmacological-grade membrane filter; pressure relief valve releases at 90-95 psi; hand pump with intake tubing; storage bag (2 or 4 liter) attaches directly to outlet of pump. Size: 9″ × 4″; Weight: 17 oz; Flow: 1 liter/90 sec; Capacity: 100-400 L.
Miniworks	$70	Similar external design to Waterworks II a slightly different ceramic filter and lacks the final membrane filter; Weight: 16 oz; Flow rate 1 liter/70 sec. Capacity: 100-400 L.
Marathon ceramics e-water siphon filter	$25-30	Same filter element as above with siphon tubing; use any two containers to siphon water through filter; Capacity 7 gal/day.

MSR filter
Claims
Removes protozoa (including *Giardia* and *Cryptosporidium*), bacteria, pesticides, herbicides, chlorine, and discoloration. Both filters meet EPA standards for removal of cysts and bacteria. Ceramic filters reduced turbidity from 68.8 NTU to 0.01 NTU. Carbon has been shown to reduce levels of iodine from 16 mg/L to <0.01 mg/L for at least 150 liters.

Comments
Excellent filter design and function. Prefilters protect more expensive inner, fine pore filters. Effective for claims; high quality control and extensive testing. No claims are made

Table 7-6
Field Water Treatment Devices—cont'd

Comments—cont'd

for viruses, although clumping and adherence remove the majority (currently 2-3-log removal, but not 4-log required for purifiers). The company is working on a microfilter that will effectively remove viruses. Until they succeed, the filter should not be considered reliable for complete viral removal from highly polluted waters in developing countries. Reservoir bag that attaches to outflow for filtered water storage is convenient. Design and ease of use are distinct advantages. Filter can be easily maintained in the field; maintenance kit and all replacement parts available. Ceramic filters can be effectively cleaned by abrading outer surface many times without compromising the filter. A simple caliper gauge indicates when filter has become too thin for reliable function. Miniworks was rated very highly in Backpacker Magazine filed tests.

Other manufacturers are incorporating Marathon ceramic filters into many different products. Gravity drip buckets are excellent products for field camps and expatriates. Iodine or chlorine can be used to assure viral destruction and the carbon will remove excess halogen, allowing long-term safe use of iodine. Siphon filter is inexpensive and compact.

Penta Pure **www.pentapure.com**
(Formerly WTC—Water Technology Corp)

Product	Price	Structure/Function
PentaPure Sport	$35	All products use PentaPure iodine resin. Drink-through sport bottle with internal (Pentacell) 3-stage cartridge: 1 micron filter, iodine resin, and charcoal filter. Filter and charcoal stages can be replaced independently. Size: 11.5″ × 3″; Weight: 8 oz; Flow: N/A; Capacity: 375 L.
Spring	$25	Drink-through sport bottle with filter and charcoal, but no iodine resin. Otherwise similar to Sport.
The following are considered "international" products. They are not marketed in the United States, but are available for export, which includes purchase for use outside the United States. They can be ordered from several companies, including TealBrook (800) 222-6614, http://www.tealbrook.com/. Availability is variable.		
Penta-Pour Bucket Ecomaster Outdoor Ecopour	$170	Gravity drip bucket with 22 L storage capacity; sediment filter (30 micron), 1 micron filter; pentacide and carbon cartridge; Size: 12″ × 30″; Weight: 3 kg; Flow: 30 L/hr; Capacity: 6,500 L.
Travel Tap, Traveler	Price not available	Pentacide and carbon cartridge. Rubber cup hose fitting on cartridge unit fits any faucet. Flow ½ gal/min; Capacity: 1,000 gallons
Outdoor 500	$1475	Expedition size hand-lever filter with steel frame; sediment filter, iodine resin, carbon block, each can be independently replaced. Size: 14″ × 9.5″ × 18.5″; Weight: 7 kg; Flow: 300 L/hr; Capacity: 30,000 L.
Outdoor M1, Survivor	Price not available	Drink-through straws; cartridge with prefilter, granular activated carbon filter sandwiched between two stages of PentPure resin; Size: 5.5″ long; Weight: 1 oz; Capacity: 100 gal (M-1), 25 gal. (Survivor)

Continued

Table 7-6
Field Water Treatment Devices—cont'd

WTC/PentaPure Iodine Resin Filters

Claims

Resin releases iodine "on demand," on contact with microorganisms; minimal iodine dissolves in water: effluent 1.0-2.0 ppm iodine. Charcoal removes residual dissolved iodine. Tested effective for bacteria, *Giardia,* schistosomiasis, viruses—including hepatitis. PentaCell tested against the new EPA protocol that requires removal of 105 bacteria, 104 viruses, and 103 *Cryptosporidium* cysts. Charcoal stage absorbs bad tastes and odors.

Comments

See discussion of iodine resins in text.

The resin is essentially inexhaustible, because the filter will become irreversibly clogged long before the resin is exhausted. However, the carbon filter may become fully absorbed with iodine and other impurities allowing iodine in the effluent. Although the amount of iodine in the outflow water is supposed to be low (1-2 ppm), higher concentrations have been measured. For long-term use, carbon filters should be changed regularly.

The company has narrowed their product line for field use and has dropped the small group hand-pump filters because there were other similar products on the market. They have also dropped the Travel Cup, a small pour through plastic cup. The Sport Bottle is handy for individual use among hikers, bikers and travelers. Pressure is generated by a combination of sucking and squeezing. Users must get used to the effort and the slower flow compared to a regular sport bottle. Drink-through straws have limited applications, mainly survival and emergency situations. The "international" products are some of the most useful ones. Penta-Pour bucket is an excellent product for expatriates and field camps. The Outdoor series would work well for stationary or vehicle-based groups. Large units are available for big groups and disaster relief. The Traveler (formerly Travel Tap) is a small, portable unit that hooks to the end of a faucet and could be very useful for expatriates and frequent travelers.

Sawyer Products **http://www.sawyerproducts.com**

Product	Price	Structure/Function
Innova BiologicWater Filter Bottle	$34	Plastic squeeze bottle with dual filtration system cartridge: prefilter contains activated charcoal and 0.2-micron hollow fiber filter, which is a cluster of microtubules. Water is drawn through the walls of the tubules either by suction or by pressure applied in squeezing the bottle. 20 oz water bottle; capacity 80 gallons, 480 refills.

Claims

GAV prefilter removes lead, chlorine, odors, taste sediment, while the microfilter removes bacteria, protozoa, and cysts. No claims for viruses; add chlorine to kill viruses.

Comments

This filter was carefully designed and tested. The potential advantage over other water bottle filters is the unique hollow fiber technology that may provide faster filtration with less pressure. Use of this product is limited to an individual or two persons sharing a water bottle. It does not avoid the two-step process for potentially highly contaminated water.

Table 7-6
Field Water Treatment Devices—cont'd

Cascade Designs **http://www.cascadedesigns.com/**
Sweetwater Filters

Product	Price	Structure/Function
Sweetwater Guardian	$60	Lexan body and pump handle; 100 micron metal pre-filter; in-line 4 micron secondary filter; labyrinth filter cylinder of borosilicate fibers removes pathogens to 0.2 micron; granular activated carbon; safety pressure relief valve; end of life indicator; outflow tubing has universal adapter that fits all water bottles; optional input adapter that attaches to sink faucet while traveling; Size: 7.75″ × 3.5″; Weight: 11 oz; Flow: 1.25 L/min (new filter); Capacity: 200 gal. Zipper carrying case with Guardian filter, viral guard cartridge and 1 L storage bag.
ViralStop	$8	A chlorine-based purifier solution; add 5 drops to each liter of filtered water, mix for at least 10 seconds, and wait 5 minutes
Walkabout	$50	Lightweight version with replaceable filter element; Size 6.5″ height; Weight: 9 oz; Flow 0.9 L/min; Capacity: 125 gal.

Sweetwater Filter
Claims
Eliminates *Giardia, Cryptosporidium,* and other critical bacterial and protozoan pathogens, pollutants, heavy metals, pesticides, and flavors. Cartridge accessory. Lighter, more compact and durable than comparable models, and easiest to clean or replace. The company recycles filter cartridges.

Comments
Well-designed filter at a reasonable price. Practical design features like universal bottle adapter. Pressure-release valve indicates when filter needs cleaning, but this can be a problem as the filter clogs. A brush is provided for cleaning and cartridges are replaceable. Rated highly in Backpacker Magazine field tests.

The iodine resin containing Viral Guard was recently removed from the market. New in-house testing of the Guardian filter with iodine resin attachment failed to inactivate Poliovirus at levels required by EPA standards under certain conditions. The failure of the viral testing was a surprise to the company, since a reliable laboratory had originally tested the product with the iodine resin and verified adequate levels of viral inactivation. It is unclear whether this indicates a problem in general with the iodine resins or with the specific design of their iodine resin filter attachment. Since they were unable to solve the problem, the company is investigating other technologies. They have developed a specially formulated chlorine solution (ViralStop) for use before filtration when high levels of contamination are possible, including viruses.

Continued

Table 7-6
Field Water Treatment Devices—cont'd

Hydro-Photon Inc — **888-826-6234** **http://www.hydrophoton.com/**

Product	Price	Structure/Function
Steri-Pen replacement element	$200	Portable, battery-operated ultraviolet water disinfection system. Disinfects up to 16 oz of clear water in less than one minute by stirring UV element in water. Uses 4 AA batteries (disposable or rechargeable: alkaline batteries provide 20-40 treatments, lithium batteries 130-140 treatments; Weight 8oz, with batteries; Length, 7"; lamp lasts 5,000 treatments. Comes with a thermoformed nylon carrying case.

Claims
Highly effective against bacteria, viruses and protozoa, including *Cryptosporidium* oocysts.

Comments
The testing for this device is sound. In general, UV light for water disinfection is well tested and widely used for water treatment in many large and varied applications; but until now, these have required a larger, fixed power and light source. The use of this portable technology is currently limited to small volumes of clear water, however the potential is great for further advances that will increase its uses in the field and make it less expensive.

One rational use of GAC is to remove the color and taste of iodine or chlorine after disinfection. If used to remove halogen, one must wait until *after* the required contact time before running water through charcoal or adding charcoal to the water. Granular activated charcoal is commonly incorporated into commercial water purification devices after the filtration or chemical disinfection steps (see Table 7-6).

CHEMICALS

Halogens (chlorine and iodine) are:

- Excellent disinfectants for bacteria, viruses, *Giardia,* and amebic cysts, except *Cryptosporidium*
- Readily available in several forms
- Inexpensive
- Can be applied with equal ease to large and small quantities of water

To achieve reliable results and reasonable taste, however, some understanding of the process is necessary.

Vegetative bacteria are markedly sensitive to halogens; viruses and *Giardia* are sensitive but require higher concentrations or longer contact times. *Cryptosporidium* cysts are extremely resistant to halogens. Little is known about *Cyclospora,* but it is assumed to be similar to *Cryptosporidium.* Certain parasitic eggs, such as *Ascaris,* are also resistant, but these are not commonly spread by water. (All these resistant cysts and eggs are susceptible to heat or filtration.) New products containing chlorine dioxide may overcome this limitation of chemical disinfectants.

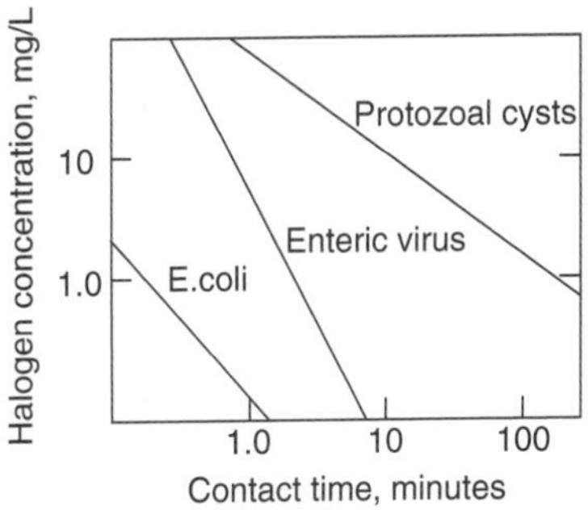

Fig. 7-1 Graph of disinfection reaction for 99.9% kill, halogen concentration versus time. Note relative susceptibility of microorganisms. Slope and position of lines vary with specific organism, disinfectant, and water temperature. (Adapted from Chang SL: WHO Bulletin 38:401,1968.)

Table 7-7
Experimental Data for 99.9% Kill with Halogens at pH 6-8

Organism	Halogen	Concentration	Time	Temperature
Giardia	Chlorine	0.5 mg/L	6-24 hr	3°-5° C (37°-41° F)
		4.0 mg/L	60 min	3°-5° C
		8.0 mg/L	30 min	3°-5° C
		3.0 mg/L	10 min	15° C (59° F)
		1.5 mg/L	10 min	25° C (77° F)
		1.5 mg/L	10 min	25° C
	Iodine	3.0 mg/L	15 min	20° C
		7.0 mg/L	30 min	3° C
Enteric viruses	Chlorine	0.5 mg/L	40 min	2° C
		0.3 mg/L	30 min	25° C
		0.3 mg/L	30 min	25° C
Polio virus	Iodine	20 mg/L	1.5 min	25° C
Escherichia coli	Chlorine	0.03 mg/L	5 min	2°-5° C
	Iodine	1.0 mg/L	1 min	2°-5° C

Primary factors determining the rate and proportion of microorganisms killed are the concentration of halogen (measured in milligrams per liter [mg/L] or the equivalent, parts per million [ppm]) and the length of time organisms are exposed to the halogen (contact time, measured in minutes) (Fig. 7-1 and Table 7-7). An increase in one allows a decrease in the other. Theoretically, for given conditions of temperature and pH, doubling contact time allows half the concentration of halogen to achieve the same results. In clear water, this principle can be used to decrease the taste of halogen. Extending contact time also adds a margin of safety.

Secondary factors are temperature of the water, organic contaminants in the water, and pH. Cold slows reaction time, so in cold water, the contact time should be increased. Alternatively, the dose can be increased in cold water. Some halogen is absorbed by organic impurities in the water, so an increased dose is required if water is cloudy (high turbidity); longer contact time may not be effective. Although clear surface water probably requires minimal halogen, some impurities (at least 1 mg/L) must be assumed, so it is prudent to use 4 mg/L as a target halogen concentration for clear water and allow extra contact time, especially if the water is cold. Water pH usually becomes a factor only in highly alkaline waters, but not in the usual case of usual surface water, which is neutral to slightly acidic.

Recommendations for chlorine and iodine disinfection of water with regard to concentration, temperature, and contact times are given in Table 7-8. Both chlorine and iodine are available in liquid and tablet form. Table 7-9 describes some commercially available halogen products.

Table 7-8
Halogen Disinfection of Water

Iodine products	**Amount to release 4 PPM in 1 L**	**Amount to release 8 PPM in 1 L**
Iodine tabs	1/2 tab	1 tab
Tetraglycine hydroperiodide	*or*	
EDWGT	1 tablet in 2 liters	
Potable aqua		
Globaline		
2% iodine solution (tincture)	0.2 ml	0.4 ml
(do not use decolorized iodine)	5 gtt	10 gtt
10% povidone-iodine solution	0.35 ml	0.70 ml
	8 gtt	16 gtt
Saturated iodine crystals in water	13 ml	26 ml
Polar Pure		

Chlorine products	**Amount for 5 ppm in 1 L**	**Amount for 10 ppm in 1 L**
Household bleach (5%	0.1 ml	0.2 ml
sodium hypochlorite)	2 gtt	4 gtt
Chlorination-Flocculation		1 tablet (8 ppm)
Chlor-floc		
AquaPure		
AquaCure		
Aquaclear	1 tablet in 2 liters	1 tablet

Contact Time in Minutes at Various Water Temperatures*

Concentration of halogen	**5° C**	**15° C**	**30° C**
2 ppm	240	180	60
4 ppm	180	60	45
8 ppm	60	30	15

gtt, Drops; *ppm,* parts per million (equivalent to mg/L); *EDWGT,* emergency drinking water germicidal tablet.

*Recent data indicate that very cold water requires prolonged contact time with iodine or chlorine to kill *Giardia* cysts. These contact times in cold water have been extended from the usual recommendations to account for this and for the uncertainty of residual concentration.

Table 7-9
Commercial Halogen Products

Extensive data exist for the effectiveness of iodine and chlorine (see text and Table 7-8) However, none of these products can be expected to kill *Cryptosporidium.*

POLAR EQUIPMENT
www.polarequipment.com

Formulation/instructions
Iodine crystals, 8 gm in 3 oz bottle; 30-50 μm fabric prefilter provided; "trap" in bottle to catch crystals when pouring off water; bottle cap is used to measure; directions and color dot thermometer on bottle (temperature affects iodine concentration in bottle); capacity: 2000 quarts; wgt: 5 oz; yields 4 ppm iodine when recommended dose is added to one quart of clean water. Warm water to 20° C (68° F) before adding iodine to shorten contact time.

Comments
Saturated aqueous solution of crystalline iodine is an excellent and stable source of iodine. Recommendations are adequate for clear, warm water; but, since it is not feasible to warm all water, extend contact time to 1 to 2 hours for very cold water. Temperature of the bottle affects the concentration of iodine in the saturated solution, which is the reason for the color-dot thermometer on the bottle. Users can adjust the dose according to the temperature, or put the bottle in an inner pocket to warm the saturated solution before use. Glass bottle can break.

Potable Aqua
Wisconsin Pharmaceuticals

Emergency Germicidal Drinking Water Tablets
Coghan Ltd.

Formulation/Instructions
Iodine-containing tablets (tetraglycine hydroperiodide) release approximately 7-8 mg iodine when added to water. One tablet is added to 1 quart of water. In cloudy or cold water, add 2 tablets. Contact time is only 10 to 15 minutes in clear, warm water, much more in cold, cloudy water (refer to table). Neutralizing tablets contain ascorbic acid. Weight: 2 oz. 50 tablets; or P.A. tablets plus neutralizing tablets

Comments
Method developed by the military for troops in the field. Advantages are unit dose and short contact time, but these concentrations create strong tastes that are not acceptable to many wilderness users. Options to improve taste include adding one tablet to 2 quarts of clear water to yield about 4 mg/L (and extend contact time), or use the neutralizer tablets. In cloudy water, use two tablets per quart (better yet, clarify water first). Ascorbic acid (vitamin C) neutralizer reduces iodine to iodide, which has no color or taste and has no disinfecting action. Aesthetically, iodine is "removed" from the water. However, iodide is physiologically active, so concerns about toxicity or physiologic activity remains. For short-term use, iodine is safe and removing the taste is a major benefit.

Sanitizer
Global Living Systems
Also available from: Chinook Medical Gear
www.chinookmed.com
(800) 766-1365

Formulation/Instructions
Chlorine crystals (calcium hypochlorite, 65% available chlorine) and 30% hydrogen peroxide in separate small plastic bottles. Achieves very high concentrations of chlorine for disinfection (30-200 ppm), then dechlorinates with peroxide, which causes formation of soluble calcium chloride (nontoxic). Excess peroxide bubbles off as oxygen. Hydrogen peroxide is also a weak disinfectant. Treated water has no chlorine taste. Highly stable if kept in cool, dry place
Total weight: 5 oz; kit treats 160 gallons.

Continued

Table 7-9
Commercial Halogen Products—cont'd

Comments
Manufactured and marketed by a cottage industry and can be very difficult to find. However, ingredients can be purchased at chemical supply (30% peroxide) and swimming pool supply (calcium hypochlorite). Sound use of chlorination and dechlorination with the minor disadvantage of two-step process. Peroxide is titrated to the estimated amount of chlorine. Measurements do not need to be exact, but it takes some experience to balance the two and achieve optimal results; 30% peroxide is extremely corrosive and burns skin, so handle cautiously. Very good technique for disinfecting large quantities. Also, the best technique for storing water on boats: high level of chlorine prevents growth of algae or bacteria during storage, then water is dechlorinated in needed quantities when ready to use.

AquaCure
Safesport Manufacturing Co
Aqua Pure World Resources

Chlor Floc
Control chemical.

Formulation/Instructions
These products are available through some outdoor equipment stores.

Tablets contain alum as flocculating agent and 1.4% available chlorine in the form of sodium dichloro-s-triazinetrione; bicarbonate causes tablet to dissolve rapidly; cloth provided for simple straining of flocculation sediment; flocculates and yields 8 mg/L free chlorine; 30 tablets individually sealed in foil packets; weight 1.6 oz.; capacity: 30 L (8 gal).

Chlor-floc and Aquapure are similar products containing sodium dichloro-isocyanurate (NaDCC) with proprietary flocculating agents and a buffering system. Cloth filter is provided. One tablet provides 8 ppm available chlorine.

Comments
This product is one of the individual field methods for U.S. military troops and has undergone extensive testing. In clear water, yields unpleasantly high chlorine levels and creates sediment. Excellent product for cloudy, colored, unpleasant smelling and tasting water. Alum is a widely used flocculent that causes suspended sediment, colloids, and many microorganisms to clump, settle to the bottom, where they can readily be filtered or strained. Most *Cryptosporidium* oocysts would be removed by the flocculation. Since chlorine reacts with contaminants, it is important to confirm some chlorine taste and smell at the end of the contact time. For added safety, prolong the contact times. May require up to 1 hour contact time in cold, polluted, and dirty water.

Aquaclear
Gal Pharm Ltd., Ireland
Imported by: BCB Survival Equipment
www.bcbin.com

Formulation/Instructions
Each tablet contains 17 mg sodium dichloro-isocyanurate (NaDCC) in paper/foil laminate. Effervescent tablet dissolved in 1 L of water releases 10 mg of free chlorine (HOCl), with 50% available chlorine in compound, released as free chlorine is used up by halogen demand. Also available in 340 mg and 500 mg of NaDSS and in screw cap tubs.

NaDSS is a stable, nontoxic chlorine compound that forms a mildly acidic solution, which is optimal for hypochlorous acid, the most active disinfectant of the free chlorine compounds. Free chlorine is in equilibrium with available chlorine that remains in compound, providing greater biocidal capacity. NaDSS is more stable and provides more free, active chlorine than other available chlorine products for water disinfection. Surface water disinfection of clear water accomplished at 10 mg/L in 10 minutes, 1 mg/L for tap water, and 2-5 mg/L for well water. Can use to wash fruits and vegetables in concentrations of 20 mg/L.

Table 7-9
Commercial Halogen Products—cont'd

Comments
Excellent source of chlorine in individually wrapped tablet form. Bulk quantities and concentrations are available for disinfection of large quantities of water for shock chlorination of tanks and other storage systems.

Micropur
www.katadyn.com

Formulation/Instructions
Silver in tablet, liquid or crystal form. Unit dosages available for small volumes of water or for big storage tanks. Most common formulation: silver-containing tablets in individual bubble packing; add one tab to 1 quart of water. Mix thoroughly and allow 2 hours contact time.

Claims
"For the disinfection and storage of clear water." "Reliably kill bacterial agents of enteric diseases but *not* worm eggs, ameba, viruses." "Neutral to taste, simple to use and innocuous." Treatment of water will ensure protection against reinfection for 1-6 months.

Comments
Silver has the advantage of having no taste, color or smell. Recently approved by the EPA to be marketed in the United States as a "water preservative" that can maintain bacteria free water for up to 6 months. Although proven antibacterial effects, silver tablets are not licensed as a water purifier in the United States. Note no claims for viruses and protozoa, because concentrations may not be adequate to kill these organisms. However, they are widely used in Europe for primary treatment of water. In addition to poorly documented effects on all different types of microorganisms, there is some difficulty controlling the residual concentration and concern over chronic effects.

Micropur Forte
Katadyn Corporation
www.katadyn.com

Formulation/Instructions
This product combines silver and chlorine in tablet or liquid form. Mix with water and allow at least 20 minutes contact time.

Claims
Chlorine ensures destruction of viruses, as well as bacteria. Effective for clear, untreated surface water. Silver maintains microbiologic purity of water for up to 6 months.

Comments
Rational combination of broad spectrum disinfection and long-term preservation for storage of water. Concentration and contact time may need to be extended for cold water and cysts, but if water is consumed right away, there is no reason to use this product, because the silver adds little advantage to chlorine alone.

Aqua Mira
McNett Outdoor Corp
www.mcnett.com
Pristine
www.pristine.ca

Formulation/Instructions
"Stabilized" chlorine dioxide generated by mixing two components (Part A: 2% stabilized chlorine dioxide, Part B: 5% food grade phosphoric acid solution). When mixed, the result

Continued

Table 7-9
Commercial Halogen Products—cont'd

Formulation/Instructions–cont'd
is 5 ppm solution of activated chlorine dioxide (ClO_2), which is then added to water. Allow 15 minutes contact time, double or longer if cold or cloudy water. Four-year shelf life. Treats up to 30 gallons of water.

Claims
Currently, limited claims in Unite States. "Kills odor-causing bacteria and improves the taste of water from rivers, lakes, streams, tap water, and more. AQUAMIRA is stabilized chlorine dioxide and contains no chlorine or iodine. AQUAMIRA's unique formula works quickly and efficiently by releasing oxygen in a highly active form to kill odor-causing bacteria without unpleasant taste or odor."

Canadian product claims complete kill of all enteric microorganisms, including bacteria, viruses, *Giardia* and *Cryptosporidium*. Imparts no taste to water and is non-toxic.

Comments
Chlorine dioxide has long been used in municipal disinfection plants, but as a gas that was not feasible for portable field use. Chlorine dioxide has been demonstrated effective against all enteric pathogens, including *Cryptosporidium* oocysts. Testing data for Aqua Mira has not yet been released in the United States, pending EPA approval as a "purifier." If this stabilized solution does generate adequate concentrations and maintains residual concentration, it will be a great addition to available methods because of its effectiveness against a broad spectrum of organisms.

Choice of Halogen

Iodine has some advantage over chlorine for field disinfection. Dilute Iodine solutions are less affected by nitrogenous wastes or pH, and most people prefer the taste at treatment levels. However, there is concern over the physiologic activity. Some alteration in thyroid function can be measured when iodine is used for water disinfection, and goiters have been associated with excessive iodine levels in water. There is the potential for hypersensitivity reactions (although these have not been described from iodinated water) and for exacerbation of preexisting thyroid problems.

Therefore iodine use is *not* recommended in the following circumstances:

- Unstable thyroid disease
- Known iodine allergy
- During pregnancy for periods longer than several weeks (because of the risk of neonatal goiter)

Despite studies documenting use of iodine for prolonged periods without problems, caution dictates against recommending iodine use for longer than several weeks to months in any individual. Although the military developed iodine tablets and still uses them in some situations, the disadvantages of unpleasant taste and color, inability to improve aesthetics of water, and alteration of thyroid function have led them to substitute chlorine tablets combined with a flocculent for many small group field applications.

Problems with chlorine or iodine use include the following:

- Taste can be unpleasant when concentrations exceed 4 to 5 mg/L
- The potency of some products (tablets and crystals) is affected by prolonged exposure to moisture, heat, and air

- Liquids are corrosive and stain
- There is some degree of imprecision because the actual residual concentration (after halogen demand) is not known

Taste may be improved by the following:

- Adding drink flavoring *after* adequate contact time
- Using GAV *after* contact time (included as a final stage in many filters)
- Reducing the concentration and increasing the contact time in clean water
- Using a technique that leaves a small residual halogen concentration in water, such as an iodine resin filter with a charcoal stage
- Removing taste by chemical means. A tiny pinch or several granules or ascorbic acid (vitamin C, available in powder or crystal form) or sodium thiosulfate (nontoxic, available at chemical supply stores) will reduce iodine or chlorine to iodide or chloride, which has no taste or color. These must be added *after* the required contact time. Note that iodide still has physiologic activity. Hydrogen peroxide will also reduce chlorine to chloride (see chlorination-dechlorination product in footnotes for Table 7-9).

Iodine Resins

Iodine resins have been incorporated into many different filter designs available for field use (Table 7-6). General testing data are convincing for iodine resins. Iodine apparently binds to microorganisms aided by electrostatic forces, but the exact mechanism of iodine transfer to organisms is not known. Organisms are effectively exposed to extremely high iodine concentrations when passing through the resin, allowing reduced contact time; however, some contact time is necessary, especially for cysts. Carbon that removes residual dissolved iodine is important to prevent excessive iodine ingestion in long-term users, but the role of residual dissolved iodine for cyst and virus destruction is not clear; some residual concentrations may be necessary. *Cryptosporidium* oocysts may become trapped in the resin, but of those passing through, half are viable at 30 minutes. Products have been redesigned with an 1 μm cyst filter, which should effectively remove *Cryptosporidium,* as well as *Giardia* and any other halogen-resistant parasitic eggs or larva. Their operation assumes that resins kill bacteria and viruses rapidly and the filter membrane removes cysts, so that no significant contact time is required for most water. Cloudy or sediment-laden water may clog the resin, as it would with any filter, or coat the resin, inhibiting iodine transfer.

The effectiveness of an individual resin matrix depends on ensuring contact of every microorganism with iodine resin (no channeling of water). Two companies recently pulled their iodine resin products from the market because repeated testing demonstrated virus breakthrough in cold, clear water with high viral loads, despite the fact that they performed well in initial premarketing tests. The companies were not able to determine whether channeling of water, a lack of residual iodine concentration in effluent water, or the need for more contact time caused the failure.

Preferred Technique

Field disinfection techniques and their effect on microorganisms are summarized in Table 7-10. The optimal technique for an individual or group depends on the number of persons to be served, space and weight available, quality of source water, personal taste preferences, and availability of

Table 7-10
Summary of Field Water Disinfection Techniques

	Bacteria	Viruses	*Giardia*/Ameba	*Cryptosporidium*	Nematodes/*Cercarea*
Heat	+	+	+	+	+
Filtration	+	+/−*	+	+	+
Halogens	+	+	+	−	+/−†

*With the exception of General Ecology FirstNeed Filter, most mechanical filters make no claims for viruses. Reverse osmosis filters should also be effective.

†Parasitic nematode eggs are not very susceptible to halogens but have a very low risk of water-borne transmission.

fuel. Unfortunately, optimal protection for all situations may require a two-step process of (1) filtration or coagulation-flocculation and (2) halogenation, because halogens do not kill *Cryptosporidium* and filtration misses some viruses. Heat is effective as a one-step process but will not improve aesthetics if the water is cloudy or poor tasting. In addition, fuel supplies may limit the use of heat. The iodine resins, combined with microfiltration to remove resistant cysts, also constitute an effective one-step process with the uncertainties previously discussed. In recognition of the need for two-stage treatment of microbiologically contaminated water, many microfilters are now packaged with a halogen. Generally the halogen is added first, with filtration as the second step.

In pristine wilderness water where there is little human or animal activity in the watershed, *Cryptosporidium* oocysts and viruses pose less risk; if present, very low numbers are likely. Heat, mechanical or iodine resin filtration, or halogens in low doses can be used. This is also the case when treating unreliable tap water. Filtration has the advantage of imparting no taste and requiring no contact time.

Water with agricultural runoff and/or sewage plant discharge from upstream towns or cities should be treated with heat or with a two-step process of filtration to remove *Cryptosporidium,* followed by halogens to ensure viral destruction. An iodine resin filter with microfiltration is an alternative. A filter containing a charcoal element has the added advantage of removing chemicals such as pesticides.

Surface water in undeveloped countries, even if clear, should be treated as contaminated with enteric pathogens. Heat is effective; simple mechanical filtration is not adequate. Halogens are reasonable but will miss *Cryptosporidium* and parasitic eggs. A two-stage process as cited previously offers added protection.

Cloudy water in developed or undeveloped counties that does not clear with sedimentation should be pretreated with coagulation-flocculation and then disinfected with heat or halogens. Filters will clog rapidly with silted or cloudy water.

When the water will be stored for a period of time, such as on a boat, motor home, or a home with rain water collection, halogens should be used to prevent the water from becoming contaminated. This can be supplemented before or after storage by filtration. Superchlorination-dechlorination is especially useful in this situation, because high levels of chlorination can be maintained for long periods, and when ready for use, the water can be poured into a smaller container and dechlorinated. If another means of chlorination is used, a minimum residual of 3 to 5 mg/L should be maintained in the water. Iodine will work for short but not for prolonged storage, since it is a poor algaecide.

On long-distance, ocean-going boats where water must be desalinated during the voyage, only reverse osmosis membrane filters are adequate.

REFERENCES

Backer HD: Field water disinfection. In Auerbach PS, editor: *Wilderness medicine: management of wilderness and environmental emergencies,* ed 4, St Louis, 2001, Mosby.

Backer HD: Effect of heat on the sterilization of artificially contaminated water (editorial), *J Travel Med* 3:1, 1996.

Backer HD: Water disinfection strategies for *Cryptosporidium, Wilderness Environmental Med* 8:75, 1997.

CDC: Surveillance for waterborne-disease outbreaks-United States, 1995-1996. *MMWR* 47(SS-50):1, 1998.

Fracker LD et al: *Giardia* cyst inactivation by iodine, *J Wilderness Med* 3:351, 1992.

Georgitos WJ, McDermott MT: An iodine load from water-purification tablets alters thyroid function in humans, *Mil Med* 158:794, 1993.

Hurst CJ, editor: *Modeling disease transmission and its prevention by disinfection,* Melbourne, 1996, Cambridge University Press.

Khan LK et al: Thyroid abnormalities related to iodine excess from water purification unites, Lancet 352:1519, 1998.

Laubusch EI: Chlorination and other disinfection processes. In *Water quality and treatment: a handbook of public water supplies, American Water Works Association,* New York, 1971, McGraw Hill.

Marchin GL, Fina LR: Contact and demand-release disinfectants, *Crit Rev Environ Control* 19:227, 1989.

McFeters GA, editor: *Drinking water microbiology,* New York, 1990, Springer-Verlag.

Marshall MM, Naumovits D, Ortega Y, Sterling CR: Waterborne protozoan pathogens, *Clin Microbiol Rev* 10:67, 1997.

Powers EM: Efficacy of flocculating and other emergency water purification tablets. Technical Report Natick/TR-93/033. United States Army Natick Research, Development and Engineering Center, Natick, MA, 1993.

CHAPTER 8

Disequilibrium: Jet Lag, Motion Sickness, and Heat Illness

Stephen A. Bezruchka

When travelers cross several time zones, go to hot climates, ascend to high altitudes, or are subject to novel motion stimuli, they may face problems of adaptation to new environmental situations. The state of disequilibrium may be uncomfortable and disabling. This chapter presents some common states of disequilibrium likely to be encountered by the traveler and suggests practical approaches to the problems.

JET LAG

When a large number of time zones are crossed quickly, the traveler's normal sleep-wake cycle is disrupted and is put into conflict with the body's underlying circadian physiologic rhythms. The traveler experiences disturbed sleep, loss of mental efficiency, and fatigue during the day—symptoms commonly known as "jet lag." Symptoms increase with the number of time zones crossed and generally begin when there is a 2-hour difference. The incidence of jet lag in travelers is almost universal, and symptoms can persist for a week or more. Circadian rhythms may take up to 2 weeks to adjust.

Specific complaints include insomnia, daytime sleepiness and fatigue, poor concentration, slowed reflexes, indigestion, hunger at odd hours, irritability, depression, a lack of resistance to infections, headache, myalgias, and dysphoria. Sleep disturbances persist longer than the other symptoms. Older people tend to have more difficulties. "Morning types," individuals who tend to go to bed earlier and awaken earlier in the day than "evening types," are more susceptible. Performance errors in pilots, reduced functioning among athletes, and decreased mental performance among diplomats are ascribed to jet lag.

Prevention and Treatment

Minimizing the effects of jet lag is best accomplished by a multifactorial approach. Few controlled studies have examined the various means of preventing jet lag, and none have compared different available modalities. Current approaches are reviewed in order of ease of use for travelers.

A nonvisual, photoreceptive, monosynaptic retinohypothalamic tract directly mediates the synchronization of the sleep-wake cycle with the light-dark cycle. Melatonin from the pineal gland may modulate this link as does the light-dark cycle. Melatonin is produced only during nighttime darkness in sighted individuals and is affected only by exposure to bright light. Resetting the circadian rhythm by timely ingestion of melatonin can reset the phase shift curve marking circadian phase position. An appropriately timed physiologic dose (0.5 mg) of exogenous melatonin can shift this phase response curve the required number of hours of time zone change. Taken in the morning, it delays circadian rhythm and advances it when taken later in the day. The actual dose required is quite low and less than the popularized panacea doses. Table 8-1 shows the timing of melatonin ingestion for eastward and westward travel beginning the day before departure and continuing for 3 days after arrival. This is time zone specific. Times for exposure to bright light are also given there, since light exposure is synergistic with melatonin. The dose suggested is the physiologic dose, but if this makes one drowsy before departure, the dose can be adjusted downward to that which does not cause unacceptable drowsiness and repeated every 2 hours to a total of 0.5 mg. Over-the-counter preparations available in the United States in health food stores are not standardized, nor can potencies be guaranteed. Liquid preparations allow titration of an appropriate dose for an individual. There are no data on long-term safety of exogenous melatonin ingestion, nor any reports of safety during pregnancy.

An alternative dosing schedule is to take melatonin at bedtime on arrival at the destination. Most trials have used large doses, 5 to 8 mg continued for 3 to 7 days after arrival. Commonly reported side effects on this regimen are drowsiness after ingestion.

Short-term pharmacologic manipulation of the sleep-wake cycle with hypnotic drugs to induce sleep is a convenient and acceptable way to manage jet lag in healthy travelers. There may not be much improvement in performance, and hypnotics do not appear to adjust circadian rhythms in humans. Zolpidem, an imidazopyridine with ω_1-benzodiazepine receptor activity, may be the best choice, as it appears to have no significant effect on next-day psychomotor performance. It may be used to treat early awakening, even while using melatonin. The short-acting benzodiazepines commonly used are triazolam, temazepam, and oxazepam. These are characterized by less daytime sedation than flurazepam (Table 8-2). The usual adult dose of hypnotics should be halved for first-time users and for geriatric patients, and travelers should be warned not to drink alcoholic beverages or to use other medications that cause drowsiness (e.g., antihistamines) concurrently. Short-term triazolam use is associated with retrograde amnesia, especially with alcohol intake. Reported dysphoric side effects (including paranoia, amnesia, suicidal ideations, and hyperexcitability) associated with chronic use of triazolam at daily doses of 0.5 mg have resulted in the United Kingdom banning it, whereas other countries such as France and Spain have limited available preparations to 0.125 mg. Triazolam is still approved for use in the United States.

Traditional advice has been to adjust the sleep schedule, beginning 3 days before departure, gradually moving bedtime closer to the customary time at the destination. For instance, if traveling eastward, a traveler would try to go to bed 1 hour earlier each succeeding night in the 3-day period before departure. If traveling westward, the traveler would try to stay up later 1 hour more each night in the pretravel period. Because it is easier to stay up later than to retire earlier, westward flights across a few meridians result in faster adaptation than eastward ones. Naps should be avoided on eastbound trips. It is useful to exercise before, during, and after the flight and to maintain good hydration.

Table 8-1
Jet Lag Treatment with Melatonin

TIME TO TAKE MELATONIN THE DAY BEFORE AND THE DAY OF DEPARTURE

Time zone change	1 to 6 hours	7 to 9 hours	10 or more hours
Travel from east to west	When you awake	When you awake	When you awake
Travel from west to east	About 3 PM	About 3 PM	When you awake

TIME TO TAKE MELATONIN ON ARRIVAL

Time zone change	1 to 6 hours	7 to 9 hours	10 or more hours
Travel from east	Day 1: when you awake	Day 1: when you awake	Day 1: when it is the same-time at departure that you took it yesterday
To west	Days 2 and 3: 1 to 2 hours later than the day before	Days 2 and 3: 1 to 2 hours later than the day before	Days 2 and 3: 1 to 2 hours later than the day before
Travel from west	Day 1: when it is the same time at departure that you took it yesterday	Day 1: when it is the same time at departure that you took it yesterday	Day 1: when it is the same time at departure that you took it yesterday
To east	Days 2 and 3: 1 to 2 hours earlier than the day before	Days 2 and 3: 1 to 2 hours earlier than the day before	Days 2 and 3: 1 to 2 hours earlier than day before

Melatonin dose is 0.5 mg (see text if this makes you sleepy)

TIME PERIODS TO BE IN AND TO AVOID BRIGHT LIGHT

Time zone change	1 to 6 hours	7 to 9 hours	10 or more hours
Travel from east to west	Get bright light later in the day	Get bright light in the middle of the day, avoid bright light later in the day	Get bright light in the morning, and avoid it the rest of the day
Travel from west to east	Get bright light in the morning	Get bright light in the middle of the day, avoid bright light later earlier in the day	Get bright light in the middle of the day, avoid bright light later in the day

Adapted from Bezruchka SA: *The pocket doctor,* Seattle, 1999, The Mountaineers.

Table 8-2
Short-Acting Hypnotics for Jet Lag

Drug*	Adult dose†	Elimination half-life
Zolpidem (Ambien)	5-10 mg PO hs	3-5 hr
Triazolam (Halcion)	0.25 mg PO hs	1.5-5.5 hr
Temazepam (Restoril)	30 mg PO hs	8-12 hr
Oxazepam (Serax)	10-15 mg PO hs	8-10 hr
Quazepam (Doral)	15 mg PO hs	39-73 hr
Flurazepam (Dalmane)	30 mg PO hs	47-100 hr

*Brand names of drugs are given for identification purposes only and do not constitute an endorsement.
†Use half the usual dose for elderly patients or first-time users.

If traveling across multiple time zones and returning after a day or two, it is better not to try to adjust to the proximate destination but to maintain the home sleep schedule. If traversing more than three time zones, scheduling a stopover of a day or more in the travel itinerary may help with readjustment of the sleep-wake cycle. Resetting the watch early on each flight to the new local time at destination is advisable for orientation. On arrival at the destination, activities should be scheduled that are appropriate for the new local time. For the first few days after arrival at a destination, major decisions should be avoided if possible, and important meetings should be scheduled at the individual's most alert time of the day at home. Vigorous physical exercise on arrival, midmorning for travel east, and late afternoon for going west helps.

The circadian clock can be shifted by exposure to bright light, although the utility of this in studies of jet lag has not been confirmed. The book *How to Beat Jet Lag* (see references) can be recommended to those wishing not to use melatonin for details on time-zone specific phototherapy regimen. Computer software is also available. To use principles of phototherapy to reset the circadian clock, the traveler should expose himself or herself to intense bright light (7000 to 12,000 lux, comparable to that of natural sunlight at sunrise). An exposure time of approximately 5 to 9 hours is needed. Light episodes before 4 AM (at the originating time zone) retard the circadian clock, whereas those after 4 AM (at the originating time zone) advance the clock. Thus travelers going eastward should expose themselves to bright light for a few hours early every morning after arrival at the destination. Those traveling westward should expose themselves to bright light in the late afternoon. Three to 4 days of such light exposure will entrain the original clock and allow it to be reset for sleeping at the destination time zone bedtime (Table 8-3).

The light level can be measured with an incident light meter used for photography, either the hand-held variety, or the meter built into a single lens reflex camera (SLR). For an ISO (ASA) 50 film, a meter reading of f:5.6 at 1/60 second indicates the brightness comparable to the required 11,000 lux. With an SLR, the film speed, aperture, and shutter speed should be set to these settings; if the meter indicates they are adequate to take a picture, the light is appropriately bright for phototherapy.

Table 8-3
Resetting the Circadian Clock with Bright Light

Direction of travel	External clock	Behavioral change	Circadian clock	Light exposure
West-to-East	Turn watch forward	Earlier bedtime; earlier awakening	Turn back circadian clock	Bright light in early morning at destination
East-to-West	Turn watch backwards	Later bedtime; later awakening	Advance circadian clock	Bright light in after-noon at destination

Wearing an eye shield on the plane, or sitting by an unshaded window at the appropriate times can contribute toward circadian clock resetting during the journey. On arrival, sunglasses should not be worn during the time exposure to bright light is necessary, and it is advisable to be outdoors when possible. When indoors, the window curtains should be open and bright room lights should be kept on during the period of phototherapy. Indoor light is much dimmer than required, but it can shift the circadian clock.

Often, travel schedules and conditions may prevent a traveler from using scheduled exposures to bright light to facilitate an adaptation to the new time zone.

Other remedies, such as the "jet-lag diet" or "anti-jet-lag" pills sold over the counter, are of questionable efficacy. The Argonne National Laboratory Jet Lag Diet tries to reset the circadian rhythm by alternative feasting and fasting beginning 3 days before departure and by timing the consumption of high-protein breakfasts and lunches, high-carbohydrate dinners, and caffeine.

MOTION SICKNESS

Motion sickness is not a true disease, but a normal response to a stimulating situation. It can be induced in anyone with a normally functioning vestibular system, given the right stimulation, but it cannot be produced by voluntary movement. People who lack vestibular function are immune.

Motion sickness as a generic term includes sea sickness, motor vehicle sickness, air sickness, and other disorders such as ski sickness, which represent a special form produced by unusual and contradictory sensory information between the visual, vestibular, and somatosensory system and is found performing winding turns on uneven ground, with insufficient visual control, especially on foggy or white-out days with reduced visibility.

One study collected data from 20,029 passengers on ferries on sea routes across the English Channel, Irish Sea, and North Sea and found that more than one third of passengers reported some symptoms of motion sickness. The incidence of illness was greater in females than males, and there was a slight decline in incidence with age. In all 21% of passengers felt "slightly unwell," 4% felt "quite ill," 4% felt "absolutely dreadful," and 7% vomited at some time. Those who traveled frequently reported

Table 8-4
Medication for Motion Sickness

Drug*	Adult dose	Side effects
Granisetron (Kytril)	2 mg PO single dose	
Odansetron (Zofran)	8 mg PO single dose	
Phenytoin (Dilantin)	200 mg PO single dose	
Cyclizine (Marezine)	50 mg PO q4-6h	Minimal sedation
Dimenhydrinate (Dramamine)	50 mg PO q4-6h	Sedation
Meclizine (Bonine, Antivert)	25-50 mg PO q6-12h	Mild sedation
Promethazine (Phenergan)	25 mg PO q8-12h	Moderate sedation
Scopolamine patch (Transderm Sc p)	1 patch applied to bare skin q72h	Dry mouth, blurry vision
Ephedrine sulfate	25 mg PO q6-12h	Cardiovascular (counteracts sedation)
Dextroamphetamine (Dexedrine)	5 mg PO qAM	Cardiovascular (counteracts sedation)

*Brand names of drugs are given for identification purposes only and do not constitute an endorsement.

less illness: this was presumed due to either habituation or self-selection. Women and people of Asian origin may be more susceptible. A past history is strongly predictive of future problems.

Nausea is a common presentation of motion sickness and may be preceded by pallor and cold sweats; eventually, vomiting occurs. Sufferers may express a desire for cool fresh air, although ambient air temperature is not found to influence susceptibility. Hypersalivation, yawning, hyperventilation, and frontal headache are reported. Drowsiness, lethargy, inhibition of gastric motility, and loss of performance proficiency are the secondary symptoms of motion sickness. Diminished gastric motility reduces the absorption of oral drugs.

Prevention

General advice includes resting before the anticipated motion and beginning with an empty stomach. Generally, high sodium foods, as well as those that are calorie dense or high in protein or fat including cheese and milk products, may be more associated with symptoms as is an increased frequency of eating. An ear plug in the nondominant side has been reported to help minimize symptoms. Seeking a place in the vehicle where motion is least, sitting in a semireclining position, and minimizing head motion, as well as looking at the horizon, help. Motion sickness may be a self-fulfilling prophecy in many, so cognitive behavioral counseling or enhancing self-efficacy with a "verbal placebo" may be useful.

Several medications are useful to alleviate the symptoms of motion sickness, especially if they are started prophylactically before the severe symptoms are manifest (Table 8-4). Antihistamines useful for motion sickness include cyclizine, dimenhydrinate, and meclizine. Cyclizine is thought to affect gastric dysrhythmias, dimenhydrinate may work as a sedative, and meclizine affects the vestibular system. Common side effects include sedation and a dry mouth. Other drugs used orally for motion sickness include promethazine (a phenothiazine derivative) and scopolamine (an anticholinergic). Drugs used to protect against radiation-induced nausea and vomiting, such as gansitron and odansetron, have found usefulness in motion sickness associated with flying jet planes and may be useful where psychomotor performance must be maintained.

Scopolamine, when given in the form of a transcutaneous drug patch, has been used but safer preparations are now available. The 0.5-mg patch is placed behind the ear, where skin permeability is highest, providing therapeutic levels of scopolamine for up to 3 days. The patch should be applied 8 hours before exposure to motion and must be worn for as long as the stimulus is present.

Initial enthusiasm for this drug has waned because side effects are common. These include dry mouth (50%), blurred vision (25%), and occasional anisocoria. Lower doses (cutting the patch into halves or quarters) may provide adequate protection and lessened side effects in some people, but this has not been studied. Drowsiness, impaired short-term memory, toxic psychosis (hallucinations, confusion, disorientation, confabulation), acute angle-closure glaucoma, or urinary retention may occur in susceptible people, especially the elderly. Side effects can become more severe after a long period of use. Anticholinergic intoxication can result after 16 or more days, especially if an allergic skin reaction develops where the adhesive patch is applied, thus allowing greater absorption of the drug. Withdrawal symptoms, including hypersalivation and increased gastrointestinal motility, are possible with prolonged use. Physiologic chemical dependency has been reported.

Sympathomimetics (catecholamine activators) can potentiate the prophylactic effects of scopolamine and antihistamines and tend to counteract the sedation caused by these drugs. Ephedrine and dextroamphetamine are effective and useful additions for prophylaxis of motion sickness when either scopolamine or an antihistamine does not work well enough (Table 8-4). Sympathomimetics should not be prescribed for patients with cardiovascular risk factors or disease because the drugs are associated with palpitations, tachycardia, and elevation of blood pressure. Patients also need to be warned about possible central nervous system (e.g., restlessness, dizziness, tremor) and gastrointestinal (e.g., anorexia, dry mouth, change in bowel habits) side effects.

Phenytoin and other anticonvulsants are being considered in the prevention of motion sickness. One study found that a therapeutic dose of phenytoin was four times more efficacious than any other single pharmacologic agent in delaying onset of artificially induced motion sickness; it was twice as effective as a scopolamine/dextroamphetamine combination. Confirmatory studies are needed. The dosage used was 15 mg/kg per day given in divided doses at 4-hour intervals over a 20-hour period before the experiment. A blood level of 9 μg/ml appears to be protective. This regimen could have useful clinical applications, as phenytoin in this study did not produce sedation or any decrease in performance.

Other drugs that have been proposed on the basis of anecdotal reports include nifedipine (calcium channel blocker) and selegiline (phenethylamine derivative). Ginger has been reported as a remedy for seasickness; however, experimental tests have yielded conflicting results, perhaps owing to variation in the type of preparation used and the experimental design.

Anecdotal reports support the use of acupressure with a commercial device (the Sea Band) to prevent motion sickness. Two studies have failed to show any beneficial response, but one group of investigators suggested that transcutaneous electrical nerve stimulation is worthy of study.

Symptoms of motion sickness may decrease with prolonged exposure to changing vestibular and optokinetic stimuli. Physical fitness is associated with an increased susceptibility to motion sickness in some individuals. Behavior modification techniques, including cognitive therapy, biofeedback, and desensitization therapy, require frequent exposure to motion over a considerable time to be effective.

Treatment

Controlled studies of different drugs to treat large patient populations experiencing the symptoms of motion sickness are lacking. Most of the reports use a variety of experimental situations to induce motion sickness in the subjects. Generally, intramuscular doses of prochlorperazine or trimethobenzamide are effective in treating the nausea and vomiting. Rectal suppositories of prochlorperazine or trimethobenzamide may be effective, but onset of action is slower because of unpredictable absorption through the rectal mucosa. In one study of motion sickness in weightless conditions simulating outer space, 50 mg of promethazine or 0.5 mg of intramuscular (IM) scopolamine were reported to be effective, but 25 mg of promethazine or 50 mg of dimenhydrinate were not.

For treatment of the secondary symptoms, IM ephedrine (25 mg) or dimenhydrinate (50 mg) are effective for dizziness, and IM metoclopramide (5 mg) aids in gastric emptying.

HEAT ILLNESS

The human body is only about 25% efficient, meaning most of our metabolic energy production is added to the body as heat. Despite being better able to tolerate heat than cold, humans continue to die in considerable numbers during heat waves around the world. In the adult, basal heat production is about 60 to 70 kcal/hr; excitement, fear, certain drugs, catecholamines, and thyroid hormones can increase heat production moderately, and physical work can produce up to 1000 kcal/hr of thermal energy.

To diffuse excess heat, skin vasodilates and blood shifts from the splanchnic circulation to the skin. Sweat forms, then skin cools as the sweat vaporizes, thus keeping a temperature gradient between heated blood and the skin, and promoting heat loss. If evaporation cannot occur because the air surrounding the skin is already saturated, sweat continues to form, but heat loss is curtailed. In these situations, extreme heat production (i.e., work) must be limited.

Children are more at risk of developing heat illness than adults because they are less efficient thermoregulators; they have a lower rate of sweating and a higher set point at which sweating starts. Children produce more metabolic heat per unit weight for a given work load and have a comparatively lower cardiac output than adults. Their larger surface area in proportion to body weight can result in greater heat absorption from the environment. Furthermore, they acclimatize more slowly than adults, and so need to reduce the intensity of activities in a hot environment for a longer period than adults.

Organizers of events in the heat have a responsibility to prevent heat illness. Plenty of hydration stations, with trained spotters for potential victims, must be provided. There must be a response system in place to deal with potential problems. Those with a fast finishing pace are especially at risk. It is appropriate to cancel events when there is a significant risk of serious heat illness from environmental factors such as when the wet bulb-globe thermometer index (WBGT) is above 25° C. There are numerous anecdotes of world-class athletes, as well as high school football players who have died as a result of heat illness.

Acclimatization

Acclimatization is the process whereby the body adapts to a hot environment. With repeated exposures to heat stress, for any given work load the cardiac output increases, there is expansion of circulating blood volume, and metabolic adaptations occur in skeletal muscle. Sweat production increases and to conserve blood volume, the sodium concentration in sweat decreases. As a result, there is less heat production for a given amount of work, but increased sweating increases the tendency to dehydration. Each liter of water lost through sweating raises rectal temperature 0.3° C, speeds heart rate 8 beats/min, and decreases cardiac output 1 L/min.

Acclimatization does not occur without work or exercise that elevates body temperature; the cardiovascular system must be capable of responding to these increased demands. A gradual increase in the time and intensity of physical exertion over 8 to 10 days is advised for those who will be active in the heat. It takes 2 weeks or more for maximal acclimatization.

Those in excellent physical condition are better able to tolerate the heat. The obese are at an increased risk of heat illness. Those with a febrile or gastrointestinal illness are at greater risk. The drugs described under heat stroke predispose to heat illness. Motor vehicle driver vigilance and other measures of performance are diminished under heat stress.

The best indication of the heat-acclimatized state is the capability to sweat profusely during heat stress. Prudent advice is to wear clothing that is lightweight and loose fitting, with only one layer of absorbent material. As much skin as possible should be exposed to facilitate sweat evaporation.

Water consumption should increase, since hypohydration is a major contributor to difficulty adapting to heat stress. Voluntary drinking replaces about two thirds of the body water lost as sweat. Individuals commonly dehydrate 2% to 6% of their body weight during hot-weather exercise even when fluids are available. Drinking on schedule makes better sense: a liter 2 hours before, a half liter 15 minutes before, and 250 ml every quarter hour during the practice or game. Weight and urine should be monitored; urine should be copious, clear, and pale. Sports drinks containing electrolytes and carbohydrates offer no advantage over cold water in maintaining plasma volume or electrolyte concentrations during exercise. Carbohydrate solutions may offer an advantage in endurance activities. Alcohol and caffeine dehydrate.

Environmental Heat Illness

Heat illness is a continuum from subtle impairment in performance to lethal heat stroke. Specific entities are described in this section.

Heat Syncope

Heat syncope includes orthostatic symptoms or fainting occurring in a person who has not undergone heat acclimatization and who is exposed to a high environmental temperature. It results because not enough salt and water have been retained and is more common in those with heart disease and those taking diuretics. The risk of heat syncope disappears as acclimatization occurs.

Heat Edema

Heat edema is seen during acclimatization and is caused by salt and water retention resulting from aldosterone production. It is seen more often in women; salt supplementation can be a precipitating factor. Heat edema vanishes as one is fully acclimatized.

Heat Tetany

Heat tetany results from hyperventilation on exposure to hot air, leading to respiratory alkalosis, paresthesias, and occasionally frank tetany.

Heat Cramps

Heat cramps are painful muscle contractions occurring in workers or athletes; they are associated with hyponatremia caused by fluid replacement of profuse sweat with free water, but not salt. Typically, the victims are acclimatized, exercising, and requiring copious sweat production to control temperature. The muscles involved are those being exercised, and symptoms tend to occur toward the end of the activity. Cramps last a few minutes and disappear spontaneously. A hot environment for the exercise is not mandatory. Salt replacement is important at the first sign of premonitory muscle twitching.

Heat Exhaustion

Heat exhaustion results from body water loss and electrolyte depletion. It is common during exercise and work in heat waves, but can occur as a result of heavy sweating while undergoing intense exercise in temperate climates. Typically postural hypotension develops immediately on termination of exercise in the heat by unacclimatized persons. Although there is a continuum, patients tend to fall into one of two categories: water depletion or salt depletion.

Early warning signs include a flushed face, hyperventilation, headache, dizziness, nausea, arm tingling, piloerection, paradoxical chilliness, incoordination, and confusion.

The water-depletion variety can occur in the very young or very old who experience dehydration but cannot act on their thirst to replenish their water losses. Soldiers, laborers in the desert, boiler-room workers, and athletes who ingest salt without adequate water are also commonly afflicted. Symptoms include thirst, fatigue, dysphoria, and impaired judgment. Examination shows dehydration and an elevated body temperature. Left untreated, heat stroke can result as the body temperature rises.

The salt-depletion variety is seen in those who replace fluid losses with water without salt; they do not experience thirst as a predominant symptom. Unlike heat cramps, salt depletion heat exhaustion tends to occur in unacclimatized individuals who exhibit systemic symptoms. Symptoms can include myalgias, nausea, vomiting, and diarrhea, as well as weakness, fatigue, and headache. Hypotension and tachycardia are seen; the body temperature is not elevated unless dehydration results from the vomiting. Replacement of sodium chloride results in rapid improvement.

Confusion is an early sign of heat injury. Delirium has been reported. Commonly, individuals with heat exhaustion suffer from both water and salt depletion; they exhibit a variety of symptoms and are often misdiagnosed as having a viral syndrome. Giving aspirin to exercising patients who develop heat exhaustion can paradoxically increase body temperature.

Treatment

When treating heat exhaustion, if hypernatremia and scant concentrated urine are present, one should assume water deficiency, calculate the water deficit, and treat. Water should be given orally if the patient is conscious and not vomiting. If shock is present, the patient should first be treated with plasma-expanding fluids; otherwise, replace volume with 5% dextrose intravenously (IV) until the serum sodium has fallen to near normal, and then add hypotonic saline to the infusion. Half the water deficit should be replaced over 3 to 6 hours. In children, give half normal saline initially until urine output is established, then decrease to quarter normal saline along with 5% dextrose. Hydration and electrolyte balance should be corrected to normal over at least 48 hours in children to avoid seizures. Severe prolonged central nervous system (CNS) symptoms may take days to resolve. Those presenting with primary salt depletion respond quickly to salty oral fluids or normal IV saline if they cannot drink.

Heat Stroke

Heat stroke results from a failure of the thermoregulatory mechanisms to meet heat stress; extreme elevations of body temperature occur, as well as end-organ damage and dysfunction. Risk factors in healthy individuals include environmental extremes (e.g., pilgrimages in Saudi Arabia, where up to 1000 cases per day may occur), salt and water depletion, infection, fever after immunization, lack of acclimatization, obesity, fatigue, and consumption of drugs that suppress sweating (e.g., anticholinergics, antiparkinsonians, phenothiazines, and antihistamines). Other drugs known to cause heat stroke include diuretics, which cause salt and water depletion; tricyclics, which increase heat production; butyrophenones, which disturb hypothalamic regulation of temperature and the ability to recognize thirst; and sympathomimetics, which increase psychomotor activity.

Diseases that are risk factors for the development of heat stroke include those compromising cardiovascular function, diabetes mellitus, hyperthyroidism, potassium deficiency, and alcoholism. Even a single bout of drinking alcoholic beverages results in some loss of acclimatization. Other conditions that result in impaired sweat production are also associated with heat stroke and include prickly heat (miliaria), healed extensive thermal burns, scleroderma, and congestive heart failure.

Prevention

Heat stroke can be prevented by encouraging the elderly and mentally ill to drink enough fluids, adjusting dosages of drugs affecting fluid balance and thermoregulation, and limiting activity in heat extremes. Those engaged in strenuous activity during hot weather need to drink more frequently and copiously than thirst dictates. Splashing in water is beneficial. Consuming 400 to 500 ml of water before exertion, and then a cup or more (300 ml) of water for every 20 minutes of exercise in the heat should be encouraged. Salt tablet consumption is not routinely recommended; the average American diet contains enough salt.

If someone feels ill or “overstressed” during exercise, he or she should stop and seek a cool area. This is especially important for driven individuals in peer group situations. After a febrile illness, individuals should be especially cautious of further heat exposure.

Clinical Features

Classic Heat Stroke

Classic heat stroke occurs in sedentary individuals exposed to several days of environmental heat stress in whom thermoregulatory mechanisms stop functioning. Heat waves in inner cities result in many casualties. It can occur at lower temperatures if the relative humidity is high. The skin is hot, dry, and flushed. Hyperthermia is invariably present, with a body temperature above 40.6° C (105° F), and some CNS disturbance must be present. Confusion may be the earliest sign, with an inability of victims to recognize their own illness. Eventually, coma may ensue. A respiratory alkalosis is usually present. Preexisting organic disease increases mortality.

Exertional Heat Stroke

Exertional heat stroke is found in males performing heavy muscular exercise on warm humid days. In the United States, it is seen in competitive long-distance runners, football players (>75 fatalities per year in the United States among amateurs), and military recruits. Victims are volume depleted and exhibit neurologic symptoms such as strange behavior, confusion, or even coma. Relative bradycardia may be seen in highly conditioned athletes with this disorder. Sweating persists in more than half the cases. These individuals present with a relatively cool, clammy skin, but with an extremely elevated core temperature (up to 44.5° C). However, by the time the individual is seen, his temperature may have dropped to the more typical febrile range, but with all the other complications present as a result of widespread organ damage: rhabdomyolysis, disseminated intravascular coagulation, lactic acidosis, hyperuricemia, and hypokalemia. A moderate to severe metabolic acidosis is seen. Few cases are seen in women. Patients who recover from heat stroke patients are more susceptible to recurrent attacks.

Differential Diagnosis of Heat Stroke in Travelers

Infections, including cerebral falciparum malaria, can occur in environments similar to those where heat stroke occurs. Encephalitis, meningitis, and typhoid fever can present with a picture similar to heat stroke. Shaking chills suggest that fever is due to an infectious etiology.

Drug-induced heat illness, especially anticholinergic poisoning, may be difficult to diagnose. Sweating suggests that anticholinergic poisoning is not present. Over half of heat stroke patients have constricted, pinpoint pupils, which also militate against anticholinergic poisoning.

Treatment

Treatment of heat stroke is a medical emergency, and delay in cooling is the single most important factor leading to death. Begin cooling at the site of collapse by disrobing, fanning, and bathing the skin with cool water. Monitor rectal temperature every 5 to 10 minutes during resuscitation. The duration of hyperthermia is the most important factor affecting survival. Reasons for delay include failure to make the diagnosis and lack of facilities to rapidly cool. Mortality is still high, at close to 10%.

Cool the Patient

The victim should be removed from the hot environment, and cooling techniques improvised depending on what is available. The classic treatment is to immerse the patient in a tub of ice water and massage the skin briskly. Although cold-induced vasoconstriction can theoretically impair heat loss, this method has been used successfully. No other technique yet proposed claims better results. Tepid or tap water may be as good as ice water for cooling and may be more comfortable. Alternatively, the patient can be wetted down with water and rubbed briskly with ice bags, keeping a large fan blowing on the patient, which may be better tolerated than ice water immersion in confused individuals. A helicopter rotor, if available, may be the best fan, used for 18 to 50 minutes. If the ice supply is limited, it should be applied to the head, neck, abdomen, axillae, and groin. Special beds (Physiological Body Cooling Unit, and the King Saud University Cooling Bed) have been constructed to allow the spraying of pressurized water at 15° C on the nude body; they were designed for use in countries where heat stroke occurs to many on pilgrimage. In evacuation, consider an open vehicle and mist sprays.

Support the Vital Signs

A heat stroke patient should be transported to a medical facility with IV rapid correction of fluid and electrolyte abnormalities; hypoglycemia, if present, should be treated. IV diazepam should be given for seizures, severe cramping, or shivering, which impair cooling. If feasible, central venous monitoring is advised to guide fluid therapy and to avoid fluid overload. If the victim is comatose, endotracheal intubation is recommended.

REFERENCES

Jet Lag

Arendt J, Deacon S: Treatment of circadian rhythm disorders-melatonin, *Chronobiol Int* 14(2):185, 1997.

Arendt J et al: Efficacy of melatonin treatment in jet lag, shift work, and blindness, *J Biol Rhythms* 12(6):604, 1997.

Avery D, Lenz M, Landis C: Guidelines for prescribing melatonin, *Ann Med* 30(1):122, 1998.

Comperatore CA et al: Melatonin efficacy in aviation missions requiring rapid deployment and night operations, *Aviat Space Environ Med* 67(6):520, 1996.

Criglington AJ, Comm B: Do professionals get jet lag? A commentary on jet lag [letter], *Aviat Space Environ Med* 69(8):810, 1998.

Houpt TA, Boulos Z, Moore-Ede MC: Midnight sun—software for determining light exposure and phase-shifting schedules during global travel, *Physiol Behav* 59:561, 1996.

Lewy AJ, Ahmed S, Sack RL: Phase shifting the human circadian clock using melatonin, *Behav Brain Res* 73(1-2):131, 1996.

Lewy AJ et al: Melatonin marks circadian phase position and resets the endogenous circadian pacemaker in humans, *Ciba Found Symp* 183:303, 1995.

Lowden A, Akerstedt T: Retaining home-base sleep hours to prevent jet lag in connection with a westward flight across nine time zones, *Chronobiol Int* 15(4):365, 1998.

Manfredini R, Manfredini F, Fersini C, Conconi F: Circadian rhythms, athletic performance, and jet lag, *Br J Sports Med* 32(2):101, 1998.

Oren DA, Reich W, Rosenthal NE, Wehr TA: *How to beat jet lag: a practical guide for air travelers,* New York, 1993, Henry Holt.

Roth T, Roehrs T, Vogel G: Zolpidem in the treatment of transient insomnia: a double-blind, randomized comparison with placebo, *Sleep* 18(4):246, 1995.

Shiota M, Sudou M, Ohshima M: Using outdoor exercise to decrease jet lag in airline crewmembers, *Aviat Space Environ Med* 67(12):1155, 1996.

Waterhouse J, Reilly T, Atkinson G: Jet-lag, *Lancet* 350(9091):1611, 1997.

Motion Sickness

Benline TA, French J, Poole E: Anti-emetic drug effects on pilot performance: granisetron vs. ondansetron, *Aviat Space Environ Med* 68(11):998, 1997.

Bruce DG et al: Acupressure and motion sickness, *Aviat Space Environ Med* 61:361, 1990.

Chelen W et al: Use of phenytoin in the prevention of motion sickness, *Aviat Space Environ Med* 61:1022, 1990.

Cheung BS, Money KE, Jacobs I: Motion sickness susceptibility and aerobic fitness: a longitudinal study, *Aviat Space Environ Med* 61:201, 1990.

Eden D, Zuk Y: Seasickness as a self-fulfilling prophecy: raising self-efficacy to boost performance at sea, *J Appl Psychol* 80(5):628, 1995.

Hausler R: Ski sickness, *Acta Otolaryngol Stockh* 115(1):1, 1995.

Jozsvai EE, Pigeau RA: The effect of autogenic training and biofeedback on motion sickness tolerance, *Aviat Space Environ Med* 67(10):963, 1996.

Knox GW et al: Phenytoin for motion sickness: clinical evaluation, *Laryngoscope* 104(8Pt1):935, 1994.

Lawther A, Griffin MJ: A survey of the occurrence of motion sickness amongst passengers at sea, *Aviat Space Environ Med* 59:399, 1988.

Lindseth G, Lindseth PD: The relationship of diet to airsickness, *Aviat Space Environ Med* 66(6):537, 1995.

Pingree BJ, Pethybridge RJ: A comparison of the efficacy of cinnarizine with scopolamine in the treatment of seasickness [see comments], *Aviat Space Environ Med* 65(7):597, 1994.

Stern RM, Uijtdehaage SH, Muth ER, Koch KL: Effects of phenytoin on vection-induced motion sickness and gastric myoelectric activity, *Aviat Space Environ Med* 65(6):518, 1994.

Stern RM et al: Asian hypersusceptibility to motion sickness, *Hum Hered* 46(1):7, 1996.

Weinstein SE, Stern RM: Comparison of Marezine and Dramamine in preventing symptoms of motion sickness, *Aviat Space Environ Med* 68(10):890, 1997.

Wood CD et al: Therapeutic effects of antimotion sickness medications on the secondary symptoms of motion sickness, *Aviat Space Environ Med* 61:157, 1990.

Heat Illness

Chung NK, Pin CH: Obesity and the occurrence of heat disorders, *Mil Med* 161(12):739, 1996.

Davis LL: Environmental heat-related illnesses, *Medsurg Nurs* 6(3):153, 1997.

Eichner ER: Treatment of suspected heat illness, *Int J Sports Med* 2:S150, 1998.

Knochel JP: Heat stroke and related heat stress disorders, *Dis Mon* 35:301, 1989.

Poulton TJ, Walker RA: Helicopter cooling of heatstroke victims, *Aviat Space Environ Med* 58:358, 1987.

Simon HB: Hyperthermia, *N Engl J Med* 329:483, 1993.

Wyon DP, Wyon I, Norin F: Effects of moderate heat stress on driver vigilance in a moving vehicle, *Ergonomics* 39(1):61, 1996.

Yaqub B, Al DS: Heat strokes: aetiopathogenesis, neurological characteristics, treatment and outcome, *J Neurol Sci* 156(2):144, 1998.

SECTION II

ADVICE FOR SPECIAL TRAVELERS

CHAPTER 9

Altitude Illness

Stephen A. Bezruchka

Altitude illness may occur even at moderate altitudes and may result in major disruption of travel plans. Self-diagnosis and treatment are the norm in many remote locations. When people with preexisting health problems desire to visit high-altitude destinations, it is reasonable to support them in undertaking such trips, provided they are strongly motivated and recognize the difficulties of coping with illness in remote locations.

ACCLIMATIZATION

Acclimatization is a complex acute and chronic process, wherein the body adapts to hypoxia by optimizing oxygen delivery to cells.

Hyperventilation

Hyperventilation is initiated by the stimulation of the carotid body in response to hypoxemia; it is the first and most important adaptation to hypoxia. Hyperventilation elevates alveolar Po_2 and produces a hypocapnic alkalosis; this limits further increases in ventilation until renal compensation by bicarbonate excretion lowers the pH closer to normal after a period of days to weeks. Hyperventilation is sustained throughout the stay at altitude. Nocturnal periodic breathing is almost universal in newcomers to altitude above 10,000 to 12,000 ft (3050 to 3650 m) and is common as low as 8000 ft (2450 m); it produces frequent awakenings, and a decrease in quality of sleep. The marked oxygen desaturation caused by periodic breathing during sleep improves with acclimatization.

Tachycardia

Tachycardia secondary to increased catecholamines is the initial circulatory response to hypoxemia. With acclimatization, the resting pulse drops. Studies looking at the coronary stress of exercise at high altitude in healthy older men show no increase over comparable exercise at lower altitudes.

Pulmonary Hypertension

Hypoxia produces pulmonary hypertension; this is thought to improve the ventilation-perfusion mismatch present at altitude. Cold and exercise act synergistically with altitude in producing pulmonary hypertension.

Cerebral Blood Flow

Hypoxia increases cerebral blood flow through vasodilation, while hypocapnia decreases it. However, the vasodilatory effect of hypoxia at high altitude overrides the effect of hypocapnia. Those who do not have a brisk hyperventilatory response to altitude may have greater vasodilation and vasogenic edema, which are often associated with headache. On the other hand, insufficient vasodilation may contribute to cerebral ischemia and ensuing complications.

Circulating Blood Volume

The hematocrit and hemoglobin rise in response to hypoxia. Initially, this is due to plasma volume contraction from diuresis; those who diurese acutely at altitude, resulting in a 2% loss in body weight, have less altitude illness. Later, erythropoietin-induced erythrocytosis occurs. Increased hemoglobin improves oxygen-carrying capacity, but if the hematocrit exceeds 60%, blood viscosity also increases.

ALTITUDE ILLNESS SYNDROMES

Problems with adaptation to altitude are multifactorial and include aberrant ventilatory control and leakage of fluid from the vascular to the extravascular space. Although individual syndromes are described next, they all may be facets of an as yet incompletely understood common pathophysiologic process.

Acute Mountain Sickness

Acute mountain sickness (AMS) occurs a few hours to days after exposure to altitude. Severe enough to limit normal activities, it is found in 15% to 30% of Colorado resort skiers, 50% of climbers on Denali (Mount McKinley), 70% of climbers on Mount Rainier, and in 25% to 50% of trekkers to the base of Mount Everest. It also occurs in those coming to intermediate altitudes (6500 ft) and prompts many to self-medicate. It is more common among those who ascend quickly, who are younger, and who have a past history of AMS. Being female does not confer an advantage. AMS is more likely in those who retain fluid at altitude and who hypoventilate (fail to hyperventilate) relative to hypoxic stress. Those who diurese are less likely to suffer. Those going to altitude with an acute infectious process such as an upper respiratory infection, diarrhea, or cough may be at greater risk of AMS and other forms of altitude illness.

Mild AMS is characterized by headache, anorexia, insomnia, nausea, and malaise. In moderate forms, there is vomiting, unrelieved headache, and decreased urine output. Features of severe AMS are ataxia (perhaps the most sensitive early sign, it may represent early high-altitude cerebral edema), altered consciousness, localized rales, and cyanosis. Peripheral edema of the hands, face, and ankles is common at altitude, especially in females, but it may be a feature of AMS. Mild AMS improves over a few days if the hypobaric stress is not aggravated by ascending. Severe AMS will usually progress unless treated aggressively.

High-Altitude Pulmonary Edema

High-altitude pulmonary edema (HAPE), a noncardiogenic pulmonary edema, occurs in 5% to 10% of those who experience AMS, but can occur without previous symptoms; 1% to 2% of those traveling above 12,000 ft (3650 m) are affected, and males predominate. It can occur at ski resorts situated at moderate altitudes. There is a high mortality rate. HAPE often occurs on the second night after ascent to altitude. Relative hypoxemia and a low hypoxic ventilatory response are present. Extremely high pulmonary artery pressures are seen in HAPE victims when compared to unaffected control subjects at altitude. There is marked ventilation-perfusion mismatch, with opening of the usually tight capillary endothelial junctions, so patchy edema is typically seen on chest x-ray. The edema fluid is very protein rich, as in adult respiratory distress syndrome. The defect that allows capillary leakage is transient, rather than due to permanent lung injury, as people who recover have gone back up to altitude on the same trip without recurrence.

Features of *early* HAPE include decreased exercise performance (earliest symptom), dry cough, fatigue, tachycardia (above resting levels for that person at altitude), rales in the right middle lobe, and tachypnea. Later there may be cyanosis, extreme weakness, productive cough, generalized rales, and dyspnea at rest. Mental obtundation, irrational behavior, and coma can be present. Atypical presentations include ataxia only, bronchospasm, or sudden death; underlying respiratory infection may possibly play a role in each of these. Fever less than 38.3° C (101° F) may be present, but by itself is not a helpful sign. Subclinical HAPE, manifested only as rales and/or as an abnormal chest radiograph, is probably common at altitude.

Risk factors for HAPE include rapid ascent, strenuous exertion on arrival, obesity, male sex, previous history of HAPE (66% recurrence rate in one study), and congenital absence of the right pulmonary artery or the proximal interruption of either pulmonary artery. Children with an concurrent inflammatory illness may be more susceptible. Individuals who have lived at high altitude can develop HAPE on reascent after going to low altitude.

High-Altitude Cerebral Edema

High-altitude cerebral edema (HACE) appears to be an end stage of AMS. It usually presents several days after the onset of mild AMS, but death has occurred within 24 hours. HACE is rare below 10,000 ft (3050 m). Vasogenic edema from a leaky blood-brain barrier may be the mechanism. Rapid ascent to significant altitudes strongly predisposes one to develop HACE. It may be more common in those who have had a significant head injury.

Clinical presentation includes impaired judgment, the inability to make decisions, irrational behavior, hallucinations, nausea and vomiting, severe headache, lassitude, truncal ataxia, and progression to coma. HAPE often can accompany HACE and vice versa. Hemiparesis and other focal neurologic signs have been reported, but these may be due to thrombosis.

High-Altitude Retinopathy

High-altitude retinopathy (HAR) is usually seen in those sleeping above 15,000 ft (4570 m). The most common presentation is asymptomatic retinal hemorrhages; these resolve spontaneously after a week or two. There may also be dilation of retinal veins, cotton-wool exudates, and disk hyperemia. Vision is affected only if one of the maculae is involved.

DIAGNOSIS OF ALTITUDE ILLNESS

Diagnosis of altitude illness in the clinical setting may be difficult if the diagnostician's judgment is also impaired by hypoxia. In addition, diagnostic tools are often not available. Goal-driven adventurers, pressured by peers and on a tight schedule, have a tendency to ascribe symptoms to causes other than altitude. Consider altitude illness in the differential diagnosis of any condition presenting at altitude.

Table 9-1
Recognition of Significant Altitude Illness

Travelers should suspect significant altitude illness in *themselves* if they have:
- A headache and feel "hung over"
- Dyspnea and a respiratory rate above 20/min at rest
- Anorexia
- Vomiting
- Ataxia
- Unusual fatigue while walking

Travelers should suspect significant altitude illness in their *companions* who are:
- Skipping meals
- Exhibiting antisocial behavior
- Stumbling
- Having the most difficulty with the activity
- Arriving last at daily destination and are the most fatigued

Table 9-1 presents signs and symptoms for recognition of significant altitude illness. Travelers going to altitude can be taught to test for ataxia by asking suspected victims of altitude illness to perform tandem walking; unaffected travelers can serve as control subjects. Walking on a narrow piece of wood close to the ground is another useful test.

The differential diagnosis of altitude illness is broad and includes dehydration, substance abuse, hypothermia, carbon monoxide poisoning (from a stove used in an enclosed tent), infection, exhaustion, and an exacerbation of a preexisting condition. Although it should be easy to exclude such conditions, mistakes are commonly made in the field.

Observing the victim's response to oxygen or to descent may help clarify the diagnosis in questionable circumstances. Groups carrying a portable hyperbaric chamber may place the victim in the bag, pressurize it for an hour, and note the response. There may be a slight placebo response to the bag, or sometimes the victim may have a claustrophobic panic reaction, but clinical judgment should clarify the situation. Sources for the currently available models are the following: Chinook Medical Gear, 3455 Main Ave, Durango, CO 81301, (800)766-1365, (970)375-1241, Fax (970)375-6343, chinook@frontier.net, http://www.chinookmed.com for the Gamow Bag; Certec, le bourge, Sourcieux le Mines, 69210 L'Arbresle, France, 33-74-70-3982, Fax 33-74-70-3766; C. E. Bartlett Pty Ltd, Ring Road, Wendouree, Victoria 3355, Australia, (61)3 5339 3103, Fax (61) 3 5338 1241, info@bartlett.net.au, http://www.bartlett.net.au for the PAC (Portable Altitude Chamber), currently the cheapest version and the easiest to get patients in and out of.

PREVENTION OF ALTITUDE ILLNESS

The keys to prevention of altitude illness are to recognize those at risk and to ensure that ascents are made slowly. Groups traveling on tight schedules, with little flexibility to wait for members to acclimatize, may generate peer pressure to climb fast. Goal-driven adventure travelers in groups may be more prone to denial; they appear to have a high incidence of problems with altitude, although confirmatory studies are lacking. Individual travelers going independently on a modest budget may be less

Table 9-2
Tips for Prevention of High Altitude Illness

1. *A slow ascent* to high altitude is most important. Because each person adapts differently to every exposure to altitude, rather than give a formula for how slow is slow enough, travelers should monitor each other for signs of high-altitude illness (see Table 9-1) no matter what the ascent rate.
2. *Climb high, but sleep low.* The sleeping altitude should rise gradually. A conservative rate of ascent is prudent, taking 2 days or more to get a sleeping altitude of 10,000 ft (3050 m). Thereafter, avoid raising the sleeping altitude more than 1000 ft (300 m) a day.
3. *Never take a headache higher to sleep.* If someone in the party develops a headache, he or she should not ascend higher to sleep, although he or she could undertake a short ascent and then descent to sleep. Be especially concerned and vigilant if a headache comes on during the day's ascent and gets worse.
4. *Failing the tandem walk test.* Anyone who fails the tandem walk test compared to controls must descend immediately to below the altitude at which symptoms first began.
5. *Carry drugs for high-altitude illness* (see Table 9-3).
6. *Avoid sedatives, tranquilizers, and narcotic analgesics.* These drugs result in hypoventilation and greater oxygen desaturation during sleep. They should be avoided at altitudes above 8000 ft (2450 m).
7. *Monitor food and water intake.* Drinking plenty of fluids is routinely recommended. The diet should be palatable and low in salt.
8. *Monitor physical activity.* Avoid strenuous overexertion for the first few days at altitude. Conscious effort to increase the depth and frequency of breathing at altitude is beneficial.
9. *Wear appropriate clothing.* Hypothermia is synergistic with the deleterious effects of altitude. Adequate clothing is necessary; the temperature drops 3.5°F for every 1000 ft (0.65° C for 100 m) of ascent.
10. *Avoid external transport to higher altitude.* When an individual is having physical problems continuing on his/her own, mechanized or animal transport to a higher altitude may lead to worsening high-altitude illness.

likely to suffer serious altitude illness. Rapid ascent, especially by flying or driving to altitude, is risky.

Physicians can advise individuals going on a commercial tour to high destinations to inquire about the availability of oxygen or a hyperbaric bag, the flexibility of the itinerary, and the availability of rescue. Are the leaders knowledgeable about altitude illness and equipped to treat it? What contingency plans are available if someone becomes severely ill? Table 9-2 describes common symptoms and signs of altitude illness. This information, outlined in more detail in the reference *Altitude Illness: Prevention and Treatment,* should be understood by all visitors to altitude.

Use of Drugs to Prevent High-Altitude Illness

Acetazolamide

This drug decreases susceptibility to AMS and reduces symptoms by speeding acclimatization. It does this by inhibiting carbonic anhydrase in the kidney and lung, thus promoting the excretion of bicarbonate and causing a slight metabolic acidosis. Acetazolamide increases minute ventilation and oxygen saturation, and decreases periodic breathing at night.

Acetazolamide should be considered for those driving or flying to altitudes of 10,000 ft (3050 m) or more, but may also be beneficial for those making slower ascents, especially those who tend to develop altitude illness. It is recommended for those who have had significant symptoms in the past, for rescue groups who must ascend quickly, and for climbers when the sleeping altitude has to be raised abruptly.

Everyone going to altitude should carry acetazolamide to treat symptoms if they occur. The dose is 125 mg twice a day, or once at bedtime. Acetazolamide can be taken on the day of ascent and continued for 2 days on arrival at altitude. It is a sulfa drug and is contraindicated in sulfa-allergic individuals. Common side effects include polyuria and paresthesias; nausea, myopia, and impotence are also seen, but less commonly. Acetazolamide may affect the taste of carbonated beverages because it decreases the hydration of carbon dioxide on the tongue. It is the only drug approved by the Food and Drug Administration (FDA) for prevention of AMS.

Dexamethasone

Dexamethasone is also effective as a prophylactic for AMS, but is not routinely recommended for several reasons. It can cause hyperglycemia, although this will probably be rare in the physically fit climbing to high altitudes. On expeditions, the euphoria induced by steroids may cloud judgment and result in denial of risks and poor decision making. Significant dysphoria may also occur on stopping the drug. There is also the possibility of rebound altitude illness when dexamethasone is discontinued. It does not facilitate acclimatization, and its mechanism is probably that of decreasing fluid leak from the microvasculature. Travelers can be advised to carry it for use in treating symptoms of cerebral edema, but it is not routinely recommended for prophylaxis.

People who need to ascend rapidly for rescue purposes may take dexamethasone in addition to acetazolamide. The standard regimen for dexamethasone is 4 mg by mouth every 6 hours, but dosing twice a day may be adequate. Dexamethasone may be of benefit to those with a history of AMS who must ascend to high altitude again, or who have an allergy or intolerance to acetazolamide. Once started, dexamethasone should not be stopped at altitude until there has been a considerable descent. Tapering of the drug may be necessary after taking it for 3 days or more, certainly if taken for more than 7 days.

Nifedipine

Nifedipine, which decreases pulmonary artery pressures, appears to be an effective prophylactic for those who are susceptible to HAPE, but it is not FDA-approved for this purpose. The prophylactic dose is 30 mg (long-acting preparation) two to three times a day. The drugs used in high-altitude illness are summarized in Table 9-3.

TREATMENT OF HIGH-ALTITUDE ILLNESS

Acute Mountain Sickness

Mild forms of AMS can be treated by staying a day or two at the altitude at which symptoms occur, then ascending cautiously. Modest exercise during the day can be encouraged. Symptomatic treatment includes mild non-narcotic analgesics for headache, and prochlorperazine for nausea and vomiting. Acetazolamide, 125 or 250 mg two or three times a day, may be started; it is especially useful for treating sleep disturbance if taken at bedtime.

Table 9-3
Drugs Used in Altitude Illness

Drug	Dose	Indications
Acetazolamide (Sulfonamide)	125 mg PO bid or 250 mg PO qhs	Prophylaxis for acute mountain sickness; treatment of mild symptoms
Dexamethasone	4 mg PO q6h	Prophylaxis for acute mountain sickness, especially for rescuers who fly into high altitudes and begin working immediately
	4-8 mg PO q6h	Treatment of high-altitude cerebral edema
Nifedipine	20 mg PO tid or 30 mg long-acting preparation PO bid-tid	Prevention of recurrent high-altitude pulmonary edema
	10 mg sublingual dose, followed by 20 mg PO tid	Treatment of high-altitude pulmonary edema (monitor blood pressure after sublingual dose)

Severe AMS calls for immediate descent, oxygen, and drug therapy. Dexamethasone at a dose of 4 mg by mouth every 6 hours may be given for severe AMS while descent is underway. Descent is a critical part of treatment: symptoms of AMS can recur with discontinuation of this drug, and progression to HAPE has occurred even after dexamethasone has been given for treatment of AMS without descent. Descent to below the altitude at which any symptoms of altitude illness first occurred may be necessary. For mild symptoms of AMS, 1 or 2 hours of simulated descent in a portable hyperbaric bag may be as effective as oxygen therapy and may, on occasion, preclude the need for actual descent. Longer periods in a portable hyperbaric bag are necessary for serious illness, and descent should be arranged. Barotitis is sometimes seen as a complication of hyperbaric therapy.

High-Altitude Pulmonary Edema

Treatment of HAPE relies on early recognition and must be expeditious to avoid death—HAPE is a medical emergency. The victim should be kept warm, given oxygen, and taken down from altitude. It is easier to descend with an ambulatory climber than with a moribund victim. A descent of 1500 to 3000 ft (500 to 1000 m) is often adequate. Strenuous exertion, however, can worsen HAPE. Descent to below the altitude at which any symptoms of altitude illness first occurred may be necessary.

The hyperbaric bag can be lifesaving. One study suggests 4 hours of stay in the pressurized chamber is beneficial for patients with HAPE.

Pulmonary vasodilators may have a useful role in improving gas exchange and the symptoms of HAPE. The greatest experience is with nifedipine, 10 mg sublingually given acutely, and 20 mg continued every 8 hours. Postural signs and symptoms in response to drug therapy must be observed if a sphygmomanometer is not available to monitor blood pressures. This is not an FDA-approved indication for nifedipine, but high-altitude travelers may wish to carry the drug for use in an emergency situation.

In serious cases of HAPE, dexamethasone is recommended when central nervous system (CNS) symptoms are present. Acetazolamide may be useful early in the course of HAPE, but it does not appear to be useful in severe cases. Diuretics and morphine were used for treatment of HAPE by early investigators, but are not currently used because the other treatments are thought to be more effective. Intravenous loop diuretics can result in hypotension and shock.

Supplemental oxygen by a continuous positive airway pressure (CPAP), positive end-expiratory pressure, or expiratory positive airway pressure delivery systems have been advocated as a temporizing measure to alleviate symptoms and increase oxygenation. These oxygen delivery systems are usually unavailable in the field situation, but a lightweight, portable CPAP mask is made (Downs CPAP Mask, Vital Signs Inc, Totowa, NJ). The CPAP mask with a 10-cm pressure valve has been successfully used in the treatment of HAPE, but pneumothorax and increased pulmonary edema can result.

Inhaled nitric oxide has been shown to improve oxygenation in those with HAPE, but its use alfresco remains untested. In a setting where it could be given, oxygen, with which there is much more experience, can as well.

With the nondescent treatment modalities available today for HAPE, there is a tendency to delay descent or cancel evacuation plans when some improvement occurs in response to initial therapy. HAPE has recurred fatally in such situations. *Descent* remains the mainstay of treatment, and should be undertaken along with hyperbaric oxygen and drug therapies.

After resolution of HAPE, some victims have reascended gradually without recurrence on that trip. Reascent should be undertaken carefully, with responsible supervision. Slow-release nifedipine, 30 mg by mouth two to three times a day, can be given prophylactically.

High-Altitude Cerebral Edema

Key principles in therapy include descent, oxygen, and dexamethasone 4 to 8 mg every 6 hours. Response to treatment may be slow. The hyperbaric bag has been used successfully, with 6 hours or more being necessary for treatment. A combination of modalities is appropriate for serious cases. Individuals who have been successfully treated for cerebral symptoms later ascended and died from a recurrence when they were no longer with the bag. Mannitol is presumed to be effective, as is endotracheal intubation with hyperventilation. Recognize that coma can persist for long periods, especially if treatment is delayed. Despite improvement, climbers with symptoms of HACE should not be allowed to reascend.

High-Altitude Retinopathy

If vision is affected, victims should descend, preferably with oxygen. Adequate hydration is important. Oxygen (or increased carbon dioxide through paper bag rebreathing) can be given for transient blindness (which is usually cortical blindness and not HAR).

PEOPLE WITH CHRONIC DISEASES GOING TO ALTITUDE

As our population ages and more recognition is given to the beneficial effects of exercise, more older people desire to travel to altitude for recreation. There are some published reports, but no controlled studies, of lowlanders with chronic diseases exposed to altitude. Not much is known about the effects of pharmaceuticals during hypoxia, and advice to patients about their medicines remains presumptive or speculative and should be given cautiously. Loss of self-esteem results from staying at home in a low-risk environment and nursing a chronic illness. In marginal clinical situations where an individual has a strong will and motivation to reach a personal goal, that person may derive great benefit from the attainment of that goal, even if it involves significant risk.

Individuals who insist on going to altitude despite medical advice to the contrary should be urged to choose an itinerary with access to easy descent and have medical help readily available. Taking oxygen along is usually impractical.

People with chronic diseases that could cause problems at altitude should first undertake an activity close to home that is similar to that planned for their trip. They should then repeat the same activity at a moderate altitude (e.g., 8000 ft) near home. If they perform well under both circumstances, they can consider that activity at even higher altitudes.

Exercise Testing for Cardiovascular Fitness

Death while exercising does not appear more common at altitude than at sea level. Deaths are more common in patients with known cardiac disease or who experience symptoms while exercising, but sudden death can occur in fit athletes as well. Exercise tests are useful in evaluating patients with known coronary disease, or who have symptoms suggestive of coronary disease. They are not useful in predicting coronary disease in asymptomatic individuals.

Preactivity exercise testing can be considered for those people 50 years of age or older who have significant risk factors for coronary artery disease, including family history, hypertension, chest pain, and ST-segment depression on the resting electrocardiogram (ECG). Those whose exercise test is positive can undergo an exercise thallium reperfusion study. If that test is positive, further studies are indicated.

Angina Pectoris

Patients with minimal symptoms of angina, who take few medicines, and who can undergo the Bruce Protocol exercise test for more than 9 minutes will probably do well at altitude. Those with moderate symptoms, who take a number of medicines, and who have exercise limitations or occasional angina at rest may tolerate some exposure to altitude. Those with severe angina and marked limitation of effort at sea level should not go to altitude, as hypoxia will increase cardiac work and precipitate severe anginal attacks.

The first 5 to 10 days at altitude are considered a dangerous period for people with cardiovascular disease, because of increased sympathetic outflow and circulating catecholamines. People with angina who are going to altitude should ascend slowly and rest for the first 2 to 3 days on arrival there. They may have decreased exercise tolerance, with earlier appearance of angina as they try to maintain their usual level of physical activity. Angina symptoms are treated with oxygen and antiangina medications; if severe, descent without exertion should be strongly considered.

Hypertension

Those with hypertension may find their blood pressures elevated at altitude. A low-salt diet and increased rest during the first few days at altitude can be advised together with self-monitoring of pressures. Some individuals may need to increase the dose of their antihypertensive drugs—this possibility should be discussed with the primary physician before departure. Beta-blockers are probably not effective at altitude because of increased sympathetic activity. Clonidine, which produces diffuse inhibition of CNS sympathetic neural outflow, and prazosin, which blocks alpha-adrenoreceptors, may be useful to control pressures. Calcium channel blockers and angiotensin-converting enzyme inhibitors also may be useful, but there are no controlled trials of any antihypertensive agents at altitude.

Postmyocardial Infarction and Postcoronary Artery Bypass Surgery

There are no data to suggest that patients with a history of myocardial infarction or coronary artery bypass surgery need to be treated any differently than those already mentioned once they have fully recovered from their acute cardiac problem.

There are no controlled studies evaluating the risk of venturing to high altitude in people with known cardiac disease. More cases are being reported of individuals sustaining cardiac events at high altitude, probably because many more are venturing higher.

Individuals with marginally controlled congestive heart failure may decompensate at moderate altitude (6500 ft) or higher, and they are difficult to assess in situ because of tachypneic and tachycardic responses to altitude. AMS and other forms of fluid retention at altitude could aggravate congestive heart failure. Such individuals should avoid altitude.

Exercise guidelines at altitude are helpful. For those with coronary artery disease, target heart rates are a better end point for activity levels at altitude than an activity prescription. Base the target heart rate on the ischemic endpoint heart rate from a symptom-limited treadmill evaluation at home altitude: 75% is the target rate for cardiac patients at altitude. A derived maximal heart rate (206-1.2 X e in years-20) may be substituted for the ischemic end point heart rate (from which the 75% target rate can be derived) in those who have not had and do not need an exercise study. The patient can test the targeted heart rate with strenuous exercise before departure.

Pulmonary Diseases

Many asthmatics report subjective improvement in their condition at altitude, perhaps because there is less dust, a lower air density, and fewer inhaled allergens. Some patients have experienced more cold- or exercise-induced bronchospasm. Such individuals should use inhaled bronchodilators before cold or exercise exposure.

Individuals with mild to moderate chronic lung disease may tolerate modest altitudes, but there is a higher incidence of AMS among this group of people. Those on home oxygen should continue and should increase the flow rate by the ratio of the home barometric pressure to the new one at destination. Altitude exposure is contraindicated for those with marked arterial desaturation and carbon dioxide retention.

Those with sleep apnea syndrome do not do well at altitude. If it is necessary to go to altitude, oxygen and acetazolamide for sleep are advised.

Neurologic Diseases

Transient ischemic attacks (TIAs) and stroke have been reported at high altitude (>16,000 ft) in young healthy individuals. Dehydration may be a contributing factor. Those experiencing a TIA at altitude should increase hydration, take an aspirin tablet a day, and descend.

People with seizures controlled by medication need to continue their anticonvulsant medicines at altitude. There does not appear to be an increased incidence of breakthrough seizures in those who maintain therapeutic levels. The seizure threshold at altitude may be lowered, so patients who have stopped taking their antiseizure medicines at sea level could have return of seizures after abrupt exposure to altitude.

Diabetes Mellitus

Insulin-requiring diabetics may experience problems regulating their insulin dose when climbing to altitude because of the day-to-day variance in energy expenditure and food intake. Blood glucose determinations should be performed more frequently than when at home doing normal work. More frequent insulin dosing with a shorter acting preparation may result in better control. Glucagon should be carried for hypoglycemic episodes (see Chapter 14). Insulin should not be allowed to freeze, and extra supplies should be carried in case of loss or breakage. Treatment of diabetic ketoacidosis at altitude has proven difficult, primarily because of problems assessing acid-base balance, and because the patient typically needs high-volume fluid resuscitation.

Sickle Cell Disease

Sickle cell disease is considered a contraindication to ascend to altitude. Altitude exposures of only 6320 ft (1925 m) are associated with an almost 60% risk of having a sickle cell crisis. Even air travel is associated with an increased risk.

The splenic infarction syndrome, with left upper quadrant pain, is more common in people with sickle cell trait rather than disease, as those with the latter have probably experienced autoinfarction of their spleens early in life. Many patients with sickle cell disease and occasional patients with sickle trait may require supplemental oxygen during air travel (this is difficult to arrange on many airlines), particularly if they have underlying pulmonary disease (see Chapter 2). All patients with sickle cell disease or trait should keep well hydrated.

Individuals with sickle cell trait and other hemoglobinopathies such as SC or beta-thalassemia, and who have normal lung function, should limit altitude exposure to 10,000 ft (3050 m), understanding that splenic infarction may occur. Those with impaired lung function may become symptomatic at lower altitudes.

GYNECOLOGIC, OBSTETRIC, AND PEDIATRIC CONCERNS AT ALTITUDE

Women taking oral contraceptives could be advised to continue them at least to moderate altitudes (<10,000 ft), since the risk of pregnancy may be greater than the increased risk of thrombosis. However, women on oral contraceptives should be advised to consider other contraceptives at higher altitudes, because of the theoretical increased risk of thrombosis and pulmonary embolism (see Chapter 12).

There are also no data regarding pregnant visitors to altitude. Studies on permanent residents at altitude show altitude-associated increase in fetal growth retardation, pregnancy-induced hypertension, and neonatal hyperbilirubinemia. It would be reasonable to limit exposure during the first trimester to 8000 ft (2450 m) for uncomplicated pregnancies.

Infants and young children born at sea level are perhaps more at risk from altitude illness than adults. However, they have been taken to altitudes over 15,000 ft (4570 m) by responsible adults without incident.

Diagnosis of altitude illness is more difficult in preverbal or young children and rapid descent is paramount if any questionable illness occurs. There are no data on the use of pharmaceuticals to prevent or treat mountain sickness in children, but acetazolamide can probably be used (see Chapter 11).

MISCELLANEOUS CONCERNS AT ALTITUDE

There is significant immune suppression in the normal human at altitudes of 10,000 ft (3050 m) or higher. B cell function and the response to active immunization are maintained, but T-cell function is impaired after exposure to simulated altitude. Anecdotally, bacterial infections at altitudes above 14,000 ft (4270 m) do not seem to respond to appropriate treatment without descent.

There are no data on the exposure of human immunodeficiency virus (HIV)-infected individuals to altitude, but pulmonary infections and infections of the gastrointestinal tract are likely to be more serious in HIV-infected travelers to altitude. Easy descent should be a readily available option in their itineraries.

Extended-wear contact lenses have been worn to 26,000 ft (8000 m) without mishap, although corneal hypoxia is a potential hazard. The use of disposable lenses obviates the increased risk of infection from improper cleaning.

Individuals who have had corneal surgery to improve eyesight have experienced markedly decreased vision with exposure to increasing altitude. Overnight stays beginning at an intermediate altitude and going higher can result in a progressive shift toward farsightedness such that those who have had radial keratotomy may have difficulty recognizing people and distinguishing features of terrain. Secondary images may be observed. Changes are noticed at altitudes of 12,000 ft (3600 m) and higher, usually after a 24-hour stay. Some people report changes at lower altitudes. Reading glasses may improve vision for those afflicted, but specific plus powers needed cannot be predicted in advance, nor do they help the secondary images. An assortment of reading glasses with different plus powers should be available for temporary correction to allow safer descents if this occurs. Those who have had such surgery should avoid hazardous routes and should always be accompanied by someone without such corneal surgery. Problems with vision at altitude have not been reported in persons who have undergone photorefractive keratectomy, nor encountered in a study of such individuals.

The use of anorexic agents (diet pills) at altitude has been associated with an increased risk of problems at altitude and is to be avoided.

DIVING AT ALTITUDE

Scuba diving in bodies of water at altitude presents new situations for potential altitude illness combined with diving disorders. The usual sea level decompression tables cannot be followed, and divers should be aware of the appropriate tables, as discussed in by Egi and Brubank.

REFERENCES

Bartsch P, Maggiorini M, Ritter M, et al: Prevention of high-altitude pulmonary edema by nifedipine, *N Engl J Med* 325:1284, 1991.

Bezruchka S: *Altitude illness: prevention and treatment,* Seattle, 1998, The Mountaineers.

Bezruchka S: High altitude medicine, *Med Clin North Am* 76:1481, 1992.

Bezruchka S: *The pocket doctor: a passport to healthy travel,* ed 3, Seattle, 1999, The Mountaineers, 1999.

Carpenter TC, Niermeyer S, Durmowicz AG: Altitude-related illness in children, *Curr Probl Pediatr* 28:177, 1998.

Durmowicz AG, Noordeweir E, Nicholas R, Reeves JT: Inflammatory processes may predispose children to high-altitude pulmonary edema, *J Pediatr* 130(5): 838, 1997.

Egi SM, Brubank AO: Diving at altitude: a review of decompression strategies, *Undersea Hyperb Med* 22:281, 1995.

Froelicher VF, West JB: Trekking in Nepal: safety after coronary artery bypass, *JAMA* 259:3184, 1988.

Grissom CK et al: Acetazolamide in the treatment of acute mountain sickness: clinical efficacy and effect on gas exchange, *Ann Intern Med* 116:461, 1992.

Hackett PH et al: Dexamethasone for prevention and treatment of acute mountain sickness, *Aviat Space Environ Med* 59:950, 1988.

Hackett PH et al: High-altitude cerebral edema evaluated with magnetic resonance imaging: clinical correlation and pathophysiology, *JAMA* 280:1920, 1998.

Hornbein TF et al: The cost to the central nervous system of climbing to extremely high altitude, *N Engl J Med* 321:1714, 1989.

Houston CS: *Going higher: the story of man and altitude,* Seattle, 1998, The Mountaineers.

Hultgren H: *High altitude medicine,* Stanford, 1997, Hultgren Publications. Order from (650)857-0891, fax (650)493-4225, hultgren@highaltitudemedicine.com

Hultgren HN: High-altitude pulmonary edema: current concepts, *Annu Rev Med* 47:267, 1996.

Hultgren HN: Coronary heart disease and trekking, *J Wilderness Med* 1:154, 1990.

Hultgren HN, Honigman B, Theis K, Nicholas D: High altitude pulmonary edema at a ski resort, *West J Med* 164:222, 1996.

Kasic JF et al: Treatment of acute mountain sickness: hyperbaric versus oxygen therapy, *Ann Emerg Med* 20:1109, 1991.

Leach J, McLean A, Mee FB: High altitude dives in the Nepali Himalaya, *Undersea Hyperb Med* 21:459, 1994.

Levine BD, Zuckerman JH, deFilippi CR: Effect of high-altitude exposure in the elderly: the Tenth Mountain Division study, *Circulation* 96:1224, 1997.

Murdoch DR: Symptoms of infection and altitude illness among hikers in the Mount Everest region of Nepal, *Aviat Space Environ Med* 66:148, 1995.

Oelz O et al: Nifedipine for high altitude pulmonary oedema, *Lancet* 2:1241, 1989.

Pollard AJ, Murdoch DR: *The high altitude medicine handbook,* Oxford, 1997, Radcliffe Medical Press.

Rabold MB: Dexamethasone for prophylaxis and treatment of acute mountain sickness, *J Wilderness Med* 3:54, 1992.

Rennie D: Will mountain trekkers have heart attacks? *JAMA* 261:1045, 1989.

Roach RC et al: How well do older persons tolerate moderate altitude? *West J Med* 162:32, 1995.

Scherrer U et al: Inhaled nitric oxide for high-altitude pulmonary edema, *N Engl J Med* 334:624, 1996.

Shlim DR, Gallie J: The causes of death among trekkers in Nepal, *Int J Sports Med* 13(suppl 1):S74, 1992.

Taber RL: Protocols for the use of a portable hyperbaric chamber for the treatment of high altitude disorders, *J Wilderness Med* 1:181, 1990.

West JR: The safety of trekking at high altitude after coronary bypass surgery (in reply), *JAMA* 260:2218, 1988.

CHAPTER 10

Diving Medicine

Alan Spira

Seen from space, Earth is a great blue orb: 70% of our planet is covered by water. It is not surprising then that humankind has had a long, intimate, sometimes turbulent relationship with the sea. We sail over ocean, sea, and lake for commerce, food, treasure, war, and exploration. The water environment has been both friend and foe; yet for all of our existence, that which lies beneath the waves has been a mystery. Only in the last 50 years we have begun to seriously explore, learn, even play in, this other world. Scuba diving has been a major factor and, as a pleasure activity, has become one of the fasting growing parts of the travel industry, as legions of travelers search the world over for exotic diving spots.

With millions of travelers scuba diving—more than 3 million a year in the United States alone—physicians need to understand the health hazards that such travelers may encounter. The underwater environment is not a forgiving one; decompression sickness, air emboli, trauma, and other risks face those who enter this world. Diving trips to remote and exotic locations are extremely common and easy today; after flying home from such a trip a diver with decompression sickness can seek out any physician anywhere on the planet. Large numbers of people are insufficiently trained in scuba and in less than adequate physical condition, leading to an increase in diving injuries and diseases. In the United States, there are approximately 800 to 900 serious accidents and 100 deaths a year.

TYPES OF RECREATIONAL DIVING

Surface Diving

Surface diving includes free diving and snorkeling. Free diving, also called breath-hold diving, the oldest type of diving, is limited by the amount of air a diver can fill his or her lungs with from the surface. The amount of time spent underwater is limited by the amount of oxygen left and retained CO_2 that stimulates breathing. Most swimmers cannot stay underwater for more than a few minutes. Snorkeling, also called skin diving, is a type of free-diving where a hollow tube allows a swimmer to breath air while facing down in water, prolonging mobility. The snorkel adds to the respiratory dead space, so there is a limit to the length and diameter of the bore that swimmers can use before the work of breathing exceeds the benefit of the snorkel.

Scuba Diving

Scuba diving is the major form of recreational diving around the world. Scuba is the acronym for **S**elf-**C**ontained **U**nderwater **B**reathing **A**pparatus. Co-invented by Jacques Cousteau and Emile Gagnan in 1943, it was originally called the *Aqualung* and is a portable supply of air carried on one's back that offers a diver tremendous freedom underwater. The primary constraint of scuba is the limited air supply, usually less than 1 hour, but this varies greatly with the diver's exertional effort and experience; 130 feet/40 meters is the generally recommended depth limit for this type of diving. Proper training courses should take several weeks of class work, pool training, and open-water practice. Weekend-long certifying courses offered by tourist resorts are usually inadequate, creating divers with insufficient training and a false sense of ability.

Scuba divers breath compressed air. The scuba tank is filled with compressed air to a pressure usually ~3000 psi. (pounds/in^2). Compressed air flows through a first stage regulator which brings the pressure down to ~100 to 160 p.s.i. above ambient pressure. The air is then guided through a second stage, a "demand" regulator, which operates when a diver inhales, opening a series of valves that releases air into the mouth at pressure similar to the diver's depth. Exhaled air is simply diverted out of the regulator into the surrounding water, with a rush of bubbles; underwater, this can be quite loud. This is also called an *open circuit scuba* system, to distinguish it from semiclosed or fully closed-circuit systems that usually contain gas mixtures other than air. This system has an inherent resistance to breathing, but modern technology has created demand regulators that deliver air at consistent low-differential pressures to minimize the extra work for the diver. Most of this chapter is dedicated to scuba-related health issues.

Technical Diving

Technical diving has been used by the military and commercial community for many years. Technical diving involves breathing gases other than air underwater of which there are several choices. Such gas mixtures offer several advantages over air, particularly in regard to less decompression sickness, but they have some serious limitations. They have become quite popular with recreational divers. Aficionados of these diving styles are often very educated and may know their diving physiology as well as the physician. There are three main types of gas mixtures:

1. Nitrox (Oxygen-Enriched Air or Enriched Air Nitrox). The benefits of nitrox include extended diving bottom times, longer repetitive dives, shorter surface intervals, less decompression illness, and less fatigue. The disadvantages of using enhanced oxygen gases include increased danger of oxygen toxicity, limitation of maximal depth possible during a dive, and the need for more sophisticated equipment, training, and dive planning. Oxygen toxicity may present with visual disturbances (such as scotomata and tunnel vision), tinnitus, dysphoria, nausea, anxiety, muscle spasms, seizures, and unconsciousness. There may not be any preceding symptoms and seizures underwater are usually fatal as a result of aspiration and drowning.

2. Heliox, a mixture of helium and oxygen, is used for deeper dives. The helium replaces nitrogen and eliminates nitrogen narcosis. High pressure neurologic syndrome (HPNS) occurs while inhaling helium under high pressure and is a neurologic disorder associated with motor problems occurring at depths greater than 600 feet of sea water (fsw)/183 meters of sea water (msw). It is manifested by tremors, dizziness, nausea, and som-

nolence when diving deeper than 500 fsw or 16 Absolute Atmospheres (ATA) (see Diving Physiology section for more details).

3. Trimix is a breathing mixture of helium, nitrogen, and oxygen, used with extremely deep dives often greater than 300 fsw/90 m. Decompression is required with this very high risk type of diving.

Scuba diving *is* a high-risk sport. There are approximately 3 million recreational scuba divers in the United States (with more than a quarter-million learning scuba annually); 1 million in Europe with more than 50,000 in the United Kingdom. In the United States annual mortality is 3 to 9 deaths/100,000. Statistically, mortality in divers is primarily drowning (60%), followed by pulmonary overpressurization syndromes (20%). Diving morbidity, far more common, can be from near-drowning, gas bubbles, barotraumas, or environmental hazards.

This chapter identifies key health concerns in diving medicine, so the travel medicine adviser can assist the diving traveler with appropriate pre-travel medical advice and can review situation in which the diving traveler needs medical care.

DIVING PHYSIOLOGY

Understanding a few fundamental physical principles aids in understanding and intelligently approaching the primary diseases of diving, not to mention promoting safe diving. There are two principle ways pressure can affect us: direct mechanical effects and metabolic effects of inspired gases. *Dysbarism,* a general term used to describe pathology from altered environmental pressure, has two main forms: barotraumas, from the uncontrolled expansion of gas within gas-filled body compartments, and decompression sickness, from too rapid a return to atmospheric pressure or prolonged breathing air under increased pressures.

On the surface of the earth every living creature is exposed to the pressure of the earth's atmosphere. When climbing mountains there is a reduction in atmospheric pressure and by physical laws, the partial pressures of the components of air are reduced. In contrast, divers are exposed to additional pressure the deeper they dive, and there are significant and important physiologic changes that occur under these circumstances. Many of the diseases that occur during and as a result of scuba diving are related to the air breathed under pressure. The primary physical factors affecting divers underwater are pressure, buoyancy, and temperature.

Recall that pressure is the amount of force acting on a unit area:

$$P = F/A$$

In the United States pressure is usually expressed as pound per square inch (psi); elsewhere, it is expressed as kilograms per square centimeter (kg/cm^2) or the Kilopascal. The pressure affecting a diver has two components: the weight of the atmosphere and the weight of the water. At sea level atmospheric pressure is equal to 14.7 psi or 1.03 kg/cm^2: This is the weight of a square inch column of air extending from the surface of the earth to the verge of outer space. It can also be expressed as 1 atmosphere (atm), 1 Pascal ($newton/m^2$), 1.013 bars, or 760 mm Hg.

Hydrostatic pressure is equal in all directions at any specific depth, because water as a liquid is incompressible. At the surface, there is 1 atmosphere of pressure on a diver. Diving gauges incorporate atmospheric pressure, so at sea level they will read 0, which is also called 1 atmosphere absolute (ATA). For every 10 meters or 33 feet (34 feet if fresh water), the hydrostatic pressure increases by an atmosphere, so at 10 meters there are 2 ATA; at 66 feet there are 3 ATA; at 99 feet or 30 meters there are 4 ATA.

Buoyancy is the next concept to consider. Archimedes discovered that any body immersed in a liquid will be buoyed up by a force equal to the weight of the liquid displaced by that body. So if the weight of a body is greater than the weight of the water it displaces, then that body will sink (negatively buoyant); if the weight of the water displaced is greater than the body displacing it, that body will float (positively buoyant). If the two weights are equal, then the body will be neutrally buoyant and thus will neither float nor sink.

The density of the water is important in determining buoyancy. Seawater is denser than freshwater: 64.0 lb/ft^3 vs. 62.4 lbs/ft^3 (or 29 kg/0.03 m^3 vs. 28.3 kg/m^3); thus bodies are more positively buoyant in seawater than in freshwater. Another factor in buoyancy is the lung volume of a diver: with fully inflated lungs, a diver displaces more water and so is more buoyant and tends to rise; a diver with deflated lungs is less buoyant and tends to sink. Other factors include amount of fat (greater body fat increases buoyancy), bone density (higher density decreases buoyancy), and neoprene wet suits, which also increase buoyancy.

The effect of temperature is discussed later in the Special Situations section.

Gas Laws

Five laws of physics are important in diving that affect the behavior of gases related to volume, pressure, and temperature of the gases.

Boyle's Law $P_1V_1 = P_2V_2$

This is the most important law of physics relevant to scuba, which explains that the volume of a gas will inversely vary with the pressure as long as the temperature is kept constant. This explains why at sea level, 1 ATA, there is 100% volume; at 33 ft or 2 ATA there is 50% volume; at 66 feet or 3 ATA volume is reduces to 33%; at 99 ft or 4 ATA the volume is now 25%; and at 132 ft or 5 ATA, the volume is 1/5 of its original volume, or 20%.

This law has physiologic consequences for the body. Although we are mostly liquid, and liquid is incompressible, humans have several areas that are air filled, such as the thorax, middle ear, sinuses, and intestines. As gases expand and contract, these areas are affected. The pressure inside any gas space must match the surrounding pressure. During descent the body gas spaces increase their pressure by decreasing their volume; on ascent these gas spaces lower their pressure by expanding their volumes.

Other pertinent gas laws include Dalton's law, which states that the total pressure of a mixture of gases is equal to the pressure of each gas independently; Henry's law, which relates the amount that a gas dissolved in a liquid at some temperature to both the partial pressure of the gas and the solubility coefficient of that gas; and Charles' law, which states that the volume of a gas is proportional to the temperature.

There are several relevant gases in diving medicine, primarily oxygen, nitrogen, carbon dioxide, helium, and carbon monoxide that affect the health and welfare of divers underwater. Air is the gas responsible for barotraumas and arterial gas emboli; nitrogen is the gas responsible for decompression illness and nitrogen narcosis.

BAROTRAUMA

Barotrauma is the damage inflicted on the body by changes in pressure, or more accurately, the pressure differences between the gas spaces and the surrounding water. It is a mechanical problem of pressures not being equal between body spaces and the hydrostatic pressures (or the diving equipment). This gradient can be positive during descent underwater with increasing pressure, or it may be negative during ascent toward the surface when the pressure within the body cavities is greater than the surrounding environment. Without equalization of pressure, it can occur in as little as 4 feet of depth.

Middle Ear

The middle ear is the most common body part affected by barotrauma, occurring in 30% to 60% of divers. Although the inner ear is fluid-filled, the middle and outer ear canal are air-filled. The middle air is separated from the outer ear by the tympanic membrane; the only way air pressure can be equalized in the middle ear is via the eustachian tube into the oropharynx (with an intact tympanic membrane).

Middle ear squeeze occurs during descent when the surrounding water pressure exceeds the air pressure in the middle ear: if the eustachian tube is closed or congested or if the pressure change is rapid, the tympanic membrane is deformed into the middle air space. As the pressure gradient is relatively greatest in the first 33 ft/10m under the surface (especially in the first 6 ft/2m), it is most likely to occur near the surface than deeper down. This unequal pressure bows the tympanic membrane, causing discomfort or a sensation of fullness; if not equalized, vascular congestion, hemorrhage, pain, and membrane rupture may follow. If the tympanic membrane ruptures and cold water rushes into the middle ear, the vestibular system is disrupted by this cold caloric stimulus; vertigo, nausea, and vomiting may ensue; and underwater this may be fatal if aspiration occurs. Hearing loss and tinnitus may also occur. Equalizing the pressure is accomplished by opening the eustachian tubes so that pressurized air from the scuba tank present in the mouth can enter the middle ear space by swallowing or other maneuvers.

Common causes for eustachian tube dysfunction include the inability to equalize as rapidly as the pressure changes; acute or chronic inflammation; allergy; anatomic deformities; prolonged use of nasal drops; frequent or acute upper respiratory infection, nasal allergies, nasal obstruction, or ear disease; and excessive smoking. Scarring of the tympanic membrane from otitis media during childhood contributes to an inflexible membrane and reduced eardrum flexibility when the pressure gradient changes; this can lead to an inability to equalize a the risk of drum rupture. It is also more difficult to equalize underwater if the diver descends head-first: when descending feet-first, drainage is more effective and easier. Underwater, if equalization is not successful, the diver must ascend until the level when equalization does occur and then redescend slowly.

A reverse squeeze is a situation where the air pressure in the middle ear exceeds that of the ambient water pressure. Air in the middle ear will expand by Boyle's law as the diver rises to the surface; if not relieved by opening the eustachian tube, the tympanic membrane will bulge outward as the water pressure decreases closer to the surface. This can also occur when a diver has taken decongestants that wear off while underwater and edema returns to the eustachian tube and middle ear before ascending.

Alternobaric vertigo is an asymmetric middle ear barotrauma during ascent, where middle ear air on either side cannot exit on ascent, with unequal vestibular stimulation, leading to vertiginous symptoms underwater. This vertigo can stop by halting the ascent or by descending again. Rarely this can lead to facial paralysis.

External ear squeeze occurs if the external auditory canal is obstructed, usually by cerumen, tight fitting hoods, or ear plugs. It may occur on ascent or descent. Pain, hemorrhage, and occasionally tympanic membrane rupture may occur.

Inner ear barotrauma can have severe consequences from round or oval window rupture with possible perilymph fistulae or cochlear hemorrhage with sensorineural hearing loss and vestibular dysfunction. Round window rupture from excessively negative middle ear pressure is more likely with overly forceful Valsalva maneuvers that increase cerebrospinal fluid and inner ear pressures. The round window is located between the middle and inner ears, and rupture often leads to tinnitus and decreased or loss of hearing. This should be suspected when tinnitus and vertigo are severe, associated with nerve deafness, and occur after a no-decompression dive. It can mimic inner ear decompression sickness (DCS), and recompression therapy may nevertheless be necessary.

Sinuses

The sinuses are the second-most common sites of barotrauma. The frontal sinuses are affected more than the ethmoids and maxillary sinuses, with pain and epistaxis the most common consequences. The ostia draining mucus from the various sinuses into the nasal cavity can easily clog with minimal inflammation, and if the pressure between the sinuses and surrounding water does not balance, barotrauma results. During descent, when most sinus barotrauma occurs, the negative pressure in the sinus cavity can tear mucous membranes from the sinus walls, which may be both painful and bloody. During ascent, the membranes are compressed and the thin skeletal walls may deform.

Upper respiratory infections, sinusitis, nasal polyps, allergies, nasal spray overuse, cigarette smoking, and anatomic abnormalities such as deviated septum can all predispose to sinus barotrauma.

Pulmonary

Pulmonary barotrauma encompasses the pulmonary overpressurization syndromes and includes thoracic squeezes and diffuse alveolar hemorrhage from rapid or uncontrolled ascents. A thoracic squeeze occurs when compression of air in the lungs reduces the volume to less than residual volume. In general, pulmonary barotrauma is uncommon, but the consequences are severe as described below.

Gastrointestinal

When a diver swallows air underwater, it expands during ascent, stretching the intestines. This barotrauma of ascent may range from uncomfortable to painful, and may be associated with increased eructation and flatulence postdive. This is most common in novice divers and those who drink carbonated beverages or eat heavily before diving. It also occurs with steep head-down angles during descent. Rarely, a hollow viscus overdistended by air, such as the stomach, may rupture from barotrauma.

Dental

Barontalgia is also called tooth squeeze. It can arise from caries, defective caps or crowns, temporary fillings, root canal therapy, periodontal abscesses, maxillary sinus congestion, or dental lesions. As a result of the gas laws, such teeth may actually implode during descent or explode on ascent. The affected tooth is often sensitive if not painful, and pain may be referred to the sinuses. The reverse is also possible; many cases of dental pain originating after flying or diving are actually sinus in origin. All divers should have good dental care and those with temporary crowns should not dive.

Mask

A mask squeeze develops as a result of not enough air pressure within the mask during descent and as a result of lower pressure, facial tissue is pulled into the mask, resulting in subconjunctival hemorrhage, periorbital petechiae, or ecchymoses. While frightful appearing, it is not serious, resolving spontaneously within days. Prevention is simply by exhaling slightly through the nose into the mask during descent. There have been reports of orbital subperiosteal hematomas, but they are rare.

PULMONARY OVERPRESSURIZATION SYNDROME

Pulmonary overpressurization syndrome (POPS) is a dysbaric illness characterized by four clinically important entities: arterial gas embolism, pneumomediastinum, pneumothorax, and subcutaneous emphysema. It is due to pulmonary barotraumas and is also called burst lung. These barotraumas arise from gas expansion during ascent that exceeds the lung's elastic ability, resulting in alveolar tissue rupture. It does not normally occur in snorkel or breath-hold diving because there is no additional gas added to decreased lung volumes at depth, as with compressed air diving. The lungs therefore can only reexpand to their original volume on ascent to the surface and not beyond that volume.

In healthy lungs, POPS most likely results when a diver breath-holds during ascent or shoots to the surface too rapidly for adequate exhalation to compensate for the degree of gas expansion. Several pathologic conditions may predispose to pulmonary barotrauma: chronic obstructive pulmonary disease, acute and chronic bronchitis, asthma with mucus plugging and bronchoconstriction, pulmonary blebs with spontaneous pneumothorax, pulmonary abscesses, and restrictive lung diseases.

Arterial Gas Embolism

Arterial gas embolism (AGE) is the most important and feared form of pulmonary overpressurization syndrome, ranking second only to drowning as the cause of death in divers. Bubbles of expanding gas rupture from overdistended alveoli into the bloodstream and immediately become emboli, lodging in arterioles and capillaries, where they cause damage. This condition becomes apparent rapidly, usually within minutes of surfacing, often with bloody froth at the mouth or chest pain; there is frequent cardiovascular collapse. Emboli may lodge anywhere. In the brain, the primary organ affected by AGE, these bubbles cause unconsciousness, vertigo, paresthesias, convulsions, paralysis or paresis, nausea, visual disturbances, headache, confusion or even personality disorders, cerebrovascular accidents, seizures, or death. In the heart they may occlude coronary vessels leading to myocardial infarction; in the spinal cord paralysis and numbness may develop. Underwater, arterial gas embolism is often fatal. Dyspnea may or may not be present. Surprisingly, 20% of AGE spontaneously resolve.

More than half of AGE cases have symptom onset within 2 minutes. Nearly all occur within 10 minutes of surfacing; many cases occur while still submerged. Uncontrolled or panic ascents and breath-holding during ascent are the most common reasons for the development of AGE.

AGE may occur in shallow dives (a matter of feet) or brief dives (lasting several seconds). The laws of physics state that the risk of air embolism is actually greatest near the surface. For example, between 99 and 66 feet, there is a change of 4 to 3 ATA, whereas between 33 feet and the surface the change is from 2 to 1 ATA—a much greater gradient, which means greater gas expansion. Each foot of seawater has a pressure of roughly 25 mm Hg, so a diver who inhales from a tank at a mere 4 feet and holds his breath to the surface has enough of a pressure gradient developed to force air across the alveolar membrane into the blood.

Pneumothorax

If the expanding gas ruptures through the alveoli and fills the pleural space, it will collapse the lung. Pleuritic chest pain and dyspnea are the most common findings. If the escaped air continues to expand as during ascent, it may push on the mediastinal structures, forcing them into the opposite hemithorax, leading to a tension pneumothorax. In this situation cardiac blood flow is impaired, resulting in hypotension, venous jugular distention, and decreased breath sounds on the opposite hemithorax. Pulmonary hemorrhage is not uncommon. Mild pneumothoraces need no treatment, as the body will reabsorb the air. Large ones requires drainage of the air with a chest tube or a Heimlich valve; a tension pneumothorax is a surgical emergency, requiring immediate removal of the trapped air with a midline needle thoracostomy in the second intercostal space of the affected side and subsequent chest tube placement. Recompression can actually worsen the situation by converting a simple pneumothorax into a tension pneumothorax if a tube thoracostomy had not yet been performed.

Anyone with a history of spontaneous pneumothorax is precluded from ever diving.

Pneumomediastinum

If the expanding gas ruptures into the mediastinal spaces, it can track up around the heart and the great vessels and even compress the trachea. Hammon's crunch is the sound of air in the precordium, which is best heard during systole. Chest pain or dyspnea may result. Without neurologic or cardiac compromise, recompression is not necessarily indicated for treatment.

Subcutaneous Emphysema

If the expanding gas ruptures under the visceral pleura, it may track under the skin with the presentation of soft-tissue crepitance, a crunching sensation when the skin is palpated. The compression of tiny air bubbles under the skin feels like the popping of bubble packing sheet. In severe cases, which may occur concurrently with pneumomediastinum, air can track up along the trachea, where swelling of the neck and face may occur, along with dysphonia or cyanosis.

DECOMPRESSION SICKNESS

Recall that air is 21% oxygen; the rest primarily consists of metabolically inert nitrogen, which is not metabolized and can accumulate in body tissues. The air a scuba diver inhales under pressure increases the amount of nitrogen absorbed into tissues; when this pressure is released, as during ascent from a scuba dive, nitrogen comes out of solution, and if it does so too rapidly, it forms bubbles in extravascular or intravascular tissues, which was first proven in the last century from work done on caisson workers (caissons are specialized engineering units used for constructing underwater tunnels and bridge abutments). This disease is also known as the bends, from the stooping posture assumed by affected caisson workers.

Decompression sickness is a very complicated pathological process but is due to nitrogen gas. Under pressure, nitrogen from inhaled air is driven by diffusion into different tissues at different rates until an equilibrium is reached. When tissue pressure is reduced, nitrogen diffuses out of cells, and this process is tissue, rate, and pressure-dependent. Nitrogen is five times more soluble in adipose than aqueous tissue and may act as a central nervous system (CNS) intoxicant or anesthetic. Tissues have a maximum concentration of nitrogen, at which point they are saturated. Under increased pressures, more gas can be driven into the tissue; this is called supersaturation.

Bubbling occurs almost continuously (shown by Doppler studies) and the amount of bubbling, time, and location (intravascular versus extravascular) determine which diseases develop. Bubbles form on decompression but do not necessarily cause overt disease. Nitrogen bubbles may form in the blood or in extravascular tissues. Bubbles in the bloodstream may act as emboli, leading to microvascular blockage and ischemia, blood sludging and induction of the complement cascade and platelet aggregation, which leads to organ or tissue dysfunction. Bubbles have been shown to accelerate the clotting process and damage the endothelium. In extravascular events, they most commonly form in fatty and aqueous tissues where they compress and deform the tissues, nerves in particular. Normally, intravascular bubbles are trapped in the pulmonary capillary bed; the lungs filter nitrogen bubbles if the number of bubbles is less than the filtering capacity.

Decompression disease from nitrogen bubbles is influenced by the pressure and the breathing gas profile. Divers are taught to make their deepest dives first because of physiologic gas loading: different tissues have different abilities to absorb and unload nitrogen—for example, fat and nerves are slow tissues in regards to nitrogen release—and gas dissolution in and out of tissue is logarithmic. After a dive one does not unload all the gas; some remains in the slow tissues (because fast tissues unload quickly) and one then enters the next dive with a gas handicap. These gas kinetics are the reason for deepest dive first. Regulation of nitrogen risk is managed through dive tables and dive computers, which are designed to limit the depth and time underwater, which would predispose to decompression illness (DCI). There are several tables in use, such as the U.S. Navy Dive Tables, the Huggins Table, and the Defense & Civil Institute of Environmental Medicine Tables. The Professional Association of Diving Instructors Recreational Dive Planner is a variant of the U.S. Navy Dive Tables that uses models meant to follow recreational patterns (such as multilevel diving), not military types, of diving. However, these tables are not infallible, and a diver can stay within the limits of the conservative U.S. Navy Dive Tables and still develop the bends.

Unlike air emboli, decompression sickness (DCS) does not occur in shallow water because it has a different etiology. Bubbles may form from too much time breathing air spent at depth so that the amount of nitrogen supersaturates tissues, or it may be from ascending at a rate at which the pressure on the gas is relieved more quickly than the body can accommodate. Unlike arterial gas emboli, these bubbles are primarily venous. Factors that lead to DCI include too rapid an ascent rate, diving for too long or at too great a depth beyond the limits of no-decompression diving limits, dehydration, age, obesity, previous injury, alcohol, and cold. The traditional rate of a diver's ascent in the water has been recommended at 60 feet/min or no quicker than bubbles ascending from the regulator. Recent research has suggested that DCI can be reduced by halving the ascent rate to 30 feet/min or even less. Bubble formation is possible even after boarding an airliner after a dive. Since standard commercial cabin pressures are not kept at sea level, pressures bubbles continue to expand as the aircraft climbs to cruising altitude.

Decompression sickness may be considered a part of DCI, according to some authorities, when arterial gas emboli are included in the definition. DCS syndromes include pain syndromes, spinal cord syndrome, cerebral syndrome, peripheral nerve syndrome, and dysbaric osteonecrosis. Generally, the sooner the onset of symptoms after a dive, the more severe the case and often the more rapid the progression. Cases involving the brain, spinal cord, heart, or lungs are medical emergencies.

The overall statistical risk of developing DCS is between 0.004% and 0.001% or an incidence according to Divers Alert Network (DAN) statistics of 1 to 2 divers per 10,000. In all 60% of all DCS symptoms occur within 30 minutes after completing a dive; 95% are seen within 24 hours after a dive. Joint pain is seen in 80% of all DCS cases, making it the most common symptoms of decompression sickness. In 41% of cases it is the first presenting symptom. Although 40% of divers have neurologic symptoms as a presenting symptom, it ultimately develops in 80% of all cases of DCS. It is advisable to view any symptom after a dive as DCS and not wait for signs to develop.

DCS is a continuum of bubble-induced injury; for convenience it is often divided into the milder DCS I and the more serious DCS II. DCS I is defined as having skin rash or muscle/joint pains only. Dermatologic findings usually include pruritis and diffusely mottled erythematous patchy rashes, as well as lividity or marbling or formication. Patches may have central cyanosis and blanch. It is often seen on the shoulders and upper thorax. Bubbles blocking the lymphatics may cause local pitting edema. Musculoskeletal symptoms are the most common feature of DCS, most often with pain that is vague and diffuse, ranging from superficial to deep and is often near a synovial joint. It is usually asymmetric and may shift in both character and in its temporal pattern. The upper extremities are the most commonly affected body parts, the shoulder being the most common site, followed by the elbows, arms, and other body parts. The pain is often characterized as dull and difficult to localize. Redness, swelling, tenderness, and increased pain with movement are not typical of DCS. There is no change with movement of a joint, but inflating a blood pressure cuff over the affected area often reduces pain when due to bubbles, but not when due to old sports or traumatic injuries.

Any neurologic, cardiopulmonary, or vestibular findings place the disease into type II. Type II DCS may be considered a diffuse, multifocal DNS disease, which can include paresthesias, hypoesthesias, paresis, paraplegia, hemiplegia, urinary retention, impaired consciousness to life-threatening coma, ataxia, seizures, and death. Among the visual disturbances seen from DCS are blurred vision, scotomata, visual field defects, and blindness, which can be confused with cerebral arterial gas embolism. Chest pain and cough may also occur with intrathoracic intravascular bubbling ("the chokes"). Hemoconcentration is also seen in both serious cases of DCS and DIC. It has recently been suggested that repeated subclinical DCS from cerebral bubbles may also lead to a condition analogous to multi-infarct dementia. Computed tomography scans have shown cerebral perfusion deficits consistently present in patients with type II DCS.

Types I and II DCS may appear simultaneously, as the disease is actually a spectrum of bubble-induced injury; there is an overlap between them, since it is a spectrum of pathology and not truly separate categories of disease. The traditional classification scheme of DCS I and DCS II appears to be frequently used incorrectly by health care professionals: 48% of divers classified as type I ultimately reported neurologic symptoms.

Spinal DCS cases are often due to bubbles in the myelin sheath, causing vasogenic edema and focal ischemia with resulting neuropathy that may resolve. In contrast, other causes such as venous plexus bubbles and hemorrhage have a poor prognosis. Spinal cord involvement is the site of the most frequent neurologic DCS involvement, and symptoms often include low back pain, abdominal pain, lower extremity weakness, and paresthesias; signs include paralysis and urinary retention. Paraplegia is more common than quadriplegia in the worst cases, often following a pattern of back and abdominal pain followed by paresthesias and loss of bladder and bowel control before the onset of paralysis. The lower thoracic spine is the most common area affected followed by lumbar and then cervical. Symptoms tend to progressively wax and wane, and there may be residual symptoms even after treatment.

Inner ear DCS is also called vestibular decompression sickness (formerly known as "the staggers") and presents with vertigo, tinnitus, hearing loss, and nausea. If these symptoms occur on descent, they are actually due to inner ear barotrauma and the dive must be aborted; oval and round window ruptures must be included in the differential diagnosis. However, if the symptoms develop during or shortly after decompression from a dive, the diver must be considered to have inner ear DCS. It is more common with decompression from deep heliox (50% oxygen, 50% helium) dives but rarely can present from shallower recreational diving depths. Individuals who suffer permanent ear injury from this condition in the past have been advised that they cannot return to diving, but recent evidence shows that in some cases after proper evaluation, diving may be permitted if proper caution is taken.

An anatomic predisposition to symptomatic decompression illness is patent foramen ovale (PFO). Approximately 20% of the population is estimated to have PFO, and nearly 40% of DCS cases have PFO. The lungs filter most of the small nitrogen bubbles formed in the venous system during a dive, which limits tissue damage. However if blood passes from right atrium to left atrium bypassing lung filtration, then bubbles may enter the arterial system where they can do great damage.

The psychologic profile of a diver may also contribute to the morbidity of DCS vis-a-vis delaying treatment. Denial is the most common factor; anxiety, panic, embarrassment, and depression may also retard or prevent a diver from presenting for therapy. DAN statistics reveal that 20% of DCS divers had symptoms before their last dive. Divers with DCS have an average delay of approximately 32 hours before calling for assistance: 50% of injured divers with mild or pain-only DCS wait more than 12 hours before seeking assistance; 20% wait longer than 96 hours. Rationalization is also a common denominator in postponing evaluation; other divers perversely view being "bent" as a measure of their experience or machismo. Many such divers refuse to seek medical care or, if they do, refuse recompression. They may return to diving prematurely, which can lead to further decompression illness or permanent damage.

NITROGEN NARCOSIS

Nitrogen under pressure acts as a narcotic. Like gaseous anesthetics, N_2 has a high affinity for lipid. Its effect is depth and descent rate-related, usually occurring at depths greater than 4 ATA (99 fsw). Jacques Cousteau called it the "rapture of the deep." Martini's law of diving equates the effect of nitrogen as being equal to a single martini for every 50 feet of depth. Symptoms increase with exercise, cold, alcohol, and fear. It can be exacerbated, even accelerated, by the ingestion of alcohol. Symptoms disappear on ascent.

SPECIAL SITUATIONS

Flying after Diving

Flying puts a diver at risk for decompression illness if the flight occurs right after diving. Most commercial aircraft keep the cabin pressure only between 5000 and 8000 feet, not at sea level, so the pressure gradient holding supersaturated nitrogen in tissues is lower than that of sea level; thus according to Boyle's law, gas bubbles expand even more. Various authorities such as the U.S. Navy, the U.S. Air Force, and DAN have recommended waiting 24 hours between one's last dive and flying, since the probability of DCS developing decreases with time after diving.

Female Divers and Diving During Pregnancy

There is no agreement as to whether women are at greater risk of developing DCS. Possible factors that could predispose women to DCS are higher fat levels (on average 10% more than males), use of birth control pills, and menses. At present, the incidence rate of DCS in women varies between 0 and 3 times that of men. Menstrual patterns and ovulation do not generally seem to be affected by recreational diving.

Pregnancy is a contraindication to diving. Potential problems include morning sickness and intensified motion sickness, reduced respiratory function, circulatory competition with the placenta, decreased fitness and endurance, increased fat and fluid leading to DCS susceptibility, and mucous membrane swelling with subsequent difficulty equalizing the ears. Although many believe that diving can induce abortion or miscarriage, an English study revealed no greater rate of spontaneous abortion in pregnant female divers compared with pregnant nondivers. In comparison, there is a real threat of fetal death in utero associated with diving closer to term. Risks to a fetus include the chance of hypoxia or hyperoxia, physical injury, and leakage of membranes leading to infection. Decompression illness may alter placental flow leading to malformation, teratogenesis, stillbirths, spontaneous abortions, and preterm labor. Maternal bubbles are likely to be filtered in the lungs; fetal bubbles, however, bypass the lungs going through the ductus arteriosus to the open foramen ovale, which can have serious consequences.

There is no evidence that diving during menses increases the risk of shark attack. However, menses can induce migraines, which are themselves a relative contraindication to diving.

Asthma

Asthma has traditionally been an absolute contraindication to scuba diving but has recently been modified to a relative contraindication for recreational divers (although it remains absolute for military and commercial diving). In Australia any evidence of asthma still precludes one from recreational diving. Allergy and infection are the two most common trigger mechanisms inducing acute smooth muscle activation and bronchial constriction. With chronic asthma there is bronchial smooth muscle hypertrophy, mucosal edema, and secretions with mucus plugs. This leads to inadequate ventilation, increased total lung capacity, and decreased compliance, especially with increased respiratory rates. Arguments against permitting asthmatics to dive include the possibility that they may develop acute airway obstruction from breathing cold, dense, and dry air through the regulator; that an attack may be brought on by the exercise of swimming, stress, or aspiration of small amounts of water while diving with resultant pulmonary barotrauma and arterial gas embolism; that bronchospasm can develop rapidly during the dive; and that airway obstruction can be localized.

The argument for permitting certain asthmatics to dive is that statistics do not support the argument against diving. In reviewing all data on asthmatics and diving, one study found that asthmatics who have normal pulmonary function at rest and whose asthma is not exercise- or cold-provoked have a risk of pulmonary barotrauma similar to that of non-asthmatic divers. A study from the United Kingdom revealed that 104 BSAC (British Sub-Aqua Club) asthmatic divers with 12,000 dives logged were without pneumothorax or arterial gas embolism. Studies from DAN indicate that asthma is not a risk factor statistically, and sophisticated statistical analyses by others have found a nonsignificant increased risk of asthmatics underwater. Other factors that support diving by asthmatics are these: (1) slower ascent rates allow for better emptying of alveoli, (2) those at risk may be more fastidious divers, (3) small airways at risk have small air volumes, (4) 90% all arterial gas emboli are from panic breath-holding or out of air or wild ascents, which are independent of lung health and are behavioral errors, and (5) asthma is not a homogeneous process.

In the United States 15 million people have been diagnosed with asthma, a prevalence of between 4% and 6%. Three million divers have asthma (prevalence of 5%), approximately equal to the general population; approximately 20 million dives are made annually. There is no question that asthmatics do dive, even with medical advice not to, so this segment of the diving population must be realistically acknowledged. The BSAC has taken the lead in changing traditional recommendations by proposing that those divers with exercise- or cold-induced asthma should not dive unless completely controlled by medications (and no bronchodilator use for at least 48 hours), whereas well-controlled allergy-induced asthma is not a contraindication for diving if there have been no recent attacks.

It has been proposed that primary care providers can screen diving candidates with a thorough history and physical examination, but any suspicions should be referred to a trained diving medicine physician. The current fit to dive versus not fit to dive categorization is today a liability—a more accurate and reasonable system would be to stratify the risk. Those with asthma and normal maximal expiratory flow rates and normal lung volumes can be diving candidates; those with acute asthma should not dive until lung and airway functions have normalized. Those suffering from acute asthma should not dive until pulmonary function has returned to normal. Asthma is thus becoming a *relative* contraindication to diving, and those with active ongoing asthma still have an absolute contraindication to diving.

Diabetes

In general, fear of hypoglycemic episodes from exercise or an insulin reaction occurring underwater with the potential sequelae of unconsciousness or seizures, and then drowning, had led most physicians to label diabetes as a contraindication to diving. It has been consistently shown that under hyperbaric conditions glucose levels fall; however, most diabetics are quite adapt at identifying and compensating for swings in serum glucose. A DAN survey revealed that although diabetics do have episodes of hypoglycemia during diving, it is uncommon. Reports from the United Kingdom suggest that diabetics may dive safely and that high partial pressures of oxygen do not lower glucose levels significantly during a dive. New-onset diabetics may be best served by not diving while those who are long-term diabetics and who are well controlled can probably dive safely. If the diver is reliable and regularly checks blood glucose levels and maintains adequate levels, then that diver may be as safe as any other diver.

Cardiovascular

Myocardial infarctions within the past year, unstable angina, arrhythmia, and congestive heart failure are contraindications to diving. If heart disease is well controlled on medications, and there are no ongoing symptoms, then it may be permissible to dive.

Atrial-septal defects disqualify one from diving. Such conditions (such as a PFO, present in 20% to 30% of the population) may allow bubbles to pass from the right to left atrium and cause cerebral air embolization. Divers with mitral valve prolapse (present in 7% to 10% of the population) need a thorough evaluation to be certain that there are no other associated problems.

Hypertension may be an absolute or relative contraindication to diving: untreated hypertension is clearly a contraindication, whereas consistently well-controlled blood pressure should not preclude a diver from enjoying the undersea world.

Postoperative Patients

Postoperative patients who are symptom-free generally may return to diving once cleared by a diving physician. There is concern that postoperative scarring may disrupt the flow of blood to the area and perhaps increase the risk of DCS, but there are no data to indicate any worse incidence of DCS. It is advisable to ensure one has maximally healed and to takes precautions not to aggravate situations that led to the surgery, such as lifting heavy tanks after spinal fusion. Those with postoperative neurologic deficits should not dive.

Patients with ostomies have no worse risk of diving disease than other divers; those with airtight Kock pouches, however, cannot dive as a result of the consequences of Boyle's law.

A unique subset of postoperative patients are those who have undergone stapes surgery. There are many reports of barotrauma after stapediaectomy, but there is no consensus among otorhinolaryngologists as to restrictions of activities that may induce barotrauma such as air travel, snorkeling, or scuba diving. Despite this lack of consensus, no significant difference has been shown in the prevalence of barotrauma. Still, it would be sensible to advise such patients that diving after stapes surgery may increase their risk of inner ear injury.

Age

Older Divers

Older divers need to have a realistic appraisal of their physical and mental capabilities. Lung disorders, heart illness, arthritis, diabetes mellitus, hypertension, and other diseases can be relative or absolute contraindications to diving. Over the age of 30, exercise capacity and strength diminish, reflexes slow, and endurance drops; cardiovascular tone gradually diminishes, neurologic decay increases, and abnormal findings may be mistaken for DCS. Those 45 years or older or those with existing disease who are considering learning to scuba dive should undergo a thorough check-up including a stress electrocardiogram and begin a comprehensive conditioning program.

Youth

The age generally allowed for diving certification is 12 years old, although sport diving has no formal age restrictions. Among the prime considerations in allowing children to dive are the level of physical and emotional maturity (including the ability to cope with crises and possible impulsive behavior, which can be extremely risky and dangerous); proper eustachian tube function (and history of frequent otitis media or upper respiratory infections), which should match adult levels by age 12; strength to handle equipment and adverse diving conditions; and equipment fit, especially of mouthpieces and face masks. Young children do not have mature sinuses, pulmonary systems, or eustachian tube function, all of which are essential to safe diving. Dental braces are not a contraindication to diving. There are insufficient data on the effect of diving on epiphyseal growth plates, so some authorities conservatively recommend waiting until long bone growth is nearly complete. Opinions vary with regard to allowing children who have tympanostomy tubes to enter the water.

Sickle Cell

Homozygous carriers should not scuba dive; the risk of sickling is too high. Heterozygotes with low hemoglobin S concentrations should beware that there is still a chance that low oxygen tension may induce sickling if the diver runs out of air underwater or if any other crisis occurs.

Mental Illness

Psychology plays a great role in diving. Divers in general need to be calm, level-headed, and able to handle the pressure and stress of the undersea environment. People with anxiety traits and depressive illness ought not to dive; those with psychoses, schizophrenia, or history of suicide attempts are precluded from diving. Panic is the primary culprit in diving emergency complications, and divers with increased anxiety traits are at higher risk for morbidity and mortality. In approximately 40% of drowning deaths the equipment is functional, with air remaining in the tank or no signs of trauma or medical problems found; the most likely explanation is that of panic. There are numerous documented cases of divers removing their regulator or making uncontrolled ascents to the surface in cases of panic. Between 19% and 41% cases of diving fatalities may involve panic. Despite the obvious significance of panic and anxiety states in the undersea environment, however, little mention is made of it in most training manuals. Anxiety may be induced by internal factors such as DCS or hyperventilation; external factors include difficult swimming conditions, entanglement in nets or kelp, visual loss (as in a cave or in a wreck), shark encounters, equipment malfunction, other divers panicking underwater, or even from simply wearing a tight wet suit. In addition, anxiety, neurosis, depression, and extroversion have all been shown to be associated with ventilatory abnormalities such as hyperventilation and hypocapnia.

Commercialization of scuba as a sport has led to an unrealistic appraisal of the dangers present, and instructors may gloss over the risks of diving. This leads to inadequate screening of potential diving candidates, casual weekend resort certification courses, and subsequent increased costs from medical care.

Epilepsy

Seizures are an absolute contraindication to diving. This remains true even if controlled with medications: break-through seizures may still occur, the diving environment may increase the risk of a seizure, and an epileptic seizure that occurs underwater is likely to be fatal. Further, the diver's buddy is put in danger, as are any possible search and rescue divers called to the scene. Additionally, antiepileptic medications have some sedative effects that are ill-advised when diving. Other possible stimuli to seizure induction underwater include hyperventilation and exposure to higher partial pressures of oxygen as with nitrox.

Exceptions to seizures precluding diving are those specific situations from infancy and childhood that include simple febrile seizures, seizures from meningitis without subsequent neurologic sequelae, and seizures from breath-holding spells or from drug/medication ingestion. If a potential diver has any history of these conditions, a full neurologic evaluation, including EEG, is necessary. If the EEG suggests any epilepsy, then that person is excluded from diving.

For divers who have suffered head trauma, if a stress EEG is normal and the patient is not on anticonvulsants, then diving may be considered 6 weeks after the trauma. This rule applies only to mild, blunt—not penetrating—injuries.

Hernia

Unrepaired inguinal hernias are a contraindication to scuba diving. If a loop of bowel becomes trapped in the inguinal canal while underwater, a surgical emergency can rapidly develop during ascent as the gas in the bowel loop expands.

The Disabled

Many disabled persons enjoy diving; for them it is only a relative contraindication. Those who undergo proper and carefully guided training after careful screening do well and benefit both physically and psychologically from diving.

Alcohol

Alcohol impairs one's judgment and predisposes to the development of DCS. One should not dive while intoxicated or during the day after alcohol ingestion.

Medications

Often overlooked, the consumption of medications can have significant effects on a diver's health. For many compounds, the actual physical effect under extremes of, or varying, pressure is unknown. The short- or long-term use of certain medications may preclude diving, such as with beta-agonists for acute asthma exacerbations, suppressive seizure therapy, or antipsychotic medications. It is wise for travelers or divers to test a medication before traveling to see whether they develop side effects. If side effects do occur, they should switch to a different medication.

Table 10-1 describes some of the more common medications.

Hypothermia

Heat is lost 25 times faster in water than on land. The body reduces blood flow to the extremities, and this peripheral vasoconstriction attempts to maintain stable body core temperature (but vasoconstriction does not

Table 10-1
Commonly Prescribed Medications

Class	Comments
Analgesics	Need for narcotic analgesic indicates process more than likely a contraindication to diving. Depresses respirations and at depth may contribute to nitrogen narcosis. For the injured or those with metabolic processes requiring analgesia, diving should be postponed until off medication and situation has resolved. Nonsteroidal anti-inflammatory drugs such as aspirin are generally safe to use but are not advised in cases of DCS for fear of inner ear bleeding. Whether this has foundation has not been proven; they are used often enough in clinical hyperbaric practice that this fear may be exaggerated. Acetaminophen (paracetamol) is generally safe.
Cardiovascular agents	Beta-adrenergic blockers are inadvisable, as they can blunt cardiac response to exercise, and topical agents used for glaucoma can also induce bronchospasm and hypotension. Vasodilators may also blunt bradycardia of diving reflex. In addition, angiotension-converting enzyme inhibitors produce dry cough, which can be problematic underwater and can also interfere with sympathetic activity with the addition of bradycardia. Cardiac glycosides such as digoxin do not appear to have additional adverse effects under hyperbaric conditions.
Birth Control Pills	Data are sparse but show no increased risk for women diving.
Insulin	Under hyperbaric conditions, insulin-dependent diabetic patients have shown lower blood glucose and plasma glucagon levels. Insulin requirements may change under such conditions, but little is still known about insulin metabolism under pressure.
Sedative-hypnotics/ CNS depressants	Absolute contraindications to diving.
Antipsychotics	Absolute contraindications to diving.
Anticonvulsants	Absolute contraindications to diving.
Antibiotics	Do not appear to cause problems while diving.
Antimalarials	Mefloquine may induce emotional instability, dizziness, or lightheadedness in some travelers. Side effects have been mistakenly attributed to decompression sickness, leading to unwarranted recompression therapy. Risk of side effects must be weighed against risk of contracting malaria and if first-time exposure, dosages should be tested before departure to identify adverse reactions. If one has taken mefloquine previously without side effects, it is logical to continue using it, even while diving. For those with side effects or first-time users, it may be better to simply use Malarone or doxycycline as an alternative.
Antihistamines/ decongestant	The traveler who requires decongestants to dive is already at increased risk from barotraumas; these agents may cause sedation, a potentially dangerous condition while underwater. However, rationale behind taking decongestants is reasonable: pseudoephedrine has been shown to decrease risk and severity of otic barotrauma. One double-blind, crossover study of a common antihistamine (clemastine fumarate) did not show any increase in sedative effects of narcosis or increased arrhythmias.
Antimotion sickness	Aside from sedation, many have side effects similar to those of antihistamines and decongestants. Drowsiness underwater is not safe. Scopolamine, probably the most effective antimotion sickness agent, has been shown to be safe with diving.

occur in the head or neck). Hypothermia can be categorized as mild, moderate, or severe. Core temperatures of 35° to 37° C (95° to 98.6° F) are considered mild and patients are alert and oriented. Core temperatures of 32° to 35° C (89.6° to 95° F) are considered moderate; these patients have apathy, mild confusion, slurred speech, poor coordination, ataxia, shivering, coordination, fatigue, muscle stiffness, and a possible paradoxical sensation of being too warm. Shivering may increase the metabolic rate sixfold. At core temperatures less than 32° C (89.6° F), severe hypothermia is present. With such low body temperatures, lethargy progresses to coma, hypotension, hyporeflexia, cold-induced diuresis, dilated pupils, and cardiopulmonary arrest. In such situations, the heart is irritable and jostling can lead to arrhythmias; one may see Osborne J waves on the electrocardiogram. The heart may also beat so slowly that it may be unnoticed. It appears that repeat cold water diving leads to acclimatization via reduced heat loss and elevated metabolic rates. In general, the average survival time in water at 0° C (32° F) is approximately 1 hour. Paradoxically, cold also has a protective effect to the heart and brain. Recovery from prolonged cold water submersion is well known in children, but less so in adults.

Adequate thermal protection is essential for every diver, and even in tropical waters hypothermia is possible. In tropical waters, divers often wear little more than swimming trunks or a bikini. If the temperature of the water is between 23° and 26° C (75° to 80° F), it might be advisable to wear a thin body suit, which also offers protection against nematocyst stings. In colder waters thermal protection is a must. Neoprene wet suits are the most common type; water trapped under the suit is warmed by the body and becomes an insulator. Dry suits offer complete isolation from water, but if torn provides no thermal protection from entering water. Divers should keep warm between and after all dives.

EVALUATION/TREATMENT

Few physicians are trained in the diagnosis and treatment of diving diseases, yet most cases of such diving-related injuries present initially to emergency departments or primary care practitioners. Since delays in initiation of proper therapy correlates with worse outcome and the ease of modern long distance travel, physicians around the world must be able to diagnose and treat DCS and arterial gas emboli.

A history must include the dive location, level of diving experience, dive profile, rate of ascent, time of onset of symptoms and variations in symptoms, and type of gas in the tank. A fundamental question is whether the injured diver was using scuba or simply snorkeling; the latter would suggest that the diver is a near-drowning victim. Although most neurologic abnormalities associated with diving are from DCS and AGE, head injury, carbon monoxide or carbon dioxide poisoning, or marine toxins must be ruled out. Cerebral bleeding such as subarachnoid or intracerebral hemorrhages should be included in the differential diagnosis. Other pertinent information includes respiratory disease history, heart conditions, CNS diseases, and alcohol or drug abuse. Signs and symptoms of AGE are usually immediate or within 10 minutes of surfacing, whereas decompression sickness may present with a delay of minutes to hours. If information is unavailable from the diver, it can be obtained from the diving buddy or the diver's computer if one was used.

Physical examination should include vital signs and evidence of pneumothorax, pneumomediastinum, subcutaneous emphysema, and ENT barotraumas. The examination must also include a thorough neurologic examination including mental status; cranial nerve examination; sensory testing for pinprick, fine touch, and proprioception; motor strength and symmetry; deep tendon reflexes; and coordination with cerebellar and spinal function testing. A proper cardiac examination should investigate for the presence of PFO, which will likely require echocardiography. Ophthalmoscopy and otoscopy are also indicated.

Laboratory tests are usually not needed, since they do not help in diagnosis or guiding therapy. Since near-drowning may complicate or be the true cause of the condition, a chest radiograph and arterial blood gas should be obtained, but should not delay or compromise recompression therapy. Radiographic tests may be of utility, but should not delay treatment.

Divers who develop otic barotrauma must be able to clear their ears before continuing a dive; if unable to do so, the dive must be aborted. If symptoms do not improve upon surfacing, referral to an otorhinolaryngologist is recommended. If there are no objective tympanic membrane findings, one should not dive until nasal and ear symptoms are gone, and the diver can easily autoinflate both ears. Systemic decongestant-antihistamines can be used as well as long-lasting nasal drops. Nasal drops should be used for less than 5 days and use of short-acting nasal sprays should be avoided because rebound congestion and mucosal dependency can develop. Many divers rely on nasal decongestants to avoid otic and sinus barotrauma. Decongestants vary greatly in their decongestant and vasoconstrictive abilities, as well as in the duration of action. Short-acting decongestants can wear off during a dive, leading to a "reverse squeeze" during ascent. Using decongestants for long periods (>5 days) can lead to the phenomenon of rebound congestion when stopping their usage. If this occurs, concurrent oral decongestants can help wean the patient off the nasal form. If there are tympanic membrane findings, a hearing test is indicated. A myringotomy is occasionally required to relieve fluid and mucus from eustachian tube obstruction. Otic antibiotic or steroid drops are of no benefit if the tympanic membrane is intact. One may return to diving only after the tympanic membrane, middle ear, and external ear have returned to normal, which may take several weeks to months of abstinence from diving and reevaluation with pneumatic otoscopy, tympanometry, and audiograms by an otolaryngologist or diving physician.

With sick or injured divers, the fundamental ABCs—airway, breathing, and circulation—should be followed. Severely ill patients and those suspected of having AGE or DCS should be transported to emergency departments or hyperbaric units at altitudes less than 300 m/1000 ft, which often requires aircraft with the capability to completely pressurize the interior. Patients should be laid in the left lateral decubitus position, not head down as previously taught (to avoid increased intracranial pressure) and given 100% oxygen by face mask at high flow rates. Nasal cannulae are usually inadequate for this condition. For patients whose symptoms resolve while breathing oxygen, observation may be sufficient; for all others, more aggressive therapy is necessary. Intravenous fluids to maintain urine output and a Foley catheter are advisable, and, since CNS injury is exacerbated by glucose, glucose-free isotonic fluids are preferred. Oral fluids can be given to fully alert patients whose airways are not in danger. If intubated, then the cuffs on both the endotracheal tube and the Foley catheter should be inflated with water, which is incompressible, so as to avoid problems in the hyperbaric chamber. Glass intravenous bottles, if used, must be vented. Aspirin, lidocaine, and use of steroids are of questionable value in treating either DCS or AGE.

The patient should be rapidly transferred to a hyperbaric unit for recompression therapy if DCS or AGE is suspected. Delay is the main factor in not obtaining full recovery. Recompression with oxygen is *the* primary treatment for AGE and DCI. Recompression will reduce bubble size, resulting in a decrease or elimination of vascular obstruction and tissue distortion. Hyperbaric or recompression chambers are artificially pressurized vessels that can accommodate one or more individuals and subject them to an increased pressure environment with intermittent, high-dose, but short-term oxygen inhalation therapy. Breathing oxygen under these conditions creates a high oxygen gradient to perfuse ischemic tissues, increases inert gas elimination, and decreases bubble size and CNS edema. Chambers may be monoplace (one or two occupants) or multiplace (multiple occupant capacity); monoplace chambers cannot accommodate all diving treatment tables, such as the air embolism treatment Table 6A (165 feet). Recompression may be with the U.S. Navy Dive Tables using 100% oxygen or the Comex Tables, which use heliox in addition to oxygen and air. The U.S. Navy Dive Tables 1 through 4 are air recompression schedules and are rarely used; Tables 5 and 6 use oxygen, although Table 5 is not commonly used. For AGE, recompression may be with the U.S. Navy Dive Table 6A using 100% oxygen or the Comex Tables; the U.S. Navy Table 6A recompresses initially to 6 ATA—a "depth" of 165 fsw.

Thorough neurologic and cardiopulmonary examinations are important both before and after hyperbaric recompression treatments for gas emboli. With prompt therapy, the majority of patients with pulmonary overpressurization syndrome have full recovery. All doubtful or unclear cases should be presumptively treated. Although hyperbaric therapy should be sought immediately, delayed recompression may still be beneficial.

U.S. Navy Dive Table 5 is used to treat DCS I. It is a shortened version of Table 6 (by 150 minutes) and is effective under naval conditions where a diving medical officer is present to do a proper neurologic evaluation (ruling out any neurologic DCS) at the time of occurrence. If DCS recurs, the diver is conveniently close by the chamber. It is efficient for military conditions and needs, as divers are under shorter treatments and are thus available sooner for more missions/assignments.

With sports scuba, time-delay factors, including denial, length of transport, and delays in getting a chamber team in once called, change these considerations. With the possibility of a neurologic symptom being present at onset but not evident to the diver, discretion is advised, so the more intensive and definitive Table 6 is used, which also reduces the risk of recurrence. As DCS is often a vague presentation, a "trial of pressure" may be attempted in the hyperbaric chamber. Response to recompression can be diagnostic. It is an error not to treat doubtful cases, since omitting a treatment may result in irreversible damage.

Table 5 may used if there are pain-only bends, with a completely normal neurologic examination, with an onset within 6 hours of reaching surface and resolution of symptoms at 60 fsw (19 msw) within 10 minutes of recompression therapy.

Table 6, the preferred treatment table for DCS, may range from 4 hours 45 minutes to 8 hours. Initially, one is "dived" (treated) to a depth of 60 fsw (18 msw or 2.8 ATA) for a specified time and then is brought up to 30 fsw (9 msw) for longer periods. The diver breathes 100% FiO_2 throughout the dive except for "air breaks" to minimize the possibility of oxygen toxicity. If symptoms in DCS Type I cases resolve within 10 minutes on O_2, then modifying the course to treatment Table 5 is permitted, although it is quite common to complete the standard Table 6 to avoid recurrence of symptoms during decompression or after treatment is finished.

In water, recompression is inadvisable, particularly when there are hyperbaric chambers nearby. Aside from the inability to administer proper medical care, hypothermia is a serious complication when underwater for prolonged periods, even in tropical waters. Rarely, in remote areas where careful supervision is present, it may occasionally be life-saving. With the availability of portable hyperbaric units, it would be preferable to evacuate a diver in a portable unit to a proper hyperbaric chamber from a remote site.

When breathing 100% oxygen under pressure, there is a risk of oxygen seizures, which are *not* a contraindication for continuing treatment. Seizures terminate after stopping oxygen flow and having the patient resume breathing compressed air for 15 minutes. Oxygen-induced seizures are not indicative of underlying epileptic disease.

The success of hyperbaric treatment for decompression illness is inversely related to the time from symptom onset to chamber treatment: the more delay between symptoms and treatment, the less resolution. Only 28.8% of patients with DCS seek medical care within 4 hours of symptom onset and 6% present more than 96 hours after onset. Up to a 20% failure rate occurs in cases of delayed treatment. On occasion, symptoms may recur after recompression therapy.

DCS can have significant long-term morbidity. Even with treatment, some divers have persistent or recurrent symptoms. Cases of spinal cord DCS are particularly resistant to treatment. The later symptoms present, the better the outcome. A DAN Report on Diving Injuries revealed that on average, 16% of patients with DCS experience symptoms for up to 3 months after treatment; 35% have been reported to remain symptomatic even 2 years after recompression treatment. Recurrent symptoms most often were reported when individuals were deprived of sleep, had long work hours, alcohol, prolonged immobilization, or psychiatric morbidity. Some residual symptoms remain lifelong.

Despite the clear relationship between delay from onset to presentation for treatment, delayed cases deserve full attention; 90% of such cases had either complete (66%) or substantial (24%) recovery. Many patients have mild to significant improvement of DCS weeks to months later.

Follow-up hyperbaric oxygen treatments are used if residual signs and symptoms remain after the initial treatment. They are continued daily until no further improvements occur. Most individuals with persistent symptoms do not require more than 5 to 10 repeat treatments.

Hypothermia requires rapid rewarming. Rewarming is best achieved by removing the diver's wet clothes, covering the diver in layers with warm blankets, applying radiant heat, giving warm oral fluids (if fully alert), rewarming with warm humidified oxygen and warmed intravenous fluids. In critical cases, warm water/saline irrigation through a nasogastric tube or Foley catheter, peritoneal lavage with warm saline, or emergency venoarterial bypass are indicated. Extracorporeal rewarming has been used successfully but requires a well-equipped medical center. One should beware of "afterdrop," a further drop in core temperature after initiating rewarming, whereby warmed blood returning to the core may deceive the hypothalamus, leading to further heat loss by reflexively dilating peripheral blood vessels. An axiom commonly heard in emergency medicine is that "No patient is dead until they are warm and dead"; resuscitative efforts must continue until core temperature is at least in the mild hypothermia range.

RETURNING TO DIVING

To return to diving, there should be no increased risk of recurrence or of worsening tissue damage.

Otic Barotrauma

After middle ear barotrauma, once all signs of abnormality have resolved, the hearing is normal, and the eustachian tubes can function, one may return to diving. However, if inner ear damage has occurred, specialized evaluation and treatment are recommended before returning to diving.

Pulmonary Barotrauma

Previously anyone who had suffered an AGE was prevented from ever diving again because of the possibility of an undetected local air trapping portion in the lungs. Now it may be that one can distinguish a "deserved" versus "undeserved" episode. If barotrauma was deserved because of violating physical laws, then theoretically one should be able to dive safely after healing has occurred. In the evaluation for pulmonary barotrauma there are several tests available. For air trapping one may use plan film radiographs or V/Q (ventilation/perfusion) scan; for shunts one can use echocardiograms; for bronchospasm one can use methacholine challenge. No test can completely rule out pulmonary pathology. The U.S. Navy dive manual recommends not diving for 4 weeks after AGE with complete resolution when treated on a short oxygen table. Navy divers are working divers, so their return to diving is shorter than civilian sport divers who should consider waiting *more* than 4 weeks before returning to diving.

DCS

Risk factors for DCS must be explored, as well as whether it is behavioral or anatomic/physiologic. One may return to diving if there was joint pain only 48 hours after complete resolution on Table 5, but only after 7 days according to Table 6. In cases of neurologic involvement, one must wait a minimum of 4 to 6 weeks after complete resolution.

MEDICAL EVALUATIONS FOR DIVING

A certain level of physical and psychologic fitness is necessary to dive safely (Table 10-2). Medical clearance is recommended for all those who desire to take up scuba diving. Evaluation for the sport scuba diver should focus on the ears, sinuses, chest/lungs, and heart, as well as the mental state. Remember that divers dive in pairs; allowing a physically or mentally unsuitable person in the water thereby endangers two lives. Situations that raise doubt should be referred to a qualified diving medicine physician for evaluation.

CONCLUSIONS

Diving is an enjoyable yet high-risk activity that can result in serious harm to the unprepared or reckless diver. Several diving injuries and illnesses may result in serious morbidity and mortality. Travel health care professionals need to be aware of the risks, be familiar with diving diseases, and able to guide their patients toward healthy diving. It is impor-

Table 10-2
Contraindications to Diving

Contraindications	Description
Absolute	History of epilepsy (except for those explained in the text); symptomatic coronary artery disease; any atria-septal wall defects; history of cerebrovascular accident; dysrhythmias; emotional instability; sickle cell trait or disease; unexplained episodes of syncope; vertiginous conditions; inability to equalize middle ear pressures; cleft palates; bullous lung disease; emphysematous lung disease; spontaneous pneumothorax; tympanic membrane perforation (unless completely healed or surgically repaired); and untreated hypertension
Relative	Asthma and diabetes as explored above; migraine headaches (whose symptoms could be misinterpreted as DCS); middle ear surgery with prosthesis; history of previous pulmonary overpressurization syndromes; hypertension; limited visual acuity; a herniated nucleus pulposus (without neurologic or physical impairments).
Temporary	Active upper and lower respiratory tract infections; pregnancy; abdominal hernias (until repaired); recent orthopedic injuries (until fully healed); and lack of physical fitness.

Table 10-3
Recreational and Professional Scuba Diving Organizations and Resources

American Canadian Underwater Certification Inc. (ACUC)
1264 Osprey Drive
Ancaster, Ontario L9G 3L2 Canada
905-648-5500 phone 905-648-5440 fax
American Nitrox Divers International (ANDI)
74 Woodcleft Avenue
Freeport, NY 11520
516-546-2026 phone 516-5446-6010 fax
Defense & Civil Institute of Environmental Medicine (DCIEM)
1133 Sheppard Ave. West
Toronto, ON M3M 3B9 Canada
1-416-635-2000 phone 1-416-635-2104 fax
Divers Alert Network
The Peter Bennett Center
6W Colony Place
Durham, NC 27705-9815
919-684-2948
International Association of Nitrox & Technical Divers (IANTD)
9628 NE 2nd, Suite D
Miami Shores FL 33138
305-751-4873 phone 305-751-3958 fax
British Sub-Aqua Club (BSAC)
16 Upper Woburn Place,
London WC1 0QW, UK
OR, Telford's Quay, Ellesmere Port
South Wirral, Cheshire L65 4FY, UK
44-0151-350-6200 phone 44-0151-350-6215 fax

Table 10-3
Recreational and Professional Scuba Diving Organizations and Resources—cont'd

International Diving Educators Association (IDEA) P.O. Box 8427 Jacksonville, FL 32239 904-744-5554 phone 904-743-5425 fax
National Association of Scuba Diving Schools (NASDS) 1012 S. Yates Road Memphis TN 38119 901-767-7265 phone 901-767-2798 fax
National Association of Underwater Instructors (NAUI) P.O. Box 14650 Montclair, CA 91763 909-621-5801 phone 909-621-6405 fax
Professional Association of Diving Instructors (PADI) 1251 East Dyer Road, #100 Santa Ana, CA 92705 714-540-7234 phone 714-540-2609 fax
Professional Diving Instructors Corporation International (PDIC) P.O. BOX 3633 Scranton, PA 18505 717-342-9434 phone 717-342-6030 fax
Scuba Schools International (SSI) 2619 Canton Court Fort Collins, CO 80525 970-482-0883 phone 970-482-6157 fax
Sub-Aqua Association (SAA) 19 Harrier Drive Canford Marina Wimborne, Dorset BH21 1XG UK
South Pacific Undersea Medical Society (SPUMS) 630 St Kilda Road Melbourne, Victoria 3004, Australia
Surf Life Saving Queensland Inc. P.O. Box 2136 Fortitude Valley Qld 4006 Australia 61 73 852-14963
United States of America Underwater Federation (USAUF) P.O. Box 13754 Gainesville, FL 32604 904-392-0584
YMCA National Scuba Program 5825-2A Oakbrook Parkway Norcross, GA 30093 404-662-5172 phone 404-242-9059 fax

tant to know the most serious health problems associated with diving, how to recognize them, and where to refer when they arise. Table 10-3 lists SCUBA diving organizations and resources.

REFERENCES

Beckman TJ: A review of decompression sickness and arterial gas embolism, *Arch Fam Med* 6:491, 1997.

Behnke AR: *The history of diving and work in compressed air. Hyperbaric and undersea medicine,* San Antonio, 1981, Medical Seminars Inc.

Bennet PB, Elliot D, editors: *The physiology and medicine of diving,* ed 4, London, 1998, WB Saunders.

Bove AA, Davis JC: *Diving medicine,* ed 3, Philadelphia, 1997, WB Saunders.
Bove AA: Medical aspects of sport diving, *Med Sci Sports Exerc* 28:591, 1996.
Cresswell JE, St Leger-Dowse M: Women and scuba diving, *BMJ* 302:1590, 1991.
Davis JC: *Medical examination of scuba divers,* ed 2, San Antonio, 1986, Medical Seminars Inc.
Davis JC, editor: *The return to active diving after decompression sickness or arterial gas embolism,* 1980, The Undersea & Hyperbaric Medicine Society: publication number 41 (RW) 11-13-80.
Divers Alert Network: *Report on diving accidents & fatalities,* Durham, 1996, Duke University Medical Center.
Divers Alert Network: *Report on diving accidents & fatalities,* Durham, 2001, Duke University Medical Center.
Donald K: Oxygen and the diver, Flagstaff, 1993, Best Publishing.
Edmonds C, McKenzie B, Thomas R: *Diving medicine for scuba divers,* Flagstaff, 1992, JL Publications.
Edmonds C, Lowry C, Pennefather J, *Diving and subaquatic medicine,* ed 3, Oxford, 1992, Butterworth Heinemann.
Kindwall EP: *Hyperbaric medicine practice,* Flagstaff, 1995, Best Publishing.
Kizer KW: Diving medicine, *Emerg Med Clin North Am* 2:513, 1984.
Kizer KW: Management of dysbaric diving casualties, *Emerg Med Clin North Am* 1: 659, 1983.
Morgan WP: Anxiety and panic in recreational scuba divers, *Sports Med* 20:398, 1995.
National Oceanic and Atmospheric Administration (NOAA) diving manual, U.S. Department of Commerce, October 1991
Oriani G, Marroni A, Wattel F: *Handbook of hyperbaric medicine,* Berlin, 1996, Springer.
PADI, Enriched air dive & resource guide, Santa Ana, Calif, 1995, Professional Association of Dive Instructors.
Shilling CW: *The diving environment: clinical significance,* Hyperbaric and Undersea Medicine, San Antonio, 1981, Medical Seminars Inc.
U.S. Navy divers handbook, Flagstaff, 1996, Best Publishing.

CHAPTER 11

Travel Advice for Pediatric Travelers: Infants, Children, and Adolescents

Sheila M. Mackell

Caring for pediatric travelers is a unique challenge to the travel medicine provider. Each facet of travel medicine has special caveats relating to the different developmental stages, sizes, and maturity levels of the infant, child, or adolescent traveler. In addition, children traveling to exotic destinations require attention to basic pediatric issues. This chapter reviews specific travel medicine issues in the pediatric population.

AIRLINE TRAVEL

Occupying children with activities during long airplane flights is intuitive for most parents. Pens, paper, playing cards, and books are essential elements of the carry-on bag. Water and snacks are helpful to have during long waits in hot airline terminals and can salvage difficult delays in customs terminals. Special meals can be ordered ahead of time for children when planning an airplane flight.

Airline regulations vary regarding children traveling alone on planes. Generally, children less than 5 years old are not permitted to travel unaccompanied by an adult. The child's age and maturity level should be taken into account when considering whether to send them alone. Nonstop flights are preferable, and contingency plans should be set up, in case delays or cancellations occur. The child should be comfortable requesting help from the flight attendants and be told what to expect during a normal flight. Education on personal and stranger safety issues is best reinforced at this time.

Children under 40 pounds are safest in airplanes if riding in an approved child restraint system. Though not required, the Federal Aviation Administration (FAA) strongly recommends their use. Holding young children on the lap or buckling them in the same seat belt as the adult carrying them is hazardous during severe turbulence, rough landings, and crash situations. Federal safety standards have found that all child restraint seats manufactured after January 1, 1981 adequately protect children under 40 pounds on an airplane. A sticker stating that all applicable FAA standards have been met for airplane travel identifies appropriate seats. Child restraint systems without this sticker are not allowed on the plane. The airline's infant-seat policy should be checked at the time reservations are made. Many airlines offer discounted seats for children using restraint systems. Choosing off-peak flights may improve the chances of getting a free individual seat for the child or infant, but purchasing a full seat is the only guarantee.

Otitis media is not an absolute contraindication to air travel. There have been no published reports to date on tympanic membrane rupture while flying. Barotrauma is a theoretical concern when middle ear equilibration fails. Have the child or infant swallow during ascent and, particularly, descent to help the eustachian tube equilibrate the middle ear. Older children can be taught pressure equalization techniques such as the Valsalva maneuver to relieve the discomfort of middle ear pressure. Administering an antihistamine before the flight may help some children, but its benefit has not been conclusively reported.

Advice on sedating children with a weight-appropriate dose of over-the-counter antihistamine may be requested by the parent(s), and can be done while waiting to board the plane. Paradoxical reactions to antihistamines occur in a small percentage of children, and are best discovered at home, before the plane trip. Prescription sedatives should be avoided. An unanticipated side effect, such as respiratory depression, can be much more serious in-flight, where medical care is unavailable.

Past recommendations have suggested that infants less than 2 weeks old should not travel by air. Studies are ongoing to address this issue, as the question of air safety for infants is a topic of public concern. The avoidance of infectious diseases between birth and 2 months old is of prime concern to parents and health care providers.

MOTION SICKNESS

Children suffering from motion sickness present particular challenges to mobile families. Nonpharmacologic treatment includes sitting susceptible children beside a window, facing forward, and avoiding heavy meals before travel. Wearing dark glasses and nighttime travel may also reduce symptoms. Ginger preparations have not been tested in children.

Acceptable and safe medications for motion sickness in children are listed in Table 11-1. Over-the-counter preparations will usually suffice for mild to moderate symptoms. The use of promethazine should be reserved for children over 2 years with severe symptoms. Any of these medications are best given 1 hour before the anticipated symptoms occur.

VACCINE SCHEDULES FOR INFANTS AND CHILDREN

Immunization against common vaccine-preventable diseases occurs routinely throughout the first 18 months of life. Routine vaccination schedules have changed yearly in the last 5 years. The varicella (Var) vaccine is recommended for all children at 12 months of age and older. The measles-mumps-rubella (MMR) is now given at 12 months. Most significant, the polio vaccine recommendation has been modified to an all-inactivated PV schedule for routine childhood polio vaccination in the United States. In countries where the oral polio vaccine (OPV) is still used, the relative risk of vaccine-associated poliomyelitis, although very low, is believed to be minimized with the sequential schedule. OPV vaccine is advised for all doses in the primary series in cases where rapid immunity is needed as a result of travel to an endemic area, or if parents refuse IPV injections. The heptavalent pneumococcal conjugate vaccine (PCV) is recommended for infants and children 2 to 23 months of age. Influenza vaccination should be considered in all children older than 6 months traveling during the influenza season.

Table 11-1
Medications for Motion Sickness

	Dose	Comments
Over-The-Counter		
Diphenhydramine	5 mg/kg/day PO divided qid	Strong sedative effect; available in liquid form
Dimenhydrinate	2-6 yr: 12.5-25 mg PO tid, to maximum 75 mg/day 6-12 yr: 25-50 mg PO tid, to maximum 150 mg/day >12 yr: 50 mg PO tid-qid Adult maximum = 400 mg/day	Available in liquid form
Meclizine	>12 yr: 25-50 mg PO once daily	Chewable tablet
Prescription		
Scopolamine (Transderm-Scop) 1.5 mg patch	>12 yr: 0.5 mg patch behind the ear every 3 days	Apply at least 4 hours before expected symptoms; wash hands after applying; do not cut patch
Promethazine	>2 yr: 0.5 mg/kg/dose PO q 8-12 hr prn	Good for severe symptoms; may cause profound sedation

Minor febrile illnesses are not a contraindication to any of the routine vaccines. Simultaneous administration of vaccines is acceptable and does not diminish antibody response. Give live viral vaccines together or, if separate, at least 30 days apart. Current recommendations for childhood vaccination are summarized in Fig. 11-1.

International travel increases the risk of exposure to communicable diseases. It is important for a young infant or child going abroad to receive as much protection as possible against preventable diseases. Unique vaccine considerations exist for children, which guide choices before travel. Routine vaccines may have to be given on an accelerated schedule, with recommendations for extra booster doses. An acceptable schedule for accelerating routine vaccines is found in Table 11-2. Some travel vaccines, such as yellow fever vaccine, have a higher rate of serious complications in the young infant and are not recommended until a certain age is attained (9 months for yellow fever vaccine). Other vaccines, such as meningococcal polysaccharide vaccine, are not optimally immunogenic in children less than 3 years old. Still others, such as hepatitis A, are not approved for use in children under certain ages owing to the presence of interfering maternal antibody that limits vaccine response.

Hepatitis A is a usually a mild disease in children less than 5 years old. These children, however, can serve as reservoirs and infect adults and caretakers. Continuing to breastfeed traveling infants offers the advantage of added gastrointestinal immunity to enteric diseases. Immunization with the hepatitis A vaccine is recommended for child travelers older than 2 years without prevaccine serology testing. Foreign-born

Table 11-2
Accelerated Routine Immunizations Schedules for Pediatric Travelers*

Vaccine	Schedule
DTaP	6, 10, 14 weeks, and 6 months after dose 3
Measles, Mumps, Rubella (Accelerated Single Measles Antigen Vaccine plus MMR Schedule)	
Single antigen measles vaccine	6-11 months of age
MMR, 2 doses	12 months of age, 1 month after first MMR
Inactivated Polio Vaccine	6, 10, and 14 weeks of age
Haemophilus Influenza Type B Conjugate Vaccine	
HbOC, PRP-T	6, 10, 14 weeks, dose 4 at 12 months
Hepatitis B Vaccine	0, 1, 2 months. Give a booster dose at 12 months

* Give as many doses as possible of a vaccine series following an accelerated schedule before departure for international travel.

2002 Recommended Childhood Immunization Schedule Footnotes

[1] **Hepatitis B vaccine (Hep B).** All infants should receive the first dose of hepatitis B vaccine soon after birth and before hospital discharge; the first dose may also be given by age 2 months if the infant's mother is HBsAg-negative. Only monovalent hepatitis B vaccine can be used for the birth dose. Monovalent or combination vaccine containing Hep B may be used to complete the series; four doses of vaccine may be administered if combination vaccine is used. The second dose should be given at least four weeks after the first dose, except for Hib-containing vaccine which cannot be administered before age 6 weeks. The third dose should be given at least 16 weeks after the first dose and at least eight weeks after the second dose. The last dose in the vaccination series (third or fourth dose) should not be administered before age 6 months.

Infants born to HBsAg-positive mothers should receive hepatitis B vaccine and 0.5 mL hepatitis B immune globulin (HBIG) within 12 hours of birth at separate sites. The second dose is recommended at age 1 to 2 months and the vaccination series should be completed (third or fourth dose) at age 6 months.

Infants born to mothers whose HBsAg status is unknown should receive the first dose of the hepatitis B vaccine series within 12 hours of birth. Maternal blood should be drawn at the time of delivery to determine the mother's HBsAg status; if the HBsAg test is positive, the infant should receive HBIG as soon as possible (no later than age 1 week).

children from developing countries may be considered for serologic testing before vaccination. Recommendations have been made from the Centers for Disease Control and Prevention for universal childhood vaccination in 11 states of the western United States where hepatitis A prevalence is high (Fig. 11-2). Parents of children less than 2 years old can be given the option of immune globulin for the infant, although it is not essential, given the mild nature of the disease in young children.

Typhoid vaccination is similarly complicated by the choices available. The oral typhoid vaccine in capsule form is approved for use in children older than 6 years. A lyophilized vaccine preparation that reconstitutes to a liquid oral suspension is available in Canada and Switzerland. This preparation can be used in children older than 3 years. The injectable typhoid Vi polysaccharide vaccine is an approved alternative in all countries for children older than 2 years. For younger infants, prudent and cautious food and water advice needs to be emphasized. The heat-inactivated phenol vaccine, although approved for use in infants at 6 months old, carries a high rate of local and systemic side effects. Its benefit should be care-

Table 11-2
Accelerated Routine Immunizations Schedules for Pediatric Travelers*—cont'd

[2]**Diphtheria and tetanus toxoids and acellular pertussis vaccine (DTaP).** The fourth dose of DTaP may be administered as early as age 12 months, provided six months have elapsed since the third dose and the child is unlikely to return at age 15 to 18 months. **Tetanus and diphtheria toxoids (Td)** is recommended at age 11 to 12 years if at least five years have elapsed since the last dose of tetanus and diphtheria toxoid-containing vaccine. Subsequent routine Td boosters are recommended every 10 years.
[3]***Haemophilus influenzae* type b (Hib) conjugate vaccine.** Three Hib conjugate vaccines are licensed for infant use. If PRP-OMP (PedvaxHib® or ComVax® [Merck]) is administered at ages 2 and 4 months, a dose at age 6 months is not required. DTaP/Hib combination products should not be used for primary immunization in infants at ages 2, 4 or 6 months, but can be used as boosters following any Hib vaccine.
[4]**Inactivated polio vaccine (IPV).** An all-IPV schedule is recommended for routine childhood polio vaccination in the United States. All children should receive four doses of IPV at ages 2 months, 4 months, 6 to 18 months and 4 to 6 years.
[5]**Measles, mumps, and rubella vaccine (MMR).** The second dose of MMR is recommended routinely at age 4 to 6 years but may be administered during any visit, provided at least four weeks have elapsed since the first dose and that both doses are administered beginning at or after age 12 months. Those who have not previously received the second dose should complete the schedule by the 11-12 year old visit.
[6]**Varicella vaccine.** Varicella vaccine is recommended at any visit at or after age 12 months for susceptible children, i.e. those who lack a reliable history of chickenpox. Susceptible persons aged ≥ 13 years should receive two doses, given at least four weeks apart.
[7]**Pneumococcal vaccine.** The **heptavalent pneumococcal conjugate vaccine (PCV)** is recommended for all children age 2 to 23 months. It is also recommended for certain children age 24 to 59 months. **Pneumococcal polysaccharide vaccine (PPV)** is recommended in addition to PCV for certain high-risk groups. See MMWR 2000;49(RR-9);1-35.
[8]**Hepatitis A vaccine.** Hepatitis A vaccine is recommended for use in selected states and regions, and for certain high-risk groups; consult your local public health authority. See MMWR 1999; 48(RR-12);1-37.
[9]**Influenza vaccine.** Influenza vaccine is recommended annually for children age 6 months and older with certain risk factors (including but not limited to asthma, cardiac disease, sickle cell disease, HIV, diabetes; see MMWR 2001;50(RR-4);1-44), and can be administered to all others wishing to obtain immunity. Children 12 years and younger should receive vaccine in a dosage appropriate for their age (0.25 mL if age 6-35 months or 0.5 mL if aged ≥3 years). Children 8 years and younger who are receiving influenza vaccine for the first time should receive two doses separated by at least four weeks.

fully weighed against the 20% to 25% incidence of systemic reactions. This vaccine is no longer in common use in many countries where the alternate typhoid vaccine preparations are available. Table 11-3 indicates the recommended ages and intervals for travel immunizations. Table 11-4 lists important vaccine interactions.

Yellow fever vaccination, an attenuated live virus vaccine, is absolutely contraindicated in infants less than 4 months old. There is a risk of encephalitis in this age group if given the vaccine. Of 18 reported cases of post-vaccination encephalitis, 14 cases were in infants. Vaccination should be delayed until 9 months old. In infants 6 to 9 months of age, the yellow fever vaccine should only be considered if epidemic exposure exists. A letter of waiver for infants and egg allergic children can be provided before travel. Intradermal testing of egg allergic travelers can be performed prior to vaccination. The vaccine is not recommended for immunocompromised individuals.

Rabies vaccination (Chapter 4; Table 11-4, this chapter) is recommended for ambulatory children who will travel extensively (1 to 3 months) or live

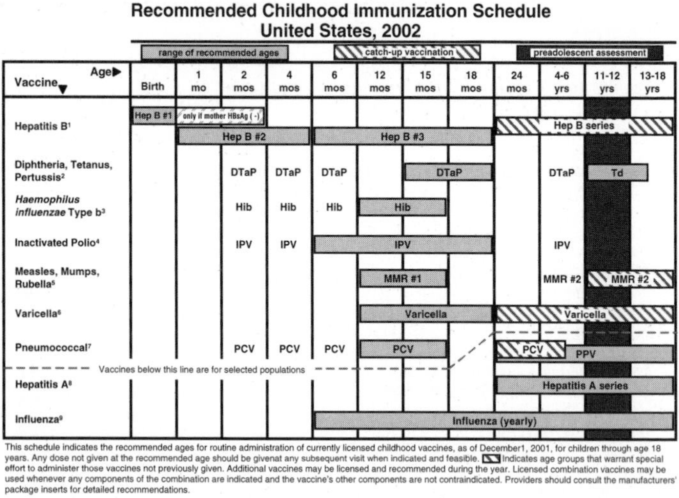
Recommended Childhood Immunization Schedule
United States, 2002
range of recommended ages
catch-up vaccination
preadolescent assessment
Vaccine
Age
Birth
1 mo
2 mos
4 mos
6 mos
12 mos
15 mos
18 mos
24 mos
4-6 yrs
11-12 yrs
13-18 yrs
Hepatitis B[1]
Hep B #1
only if mother HBsAg (-)
Hep B #2
Hep B #3
Hep B series
Diphtheria, Tetanus, Pertussis[2]
DTaP
DTaP
DTaP
DTaP
DTaP
Td
Haemophilus influenzae Type b[3]
Hib
Hib
Hib
Hib
Inactivated Polio[4]
IPV
IPV
IPV
IPV
Measles, Mumps, Rubella[5]
MMR #1
MMR #2
MMR #2
Varicella[6]
Varicella
Varicella
Pneumococcal[7]
PCV
PCV
PCV
PCV
PCV
PPV
Vaccines below this line are for selected populations
Hepatitis A[8]
Hepatitis A series
Influenza[9]
Influenza (yearly)
This schedule indicates the recommended ages for routine administration of currently licensed childhood vaccines, as of December1, 2001, for children through age 18 years. Any dose not given at the recommended age should be givenat any subsequent visit when indicated and feasible. Indicates age groups that warrant special effort to administer those vaccines not previously given. Additional vaccines may be licensed and recommended during the year. Licensed combination vaccines may be used whenever any components of the combination are indicated and the vaccine's other components are not contraindicated. Providers should consult the manufacturers' package inserts for detailed recommendations.

Fig. 11-1 Recommended childhood immunization schedule United States, 2002.

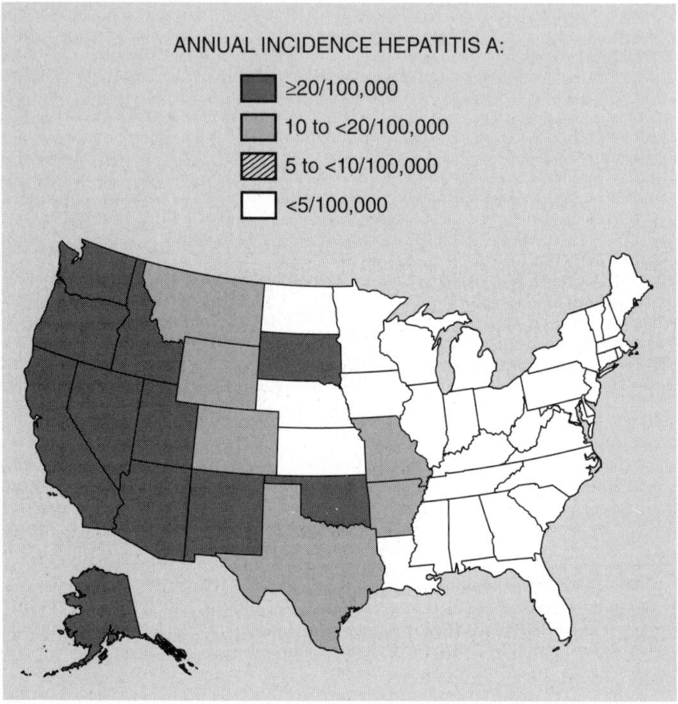

Fig. 11-2 Increased Hepatitis A in western United States.

Table 11-3
Travel Vaccinations for Children

Vaccine	Age	Primary series	Booster interval; comments
Cholera, oral (CVD103-HgR)*†	>2 yr	1 dose oral, in buffered solution	Optimal interval not established, manufacturer recommends 6 mo
Hepatitis A	>2 yrs	Havrix (GSK): 2 doses (0.5 ml IM) at 0, 6-18 mo later VAQTA (Merck): 2 doses (0.5 ml IM) at 0 and 6 mos	See text
Immune globulin	Birth	0.02 ml/kg IM	Lasts 6 wks; see text
Japanese B encephalitis	>1 yr	1-3 yr: 3 doses (0.5 ml SC) at 0, 7, 14 or 30 days >3 yr: 3 doses (1.0 ml SC) at 0, 7, 14 or 30 days	3 yr
Meningococcal meningitis	>2 yr	1 dose (0.5 ml SC)	Boost after 2-3 yrs if first dose was given before 4 years old
Plague vaccine	>18 yr	Not for use in children	
Rabies vaccine	Any age	3 doses (1 ml IM, deltoid [or anterolateral thigh in infants], or 0.1 ml ID) at 0, 7, 21 or 28 days	Only HDCV approved for intradermal use
Typhoid, Ty21a†, oral	>3 yr* >6 yrs	3 doses: 1 sachet PO in 100 ml water every other day 4 doses: 1 capsule PO every other day	Liquid vaccine* booster : 7 yr Capsule vaccine booster : 5 yr
Typhoid, Vi polysaccharide, parenteral	>2 yr	1 dose (0.5 ml IM)	Boost after 2 yr for continued risk of exposure
Typhoid, heat-phenol inactivated, parenteral	>6 mo	6 mo-10 yr: 2 doses (0.25 ml) SC at 0 and >4 weeks >10 yr: 2 doses (0.5 ml) SC at 0 and >4 weeks	Boost every 3 years. Less reaction if given intradermally; see text
Yellow fever‡	>9 mos	1 dose (0.5 ml SC)	10 yr; see text

* Not approved in the United States. Available in Canada and Switzerland.
† Caution, may be contraindicated in patients with any of the following conditions: pregnancy, leukemia, lymphoma, generalized malignancy, immunosuppression resulting from HIV infection or treatment with corticosteroids, alkylating drugs, antimetabolites, or radiation therapy.
‡ See manufacturer's package insert for recommendations on dosage.

Table 11-4
Vaccine Interactions

Vaccine	Interaction	Precaution
Measles-Mumps-Rubella (MMR) vaccine and Varicella vaccine	Immune globulin or other antibody containing blood products	Give vaccines at least 2 wk before immune globulin (IG), or 3-11 mo after IG, depending on dose and product received.
Oral typhoid vaccine	Antibiotics	Delay vaccine administration at least 24 hrs after antibiotics.*
Oral typhoid vaccine	Mefloquine malaria chemoprophylaxis	Schedule an interval of at least 24 hr between an oral typhoid dose and a mefloquine dose
Oral typhoid vaccine	Proguanil	Do not administer concurrently.
Rabies vaccine (HDCV) intradermal series	Chloroquine malaria chemoprophylaxis, and possibly mefloquine	Complete intradermal rabies vaccine before starting chloroquine; use the rabies vaccine IM series if the 3-wk interval is not possible.
Virus vaccines, live (MMR, OPV, Varicella, yellow fever vaccine)	Other live virus vaccines	Give live virus vaccines on the same day, or separate the doses by at least 1 mo.
Virus vaccines, live (MMR, OPV, Varicella, yellow fever vaccine)	Tuberculin skin test (PPD)	Do the skin test before or on the same day as receipt of a live virus vaccine, or 4-6 wk after: virus vaccines can impair the response to the PPD skin test.
Varicella	Salicylates	Avoid salicylates 6 wk after vaccine due to theoretical risk of Reye's syndrome

From Conner N, Jong EC: Immunizations for international travelers. In Bia F, editor: *Travel medicine advisor,* Atlanta, 2002 (in press); American Health Consultants, and CDC: *Health information for international travel 2001-2002,* Atlanta, 2001, DHHS.

*These recommendations are based on theoretical considerations; efficacy studies are in progress.

in rural villages in countries where rabies is endemic. The initial treatment of animal bites with soap and water first aid measures must be emphasized, along with the importance of obtaining postexposure rabies prophylaxis within 24 hours.

A tuberculosis (TB) skin test is recommended for children before, if the TB status is unknown, and after extended travel in tropical and developing countries. BCG vaccine administration in the United States is controversial. Some advocate its use for infants less than 1 year old if high-risk travel to rural, endemic areas is planned. BCG vaccine decreases the incidence of TB meningitis in this age group. Official United States recommendations for BCG vaccine administration are limited to (1) continuous exposure to an untreated or ineffectively treated person with infectious TB or multidrug-resistant (MDR) TB when the child cannot be removed from the environment, or (2) health care workers in settings of a high percentage of MDR TB and an unsuccessful TB control program. It is contraindicated in immune-deficient persons.

MALARIA PREVENTION

Personal Protective Measures

Malaria is transmitted by biting female anopheline mosquitoes, which feed mainly between the hours of dusk and dawn. The risk of exposure to malaria in an infant or child can be greatly reduced by the following maneuvers: (1) limit outdoor exposure during the hours between dusk and dawn; (2) wear protective clothing that covers most of the body when outdoors (a hooded "bug suit" that covers head, arms, body, and legs can be made out of mosquito netting, or is commercially available); (3) use DEET-containing (diethyltoluamide) insect repellent of 35% or less, sparingly, on exposed areas of skin when outdoors (see Chapter 1); (4) spray a permethrin-containing insecticide on external clothing (see Chapter 1); and (5) sleep under a permethrin-impregnated mosquito net at night (see Appendix for vendors and Chapter 1). The use of permethrin-impregnated bed nets has been studied in many rural malarious areas, with a dramatic decrease in the transmission of malaria, even when chemoprophylaxis is not being used.

The active ingredient in recommended mosquito repellants is DEET. DEET has been approved by the Environmental Protection Agency (EPA) for use in humans, but with specific warnings and directions. Child safety claims were removed from labeling in 1998. Brief exposure, following the label directions, is not believed to pose a health concern. DEET is recommended for use in children at concentrations of 35% or less. Although rare, reported toxicities include seizures, subacute encephalopathy, and local skin or eye irritation. Advise parents to apply it sparingly, avoiding the palms, and do not allow children to handle it directly. It should not be applied under clothing and should be washed off once indoors. A patch test on the antecubital fossa can identify children with skin sensitivity. Combination DEET/sunscreen products have not received EPA approval pending further assessment of potentially unnecessary DEET exposures. Specific EPA updates can be obtained at the website: http: www.epa.govpesticides and at the National Pesticide Telecommunications Network at 1-800-858-7378. If using both products, apply the sunscreen product to the skin first, then the insect repellent.

Some insect repellants containing citronella, lemon eucalyptus, and neem oil, and the Avon bath oil, Skin-so-Soft, have been shown to have limited effectiveness as repellants but no significant action against the

Anopheles mosquito that transmits malaria. Their use is not recommended for insect protection when traveling to malarious areas.

In general, protecting the traveling child from insect bites will decrease exposure to malaria and other serious infections spread by biting insects. Many of these infections, including dengue fever, encephalitis, filarial diseases, leishmaniasis, trypanosomiasis, and cutaneous myiasis, are not vaccine-preventable, so minimizing exposure is critical. The scratching of mosquito bites also predisposes children to impetigo in the tropics.

Chemoprophylaxis

Chloroquine is used to prevent chloroquine-sensitive malaria. Chloroquine can be used in any sized infant; however, its pill form makes dosing small infants difficult. Chloroquine can be obtained abroad as a pediatric suspension, but is not available in the United States or Canada in this form.

Mefloquine, the drug used for prevention of chloroquine-resistant malaria, is given to children using a weight-adjusted dose. It is currently recommended for use in infants weighing more than 5 kg. Contraindications to the use of mefloquine (seizure disorders, cardiac conduction defects, and neuropsychiatric disorders) are identical to those for adults. Doxycycline cannot be used in children less than 8 years old owing to dental staining. A new fixed-drug combination, atovaquone/proguanil is highly effective as chemoprophylaxis against chloroquine malaria, and may be used in infants weighing >11 kg. Primaquine phosphate is used for eradication of latent incubating *Plasmodium vivax* or *Plasmodium ovale* malaria parasites in the liver after intense exposure in endemic areas (Table 11-5 and Chapter 5). No studies have been done on loading doses of antimalarials in children, and such practices are not recommended in pediatric age groups at this time. A summary of antimalarial drugs and pediatric dosing is found in Table 11-5.

Children less than 6 years old usually have difficulty swallowing pills. Parents of the traveling child can purchase a "pill splitter" available in many pharmacies. After splitting a mefloquine or chloroquine tablet into the appropriate-size pieces, the tablet fragment can be crushed to a fine powder with the back of a spoon or with a "pill crusher" also available in many pharmacies. The correct dose of powdered medication can then be mixed into a spoonful of chocolate syrup or jelly (to mask the bitter taste) and given to the child. For older children, the portion of a crushed pill can be embedded in a candy bar or other sweet food. For infants weighing between 5 and 10 kg, one-fourth tablet can be finely crushed and mixed in a measured aliquot (10 ml) of breast milk or formula. The calculated milliliter dose can then be given by syringe, with the remainder being discarded.

Alternatively, if the correct dose for weight is calculated and prescribed, a pharmacist can pulverize the medication and dispense the proper weekly dose (with the addition of inert filler) into capsules. The capsules can be opened up and suspended into a spoonful of chocolate syrup for the weekly dose. Feedback from pharmacists and parents indicates that pediatric doses are much more difficult to prepare from the commercial enteric-coated tablets of chloroquine (500 mg). Generic chloroquine phosphate tablets (250 mg), if available, lend themselves more readily to pediatric preparations.

Antimalarial drugs are not secreted in the breast milk at therapeutic levels, so nursing infants of mothers taking antimalarials must also be given appropriate chemoprophylaxis. Parents should be warned that antimalarial drugs are extremely toxic and that the tablets should be stored in childproof containers out of reach of small children. Ingestion of one 500 mg

Table 11-5
Drugs Used for Malaria Chemoprohylaxis in Children

Drug	Dose	Comments
Chloroquine phosphate (Aralen)	8.3 mg/kg/wk (salt) = 5 mg/kg(base)*; max 500 mg/wk (salt), 300 mg/wk (base)	Use 250 mg tablets if available; very bitter; liquid preparation available in some countries
Hydroxychloroquine sulfate (Plaquenil)	6.5 mg/kg/wk (salt) = 5 mg/kg (base)*; max 400 mg/wk (salt), 310 mg/wk (base)	200 mg tablet; liquid preparation may be available
Mefloquine (Lariam)	**Weight** / **Dose*** 5-15 kg: 5 mg/kg/wk 15-19 kg: 1/4 tab q wk 20-30 kg: 1/2 tab q wk 31-45 kg: 3/4 tab q wk >45 kg: 1 tab q wk	250 mg tablet; no liquid form available
Atovaquone/proguanil (Malarone)	**Weight** / **Dose**† 11-20 kg: 1 tab/day 21-30 kg: 2 tabs/day 31-40 kg: 3 tabs/day >40 kg: 4 tabs (1 adult tab)/day	62 mg atovaquone and 25 mg proguanil pediatric tablet
Doxycycline (Vibramycin, Daryx, others)	2 mg/kg/day, up to 100 mg/day‡	100 mg tablet; contraindicated in <8 yr old
Primaquine phosphate	0.5 mg/kg salt = 0.3 mg/kg base daily × 14 days	26.3 mg (15 mg base) tablet; must check G6PD status; postexposure terminal prophylaxis for *P. vivax*

G6PD, Glucose-6-phosphate dehydrogenase.
*Start 1 wk before entering malarious area and continue 4 wks after returning.
†Start 1-2 days before entering malarious area and continue 7 days after returning.
‡Start 1-2 days before entering malarious area and continue 4 weeks after returning.

(salt) tablet of chloroquine resulted in death of a 12-month-old toddler. Chloroquine overdose in children has a reported 80% mortality rate.

Drug dosing for standby therapy of malaria in children can be found in Chapter 5. Parents should be urged to seek medical evaluation of any ill child and not to treat this potentially life-threatening disease without medical guidance.

DIARRHEA PREVENTION AND TREATMENT

Prevention of diarrhea in children is especially important during travel in hot, tropical climates, since children rapidly become dehydrated during diarrheal illnesses. Safe food and water selection is the same as for travelers in general, and is outlined in Table 6-2 and discussed in detail in Chapter 6. Breast milk is ideal for the traveling infant. Other milk should be boiled, pasteurized, or irradiated. Ultra-high temperature labeled milk, sterilized by flash heating to 137° C for 2 to 4 seconds, is also an available alternative that does not require refrigeration until opening. In addition to preventing diarrheal illness, meticulous attention to safe food and water selection will also decrease exposure to intestinal parasites. The worldwide burden of *Ascaris* and hookworm is carried mainly by children through ingestion of these pathogens. Hand washing, especially before eating, nail trimming, and wearing shoes are simple ways to interrupt transmission of these common parasites.

Preventing dehydration by oral rehydration with appropriate fluids is the first-line treatment of diarrhea in children. The World Health Organization's recipe for oral rehydration solution (ORS) is recommended. The molecular basis for ORS relies on a 1:1 ratio of sodium to glucose transport at the intestinal epithelial level. A powdered formula is commercially available in inexpensive foil packages that can be suspended in 1 L of purified water to yield the correct solution (see Chapter 6). Cereal-based oral rehydration therapy is also available. The rice cereal base offers a lower osmolarity and provides continued nutrition during the illness. Once the starch base is absorbed, twice the amount of glucose is released to promote intestinal reabsorption of electrolytes. In patients with cholera, the cereal-based ORS has been shown to provide clinically significant reductions in 24-hour stool output compared with standard ORS. In acute, noncholeric diarrhea, the effect is less pronounced. ORS should be used in place of milk-based formula and other fluids until the child is fully recovered from the initial dehydration phase of the illness. One half to 1 cup of ORS is recommended for each diarrheal stool passed in a 10 kg child. Practical recommendations for giving the required volume of ORS include using a syringe or a spoon, adding presweetened drink mix as some of the glucose source for both the color and flavor, and making it into frozen treats. The only contraindications to ORS are intractable vomiting, ileus, and abnormal level of consciousness. Slow and steady administration of oral fluids to the vomiting child avoids overdistention of the stomach. Parental education regarding early signs of dehydration (decreased urine output and tears) and quantities of ORS to use is an important part of counseling about travelers' diarrhea (TD).

Recommendations regarding medications used for prevention and treatment of pediatric TD differ from those for adults. Bismuth subsalicylate (BSS) and antibiotics are not recommended for prevention of TD in pediatric patients. BSS may be considered for symptomatic treatment of watery diarrhea in infants and small children. It should be avoided if fever or bloody diarrhea is present. The use of BSS is contraindicated in persons with aspirin allergy. It should not be used in children and teenagers who have varicella or influenza, or who have had recent exposure, because of the theoretical risk of Reye's syndrome. Each tablespoon (15 ml) of commercial BSS suspension (Pepto-Bismol) contains 130 mg of salicylate. Several studies have reported that relief of diarrhea was safely obtained in hospitalized infants and young children with a weight-adjusted dose of BSS equal to 100 to 150 mg/kg/day given orally in 5 doses for up to 5 days without adverse side effects. Both the salicylate and the bismuth levels were well below toxic ranges.

Antimotility medications (loperamide, diphenoxylate) are not recommended in infants or young children. One investigation on the use of loperamide at the standard dosage (0.2 mg/kg/day) in infants and young children did not show a statistically significant difference in duration or outcome of illness when compared to placebo. In another study, high-dose loperamide (0.8 mg/kg/day) was shown to reduce stool output in hospitalized infants. Adverse central nervous system events, abdominal distention, and ileus have been reported in infants and young children taking loperamide. This evidence precludes routine recommendation for its use as a self-administered medication in children less than 6 years old. Because it is readily available to parents over the counter, discussion of its indications and side effects is warranted in pretravel counseling. Loperamide may be considered for occasional use in older children if symptoms of dysentery are absent and a prolonged journey is necessary.

Bulking agents such as kaolin and pectin have little effect on overall disease and are not recommended. Probiotics including various species of the genus *Lactobacillus* are being studied for their effect in children. In the study by Oberhelman et al., there was a protective effect against diarrhea in nonbreastfed infants 18 to 29 months old fed *Lactobacillus* GG daily. The role of these supplements in traveling children has not been delineated, but it points to an interesting direction in diarrhea prevention.

Safety and efficacy influence antibiotic treatment of TD in infants and young children. Choices for treatment in children differ from those for adults. The antibiotics that are considered safe for pediatric use are not necessarily effective against some of the emergent drug-resistant strains of bacterial pathogens implicated in TD (Chapter 6). Among the antibiotics that might be used against bacterial enteric pathogens, ampicillin, amoxicillin, trimethoprim/sulfamethoxazole (TMP/SMX), erythromycin and azithromycin are considered suitable for pediatric use (Table 11-6). Ampicillin and amoxicillin, however, are unlikely to be effective against common pathogens of TD. Growing resistance to TMP/SMX worldwide precludes assurance of cure. It is no longer marketed in the United Kingdom because of concerns about Stevens-Johnson syndrome. Furazolidone covers resistant strains of *Escherichia coli* and can treat some strains of cholera. The *Vibrio cholerae O139* strain, currently epidemic in parts of Asia and South America, is resistant to furazolidone.

Quinolones are not currently approved by the U.S. Food and Drug Administration (FDA) for use in children less than 18 years old. Compassionate use experience with quinolones in children has not borne out the potential risk of the joint toxicity seen in experimental animals. A reexamination of recommendations on pediatric use is anticipated in the next 2 years. Many advocate that the benefits of a 3-day course of quinolones in children outweigh the risks for this potentially severe disease. Nalidixic acid, a nonfluorinated quinolone, has a long history of use in children for urinary tract infections. It is used in many countries for pediatric TD and is effective against some strains of *E. coli* and *Shigella* resistant to other drugs. Arthropathy has not been reported in children taking nalidixic acid. However, it has the same theoretical contraindications as fluoroquinolones, and is not approved by the FDA for use in children less than 18 years old unless the potential benefit justifies the risk. Obtaining informed consent is recommended if quinolones are prescribed for pediatric patients.

Given these constraints, a practical recommendation is to prescribe a therapeutic course of azithromycin in the travel medical kit for first-line antibiotic treatment of pediatric diarrhea. There have been no studies done to date to evaluate the duration of treatment needed for pediatric travelers diarrhea. A three day course of treatment is standard practice. If a second-line drug is deemed necessary because of allergy, parental anxiety, location, or duration of travel, a course of furazolidone can be given. If *Campylobacter* coverage is desired, erythromycin or azithromycin is preferable. Advantages and disadvantages of different antibiotics are listed in

Table 11-6
Antibiotic Choices for Travelers' Diarrhea in Children

Drug	Dose	Liquid Form	Cost	Coverage	Comments
Trimethoprim/Sulfamethoxazole	>2 mo old: 8-10 mg/kg/day of trimethoprim divided bid	Yes	Inexpensive	No coverage for resistant *Escherichia coli, Campylobacter,* and *Shigella*	Risk of Stevens-Johnson syndrome
Erythromycin	50 mg/kg/day divided qid	Yes	Inexpensive	Covers *Campylobacter*	Gastrointestinal side effects can be significant
Furazolidone	5-8 mg/kg/day divided qid	Yes	Intermediate	Less resistance among enterotoxigenic *E.coli* resistance; covers some Vibrio *cholerae**; covers *Giardia,* but 10-day course needed	Oral suspension available
Azithromycin	10 mg/kg/day	Yes	Expensive	In vitro gram-negative coverage; covers quinolone resistant *Campylobacter*	Convenient daily dosing

*See text.

Table 11-5. Alternatively, parents should be informed that if prompt improvement after first-line treatment does not occur, medical evaluation is indicated. The proposed treatment plan should be discussed in detail with the parents. Any medications prescribed should be labeled with the indication for use. Families should be instructed to seek medical care for the child with severe dehydration, vomiting that prevents oral rehydration, fever lasting longer than 24 hours (especially in malarious areas), grossly bloody stools, and symptoms that continue or become worse.

Dietary energy intake improves nutritional outcome in pediatric diarrheal disease. Early enteral feeding stimulates intestinal cell renewal. Parents can continue breastfeedings or restart full strength lactose-free or lactose-reduced formula in bottle-fed infants as soon as rehydration has occurred. Cow's milk products should be reintroduced gradually. The incidence of true postdiarrheal lactose intolerance varies. Severe rotaviral illness is the pediatric enteritis most likely to be associated with lactose intolerance and malabsorption, with rates reported as high as 60% to 80%. Most infants with mild-to-moderate rotaviral illness can return directly to cow's milk-based formula. Well-tolerated foods include the "BRAT" diet: bananas, rice, applesauce and toast. Starches, cereals, yogurt, fruits, and low-fiber vegetables are good alternatives. Foods high in simple sugars should be avoided in favor of complex carbohydrates until intestinal recovery has occurred.

GENERAL SAFETY FOR TRAVELING CHILDREN AND ADOLESCENTS

Toddlers should be carefully labeled with identification that is carried in a waistpack or affixed to their clothing. The child's name, birth date, citizenship, and passport number should be included, along with the telephone number and address of the appropriate consulate or embassy in the destination country. An active, curious toddler can easily wander off in a crowded airport, train station, or market. The use of a chest harness on the child with a tether to an accompanying parent or adult is strongly recommended.

In many developing countries, the car seat will need to be fastened to the automobile or bus seat for the small child who will do extensive land travel. A nylon webbing strap or a length of climbing rope should be taken along to use with the car seat.

Accidental poisoning occurs commonly at home, even with close supervision, and increased vigilance is needed during travel. Contents of the travel medical kit, particularly antimalarial medications, are potential sources of poisoning when a toddler explores a new environment. All medications should be kept in childproof containers and out of the reach of small children. New accommodations need careful inspection to make sure that contact with matchbooks, chemicals, cleaning solutions, and insecticide pads or coils can be supervised at all times, or that these items are removed from easy access. Poisonous plants should be removed from easy reach. Electrical outlet covers should be used. Supervision around swimming pools is vital.

All travelers to tropical and developing countries need advice about rabies prevention. The natural curiosity and friendliness that many children have toward animals should be discussed with parents. Children should be monitored closely to prevent animal contact while traveling. Older children should be warned to be cautious with all animals. Animal bites, particularly dog bites, in tropical and developing countries can be quite dangerous. In addition to the physical trauma and risk of bacterial wound contamination, rabies infection is of primary concern.

ALTITUDE

Children who accompany their parents to high-altitude destinations are at risk of developing altitude-related illnesses. The diagnosis of altitude illness is more difficult to recognize in young children. Nonspecific symptoms that cannot be verbalized, like irritability, anorexia, and headache, mark the onset of potential altitude illness. Rapid decent is critical if any questionable illness or behavioral change occurs. Several small studies have shown that infants and young children born at sea level are perhaps more at risk of high altitude pulmonary edema than adults. Viral respiratory illnesses appear to increase this risk. Children with chronic lung disease, cardiac lesions with increased pulmonary blood flow, or sickle cell disease have been shown to have a predisposition to develop altitude illness.

Precautions against altitude illness in children are identical to those for adults: acclimatization by slow ascent and sleeping at altitudes below maximum daily altitudes. If air travel to altitude precludes slow acclimatization, rest and avoidance of dehydration and overexercise in the early stages of the trip are best advised. Preventive medications, such as acetazolamide, have not been conclusively studied in children. For older children and adolescents who have demonstrated past severe acute mountain sickness, a weight-adjusted dose of acetazolamide can be considered. Likewise, there are no data on the use of pharmaceuticals to treat mountain sickness in children.

Infantile subacute mountain sickness is a distinct clinical entity that has been described in a small group of infants and young children several months after relocating from sea level to Tibet. Muscular hyperplasia of the pulmonary vascular bed appears to occur in an unpredictable subset of these children. The resultant pulmonary hypertension and right heart failure are severe enough to cause death. It is thought to be a complete failure of acclimatization.

MISCELLANEOUS ISSUES FOR YOUNG TRAVELERS

Diaper availability may be limited in some developing countries. The need to bring along an appropriate supply of cloth diapers seems obvious, but may prompt logistical considerations. Diaper liners can be helpful for disposal of stool when in remote locations. Advise families traveling to Africa about the Tumbu fly. Cloth diapers dried in the sun can have fly eggs deposited on them and later result in larval myiasis when used. Although work intensive, ironing cloth diapers and other articles of clothing dried in the sun will kill the eggs and ensure safety.

Toilet training can be interrupted when a change in routine occurs. Lowering adult expectations of traveling toddlers is wise. Older children may be reluctant to use unfamiliar toilets, so carrying an extra change of clothing and toddler pants is recommended. Using the toilet on the airplane just before deplaning avoids the problem of unavailability or phobia of facilities in overseas terminals.

Children are vulnerable to the cumulative effects of sun exposure and damage. Lifetime risk of malignant melanoma and nonmelanoma skin cancers is related to sun exposure that occurs before the age of 18 years. Sunburns in childhood magnify the risk. Avoiding midday exposure, when the sun is strongest, is recommended. Clothing and brimmed hats are the first lines of defense. Clothing made from tightly woven fabric that absorbs ultraviolet light is available commercially. Standard clothing, however, affords considerable protection. Sunscreens with a sun protection factor (SPF) of 15 or greater should be used on exposed skin. SPF 15 provides 93% protection from ultraviolet B rays, whereas SPF 30 provides almost 97%. Sunblocks containing zinc oxide or titanium dioxide offer the advantage of a physical barrier, rather than chemical protection. Any sunscreen should be applied liberally to children older than 6 months at least 30 minutes before exposure. Concern over excessive body surface area for sunscreen absorption has led to the recommendation that infants less than 6 months rely solely on sun avoidance. Reapplication is necessary every 2 hours and less frequently with waterproof varieties. Waterproof sunscreens are effective for at least 80 minutes in water. When traveling overseas, advise bringing an adequate supply of sunscreen, should it be unavailable while away. Sunglasses that block ultraviolet rays are also recommended to protect the retinas of children's eyes.

Many high schools send groups of students abroad for work or study. The adolescent traveling without a parent should be counseled, in a private session, regarding preventive measures against human immunodeficiency virus infection and other sexually transmitted diseases. Providing information on abstinence and safe sex practices, as well as advising against any tattoos or body piercings abroad, should be part of preparing these travelers.

A suggested medical kit for travel with children is found in Table 11-7. Any essential medications, especially for asthma, anaphylaxis, or chronic

Table 11-7
Recommended Medical Kit for Travel with Children

Medical card with age, weight, any important medical history, allergies, blood type, if known immunization records

Over-the-counter medications:
- Acetaminophen
- Ibuprofen
- Antihistamine (e.g., diphenhydramine)
- 1% hydrocortisone cream
- Cough suppressant
- Antibacterial skin ointment
- Bismuth subsalicylate/loperamide, depending on age
- Antifungal cream

Prescription Medications:
- Any regularly taken, with adequate supply
- Antibiotic treatment dose for traveler's diarrhea
- Antimalarial medication, if indicated

Consider:
- Antibiotic if child has recurrent otitis
- Injectable epinephrine kit, if history or severe allergic reaction to insect stings or foods
- Antibiotic eye drops
- Medication for motion sickness, if susceptible

First aid supplies/Miscellaneous:
- Thermometer, safety pins, colorful adhesive bandages, ACE wrap
- Sunscreen, lip balm
- Disposable wipes
- Syrup of Ipecac, and/or a bottle of charcoal mixed with Sorbitol, with instructions on use
- Oral rehydration salts
- Mosquito repellant
- Povidone iodine solution

For wilderness adventures, add:
- Thermal reflective blanket
- SAM splint

disease, should be labeled and carried on board the airplane. Any child with a chronic disease should have a visit, or at least a telephone consultation, with the regular provider before travel. Children with asthma need to update their asthma management plan. It is advisable to review the management of asthma exacerbations and carrying an adequate supply of inhalers and prednisone. Evacuation insurance is a prudent purchase for all travelers, since medical evacuations are not a standard part of U. S. health plans.

REFERENCES

A spectrum of sun protection, *Consumer Reports* May 1998, pp 20-23.

Bowie MD, Hill ID, Mann MD: Loperamide for treatment of acute diarrhea in infants and young children. A double-blind placebo-controlled trial, *S Afr Med J* 85(9):885, 1995.

Carpenter TC, Niermeyer S, Durmowicz AG: Altitude-related illness in children, *Curr Probl Pediatr* 28(6):177, 1998.

CDC: Yellow Fever Vaccine Recommendations of the Immunization Practices Advisory Committee (ACIP), *MMWR* 39:RR-06, 1990.

CDC: The management of acute diarrhea in children: oral rehydration, maintenance, and nutritional therapy, *MMWR* 41:RR-16, 1992.

CDC: The role of BCG vaccine in the prevention and control of tuberculosis in the United States: a joint statement by the Advisory Committee on Immunization Practices and Advisory Council for the Elimination of Tuberculosis, *MMWR* 45(no.RR-4):1, 1996.

CDC: *Health information for international travel, 2001-2002, Atlanta, 2001,* US Department of Health and Human Services.

DuPont H, Steffen R: *Textbook of travel medicine and health,* ed 2, Ontario, 2001, BC Decker.

Figueroa-Quintanilla D et al: A controlled trial of bismuth subsalicylate in infants with acute watery diarrheal disease, *N Engl J Med* 328(23):1653, 1993.

Gore SM, Fontaine O, Pierce NF: Impact of rice based oral rehydration solution on stool output and duration of diarrhea: meta-analysis of 13 clinical trials, *BMJ* 304(6822):287, 1992.

Gore SM, Fontaine O, Pierce NF: Efficacy of rice-based oral rehydration, *Lancet* 348(9021):193, 1996.

Hampel B, Hullman R: Ciprofloxacin in pediatrics: worldwide clinical experience based on compassionate use—safety report, *Pediatr Infect Dis J* 16(1):127, 1997.

Heath D: Missing link from Tibet, *Thorax* 44(12):981, 1989.

Jong EC, Montella KR: Travel advice for pregnant women, infants and children. In Jong EC, McMillan R, editors: *The travel and tropical medicine manual,* ed 2. Philadelphia, 1995, WB Saunders.

Kelly JC, Wasserman GS: Chloroquine poisoning in a child, *Ann Emerg Med* 19(1):47, 1990.

Lobel HO, Kozarsky PE: Update on prevention of malaria for travelers, *JAMA* 278(21):1767, 1997.

McCarthy VP, Swabe GS: Chloroquine poisoning in a child, *Pediatr Emerg Care* 12(3):207, 1996.

Motala D, Hill ID, Bowie MD: Effect of loperamide on stool output and duration of acute infectious diarrhea in infants, *J Pediatr* 117(3):467, 1990.

Nuutinen M, Turtinen J: Growth and joint symptoms in children treated with nalidixic acid, *Pediatr Infect Dis J* 13(9):798, 1994.

Oades PJ, Buchdahl RM, Bush A: Prediction of hypoxaemia at high altitude in children with cystic fibrosis, *BMJ* 308(6920):15, 1994.

Oberhelman RA et al: A placebo-controlled trial of Lactobacillus GG to prevent diarrhea in undernourished Peruvian children, *J Pediatr* 134(1):15, 1999.

Peltola H, Ukkonen P, Saxen H, Stass H: Single-dose and steady-state pharmacokinetics of a new oral suspension of ciprofloxacin in children, *Pediatrics* 101(4 Pt 1): 658, 1998.

Peter G, editor: *Red Book: Report of the Committee on Infectious Diseases,* ed 24, Elk Grove Village, IL, 1997, American Academy of Pediatrics.

Pickering LK: *2000 Redbook: report of the committee on infectious diseases,* ed 25, Elk Groove Village, IL, 2000, American Academy of Pediatrics.

Pickering LK, Feldman S, Ericsson CD, Cleary TG: Absorption of salicylate and bismuth from a bismuth subsalicylate-containing compound (Pepto-Bismol), *J Pediatr* 99(4):654, 1981.

Pitzinger B, Steffen R: Incidence and clinical features of traveler's diarrhea in infants and children, *Pediatr Infect Dis J* 10:719, 1991.

Rakita R, Jacques-Palaz K: Intracellular activity of azithromycin against bacterial enteric pathogens, *J Antimicrob Agents Chemother* 38:1915, 1994.

Schaad UB, Wedgwood-Krucko J: Nalidixic acid in children: retrospective matched controlled study for cartilage toxicity, *Infection* 15(3):165, 1987.

Scoggin CH et al: High-altitude pulmonary edema in the children and young adults of Leadville, Colorado, *N Engl J Med* 297(23):1269, 1977.

Statement on oral cholera vaccination, *Can Commun Dis Rep* 24:1, 1998.

Sui GJ et al: Subacute infantile mountain sickness, *J Pathol* 155(2):161, 1988.

Sun-protection behaviors used by adults for their children—United States, 1997, *MMWR* 47(23):480, 1998.

Theis MK et al: Acute mountain sickness in children at 2835 meters, *Am J Dis Child* 147(2):143, 1993.

Truhan AP et al: Sun protection in childhood, *Clin Pediatr (Phila)* 30(12):676, 1991.

CHAPTER 12

Travel Advice for Women

Susan Anderson

Travel health issues for women will vary according to the life stage and lifestyle of the women. Issues differ depending on whether the woman is in her second trimester of pregnancy or about to go on her first solo journey at age 80. To adapt the standard pretravel health recommendations to the needs of a female traveler, one needs to consider potential gender- and age-related issues with regard to susceptibility and long-term sequelae of parasitic and other infectious diseases, safety of immunizations during pregnancy, and adaptation of the medical kit for health concerns particular to the life stage of the woman. Other gender-related issues that may be important relate to environmental risks such as altitude or climate, or sports-related concerns.

Until recently researchers have paid little attention to either sex or gender issues in the field of tropical disease. If differences were considered at all, the focus was clearly on women's reproductive lives, assessing the effects of tropical disease on fertility and pregnancy outcomes. Gender and life stage issues are important when considering risks for travel and tropical diseases, possible complications, available treatment, and response to treatment. They are also important when considering preventive measures including vaccines and chemoprophylaxis. Biologic differences between men and women may affect the course of tropical disease, long-term sequelae, or response to treatment.

These issues are important to consider when we counsel female travelers about possible risks of disease before travel. For example, are the immunizations and medications recommended for a specific itinerary contraindicated in pregnancy? Can a woman on estrogen replacement trek safely over an 18,000-mile pass? Do the antimicrobial agents prescribed for malaria chemoprophylaxis or for self-treatment of traveler's diarrhea interfere with the efficacy of the oral contraceptive pill? What is a woman's risk of female genital schistosomiasis and future infertility if she is a Peace Corp volunteer working on a water conservation project for 2 years in a schistosomiasis endemic country?

GENDER-RELATED ISSUES IN TROPICAL DISEASE

Although there is a growing amount of research in developed countries with regard to the interrelationships between gender and health, few studies in developing countries have focused on gender differences with regard to the biomedical, social, or economic impact of tropical diseases, much less their impact at the personal level. For this reason the World Health Organization (WHO) section of Tropical Diseases Research (TDR) formed the Gender and Tropical disease Task Force to stimulate research on gender determinants and consequences of tropical disease. These include differences in exposure to disease, intensity of infection and morbidity, length of incapacity, care received or given during illness, access to and use of health services and impact of illness on productive and reproductive capacity social activities and personal life. The focus of WHO is on women living in endemic countries. We also need to consider the possible gender-related effects of tropical disease on female travelers living in endemic areas for extended periods and/or female adventure travelers involved in high-risk activities.

Differences between female and male prevalence rates are difficult to measure, as cases in women are more likely to be undetected. When incidence rates in women and men are equal, there are still significant differences between the sexes in both the susceptibility and impact of tropical disease. Even when tropical diseases are shared by both sexes they may have different manifestations, natural histories, or severity. For example exposure to malaria is similar in women and men, with a slightly higher incidence in men. Biologically, however, a woman's immunity is compromised during pregnancy, making her more likely to become infected and implying a different severity of the consequences. Malaria during pregnancy is an important cause of maternal mortality, spontaneous abortion, and stillbirths.

Likewise schistosomiasis is shared by both sexes, but genital schistosomiasis in women has been associated with a wide range of pathobiologic manifestations such as infertility, abortion, and preterm delivery. Changes in the female genital epithelium may be classified as hypertrophic with formation of polyps and papillomas or sclerotic with formation of fibrous tissue. Women may have lesions of the vulva, vagina, cervix, uterus, and fallopian tubes. Two cases of schistosomiasis prompted an investigation of the occurrence and risk factors for schistosomiasis among expatriates in Malawi by the Centers for Disease Control and Prevention (CDC). Of 917 persons serologically tested, 302 (33%) had schistosomal antibody detectable by immunodot blot; of these 292 (93%) had antibody to *Schistosoma haematobium.*

Parasitic infection as the only or concomitant cause of infertility in returned travelers has been rare; however, a recent case report found the microfilariae of *Mansonella perstans* in the aspirated follicular fluid of a former woman traveler who underwent in vitro fertilization with embryo transfer because of tubal pathology. She was also found to have a *Schistosoma* infection. Thus physicians may be confronted more often with parasitic infections causing infertility, not only in patients originating in tropical countries but also in Western women as a result of a tendency to travel and work in exotic and subtropical countries.

Further research is needed to clarify the general question of sex differences in susceptibility and differential severity of the sequelae of tropical disease infection. See Table 12-1 for examples of gender-specific effects of infection with parasitic diseases.

These issues are important when we advise women on pretravel issues, especially the long-term or adventure traveler. Knowledge of gender-specific risks for tropical disease is also important when we evaluate returned female travelers and recent female immigrants to the Untied States for health problems related to their history of travel and/or living in an endemic country.

Table 12-1
Tropical Disease Infections: Issues Specific to Women

Parasite	Issues specific to women
Intestinal Nematodes	
Ascariasis	Adult worms can invade the female genital tract cause tubo-ovarian abscess, pelvic pain, and infertility
Enterobiasis (pinworm)	Migrant females can ascend vagina to the pelvic peritoneum and can cause vaginitis and pelvic inflammatory disease
	Pregnancy can exacerbate symptoms of vaginitis and pruritis vulva
Strongyloidiasis	Lactation is contraindicated; larvae may be passed in milk to infant
Tissue Nematodes	
Wucheria bancrofti	Adult worms inhabit lymphatics and regional lymph nodes
	May affect breast, vulva, and pelvic organs
Brugia malayi	Adverse effect on fertility and lactation
	Elephantitis of vulva may obstruct labor and necessitate C-section
	Pregnancy may exacerbate edema and chyluria
	May be associated with hydramnios
	Microfilaria can invade placenta and the fetus
Trichinella spiralis	May disrupt menstrual cycle
	May cause abortion, premature labor, stillbirth, ? intrauterine infection
Trematodes	
Schistosomiasis	Pregnancy
	Acute and chronic inflammation of the fallopian tubes/ovaries can lead to salpingitis, infertility, ectopic pregnancy
	Lesions of the cervix, vagina, vulva may impede intercourse
	May need surgery before vaginal delivery

GENERAL HEALTH ISSUES OF WOMEN TRAVELERS

Basic questions related to health include the following: What is the woman's reproductive stage of life? Is she using contraception? Is her contraceptive method appropriate for her travel itinerary? Does she have emergency contraception? Is she prepared to treat the usual women's health problems such as urinary tract infections (UTIs), vaginitis, and menstrual cramps? If menopausal does she have estrogen replacement therapy or herbal medications for symptoms? What does she have for stress reduction? A format for obtaining a pretravel health history for women is given in Table 12-2.

Menstruation

Women between 12 and 55 years old menstruate on the average of once a month, with a high degree of variability among women. During travel, a

Table 12-2
Pretravel History for Women

Current Age
Menstrual History
- Date of last menstrual period
- Irregular menses/dysfunctional uterine bleeding (DUB)
- Menstrual products: tampons, pads, alternative options
- Premenstrual syndrome (PMS)
- Postmenopausal
  - Symptoms
  - Issues regarding estrogen replacement therapy (ERT)

Reproductive History
- Previous pregnancies, births, abortions
- Need for contraception/emergency contraception
- Pregnancy issues during travel

Sexually Transmitted Infections
- Men partners
- Women partners
- Both
- Diagnosis and treatment card
- ?HIV prophylaxis for high-risk encounters

Health Maintenance
- Vital signs: blood pressure, heart rate, and respirations
- Breast self-examination
- Mammogram

woman should be prepared for either the worst menstrual period of her life with more cramping and more bleeding than usual or for her periods to actually cease. Menses may cease or become irregular during travel for a number of reasons, not just because of pregnancy. For example, the mere stress of traveling, including changes in sleep patterns, diet, activity, illness, and time zones, can easily disrupt a woman's menstrual cycles. A woman should be taught about the possible changes and how to evaluate them. She should keep a record of her menstrual periods before travel and continue during travel.

It is important to carry enough disposable sanitary napkins or tampons for the whole trip, since they are not available in many countries. Recently a number of new products have been developed including disposable menstrual cups and a rubber device that may be reused for up to 10 years. Towelettes and plastic bags to dispose of sanitary supplies are also useful. Recommendations can be made regarding measures to take depending on whether she uses oral contraceptives, her previous history, and the result of a self-pregnancy test. A woman should be warned that just because she is not menstruating while traveling does not mean she is not ovulating. She still needs a method of contraception to prevent an unplanned pregnancy. Self-pregnancy tests are also important in the evaluation of a sexually active woman of reproductive age to help determine whether her abdominal pain and/or abnormal vaginal bleeding could be related to a pregnancy or some other cause.

Medication for menstrual cramping and other symptoms of premenstrual syndrome should also be carried in the medical kit.

Urinary Tract Infections

Women are prone to UTIs during travel as a result of multiple factors including dehydration, less frequent urination because of a lack of convenient toilets, fewer available facilities for hygiene, an increase in sexual activity, and other changes in exercise, diet, and clothing. Preventive measures include instructions for female travelers to stay well hydrated and to urinate wherever there is convenient access to a public toilet whether or not the bladder is full. The ideal outfit for a woman would be a free-flowing skirt or similar attire that would make it easy to urinate in the squatting position whether in a pit toilet or anywhere outdoors. A woman might want to practice this technique a few times so she will have the confidence that she can get in and out of the position innocuously to urinate in public without embarrassment. A number of plastic and paper funnel devices have been designed so that a women may urinate in the standing position. These require some practice to avoid urinating on oneself. They are especially useful in extremes of cold weather and altitude when a woman might not want to wear a skirt or pull down her pants. To maintain hygiene in unexpected places, it is important to carry a supply of paper tissues or toilet paper and some packets of premoistened towelettes in a fannypack or backpack. If an older woman is experiencing vaginal dryness and urinary frequency or urgency without dysuria, recent data suggest that estrogen vaginal creams or even an oral contraceptive pill intravaginally once a week may decrease urogential dryness and frequency symptoms.

If a woman experiences increased frequency, urgency, and dysuria, she should be advised how to diagnose and treat herself for a UTI with an antibiotic and an analgesic.

If an older women has a problem with stress incontinence or bladder control, she should consult with a physician specializing in female urinary tract problems in advance of the anticipated trip. For minor problems a women can be taught to do Kegel exercises and bring a supply of panty liners.

Vaginitis

Women are at risk for vaginitis during travel, secondary to many of the same reasons as for UTI. One of the most common causes of vaginitis is *Candida albicans.* This organism usually causes a thick cottage cheese-like white discharge with vulvar and vaginal itching. The risk of yeast vaginitis may be greater if doxycycline is used for malaria chemoprophylaxis or if other broad-spectrum antibiotics are used for the treatment of traveler's diarrhea or some other infectious problem such as infections of the respiratory or urinary tract.

Several topical preparations against yeast are available over the counter including nystatin, miconazole, and chlortrimazole vaginal creams or troches. Prescriptions for resistant cases can be recommended such as terazole vaginal cream (3 days) or fluconazole (150 mg as a single oral dose). Many women would prefer to use the oral medication, as the vaginal creams can be messy during travel. Other women feel the vaginal creams help with the symptoms of itching. A hydrocortisone cream may also be used if needed for vulvar itching. Any persistent symptoms should be evaluated by her gynecologist when returning home. Even if a woman has never had vaginitis, it is important to prepare her for the possibility, especially for extended travel. Another common cause of vaginal discharge is bacterial vaginosis. This is caused by overgrowth of the bacteria in the vagina, which can be due to many of the same causes listed previously. The discharge is usually more of a grayish color with a fishy odor. Bacterial vaginosis is treated with metroniadazole or clindamycin vaginal cream or oral tablets. If a female traveler has a new discharge and pelvic pain after a new sexual encounter, she may have a sexually transmitted disease and should follow the recommendations discussed in Chapters 36 through 39.

Contraception

Contraceptive advice should be included in the pretravel counseling for all women of reproductive age at risk for pregnancy. It should also be included in the pretravel counseling for men who might put women at risk for pregnancy. This is especially important if the man's partner might be in a country where she might not have easy access to contraception.

The number of women traveling who become pregnant as a result of a lack or misuse of contraception is much higher than would be expected. If a woman is already using contraception, the method should be evaluated for its ease of use and reliability during travel along with any special recommendations concerning its use during travel. If a women wishes to try a new contraceptive method, ideally she should begin months before travel, especially if she is planning to be overseas long term or will be living in a remote area. Back-up plans for what the woman should do if she loses her present method should be discussed. For example, if she is on oral contraceptives and the packages are lost or stolen what should she do? The International Planned Parenthood Federation (IPPF) keeps a worldwide guide to contraceptives and an address list of family planning agencies. A woman's itinerary can be reviewed and the possible alternatives can be looked up in the Directory. The Federation address is IPPF, 120 Wall Street, 9th Floor, New York, NY 10005. There are a variety of new methods including barrier and hormonal methods. There is also a "fancy personal computer" for the high-end traveler. Table 12-3 lists common contraceptive methods.

Special Considerations for Women on Oral Contraceptives

Women should be advised to take extra supplies of their oral contraceptives with them, since it may be difficult to find the exact brand in another country. An empty package should be kept in case she needs help from the local pharmacist to find an alternative. It may be difficult to remember to take an oral contraceptive pill when traveling because of changes in time zones and schedule. It is advised that the woman set a special wristwatch alarm, dedicated to oral contraceptive dosing control, for every 24 hours. This is especially important with the low dose combined and progestin only pills. Another problem is pill absorption during illness. Nausea and vomiting and/or diarrhea may cause decreased pill absorption. If vomiting occurs within 3 hours of taking a pill she should take another one. If nausea and vomiting and/or diarrhea are persistent, the woman should consider using another contraceptive method for the rest of the month. Another option might be to insert the oral contraceptive pill in her vagina for absorption. A number of studies have supported the use of vaginal absorption of oral contraceptives in either the pill or the ring form as a method of contraception or estrogen replacement.

Text continued on p. 196

Table 12-3
Common Contraceptive Choices

Methods	Mechanism	Advantages/disadvantages	Travel issues
Barrier Methods			
Spermicides creams, jellies, foams, melting suppositories, sponges, foaming tablets, films	Surface active agents which damage the cell membranes of sperm, bacteria and viruses	Chronic exposure may cause mucosal injury that increases risk for HIV transmission	Easy to carry Readily available Bring own supplies Female controlled
Cap	Mechanical barrier Requires spermicide	Requires clinician fitting Can use for up to 48 hours Needs practice to use Small risk for TSS	Easy to carry Rubber may deteriorate in heat and humidity
Sponge	Polyurethane sponge containing nonoxynol-9 protects for 24 hr no matter how many times intercourse occurs Leave in place for 6 hours after intercourse	One size Over the counter Moisten with water before use and insert Loop for removal Do not wear longer than 24-30 hr owing to risk for TSS	Easy to carry, use Use bottled water for moistening in countries with questionable water supply
Diaphragm	Domed-shaped rubber cup Must use with spermicide Protection for 6 hr	Requires clinician fitting Insert extra spermicide with repeated intercourse After use leave in for 6 hr	Carry in climate-resistant case Spermicide may not be available in developing countries
Condom			
Female condom (Reality)	Polyurethane pouch Spermicide not required One use only	Can be inserted 8 hours prior	Female controlled Bring supply from United States Does not deteriorate in heat and humidity

Male condom	Latex	Possible allergy Do not use oil-based lubricants	Male controlled Quality varies country to country Bring supply from United States of latex and polyurethane types
	Polyurethane	Thinner/stronger, more resistant to deterioration Can use oil based lubricants	
	Lambskin/natural	Small pores permit passages of viruses-hep B, HSV, HIV Use only for contraception Brands and materials differ in quality	May break down in heat and humidity. Carry in special case Use EC if condom breaks or slips and no backup method in place (OCP/diaphragm/sponge/etc) Store in cool, dry place
Hormonal Methods			
Progestin only pills	Inhibition of ovulation (may occasionally ovulate) Thickened and suppressed cervical mucus Suppression of midcycle LH and FSH	Use if cannot take estrogen Take same type of pill every day (no pill-free week) Decreased menstrual cramps, less bleeding Can use when breastfeeding Older women, smokers can use	Need to be prepared for irregular bleeding MUST take pill at same time every day (set alarm watch to help with time zone changes) MUST use additional method for protection against STDs
Combined pill Estrogen and progesterone	Inhibition of ovulation Many different types Monophasic Triphasic	Increased menstrual cycle regularity Less blood loss Less cramping Less ectopic pregnancy Less PID Fewer cysts Fewer fibroids Less endometriosis If nausea and vomiting need to take back up method or consider placing pill in vagina for absorption May use as EC; check instructions	Convenient, effective, easy to carry Need to take every 24 hours May use to delay menses by starting next package of active pills after 3 weeks of previous package Consider drug interactions Bring supply from United States; research availability of OCP and or other method to use if OCP lost or stolen See IPPF guide to Hormonal Contraception

Continued

Table 12-3
Common Contraceptive Choices—cont'd

Methods	Mechanism	Advantages/disadvantages	Travel issues
Hormonal Methods—cont'd			
Depo-Provera	IM 150 mg dose administered every 3 months blocks LH surge and ovulation	Side effects: Weight gain, menstrual irregularities, acne, mood changes, decreased libido, osteoporosis, good for women who can't take estrogen	Use when there are compliance issues (e.g., unable to remember OCP) Need dose every 3 months (may be difficult to get if traveling) Need to be prepared for irregular bleeding
Norplant 1 and Norplant 2	6 or 2 thin permeable Silastic capsules which contain the synthetic progestin levonorgestrel	Menstrual irregularities Implants difficult to remove, may be broken No protection against STDs Side effects: Weight gain, acne, alopecia Contraindications include thrombophlebitis, liver disease, liver tumors, breast cancer, and pregnancy	Long-term protection 3-5 years May be difficult to remove when traveling Need to be prepared for irregular bleeding Amenorrhea may be positive side effect, need fewer menstrual supplies
Transdermal patch (Evra)	One patch/wk × 3 wk, followed by 1 wk patch free Each 20 cm^2 patch contains 6 mg progesterone norelgestromin and 0.75 mg ethinyl estradiol	Side effects and contraindications similar to combined OCP Good alternative to remembering daily dose of pill	More reliable in traveling across multiple time zones Absorption not affected by GI illness
Vaginal ring (Nuvaring)	Flexible, colorless vaginal ring used for 3 wk followed by 1 wk ring free Releases combinatin of progestin with estrogen for absorption across vaginal wall	Side effects and contraindications similar to combined OCP Ring can be removed for up to 3 hr without losing efficacy (e.g., intercourse)	More reliable in traveling across multiple time zones Absorption not affected by GI illness

IUD			
Only 2 approved for use in United States (others available worldwide)	Inhibition of sperm migration, fertilization and ovum transport Creates spermicidal environment by provoking a sterile inflammatory reaction that is toxic to sperm and implantation	Main risk of IUD induced infection: -at insertion -more than one partner Medical risks: -history of PID -STD/HIV risk factors -pregnancy -abnormal bleeding -impaired immunity History of ectopic pregnancy -impaired coagulation (ITP, Coumadin) -anemia <28% -anatomic difficulty (fibroids, other)	Great for some women -parous -one sexual partner -no other risk factors as listed Need to know how to check for string
Progesterone T Replace every year	T-shaped IUD composed of ethylene/vinyl copolymer contains titanium dioxide Vertical stem holds progesterone dispensed in silicone fluid.		Need to know what to do in case of emergency Back-up method if falls out Need to protect against STDs
Copper T 380A Replace every 10 years	T-shaped polyurethane frame holding 380 mg of exposed surface of copper		Good for 10 years Need fewer supplies
Future Methods of Contraception Presently in Clinical Trials and/or Available in Other Countries			
Mechanical Barrier Methods	Mechanism and use		Travel Issues
Lea's Shield (available in Canada and Europe)	Silicone rubber cap one size fits all oval bowl that looks like a loose-fitting cervical cap Recommended for use with spermicidal jelly Does not require clinician fitting Has a loop for easy removal Should be left in place for at least 8 hours after intercourse Can be worn for 48 hours Replace one a year		Easy to transport Carry in climate-resistant case Rubber may deteriorate in heat
Fem Cap	Silicone rubber sailor hat shaped cap is intended for use with or without spermicide Two sizes being tested; clinician fitting required Can be worn up to 48 hours Phase III clinical trials involving 800 women at 10 university health centers; 5% failure rate		Easy to carry Use Do not need spermicide

Continued

Table 12-3
Common Contraceptive Choices—cont'd

Future Methods of Contraception Presently in Clinical Trials and/or Available in Other Countries—cont'd		
Gyneseal (Made in Australia)	Unique two-part chamber designed in Australia as either a menstrual blood collection device (like a tampon) and/or a contraceptive barrier Inner diaphragm-shaped chamber drains through a one-way valve into an outer collection chamber that clings by suction to the vaginal vault. Inner part seals to the outer part so that blood or secretions do not stay in contact with the cervix and do not leak into the vaginal vault	Could be used during menstrual periods and for contraception Less to carry!
Oves (Made in France)	Shaped like the Prentiff cervical cap Disposable device made of thinner, softer silicone rubber designed for one time use with spermicide Dow chemical recently acquired rights to product May be developed as a vehicle to deliver medicines transvaginally rather than as a contraceptive device Vaginal mucosa provides a good adsorptive surface for administering medicines (used by women taking EC or chemotherapy who experience so much nausea they can't take their oral medicines; can place pills high in vagina and achieve good systemic levels)	Disposable Need enough for entire trip *May also be used to promote vaginal absorption of medicine in case of nausea and vomiting*
Protectaid Sponge (Available in Canada)	Soft polyurethane sponge impregnated with a F-5 gel dispersing agent and 3 spermicides Works as a physical barrier, protecting the cervix Chemical action of spermicides Reservoir of gel (continuous release) Absorption of semen, no leakage Leave in for at least 6 hr after intercourse Can be kept in for 12 hours May have repeated acts of intercourse during that period	Easy to use Easy to carry in individual packets Available without a prescription
Disposable diaphragms	Two diaphragms that release spermicide are being tested in clinical safety trials They may be used up to 24 hours with multiple acts of intercourse	Easy to use No spermicide required

"Computerized" Natural Family Planning		
Persona	Hand-held monitor. Computer reads, stores, and analyzes hormonal cycle data from urine tests to give feedback on safe sex times. Becomes more accurate with time as computer gets to know your cycle Uses urine test to monitor hormone level	Available from UK $185.00
Bioself Fertility Indicator	Electronic fertility indicator Identifies both period of maximum fertility (most favorable days for conceiving a child) and the infertile period during which contraception is not possible	$100.00
Lady Comp	Microcomputer equipped with a thermic sensor that allows the user to measure the body's basal body temperature in the mouth first thing in the morning A sophisticated program takes charge to determine actual fertility of the day based on the measurement of the last 10 years Provides an indication of currents fertility, a prognosis for fertility for next 6 days, a prognosis for impregnation, and prognosis of menstruation	Available for $700.00 From German manufacturer
Baby Comp	Microcomputer similar to above that can be used for contraceptive purposes to assess least fertile days or for help in conceiving on most fertile days	$900.00 from German manufacturer
Clear Plan Fertility Monitor	Identifies a women's fertile days about 6 per month. Allows women to avoid or maximize chance of pregnancy	$200.00
PFT 1-2-3- KIT	Combines a powerful compact microscope with multicolored slides to distinguish fertile days from nonfertile days Used to pinpoint ovulation enabling her to avoid or achieve pregnancy	

Adapted from Contraceptive Report 1994, Contraceptive Technology 1998, Web sites on Contraception.

HIV, Human immunodeficiency virus; *TSS,* toxic shock syndrome; *HSV,* herpes simplex virus; *EC,* emergency contraception; *OCP,* oral contraceptive pill; *LH,* luteinizing hormone; *FSH,* follicle-stimulating hormone; *STD,* sexually transmitted disease; *PID,* pelvic inflammatory disease; *IPPF,* International Planned Parenthood Federation; *ITP,* idiopathic thrombocytopenic purpura.

Women should be reminded to take adequate supplies abroad because obtaining the same brand while traveling can be difficult and time consuming. Many low-income countries may have only higher dose contraceptives. The IPPF book on Hormonal Contraception can be used to see what might be available according to the woman's itinerary.

Potential Drug Interactions Between Oral Contraceptives and Other Medications

The potential interaction between oral contraceptives and other medications has been the subject of many recent studies and case reports. Some of the interactions are well documented and therapeutically relevant; others are not well substantiated and are controversial. Drug interactions can exist in both directions. Oral contraceptives can be affected by other drugs (hormone levels either increased, leading to greater effects, or decreased, leading to possible pregnancy), or they can interfere with the metabolism of other agents. Potential mechanisms underlying these interactions include hepatic microsomal enzyme induction or inhibition, interference with the enterohepatic circulation of steroid metabolites, interference with absorption from the gastrointestinal tract, and alterations in protein binding. In addition there is much individual variation in the way that women metabolize oral contraceptives; age, individual pharmacokinetics, diet, body size, physical activity, and neuroendocrinologic conditions all make it difficult to predict exact drug levels in an individual women.

Drug Interactions That May Affect Oral Contraceptive Efficacy

The main concern with travelers is whether antibiotics affect oral contraceptive efficacy. Antibiotics have been shown in animal studies to kill intestinal bacteria responsible for the deconjugation of oral contraceptive steroids in the colon. Without such deconjugation and subsequent reabsorption, decreased hormone levels result leading to a decrease in hormone efficacy. Despite numerous case reports of penicillins, tetracyclines, metronidazole, and nitrofurantoin causing contraceptive failure in humans, no large studies have demonstrated that antibiotics other than rifampin lower steroid blood concentrations. To date there are no known drug interactions between oral contraceptives and malaria chemoprophylaxis.

Contraceptive Failure: Emergency Contraception

The potential for being or becoming a pregnant traveler exists for most women of reproductive age. Contraceptive failures are common. Condoms break, diaphragms slip, contraceptive jelly runs out, oral contraceptives may be missed due to changes in time zones, malabsorption of the pill may occur as a result of vomiting and diarrhea, or the oral contraceptive may have decreased efficacy in smokers or when combined with certain medications. The contraceptive method may also be lost or stolen. A woman may experience a rape or assault.

Emergency contraception is defined as a method of contraception that a woman can use after unprotected intercourse to prevent pregnancy. It mist be used within 72 hours to be effective. Thus it is important for the travel medicine clinician to include a prescription for emergency contraception for women who may be at risk for pregnancy. In 1997, the Food and Drug Administration (FDA) approved six brands of oral contraceptives to be used in preventing pregnancy when taken within 72 hours of unprotected intercourse. There are a number of options. The easiest method for a female traveler is either the combination contraceptive pill (Yupze) regimen or the progestin-only minipills (Levonorgestrel) regimen.

Two doses (totaling 200 µg of ethinylestradiol [EE] and 2.0 mg norgestrel OR 1.5 mg levonorgestrel) should be taken 12 hours apart as soon as possible after unprotected intercourse. Treatment is most effective if initiated within the first 12 to 24 hours and is unlikely to work if more than 72 hours later. Nausea and vomiting are common with the combined pill regimen, so antiemetics may be prescribed such as Compazine or Phenergan or over-the-counter diphenhydramine to be taken 30 minutes before the second dose. An extra dose of pills might be provided for the woman in case she vomits within 1 to 3 hours after taking the first dose (Table 12-4).

Recent data from a multicenter WHO trial suggests that in terms of efficacy and side effects, levonorgestrel may be a better option for EC than the combined pill regimen. Side effects of the oral EC methods are generally confined to nausea in 50% of women using the combined pills and vomiting in 18%. There are fewer gastrointestinal side effects with the levonorgestrel-only pills: 23% of women have nausea and about 6%

Table 12-4
Emergency Contraceptive Methods

Combined pill*	No. pills per dose	Ethinyl estradiol per dose (µg)	Levonorgestrel per dose (µg)	Instructions for combined pill regimens
Preven Kit	2 light blue	100	0.5	Two doses 12 hr apart
Ovral	2 white	100	0.5	Within 72 hr of unprotected intercourse
Lo-Ovral	4 white	120	0.6	May need anti-nausea medications
Nordette	4 orange	120	0.6	
Levelen	4 orange	120	0.6	
Levora	4 white			
TriLevelen	4 yellow	120	0.5	
Triphasil	4 yellow	120	0.5	
Trivora	4 pink			
Alesse	5 pink	100	0.5	
Progestin Only				
Ovrette	All 20	0	0.75	See below
Levonorgestrel	1 white	0	0.75	Two doses (.75 µg) 12 hr apart within 72 hr
(Postinor)	1 white			
(Plan B)		0	0.75	

From Task Force on Postovulatory Methods of Fertility Regulation: *Lancet* 352:428, 1988.
*Much lower incidence of nausea and vomiting without combined pill regimen.

vomit. Antiemetics may be prescribed before each dose, although there are no data to support this practice. Withdrawal bleeding should occur within 21 days of taking EC. If it does not the woman should perform a pregnancy test. If she is pregnant, there are no data to indicate an adverse effect on a pregnancy carried to term after EC use.

EC is not an abortifacient. Data suggest that the primary mechanism of action of EC is to delay or prevent ovulation. Since it is also effective after ovulation, several other mechanisms have been hypothesized including interference with corpeus luteum function, change in cervical mucus, alternation in tubal transport or the endometrium, or inhibition of fertilization; but none have been proven.

Mifepristone (RU-486) is probably more effective, safer, and has fewer side effects then either levonorgestrel or the Yuzpe regimen. It is widely available in China and may be available in other countries soon.

Worldwide there is great variability in the availability of emergency contraception. In case a women loses her prescription or it is stolen, it would be important to advise her of the methods that might be available in the areas she is traveling to. This might be done by checking with the Consortium for Emergency Contraception *http://www.path.org/cec.htm* (Table 12-5).

An additional information resource is the toll-free Emergency Contraception Hotline: 1-888-NOT-2-LATE or http://opr.princeton.edu/ec/

If a traveler becomes pregnant and wishes to terminate the pregnancy, it may be best for her to return home depending on where she is. More than half of the 128 countries listed by the IPPF prohibit abortion except in extreme circumstances such as rape and life-threatening illness.

Sexually Transmitted Diseases

Sexually transmitted diseases (STDs) are of special importance to women owing to the gender-related pathophysiology of most of them, as is evidenced by the increased rate of transmission from an infected male to an uninfected female combined with an increased rate of serious sequelae in women.

To prevent contracting an STD, one should avoid casual sex or practice safe sex by using condoms no matter what other means of contraception is being used simultaneously. High quality latex condoms are an essential part of the personal medical kit of modern adult travelers regardless of gender and regardless if sexual activity during travel is planned or unplanned. A female condom made out of polyurethane is an effective alternative for persons allergic to latex. Travelers may be provided with an STD signs and symptoms card for self-diagnosis and possible treatment.

HIV prophylaxis for a high-risk exposure resulting from unprotected intercourse is important for female travelers to know about and to get access to if needed. There is an increased rate of HIV transmission from an infected male to an uninfected female, which is estimated to be at least equivalent to a needle stick. Thus postexposure HIV prophylaxis must be considered. In certain cases a woman might want to be given a 7-day supply of antiviral drugs to carry with her and to use in an emergency situation until the situation can be further evaluated and/or more medication can be obtained. The woman may also choose to return home. The average wholesale cost of the two-drug exposure regimen for 28 days is approximately $500. Adding a protease inhibiter adds $500 to $600. These medications are not available in most developing countries.

Table 12-5
Emergency Contraception (EC) Available Worldwide

Argentina	Immediate Yuzpe regimen
Brazil	Postinor 2 approved 1999
Bulgaria	Postinor 4 and Postinor 10 levonorgestrel regimens
Czech Republic	Postinor 4 and Postinor 10 levonorgestrel regimens
Denmark	Tetragynon Yuzpe regimen
Finland	NeoPrimovlar Yuzpe regimen
France	Tetragynon Yuzpe regimen approved 1998 Levonorgestrel regimen approved 1998
Germany	Tetragynon Yuzpe regimen approved 1998
Hong Kong	Postinor 4 and Postinor 10 levonorgestrel regimens
Hungary	Postinar 4 Postinor 10 and Postinor 2 levonorgestrel regimens
Jamaica	Postinor 4 and Postinor 10 levonorgestrel regimens
Kenya	Postinor 4 and Postinor 10 levonorgestrel regimens
Malaysia	Postinor 4 and Postinor 10 levonorgestrel regimens
Netherlands	Lynoral high dose estrogen regimens
New Zealand	Oral contraception-4 Yupze regimen marketed but then withdrawn due to legislation; need for a physician prescription
Nigeria	Postinor 4 and Postinor 10 levonorgestrel regimens
Norway	Tetragynom Yuzpe regimen
Pakistan	Postinor 4 and Postinor 10 levonorgestrel regimens
Poland	Postinor 4 and Postinor 10 levonorgestrel regimens
Singapore	Postinor 4 and Postinor 10 levonorgestrel regimen
Slovakia	Postinor 4 and Postinor 10 levonorgestrel regimens
South Africa	E-Gen-C Yuzpe regimen launched August 1997, levonorgestrel regimen expected in early 1999
Soviet Union	Postinor 4 and Postinor 10 levonorgestrel regimens
Sri Lanka	Postinor 2 levonorgestrel regimen launched 1998
Sweden	Tetragynon Yuzpe regimen
Thailand	Tetragynon Yuzpe regimen
United States	Preven Yuzpe regimen launched 1998
United Kingdom	Oral contraception-4 Yuzpe regimen launched 1985
Uruguay	Postinor 4 and Postinor 10 levonorgestrel regimens
Vietnam	Postinor 4 and Postinor 10 levonorgestrel regimens

List of countries for which EC has been registered as a dedicated product.

Gynecologic Concerns at Altitude

Women taking oral contraceptives could be advised to continue them at least to moderate altitudes (<10,000 ft [3050 m]), since the risk of pregnancy may be greater than the increased risk of thrombosis. However, women on oral contraceptives should be advised to consider other contraceptives at higher altitudes because of the theoretical increased risk of thrombosis and pulmonary embolism.

Estrogen replacement therapy is actually a physiologic dose of estrogen (estimated to be less than one-third that of the estrogen in low dose oral contraceptives) and therefore not contraindicated at altitude.

Personal Security and Safety Issues

If possible women should take a self-defense course before travel. Other advice might include the following: assess risks in new areas carefully, dress moderately respecting local customs, talk to other travelers, use common sense, and avoid walking in unknown areas at night. Individuals may carry pepper spray or personal alarm to scare, depending on regulations at destination.

Recommendations for a Woman's Medical Kit

Women travelers, especially those embarking on adventure travel itineraries, or planning extensive travel abroad, may find it beneficial to augment the basic travel medical kit (see Chapter 1) with supplies and medications specific to a given woman's life stage and reproductive health (Table 12-6).

Table 12-6
Medical Kit for Women

- Menstrual supplies
  - Calendar to keep track of menses
  - Supplies/devices
    - Pads, tampons, menstrual cups, etc
    - Towelettes/plastic disposal bags
  - Premenstrual syndromes (PMS)
    - Ibuprofen, other
  - Dysfunctional uterine bleeding
    - Premarin, estradiol
    - Oral contraceptive pills
    - Ibuprofen, other
- Urinary tract infections
  - Ciprofloxacin
  - Pyridium
  - Optional: urinary dipstick to check for leukocytes and nitrites
- Urinary voiding
  - Toilet tissue, towelettes
  - Funnels—paper or plastic
- Vaginitis caused by *Candida*
  - PH paper: pH < 4.5
  - Acidophilis dietary supplements
  - Vaginal creams: miconazole vaginal cream
  - Vaginal suppositories: Mycostatin
  - Oral medication: fluconazole
  - Mild soaps
- Hydrocortisone cream for pruritus
- Loose-fitting clothes
- Bacterial vaginosis
  - pH paper: pH > 4.7
  - Vaginal creams-Metrogel, clindamycin
  - Oral-metronidazole, clindamycin
- Trichomoniasis
  - Metronidazole
- Contraception
  - Chart to keep trace of pills if using them, menstrual periods
  - Timer: special wrist watch "alarm" to use for OCP dosing when changing time zones, traveling
  - Male/female condoms
  - Diaphragm/cap/sponge
  - Spermicides-contraceptive creams, jellies, films

Summary

Pretravel and posttravel evaluation of women should consider the life stage and lifestyle of the woman along with possible gender and age-related issues relating to risks, prevention, and treatment of travel and tropical diseases. More research and data are needed in this area.

TRAVEL DURING PREGNANCY

Pregnant women of all ages and at all stages of pregnancy are traveling for business, professional, and personal reasons. Clinicians who advise pregnant women should be able to assess the risks involved in short- and long-

Table 12-6
Medical Kit for Women—cont'd

- Emergency Contraception
  - Review options in country of destination
  - Combined pill regimen or levonorgestrel regimen
  - Antiemetic tablets or rectal suppositories
- Emergency postexposure HIV prophylaxis for high-risk unprotected sexual encounter
- Pregnancy Tests
  - Carry extras, depending on length of trip
- Sexually Transmitted Infections
  - Preventive measures: condoms, dental dams, Saran wrap, gloves, barrier methods
  - Magnifying glass
  - Chart for identifying basics, recommendations for treatment
  - Medications for treatment
- Perimenopausal/menopausal Issues
  - Vaginal dryness: estrogen creams
  - Menstrual cycle irregularity: consider low-dose OCP
  - Stress incontinence: vaginal moisturizers and lubricants, Kegel exercises
  - Hot flashes and night sweats
  - Estrogen replacement therapy (ERT)
  - Vitamin E
  - Clonidine patch or pill
- Insomnia
  - Avoid stimulants (caffeine, other), exercise, eat food with tryptophan
  - Irritability/Moodiness: exercise, ERT/antidepressants
  - Osteoporosis: weight-bearing exercise, calcium, vitamin D, medications
  - Headaches: may be triggered by changes in hormones
  - Alternative products: (unclear benefit, studies underway) quai, ginseng, black cohash, Vitex/chasteberry, melatonin, St. John's wort, wild yams (contains diosgenin the starting point for the synthesis for progestins, human body does not have enzyme to convert progesterone from yams)
- Pregnancy Supplies
  - Blood pressure cuff
  - Urine protein/glucose strips
  - Leukocyte esterase strips
- Personal Safety
  - Alarms
  - Pepper spray
  - Lessons in self defense before trip

OCP, Oral contraceptive pill; *HIV,* human immunodeficiency virus.

term travel. This is especially important when a woman is planning an extended period of travel and/or travel to a remote area in which no medical facilities may be available. The woman's itinerary should be reviewed and assessed for risks relating to a destination or a specific activity that may be a risk to the mother or fetus. If risks are involved, the pregnant traveler should be fully informed so that she can make the best possible decision and/or consider alternatives. A number of gestation-related changes are important to consider when counseling a pregnant woman including effects on the immune system and circulatory, respiratory, and metabolic functions. For example infections such as malaria, typhoid, or amebiasis may have more severe or even fatal complications in a pregnant women because of her suppressed immune status during pregnancy.

Basic Questions to Answer When Counseling Pregnant Women

Pregnant women anticipating travel to remote places need to have the following information before confirming their itinerary:

1. What medical, obstetric, social, and demographic risks are associated with travel?
2. Are the required and recommended immunizations for the itinerary safe in pregnancy?
3. What drugs against malaria and other parasitic illnesses are safe in pregnancy?
4. What prophylactic or therapeutic measures against traveler's diarrhea are safe in pregnancy?
5. What medical services are available in the area(s) of destination?
6. What does her American health insurance cover if she is out of area for delivery or pregnancy-related complications?
7. What are signs of serious pregnancy-related illness for which emergency medical help should be sought?
8. What are some general guidelines to follow for the medical management of illness that will safeguard the pregnant woman and her fetus?

First, the past medical and obstetric history should be reviewed with the woman in conjunction with her obstetrician. See Pretravel Evaluation for Pregnant Women Table 12-7. In general travel during the last month of pregnancy and travel that may pose a serious risk to the mother should be avoided. Possible risk factors and relative contraindications to travel are listed in Table 12-8. If a woman has had a previous adverse pregnancy outcome or has had a difficult time becoming pregnant and is in her late 30s or 40s, she should weigh the possible risks carefully.

The complete itinerary should be evaluated with attention to both quality of medical care possible during transit and at the final destination. Access to high-quality care during travel is essential in case of preterm labor or an unexpected complication of pregnancy. The itinerary should also be reviewed for possible risks such as exposure to chloroquine-resistant *falciparum* malaria or the need to travel over a 14,000 pass. The potential exposure to specific health risks may be improved by adjusting certain destinations and activities on the trip route.

It is important for a woman to check with her insurance plan regarding health insurance coverage. Many insurance plans do not cover pregnant women overseas, and many have gestation cutoff dates for travel beyond which they will not cover delivery out of the area. She may have to buy additional coverage if the trip is necessary. Pregnant travelers should carry a copy of their medical records (including blood type and Rh) in case of an emergency.

Table 12-7
Pretravel Evaluation for Pregnant Woman

Step	Content
History	Review past medical and past obstetric and gynecologic history
Physical examination	Obstetrician to assess gestational age, fetal growth performance, coexistent medical, obstetric, social and demographic risks
Laboratory tests	Serology for hepatitis B, CMV, measles, rubella, chickenpox, toxoplasmosis depending on history
Review planned itinerary	Access to care and health insurance coverage
	Risk/benefit analysis for mother and fetus for exposure to:
	Infectious disease: usual and exotic
	Recommended immunizations
	Recommended chemoprophylaxis against malaria
	Risk of treatment if acquire the disease
	Environmental risks
	Water/Food
	Transportation
	Insects
	Altitude
	Scuba
	Heat
	Sports activity
	Other
Specific recommendations	Immunizations
	Environmental risks
	Transportation
	Insects
	Water/Food
	Altitude
	Medical kit: include copy of medical history including blood type and Rh factor

CMV, Cytomegalovirus.

Cultural aspects of traveling while pregnant or nursing should also be considered. In some countries, a women who is 8 months pregnant may not be taken seriously as the chief spokesperson for a company in an important negotiation. Similarly, breastfeeding an infant at an important meeting may not be conducive to playing boardroom politics.

Transportation Risks During Pregnancy

Airlines

Most airlines do not allow pregnant women to travel if they are at more than 35 to 36 weeks of gestation without a letter from a physician. Commercial aircraft cruising at high altitudes are able to pressurize only to 5000 to 8000 ft above sea level. Women with moderate anemia (Hgb <8.5 g/dl) or with a compromised oxygen saturation may need oxygen supplementation. Women with sickle cell disease may experience a crisis during the de-

Table 12-8
Relative Contraindications for Travel During Pregnancy

Medical Risk Factors
Congenital or acquired heart disease (especially valvular disease or congestive heart failure)
History of thromboembolic disease
Medical disease requiring ongoing assessment and medication
Anemia (hemoglobin <8.5 g/dl)
Chronic lung disease including asthma

Obstetric Risk Factors
History of miscarriage
Threatened abortion or vaginal bleeding during present pregnancy
Incompetent cervix
Premature labor, premature rupture of membranes, or placental abruption or separation with prior pregnancy
History of ectopic pregnancy (should be ruled out before travel with ultrasound)
History of or present placental abnormalities
Multiple gestation in present pregnancy
History of toxemia, hypertension, diabetes with any pregnancy
History of infertility or difficulty becoming pregnant
Primigravida >35 or <15 years old

Travel to Destination That May Be Hazardous
High altitude
Scuba
Areas endemic for or where epidemics are occurring of life-threatening food or insect-borne infections
Areas where chloroquine-resistant *Plasmodium falciparum* is endemic
Areas where live vaccines are required and recommended

From CDC *Health Information for International Travel*, 2001-2002.

saturation. Even those with sickle cell trait may experience hematuria or renal microthrombosis during desaturation. The fetal circulation and fetal hemoglobin protects the fetus against desaturation during airflight.

Certain precautions should be taken by pregnant women during flight. An alteration in clotting factors and venous dilation during pregnancy predispose pregnant women to superficial and deep thrombophlebitis or "economy class syndrome." Pregnant women have a rate of acute iliofemoral venous thrombosis that is six times more frequent among pregnant women than nonpregnant women. Contributing factors to this risk to this may be (1) compression on the inferior vena cava and iliac veins by the enlarged uterus and/or (2) an increase in the coagulation factors and fibrinolysis inhibitors. The pregnant traveler should request an aisle seat and should walk in the aisles at least once an hour during long airplane flights whenever it is safe to do so to increase the circulation. General stretching and isometric leg exercises should be encouraged on long flights.

The low humidity of pressurized flights leads to significant insensible water loss. Cabins are maintained at 8% humidity. Hydration is crucial for placental blood flow. Women should be encouraged to drink nonalcoholic beverages. Seat belts should be worn low around the pelvis and should be worn throughout the flight.

Intestinal gas expansion can be particularly uncomfortable for the pregnant traveler. She should avoid gas-producing foods and airline food. Women should bring their own healthy snacks and bottled water. Airport security machines are generally safe during pregnancy. These are magnetometers and are not harmful to the fetus.

Jet lag is an important phenomenon for travelers heading eastward over several time zones. Pharmacologic therapy for jet lag is not recommended during pregnancy. Pregnant women should get enough fluids, food, and rest whether or not they use planned schedules to avoid jet lag. A program of daily exercise and alteration of sleep pattern that can minimize disturbances in circadian rhythm and mentation that occur as a result of jet lag are recommended. Melatonin has not been found to cause toxicity during pregnancy, but it has not been well studied.

Automobile Travel

A pregnant women should not sit for prolonged periods when traveling in an automobile or bus because of the risk of venous stasis and thromboembolism as previously discussed. Varicose veins of the perineum and legs are also common pregnancy-related problems exacerbated by prolonged sitting or a supine posture. Thus pregnant women should wear elastic hose and avoid prolonged periods of immobilization. The usual recommendation is driving for a maximum of 6 hours a day with stopping at least every 1 to 2 hours for 10 minutes to walk and increase venous return from the legs.

Motor vehicle accidents account for most severe blunt trauma to pregnant women. The American College of Obstetricians and Gynecologists (ACOG) has recommended that pregnant women wear three-point restraints when riding in automobiles. Travelers should be warned that in many parts of the world, taxicabs and other automobiles and buses do not have safety restraints.

Sea Travel

Sea voyages can exacerbate the nausea and vomiting associated with pregnancy. Most cruise liners will carry pregnant women up to the seventh month of pregnancy and have reasonably well-equipped medical facilities abroad. Caution must be observed when walking on deck to avoid accidents caused by the motion of the ship and the general imbalance imposed by pregnancy.

Classification of Drugs and Vaccines Used in Pregnancy by the FDA

It is particularly important to consider possible adverse outcomes on the mother or the fetus before use of any medication. For a comprehensive review the reader is referred to an excellent text by Briggs et al, *Drugs Pregnancy and Lactation.* The Organization of Teratology Information Services can be used for referral to the nearest service (801) 328-2229. Drugs commonly used by travelers may be classified under the following areas.

FDA Use-in-Pregnancy Ratings

The FDA has established a system that classifies drugs on the basis of data from humans and animals ranging from class A drugs, which are designed as safe during pregnancy, to class X drugs, which are contraindicated in pregnancy because of proven teratogenicity. The system has resulted in ambiguous statements that may not only be difficult for physicians to interpret and use for counseling but may cause anxiety among women. It is also been found that the classification is not updated when new data are available.

Category A	Adequate and well-controlled studies in women show no risk to the fetus
Category B	No evidence of risk in humans. Either studies in animals show risk, but human findings do not, or, in the absence of human studies, animal findings are negative
Category C	Risk cannot be ruled out. No adequate and well-controlled studies in humans, or animal studies are either positive for fetal risk or lacking as well. Drugs should be given only if the potential benefit justifies the potential risk to the fetus.
Category D	There is positive evidence of human fetal risk. Nevertheless, potential benefits may outweigh potential risks.
Category X	Contraindicated in pregnancy. Studies in animals or humans or investigations or postmarketing reports have shown fetal risk that far outweighs any potential benefit to the patient.

The Teratology Society has proposed that the FDA abandon the current classification in terms of a more meaningful evidence-based narrative statements. Other countries such as Sweden, Australia, the Netherlands, Switzerland, and Denmark have different classification systems based on a hierarchy of estimated fetal risk.

The clinician must help the pregnant woman to weigh the risk/benefit ratio of travel on both the developing fetus and maternal health. This includes evaluating the risks for the woman or her fetus with regard to the recommended immunizations, need for chemoprophylaxis, and exposure to malaria, traveler's diarrhea, or other parasitic and infectious diseases and environmental concerns. If the women must travel, physicians and other health practitioners involved in travel advice should be aware of the following guidelines and precautions that will help to ensure the safety of the mother and her unborn traveler.

Travel Vaccines in Pregnancy

Vaccines given for international travel should reflect the actual risks of disease and the probable benefit of the vaccine. If a woman is pregnant the risk/benefit ratio of each immunization should be carefully reviewed with regard to its potential effect on the fetus versus risk of contacting the actual disease and its subsequent effect on the mother or fetus.

Toxoid vaccines such as tetanus and diphtheria vaccines; inactivated vaccines such as inactivated polio vaccine, inactivated typhoid vaccine and hepatitis A and B vaccines, viral influenza vaccine, rabies vaccine, and Japanese encephalitis vaccines; polysaccharide vaccines such as meningococcal and pneumococcal vaccines; and immune globulin or specific globulin preparations are all probably safe in pregnancy. These vaccines are classified as Pregnancy Category B or C because there are insufficient scientific data to evaluate the safety and use of these vaccines in pregnancy. If possible all vaccines should be deferred during the first trimester. Indications for vaccination during pregnancy are listed in Table 12-9.

Live, attenuated-virus vaccines are generally contraindicated in pregnant women or those likely to become pregnant within the next 3 months after receiving vaccine(s). Measles, mumps, and rubella vaccines are absolutely contraindicated during pregnancy. Yellow fever and oral polio vaccines may be given if exposure is unavoidable.

Table 12-9
Use of Vaccines During Pregnancy

Vaccine		Use
Hepatitis A	Inactivated virus	Data on safety in pregnancy are not available; the theoretical risk of vaccination should be weighed against the risk of disease
Hepatitis B	Recombinant or plasma-derived	If indicated
Immune globulins, pooled or hyperimmune	Immune globulin or specific globulin preparations	If indicated
Influenza	Inactivated whole virus or subunit	If indicated
Japanese encephalitis	Inactivated virus	Data on safety in pregnancy are not available; the theoretical risk of vaccination should be weighed against the risk of disease
Measles	Live attenuated virus	Contraindicated
Meningococcal meningitis	Polysaccharide	If indicated
Mumps	Live attenuated virus	Contraindicated
Pneumococcal	Polysaccharide	If indicated
Polio, inactivated	Inactivated virus	If indicated
Rabies	Inactivated virus	If indicated
Rubella	Live attenuated virus	Contraindicated
Tetanus-diphtheria	Toxoid	If indicated
Typhoid (ViCPS)	Polysaccharide	If indicated
Typhoid (Ty21a)	Live bacterial	Data on safety in pregnancy are not available
Varicella	Live attenuated virus	If indicated
Yellow fever	Live attenuated virus	If indicated

From CDC: *Health Information for International Travel*, 2001-2002, Atlanta, DHHS, 2001.

Certain travel vaccines are discussed next in the context of the pregnant traveler. The reader should consult Chapter 4 for a detailed review of vaccines for travelers.

Cholera

The killed bacterial cholera vaccine widely used in the past is not contraindicated in pregnancy. However, it is of fairly low efficacy and is no longer recommended. Two new oral killed cholera vaccines are available outside the United States. Until the safety and efficacy of these vaccines have been established, no clear recommendations can be made. A live attenuated oral cholera vaccine (CVD 103 HgR strain) is available in Canada and several European countries, and its availability in the United States is anticipated. Pregnancy information is not available, but because the vaccine contains live organisms, it should *not* be used in pregnancy. The cholera toxin B-subunit-whole-cell vaccine (BS-WC) is discussed in Chapter 4.

Hepatitis A Vaccine

Hepatitis A virus (HAV) infection of the mother is not associated with perinatal transmission; however, placental abruption and premature delivery of an infected infant have been reported during acute HAV infection. The safety and efficacy of the inactivated hepatitis A vaccines in pregnant women have not been established, and the vaccine is classified as FDA pregnancy category by the manufacturer. Because this is not a live virus vaccine, the main concern is a febrile response. If a high-risk itinerary is planned, hepatitis A vaccine or immune globulin should be given. Serology should be checked before travel if the patient was born or has lived in developing countries (see Chapter 4).

Hepatitis B Vaccine

Hepatitis B vaccine is recommended for a pregnant women if she is a long-term traveler planning delivery overseas; there is a possibility she will be sexually active with a new partner; or she is working in a health care clinic, refugee camp, or similar setting. Hepatitis B vaccine should be considered in all sexually active women including pregnant women visiting areas where blood is not routinely screened for hepatitis B. Hemorrhage after miscarriage or delivery could require transfusion with possible infected blood. If the mother carries the hepatitis B surface antigen or e antigen, the newborn should receive the hepatitis B vaccine and hyperimmune globulin at birth. Ideally all pregnant women should be screened for hepatitis B carriage and immunity. The current practice is to screen for hepatitis B surface antigen (HbsAg) only. Infants born to mothers who are carriers of HbsAg should immediately be given hepatitis immune globulin (HBIG) and vaccinated as well. Hepatitis B vaccine (recombinant) series can be administered to pregnant women who are at risk and have negative serology for past infection, preferably after the first trimester. Immunization for HBV also prevents hepatitis D.

Japanese Encephalitis Vaccine

The safety of the Japanese encephalitis vaccine in pregnant women has not been determined. If travel to an at-risk area is not mandatory, travel should be delayed.

Meningococcal Vaccine

Meningococcal vaccine in the United States is a tetravalent vaccine from serogroups A, C, Y, and W135. It is recommended for travelers to high-risk areas including the sub-Saharan African epidemic belt for meningococcal disease from December through June or in epidemic foci such as Kenya, Uganda, Tanzania, Nepal, and India year round. In a number of other countries only bivalent vaccine from serogroups A and C is commonly used. An A and C bivalent vaccine has been evaluated in pregnant women and infants during an epidemic of meningitis in Brazil and appeared to be safe.

Polio

The pregnant traveler needs adequate protection against polio. Paralytic disease may occur with greater frequency when infection develops during pregnancy. Anoxic fetal damage with maternal poliomyelitis has been reported. There is a 50% rate mortality in neonatal disease contracted transplacentally during the third trimester. If she has received the primary immunization and the last dose was within 10 years, she is considered protected (although some experts would recommend a booster within 5 years if traveling to a highly endemic area). Presently it is recommended that the enhanced potency inactivated vaccine be given to pregnant women for travel to endemic areas. Oral polio vaccine may be administered if inactivated polio vaccine is not available in a high-risk situation. Several thousand pregnant women in Finland received the oral polio immunization during a nationwide immunization campaign. There was no increase in the occurrence of congenital malformations.

Rabies Vaccines (Diploid Cell Culture)

Rabies vaccine may be given during pregnancy for preexposure or postexposure prophylaxis. A recent review of the literature found 24 cases of pregnant women exposed to rabid animal bites. The exposures occurred during all trimesters. The women received equine rabies immune globulin and vero cell vaccine or duck embryo vaccine. Among the infants, two were born prematurely and there was one spontaneous abortion. There were no physical or mental abnormalities except in a case described where the child did well after surgical repair of transposition of the great vessels. In this case the bite occurred after the heart would have been formed embryologically, so the congenital malformation was not thought to be vaccine related.

Vaccination preexposure or postexposure to rabies is considered safe with modern tissue culture-derived rabies vaccine products. If a woman is high risk or visiting an endemic country for more than 30 days, she should receive preexposure vaccination. Postexposure vaccination should be administered as soon as possible after a scratch or bite of an infected mammal including monkeys and bats. In a mother with rabies, a viable infant should be delivered as soon as possible and given rabies hyperimmune globulin and the postexposure vaccine regimen.

Typhoid Vaccines

Three vaccines are available for the prevention of typhoid. Information is not available on the safety of any of these vaccines during pregnancy. Of the three, the Vi capsular polysaccharide parental vaccine is recommended during pregnancy only if clearly indicated. The older heat/phenol inactivated parental typhoid vaccine should be avoided in pregnancy owing to the known risk of fever and systemic effects associated with this preparation. The live-attenuated Ty21A bacterial oral vaccine is not recommended on theoretical grounds.

Yellow Fever

Yellow fever vaccine is a live virus vaccine and should not be given to pregnant women unless travel to an endemic area is unavoidable. In these instances the vaccine should be given.

The yellow fever vaccine (17d vaccine) was administered to 101 pregnant women during the 1986-1987 outbreak in Nigeria without any untoward effects to the fetus or the mother. Antibody responses of pregnant women and mothers who were vaccinated mainly during the last trimester were much lower than those of nonpregnant women vaccinated with yellow fever in a comparable control group. A recent study of women immunized inadvertently during pregnancy found one apparently well neonate with yellow fever viral-specific immunoglobulin M antibody indicating vaccine-related congenital exposure. No congenital abnormalities have been reported after administration of the vaccine during pregnancy.

If a pregnant women is traveling to an endemic area, based on the degree of exposure and risk for yellow fever, a waiver may be given if the risk is low and the vaccination is for international requirements only. If travel to a high-risk area is necessary, the benefits of the vaccine far outweigh the small theoretical risk to the fetus and the mother.

Drugs Against Malaria and Other Parasitic Diseases in Pregnancy

Prevention of malaria in travelers, including pregnant women, is discussed in detail in Chapter 5. In brief, the *weekly doses* of chloroquine phosphate used for chemoprophylaxis of chloroquine-sensitive strains of malaria appear to be safe during pregnancy. Chorioretinitis has been reported in newborns of mothers given daily doses of chloroquine and is a theoretical risk.

The chemoprophylaxis of malaria in areas where chloroquine-resistant malaria is present is more of a problem for the pregnant traveler, because of concerns about the safety of the other antimalarial drugs with regard to fetal growth and development. In a double-blind, placebo-controlled study of mefloquine (MQ), antimalarial prophylaxis in the second and third trimester of pregnancy in a highly endemic area along the Thai-Myanmar border, MQ gave more than 86% protection against *Plasmodium falciparum* and complete protection against *Plasmodium vivax* infections while posing little risk to the fetus. Weekly MQ prophylaxis was well tolerated except for transient dizziness associated with the initial loading dose (10 mg/kg) used in this study. A loading dose MQ for pregnant women is not recommended in clinical practice at this time.

The Centers for Disease Control and Prevention (CDC) has issued a statement that MQ can be used if needed during the second and third trimester for malaria prophylaxis. MQ use in pregnancy has been monitored by the CDC registry, and recently trends have been noted. In a few studies there was a significant excess of stillbirths in the MQ group. An increase in the number of spontaneous abortions was also noted in the Somalian armed forces with inadvertent use of MQ during pregnancy. However, a growing number of pregnant women, in highly endemic areas for multidrug-resistant *falciparum* malaria, have received MQ for treatment in the first trimester of pregnancy followed by weekly doses for prophylaxis without any evidence of congenital malformation or perinatal pathology. Until more data are available, the use of MQ for malaria prophylaxis in the first trimester of pregnancy remains a matter of individual risk/benefit analysis. See Chapter 5 for a details consideration of alternative chemoprophylactic regimens for chloroquine-resistant *P. falciparum* malaria.

Treatment of diagnosed malaria during pregnancy is indicated because the potential adverse effects of the antimalarial drugs to the mother and fetus are far outweighed by the potential morbidity and mortality of untreated malaria. Maternal malaria can cause profound anemia; predispose to serious intercurrent illness; cause intrauterine infection and placental insufficiency; and contribute to intrauterine growth retardation, prematurity, low-birth weight, abortion, and stillbirth. The treatment of malaria is discussed in detail in Chapter 17.

Prevention of Traveler's Diarrhea During Pregnancy

Antimicrobial prophylactic therapy is not recommended for prevention of traveler's diarrhea. Preventive measures should include boiling water or purifying it chemically; drinking only bottled carbonated water, bottled or canned fruit juices or soft drinks, and hot liquids; using great caution to avoid using ice; and not eating fresh salads or raw vegetables. The iodine-based methods of chemical water purification (Chapter 7) are probably safe during pregnancy for short-term (less than 3 weeks) travel. However, prolonged use of iodine-treated water by a pregnant woman could result in adverse effects on the fetal thyroid gland.

Treatment of traveler's diarrhea is somewhat difficult. The typical illness causes several weeks of watery diarrhea and is self-limited, but can lead to significant weakness and malaise in both the pregnant and non-pregnant traveler. Bismuth subsalicylate (Pepto-Bismol) has been used without complication in pregnant women but has relative contraindications. Bismuth in large doses is a known teratogen in sheep, and in humans salicylates have been both teratogenic and the cause of fetal bleeds throughout pregnancy. The antiperistaltic medications loperamide and diphenoxylate have been used without complication in pregnant women and are not known teratogens. Diphenoxylate has a known, and loperamide a theoretical, narcotic-like effect, which could cause respiratory depression if given to the mother in high doses toward term. Both these antiperistaltic agents should be used with caution for control of frequent watery diarrhea and intestinal cramps in the traveler (Chapter 6).

The usual antibiotic of choice for treatment of traveler's diarrhea is one of the fluoroquinlones; however, these are contraindicated during pregnancy because of an association with fetal cartilage abnormalities in animal studies. Resistance to trimethoprim/sulfamethoxazole (Bactrim, Septra, co-trimoxazole) is widespread among bacterial pathogens causing diarrhea; however, this antibiotic combination is considered generally safe in the second trimester of pregnancy and could be tried as initial antibacterial therapy by a pregnant woman who was not allergic to sulfa drugs. Trimethoprim in large doses has been shown to be teratogenic in the first trimester, with defects including cleft palate, limb defects, and micrognathia in rats and rabbits. It is a folic acid inhibitor and so has theoretical contraindications as well. Sulfamethoxazole, although not teratogenic, is contraindicated toward term particularly after 32 weeks, since it competes with bilirubin for protein binding sites and can be a cause of hyperbilirubinemia and kernicterus in the newborn. In addition, it can cause hemolysis in the glucose 6-phosphate dehydrongenase-deficient neonate. Both drugs are excreted in breast milk at greater than 50% maternal levels; thus the contraindications are significant for lactating women as well. One other option that might have some use in pregnancy for the treatment of enteric pathogens is azithromycin (Zithromax), although it is relatively expensive. Doxycycline is known to stain both fetal teeth and bones and is contraindicated in pregnant women and neonates.

In summary, it appears that the safest course for pregnant women is to take all preventive measures possible, and if diarrhea occurs, to have with them a supply of loperamide oral rehydration solution (see Chapter 6) and trimethoprim/sulfamethoxazole or azithromycin. If fever or bloody diarrhea occurs, immediate medical care should be sought.

Other Parasitic Diseases

All travelers can decrease the risk of acquiring parasitic infections in tropical areas by following general insect precautions (Chapter 1), by selecting safe food and water (Chapters 6, 40, and 41), and by wearing shoes in rural areas (Chapter 40).

The effects of parasitic disease, including protozoan, nematode, trematode, and cestode infections, on pregnancy and the fetus are summarized in Table 12-10. There are no absolutely safe antiparasitic drugs for use during pregnancy. Decisions for medical intervention must be made on the basis of serious risk on either fetal or maternal health by the disease itself. It is important to note that in the case of mild infection (light parasite loads), it is best to delay treatment until the postpartum period.

There are subtle changes in maternal cell-mediated immunity (CMI) during pregnancy presumably related to the need to inhibit the rejection of the fetoplacental unit. Infectious pathogens cleared or contained by the CMI may produce a more aggressive clinical course in a pregnant women. Leprosy may shift toward the lepromatous pole from the tuberculoid pole. Amebiasis may lead to fulminant disease. Women infected with the cutaneous form of leishmaniasis show greater risk of progression to invasive disease; some experts recommend termination of the pregnancy. There is no change in preexisting humoral immunity or the capacity to produce antibodies in response to infection or immunization during pregnancy.

Table 12-10
Potential Effects of Parasitic Infections on Reproduction*

Parasitic infections	Impaired fertility	Failure to carry to term	Fetal infection
Protozoans			
Entamoeba histolytica	X	X	X
Giardia lamblia	X	X	X
Leishmania species	X	X	X
Plasmodium species (malaria)	X	X	X
Trypanosoma species	X	X	X
Toxoplasma gondii		X	X
Pneumocystis carinii		X	X
Intestinal Nematodes			
Ascaris lumbricoides	X	X	X
Enterobius vermicularis (pinworm)	X		
Trichuris trichiura (whipworm)			
Hookworm species	X	X	X
Extraintestinal Nematodes			
Strongyloides stercoralis	X	X	
Trichinella spiralis	X	X	X
Filaria species	X	X	X
Trematodes			
Schistosoma species	X	X	
Clonorchis sinensis	X	X	
Paragonimus westermani	X	X	
Cestodes			
Echinococcus species	X	X	
Taenia species	X	X	

Adapted from MacLeod CL, Lee RV. In Burrow GN, Ferris TF, editors: *Medical complications during pregnancy*, ed 2, Philadelphia, 1988, WB Saunders.
*See text for discussion.

Treatment of giardiasis and amebiasis is discussed in Chapter 26. Metronidazole, which has a theoretical risk of transplacental carcinogenesis, has been used in severe dysentery related to infection with *Giardia lamblia* or *Entamoeba histolytica* without adverse fetal effects. Quinacrine or furazolidone (Chapter 26) can be considered for treatment of giardiasis during pregnancy, as they pose less hypothetical risk than metronidazole. Quinacrine may not be tolerated, however, owing to common side effects of severe nausea and vomiting. Tinidazole (Fasigyn) is the treatment of choice for Giardia and amebiasis. However, tinidazole is not marketed in the United States or Canada. There is no official recommendation for the use of tinidazole during pregnancy.

The impaired fertility and failure to carry to term noted for the helminthic (worm) parasite infections in Table 12-11 are generally not seen in travelers who have acquired infections with small numbers of worms. However, heavy infections with parasites acquired after intensive exposure in endemic areas over years may be of concern; these are most likely to be seen in natives or refugees of such areas moving to temperate zones such as the United States. However, as more women travelers are living in endemic areas for work or recreation, the incidence in these women may increase.

Indications for treatment of intestinal nematodes during pregnancy are summarized in Table 12-11. In the case of disease caused by chronic parasite infections, the symptoms and dysfunction may not be reversible even after appropriate treatment of the parasites. It should be noted that

Table 12-11
Indications for Treatment of Intestinal Nematodes During Pregnancy*

Parasite	Ineffective stage	Mode of transmission	Adult habitat	Indications for treatment during pregnancy
Enterobius vermicularis (pinworms)	Egg	Ingestion	Cecum	None
Trichuris trichiura	Egg	Ingestion	Colon	Rectal prolapse; blood loss
Ascaris lumbricoides	Mature egg	Ingestion	Small intestine	Worm obstruction
Hookworm: *Necator americanus* *Ancylostoma duodenale*	Larvae	Skin penetration	Small intestine	Heavy infestation: anemia or malnutrition not responding to supportive therapy
Strongyloides	Larvae	Skin or colon mucosa penetration	Small intestine	Presence of infection

Adapted from Lee RV. In Burrow GN, Ferris TF, editors: *Medical complications during pregnancy,* Philadelphia, 1982, WB Saunders.
*See text for discussion.

women with known intestinal parasites should receive regular prenatal care, including monitoring of the maternal hematocrit, and prenatal vitamins containing folate and B_{12}.

Other Infections

Lyme disease, caused by a tick-vectored spirochete, *Borrelia burgdorferi,* occurs in people who hike, camp, hunt, and travel to endemic areas, most notably the northeastern United States. However, Lyme disease has been reported in Europe, North Africa, Asia, and Australia; and potential tick vectors are found worldwide.

Lyme disease during pregnancy is associated with an increased risk of spontaneous abortion, premature labor, and intrauterine growth retardation. In one retrospective review of 19 cases of *B. burgdorferi* infection during pregnancy, five women experienced adverse fetal outcomes including one intrauterine fetal death. In an endemic area of Italy, 12% of 49 women suffering spontaneous abortion and 6% of 49 women experiencing normal vaginal delivery had serologic evidence of *B. burgdorferi* infection. Larger seroepidemiologic studies in the United States and Europe of infants from endemic and nonendemic areas could find no association between congenital malformations and antibody to *B. burgdorferi* in cord blood. Considering the widespread prevalence of infection in endemic areas, the rarity of adverse fetal outcome suggests that transplacental infection is unusual or that fetal infection is rarely injurious.

Treatment with using penicillin G or amoxicillin, 500 mg three times a day for a minimum of 3 weeks, is recommended for all women with early or confirmed infection or tick bite during pregnancy in a high-risk area.

Exercise and Sport-Related Risk

In general, a pregnant woman should avoid any vigorous physical activities that she did not regularly participate in before pregnancy. The American College of Obstetrics and Gynecology (ACOG) guidelines state that a pregnant women should tailor their exercise to their needs and abilities. The woman should exercise within a comfort zone. If the woman is healthy and accustomed to vigorous exercise, there is no reason that she cannot exceed the ACOG guidelines as long as she does not become hyperthermic, hypoglycemic, or dehydrated.

The effects of altitude is discussed in Chapter 9. There are limited studies on short-term exposure in pregnancy. Altitude-associated effects such as fetal growth retardation, pregnancy-induced hypertension, and neonatal hyperbilirubinemia have been documented in studies on permanent residents at altitude. A healthy, nonacclimatized, sedentary pregnant women should not exceed an altitude of 2500 meters (8250 ft) during the first 4 to 5 days of short-altitude exposure during the first trimester. If she wishes to combine this with a recreational activity such as climbing or skiing she should do so at a lower level. Preferably a pregnant women should spend a few days at rest at altitude before exercise to allow for adaptive mechanism to come into play. Elite athletes, skiers, and mountain climbers should discuss their risk with their personal physician. There may be no contraindication to short-term moderate exercise at 8000 to 11,000 ft. Changes in the pregnant woman's center of gravity and joint laxity may increase her risk of an injury. It is probably best not to ski or hike in remote areas owing to lack of access to emergency care.

Scuba diving is not recommended, since the fetus is not protected from decompression problems and is at risk from malformation and gas embolism after decompression disease. If a woman inadvertently completes a dive before she knows she is pregnant, the present evidence is not to recommend an abortion, since several normal pregnancies have been documented. Snorkeling can be practiced during pregnancy, but scuba should be discontinued until after the birth. Water skiing or other water sports that might force water and air in the vagina or injure the uterus are generally contraindicated for all pregnant women.

Maternal hyperthermia may lead to neural tube defects, so exposure to excessive heat during hot tubs, sauna, or heavy exertion in hot weather is not recommended. All exercising women should pay particular attention to adequate hydration to maintain placental blood flow.

Medical Service Available in the Area of Destination

Travel during the last 4 weeks of pregnancy should be limited to travel that is absolutely necessary, to avoid delivery in a strange hospital with no medical records available. Domestic airlines regulations stipulate that no travel at greater than 36 weeks' gestation is allowed, and most foreign airlines have a cutoff of 35 weeks' gestation. In addition, a note signed by the patient's physician specifying the expected date of confinement is required by most airlines. Pregnant travelers should ask their own doctors for referral to colleagues in the destination countries. Listings of medical services available can be obtained from some travel agencies and airlines. A list of English-speaking physicians around the world is available from the International Association of Medical Assistance to Travelers (IAMAT) (see Appendix).

Health Insurance Coverage When Out of Area

This consideration is extraordinarily important. Each health insurance company has different stipulations about coverage when out of area. Many have gestational date cutoffs for travel, beyond which they will not cover delivery out of area, and this information should be ascertained before departure.

Signs of Serious Pregnancy-Related Illness for Which Emergency Medical Help Should Be Sought

These signs should be learned before departure. Travel should be avoided, particularly in the last trimester, if multiple births are expected or if there is a history of pregnancy-induced hypertension or bleeding. Home blood-pressure cuffs and urine dipsticks for urine sugar and protein should be carried by pregnant women traveling to remote places during the third trimester. Signs of serious pregnancy-related illness for which medical attention should be sought include:

1. Bleeding
2. Severe abdominal pain
3. Contractions
4. Hypertension
5. Proteinuria
6. Severe headache or visual complaints
7. Severe edema or accelerated weight gain
8. Suspected rupture of membranes

REFERENCES

ACOG committee opinion: Air travel during pregnancy, *Int J Gynaecol Obst* 76:338, 2002.

Agostini R: *Medical and orthopedic issues of active and athletic women,* Philadelphia, 1994, Hanley & Belfus.

Anderson S: Women's health and travel. In Zuckerman J, Zuckerman A: *Principles and practice of travel medicine,* Sussex, England, 2001, John Wiley & Sons.
Artal R: Exercise and pregnancy, *Clin Sports Med* 2:363, 1992.
Ballagh SA et al: Dose finding study of a contraceptive ring releasing norethindrone acetate/ethinyl estridiol, *Contraception* 50:535, 1994.
Balocco R: Mefloquine prophylaxis against malaria for female travelers of childbearing age, *Lancet* 340:309, 1992.
Barry M, Bia FJ: Pregnancy and travel, *JAMA* 261:728, 1989.
Bia FJ: Medical considerations for the pregnant traveler, *Infect Dis Clin North Am* 6:371, 1992.
Bjarnadottir R et al: Comparison of cycle control with a combined contraceptive vaginal ring and oral levonorgestrel/ethinyl estradiol, *Am J Obstet Gynecol* 186(3):389, 2002.
Briggs GG, Freeman RK, Yaffe SJ: *Drugs in pregnancy and lactation: a reference guide to fetal and neonatal risk,* ed 4, Baltimore, 1994, William and Wilkins.
Burrow GN, Ferris TF, editors: *Medical complications during pregnancy,* Philadelphia, 1998, WB Saunders.
Burtin P et al: Safety of metronidazole in pregnancy: a meta-analysis, *Am J Obstet Gynecol* 172:525, 1995.
Camporeri EM: Diving and pregnancy, *Semin Perinatol* 20:292, 1996.
CDC: *Health information for international travel 2001-2002,* Atlanta, 2001, DHHS.
Chabala S, Williams M, Armenta R, Ognjan AF: Confirmed rabies exposure during pregnancy: treatment with human rabies immune globulin and human diploid cell vaccine, *Am J Med* 91:423, 1991.
Chompootaweep S et al: The use of two estrogen preparations (a combined pill versus conjugated estrogen cream) intravaginally to treat urogential symptoms in postmenopausal Thai women: a comparative study, *Clin Pharmacol Ther* 64: 204, 1998.
Cook GC: Use of antiprotozoan and antihelminthic drugs during pregnancy: side effects and contraindications, *J Infect* 25:1, 1992.
Coutinho EM et al: Comparative study on intermittent versus continuous use of a contraceptive pill administered by the vaginal route, *Contraception* 51:355, 1995.
Cruikshank DP, Wigton TR, Hays PM: Maternal physiology in pregnancy. In Gabbe SG, Niebyl JR, Simpson JL, editors: *Obstetrics: normal and problem pregnancies,* ed 3, New York, 1996, Churchill Livingstone.
Cunningham FG, MacDonald oral contraception, Grant NF: Antepartum management of normal pregnancy: prenatal care. In Cunningham FG, Williams JW, editors: *Williams obstetrics,* ed 20, Stamford Conn, 1997, Appleton and Lange.
Dolan G et al: Bed nets for the prevention of malaria and anemia of pregnancy, *Trans R Soc Trop Med Hyg* 87:620, 1993.
Drugs for parasitic infections, *Med Lett* 40:1, 1998.
Feldmeier H et al: Female genital schistosomiasis: new challenges from a gender perspective, *Trop Geographic Med* 47:S2, 1995.
Fesharek R, Quast U, Dechert G: Postexposure rabies vaccinations during pregnancy, *Vaccine* 8:409, 1990.
Garcia-Moreno C: *Gender and health: a technical paper,* World Health Organization, 1998, Geneva.
Gilstrap L, Faro S: *Infections in pregnancy,* New York, 1997, John Wiley and Sons.
Glasier A: Emergency postcoital contraception, *N Engl J Med* 337(15):1058, 1997.
Glasier A: Emergency contraception in a travel context, *J Travel Med* 6:1, 1999.
Golenda CE et al: Gender-related efficacy difference to an extended duration formulation of topical N,N-Diethyl-m-Tolumamide (DEET), *Am J Trop Med Hyg* 60(4):634, 1999.
Harjulehto-Mervaala T et al: Oral polio vaccination during pregnancy: no increase in the occurrence of congenital malformations, *Am J Epidemiol* 138:407, 1993.
Hatcher RA et al: *Contraceptive technology,* New York, 1998, Ardent Media.
Hawkes S, Hart G: Sexual health of travelers, *Infect Dis Clin North Am* 12:413, 1998.
Heimer G, Samsioe G: Effects of vaginally delivered estrogens, *Acta Obstet Gynecol Scand Suppl* 163:1, 1996.
Huche R: Physical activity at altitude in pregnancy, *Semin Perinatol* 20(4):303, 1996.

Huch R et al: Physiologic changes in pregnant women and their fetuses during jet travel, *Am J Obstet Gynecol* 154:996, 1986.
Hulgren H: *High altitude medicine,* Stanford, Calif, 1997, Hulgren Publications.
Katz M, Gerberding JL: The care of persons with recent exposure to HIV, *Ann Intern Med* 128:306, 1998.
Koren G, Pastuszak A, Ito S: Drugs in pregnancy, *N Engl J Med* 338:1128, 1998.
Lee RV, Barron WM, Cotton DB, Coustan DR, editors: *Current obstetric medicine,* vol 1, St Louis, 1991, Mosby-Year Book.
Lurie P et al: Postexposure prophylaxis after nonoccupational HIV exposure: clinical, ethical, and policy considerations, *JAMA* 280(20):1769, 1998.
Maccato M, Hammill H: Travel recommendations during pregnancy and breast feeding, *Pediatr Infect Dis J* 3:18, 1992.
MacLeod CL: The pregnant traveler, *Med Clin North Am* 76:1313, 1992.
MacLeod C, Lee R: Parasitic Infections. In Burrow G, Ferris TF, editors: *Medical complications during pregnancy,* ed 3, Philadelphia, 1988, WB Saunders.
Choice of contraceptives, Med Lett 37:9, 1995.
Miller RW: Effects of prenatal exposure to ionizing radiation, *Health Phys* 59:57, 1990.
Mishra L, Seeff LB: Viral hepatitis A through E, complicating pregnancy (review), *Gastoenterol Clin North Am* 21:873, 1992.
Moore J, Becker C: *Prevention of STD and HIV infection among Peace Corps volunteers: research recommendations,* Atlanta, 1993, Centers for Disease Control and Prevention.
Alternative feminine hygiene, *Ms. Magazine,* March 1993.
Nasidi A et al: Yellow fever vaccination and pregnancy: a four year prospective study, *Trans R Soc Trop Med Hyg* 87:337, 1993.
Nosten F et al: Mefloquine prophylaxis prevents malaria during pregnancy: a double bind, placebo controlled study, *J Infect Dis* 169:595, 1994.
Perlman D: Morning after HIV experiment starts in SF project to offer drugs, counseling, *San Francisco Chronicle,* October 14,1997, A2.
Phillips-Howard PA et al: Safety of mefloquine and other antimalarial agents in the first trimester of pregnancy, *J Travel Med* 5(3):121, 1998.
Phillips-Howard PA, Wood D: The safety of antimalarial drugs in pregnancy, *Drug Safety* 14:131, 1996.
Pinkerton SD, Holtgrave DR, Bloom FR: Cost-effectiveness of post-exposure-prophylaxis following sexual exposure to HIV, *AIDS* 12(9):1067, 1998.
Rogerson SJ, Beeson JG: The placenta in malaria: mechanisms of infection, disease and fetal morbidity, *Ann Trop Med Parasitol* 93(suppl 1):S35, 1999.
Samuel B, Barry M: The pregnant traveler, *Infect Dis Clin North Am* 12(2):325, 1998.
Sibai BM, Odlind V, Meador ML, et al: A comparative and pooled analysis of the safety and tolerability of the contraceptive patch (Ortho Evra/Evra), *Fertility & Sterility* 77(2 Suppl 2):S19, 2002.
Smoak BL et al: The effects of inadvertent exposure of mefloquine chemoprophylaxis on pregnancy outcomes and infants of US Army servicewomen, *J Infect Dis* 176(3):831, 1997.
Sylvia BM, McMullen P, Levine E, et al: Prenatal care needs availability, accessibility, use and satisfaction: a comparison of military women within and outside the continental United States, *Mil Med* 166:443, 2001.
Task Force on Postovulatory Methods of Fertility Regulation: Randomized control trial of levonorgestrel versus the Yuzpe regimen of combined oral contraception for emergency contraception, *Lancet* 352:428, 1998.
Tsai TF, Paul R, Lynberg MC, Letson GW: Congenital yellow fever infection after immunization in pregnancy, *J Infect Dis* 168:1520, 1993.
Vanhauwere B, Maradit H, Kerr L: Post-marketing surveillance of prophylactic mefloquine (Lariam) use in pregnancy, *Am J Trop Med Hyg* 58(1):17, 1998.
Vlassof C: The gender and tropical disease task force of TDR: achievements and challenges, *Acta Trop* 67:173, 1997.
Zacur H et al: Integrated summary of Ortho Evra/Evra contraceptive patch adhesion in varied climates and conditions, *Fertility & Sterility* 77(2 Suppl 2):S32, 2002.

CHAPTER 13

Travel and HIV Infection

Mary E. Wilson and Vito R. Iacoviello

All travelers fall into one of two categories: infected with human immunodeficiency virus (HIV) or at risk for HIV infection. Issues related to HIV should be addressed as a routine part of pretravel preparation. This chapter reviews travel preparation for the HIV-infected person and identifies potential sources of HIV infection during travel and interventions to prevent exposure to HIV.

THE HIV-INFECTED TRAVELER

HIV-infected persons require special preparation for travel to many geographic areas. The reasons are many: risk of infection with many common and unusual pathogens is increased; usual therapy may fail to cure infection; manifestations of infection may be atypical; reactions to drugs are common and may mimic other diseases; immune response to vaccines may be diminished; and political, social, and legal issues may complicate movement from one country to another. With the introduction of highly active antiretroviral therapy, many HIV-infected persons remain healthy and active and are traveling. This raises additional issues about potential drug-drug interactions and the need for regular laboratory monitoring. Table 13-1 lists drugs commonly used by HIV-infected persons and indicates potential interactions with drugs commonly used by travelers.

Infectious Disease Risks

Travelers encounter pathogens that are absent or uncommon in their country of residence. In addition, their risk of infection with ubiquitous pathogens such as *Salmonella* species is greater during travel than during day-to-day life at home. Many of these pathogens cause increased morbidity and mortality in HIV-infected persons. Three general groups of infections merit special attention: enteric infections, respiratory infections, and vector-borne infections.

Enteric Infections

Pathogens that enter via the gastrointestinal tract pose considerable threat to the HIV-infected traveler. Both intestinal mucosal and systemic defenses against gut pathogens are compromised in HIV-infected persons. Decreased gastric acid and diminished local immune response mean that a smaller inoculum may be needed to establish infection in an HIV-infected person. Once established, infection may be more severe and

Table 13-1A
Selected Drug-Drug Interactions for HIV-Infected Travelers*

Medication	Interacting medication/drug	Precaution/recommendation
Abacavir	Alcohol	Increases abacavir concentration
Amprenavir	Sulfonamides	Cross-hypersensitivity possible
	Astemizole, rifampin, triazolam, cisapride	Co-administration contraindicated
	Amiodarone, quinidine, warfarin	Closer drug monitoring suggested
	Tricyclic antidepressants	Closer drug monitoring suggested
	Rifabutin	Decrease rifabutin dose by 50%
	Oral contraceptives	Efficacy may be reduced
	Viagra (sildenafil)	Probable increase in levels and side effects.
	Antacids, didanosine	Separate by at least 1 hour
	Delavirdine, ritonavir, cimetidine	Possible increase in amprenavir concentrations
	Efavirenz, nevirapine	Possible decrease in amprenavir concentrations
Delavirdine	Alprazolam, astemizole, quinidine, rifabutin, rifampin	Co-administration contraindicated
	Terfenadine, triazolam	Co-administration contraindicated
	Antacids, didanosine	Separate by 1 hour
	Clarithromycin	Decrease clarithromycin dose 50%
	Dapsone	Increases delavirdine concentrations
	Indinavir	Change indinavir to 600 mg q8h
	Warfarin	Avoid or monitor closely, increases delavirdine concentration
Didanosine	Quinolones, dapsone, ketoconazole	Take 2 hours apart
Efavirenz	Nelfinavir	Increased nelfinavir levels
	Indinavir, amprenavir, clarithromycin	Decreased levels of these drugs
	Indinavir, astemizole, terfenadine, cisapride,	Co-administration contraindicated
	Triazolam, rifampin	Co-administration contraindicated
	Rifabutin	Decrease rifabutin dose 50%
	Ketoconazole	Decrease indinavir to 600 mg po q8h
Kaletra (lopinavir/ ritonavir)	Multiple	See ritonavir
Lamivudine	Trimethoprim/sulfamethoxazole (T/S)	Increased lamivudine concentration
Nelfinavir	Ketoconazole	Increased nelfinavir levels
	Rifampin	Decreased nelfinavir levels
	Terfenadine, astemizole, cisapride, triazolam	Co-administration contraindicated
	Oral contraceptives	Decreased levels of oral contraceptive
Nevirapine	Oral contraceptives, indinavir, saquinavir	Decreased levels of these drugs
	Rifampin, rifabutin	Decreased nevirapine levels
	Ketoconazole, itraconazole, clarithromycin, erythromycin	Increased nevirapine levels
Ritonavir	Alprazolam, amiodarone, astemizole, bupropion, cisapride, diazepam, flurazepam, piroxicam, propoxyphene, quinidine, rifabutin, terfenadine, triazolam	Co-administration contraindicated
	Oral contraceptives, theophylline	Decreased levels of these drugs

Continued

Table 13-1A
Selected Drug-Drug Interactions for HIV-Infected Travelers*—cont'd

Medication	Interacting medication/drug	Precaution/recommendation
Saquinavir	Astemizole, terfenadine	Avoid co-administration
Stavudine	Dapsone, ethionamide, iodoquinol, metronidazole, isoniazid	Potential additive toxicity, specifically neuropathy
Tenofovir	Didanosine	Increased concentration; no need to adjust dose
Zalcitabine	Dapsone, ethionamide, iodoquinol, metronidazole, isoniazid	Potential additive toxicity, specifically neuropathy
Zidovudine	T/S, pyrimethamine, atovaquone, fluconazole, probenecid	Potential increased toxicity, may increase zidovudine levels
	Dapsone	Potential additive hematologic toxicity

*For full discussion of drug interactions please see pharmaceutical company package insert.

Table 13-1B
Potential Drug Interactions of Frequently Used Travel-Related Medications*

Drug	Potential interaction with HIV medication
Acetozolamide	No specific contraindications
Chloroquine	No specific contraindications
DEET	No specific contraindications
Doxycycline	No specific contraindications
Loperamide	No specific contraindications
Mefloquine	No clinical data, from anecdotal experience no adverse events noted with nelfinavir
	No clinical data or formal pharmacologic data available with ritonavir; therefore co-administration could result in increased or decreased levels of either drug
	No formal pharmacologic data available for indinavir
Pepto-Bismol (bismuth subsalicylate)	No specific contraindications
Trimethoprim-Sulfamethoxazole	Zidovudine-potential additive toxicity
	Lamivudine-increased lamivudine concentrations
Quinolones	Administer quinolone at least 2 hours before didanosine

*Information obtained from pharmaceutical company package insert and communication with company representatives.

difficult to cure. Infections with *Salmonella, Shigella,* and *Campylobacter* species tend to be bacteremic, chronic, and relapsing. Salmonellosis is often characterized by recurrent bacteremias. Campylobacteriosis, cryptosporidiosis, and microsporidiosis may extend into the biliary tree. Table 13-2 summarizes some of the enteric infections frequently encountered by travelers and indicates morbidity in HIV-infected persons relative to the general population.

Respiratory Infections

Respiratory tract infections are common during travel, although the etiology is usually undefined. Several outbreaks of influenza in travelers have been documented. It is uncertain whether influenza per se causes increased morbidity in HIV-infected persons; however, HIV-infected persons are at increased risk for invasive infections with two bacterial pathogens, *Streptococcus pneumoniae* and *Haemophilus influenzae,* that commonly complicate influenza. Legionnaires' disease has infected travelers staying at resort hotels and using spa facilities in several locations including Europe and the Caribbean. Recent outbreaks of influenza and legionellosis on cruise ships document another possible place of transmission.

Table 13-2
Enteric Infections in Travelers

Disease	Estimated incidence in travelers*	Estimated morbidity/mortality in HIV-infected persons†
Amebiasis	Uncommon in most areas	Same or increased
Campylobacteriosis	Common	Increased
Cholera	Rare	Probably increased
Cryptosporidiosis	Probably common	Increased
Cyclospora	Probably common	Possibly increased
Escherichia coli diarrhea	Common	Possibly increased
Giardiasis	Uncommon in most areas	Same or increased
Isosporiasis	Uncommon in most areas	Increased
Microsporidiosis	Unknown	Increased
Salmonellosis	Common	Increased
Shigellosis	Common	Increased
Typhoid fever	Rare or uncommon in most areas	Increased
Vibrio parahaemolyticus and other noncholera *Vibrio* species	Uncommon	Possibly increased

Adapted from Wilson ME, von Reyn CF, Fineberg HV: Infections in HIV-infected travelers: Risks and prevention, *Ann Intern Med* 114:582, 1991.

**Common* indicates pathogens reported to cause at least 5% of cases of diarrhea in travelers in multiple studies in different geographic areas; *uncommon* refers to pathogens causing less than 5% of diarrheal cases. *Rare* describes infections not found as a cause of diarrhea in most studies of travelers. For nondiarrheal illnesses, *rare* indicates incidence in travelers is less than 10 cases per 100,000 per month.

†Estimated morbidity and mortality in HIV-infected persons represents a composite of greater frequency and severity of disease in HIV-infected persons relative to normal hosts.

Two geographically focal fungal infections, histoplasmosis and coccidioidomycosis, can be progressive and disseminated in HIV-infected persons. Infection occurs via inhalation of airborne organisms. The endemic area for coccidioidomycosis includes the southwestern United States, parts of Mexico, and Central and South America. Although the largest number of cases of histoplasmosis has been in the United States, cases have been reported from all continents. Another soil-associated fungal pathogen, *Penicillium marneffei,* found in Southeast Asia and China, is increasingly being found as a cause of disease (pulmonary and skin findings are common) in HIV-infected persons, especially in northern Thailand where more than 1000 cases have now been diagnosed. Travelers to the area who have become infected have manifested symptoms as early as 4 to 5 weeks and as late as 10 years or more after exposure.

HIV-infected persons are exquisitely susceptible to tuberculosis. Among HIV-infected persons with latent tuberculosis, about 10% per year develop active infection. The likelihood of exposure to tuberculosis in many developing countries (where annual incidence rates may exceed 100/100,000 population) is substantially higher than in the United States (annual incidence rates less than 10/100,000 population). Rarely, transmission has also been documented during travel (e.g., airplane, bus, train, boat). Tuberculin skin testing (intermediate-strength purified protein derivative) should be done on all HIV-infected persons, regardless of travel plans (see Chapter 22). An induration of 5 mm is considered positive in HIV-infected persons. The skin test should be repeated after prolonged stays in high-incidence areas, which include many parts of Africa and Asia. A infection of 4 to 12 weeks after exposure is generally required for development of delayed-type reactivity to the tuberculin test. HIV-infected persons may want to avoid prolonged stays (and especially repeated or long periods in indoor congregate settings with poor ventilation) in areas of the world where tuberculosis rates are high and multidrug resistance common.

Sinusitis is common in HIV-infected persons, especially in patients with CD4 counts less than 200/mm^3. Sinusitis tends to be severe, recurrent, and difficult to treat; it often involves multiple sinuses, including posterior sinuses. Changes in air pressure associated with air travel may convert previously asymptomatic or minimally symptomatic infection into acute, severe sinusitis. Use of decongestants, especially before descent, may lessen the risk. Reviewing the history for symptoms of current or past disease may help identify persons at increased risk, although symptoms are often nonspecific.

Vector-Borne Infections

Scientific studies have failed to show a major biologic association between HIV-1 and *falciparum* malaria. On the other hand, many case reports and studies show that HIV infection changes the clinical course of visceral leishmaniasis and probably also cutaneous leishmaniasis. In visceral leishmaniasis, mortality is high, often reflecting delayed diagnosis. Typical clinical features, such as splenomegaly and hyperglobulinemia, may be absent; and antibodies, often sought for diagnostic purposes, may be absent or delayed in appearance. Infection may first become manifest months or years after exposure in endemic areas; these include popular tourist destinations, such as Spain and other parts of southern Europe (see Chapter 34). Interactions between HIV and trypanosomiasis are less well characterized. A few reports document acute meningoencephalitis and central nervous system (CNS) mass lesions caused by *Trypanosoma cruzi* (American trypanosomiasis or Chagas' disease) in HIV-infected persons (see Chapter 23). As with visceral leishmaniasis, late reactivation may also be a feature of American trypanosomiasis. Because few travelers stay in accommodations where they are at risk for being bitten by infective reduviid bugs, reports of American trypanosomiasis in visitors to endemic areas have been rare. Fatal seronegative ehrlichiosis (a tick-borne infection) has been reported in an HIV-infected person. Babesiosis may also be more severe.

Preparation of the HIV-Infected Traveler

The approach to the HIV-infected traveler involves a series of steps, as outlined in Table 13-3. Depending on the destination and circumstances, some steps may be omitted or abbreviated. Evaluation and preparation of the HIV-infected traveler in most instances will require extra time. An early step is to review the feasibility of the planned travel. Essential to the evaluation is an estimate of the stage of HIV disease; this will help assess the types of infections and other complications that are most likely. A recent CD4 count and viral load measurement are generally the most helpful. Although some infections (e.g., *S. pneumoniae, Mycobacterium tuberculosis, Salmonella* species) occur with increased frequency even in early HIV infection, many infections that may require sophisticated medical facilities for diagnosis, such as *Pneumocystis carinii* pneumonia and CNS toxoplasmosis, are seen primarily in persons with CD4 counts less than $200/mm^3$. Destination and duration of stay will affect recommendations. For persons with late-stage infection or those planning a prolonged stay, it is especially important to identify medical resources before departure. All travelers should have medical insurance that will provide coverage during the trip. For travel to developing countries (or any place where good medical facilities may be unavailable), travelers should also have special insurance that will cover evacuation in the event the local medical facilities are inadequate to provide good care for an acute illness or injury. It may be necessary to arrange in advance for the continuation of special therapy or laboratory testing.

As of January 1999, more than 60 countries required HIV testing for some foreigners before entry into the country. Specific regulations vary among countries and change over time. Different groups for which HIV screening was required by various countries as of 1999 included applicants for long-term residence or for citizenship, foreign students, entertainers, and foreigners seeking permits as unskilled laborers. Require-

Table 13-3
Preparation and Education Before Departure

Review feasibility of planned travel
Identify medical resources abroad
Anticipate legal and immigration issues
Review itinerary and area-specific risks
Educate regarding risk reduction (e.g., prudent dietary habits)

ments for testing are often tied to duration of expected stay. Knowledge of updated regulations in the destination countries can help avoid embarrassing, disruptive, and unpleasant experiences. U.S. test results are accepted in some countries, but not in others. In some countries, entering travelers can be required to undergo testing at the demand of government officials. This evokes all of the concerns about quality control in testing, reliability of confirmatory tests, and sterility of needles and syringes.

One goal of a pretravel visit is to identify specific risks, assess their magnitude, and educate the traveler in ways to reduce them. Destination-related risks for the HIV-infected traveler may influence decisions about whether to undertake all or part of a proposed trip. The health care provider should review area-specific risks and consider available means to reduce them. Guidelines for prevention of disease and bureaucratic difficulties should be provided, preferably accompanied by written information. The traveler will have to decide whether the estimated risks are worth taking. Under some circumstances, the traveler may decide to change an itinerary if risk of serious disease cannot be eliminated or reduced.

For the long-term traveler it is essential to assess the need for periodic laboratory testing and the availability of specialized tests, such as routine chemistries and hematology studies but also T-cell subsets and viral quantitation, in the destination country. Also to be reviewed is the feasibility of appropriate storage of the drugs, especially if the destination is a tropical, developing county, where refrigeration may be unavailable or erratic. Some drugs are sensitive to moisture (e.g., indinavir), ritonavir (Norvir) capsules require refrigeration, and delavirdine should be stored at 68° to 77° F. In general, a patient should be on a stable regimen for at least 8 weeks before departure. Patients on a stable regimen usually require monitoring tests every 4 months, although this can be extended to 6 months in selected patients. The physician and patient can work together to develop an antiretroviral regimen with less stringent storage requirements, a manageable dosing schedule, and less stringent hydration requirements.

Immunoprophylaxis

Preventive strategies for travel-associated infectious diseases include immunoprophylaxis and chemoprophylaxis. With respect to vaccines, two basic questions are relevant. What extra vaccines should be given or considered because of the increased need for protection? What routine vaccines should be avoided or given with caution to the HIV-infected person because of increased risk of adverse events from the vaccines?

For each of the vaccines, efficacy and safety should be considered. In general, administration of vaccines to HIV-infected persons leads to antibody levels that are lower and less durable. The immune response tends to reflect the degree of HIV-induced immunosuppression. Response may be poor and less durable in persons with late-stage infection. In HIV infection, both cellular and humoral immunity are compromised; presence of measurable antibodies may not reflect protection.

Serious adverse events associated with vaccine administration in HIV-infected persons have been rare despite early concerns about the use of live vaccines. Although a number of studies have documented transient increases in plasma levels of HIV RNA after vaccination with influenza and pneumococcal vaccines and tetanus toxoids, there has been no clear evidence that the antigenic stimulus from vaccines leads to a sustained increase in HIV replication or hastens progression of HIV disease. Not surprisingly, antibody response varies with the vaccine and among individuals.

Four general recommendations follow from these observations are: (1) The potential benefits from many of the vaccines seem to outweigh their risks; (2) one may want to measure antibodies to assess response to vaccine; (3) administration early in HIV infection is more likely to be efficacious; and (4) where different routes or schedules are available, the most immunogenic should be used. Although yellow fever vaccine is the only one required for entry into some countries, many others are prudent. (Meningococcal vaccine required for travel to Saudi Arabia during the Haj is safe to give even in late-stage HIV vaccine.)

Routine Vaccines

Table 13-4 lists vaccines to consider giving an HIV-infected person before travel. These assume the patient received the full primary series of immunization with vaccines usually given in childhood. The pretravel visit offers an opportunity to review routine vaccines. Annual influenza vaccination is recommended for HIV-infected persons, even when no travel is planned. Because influenza occurs during April through September in the Southern Hemisphere and throughout the year in tropical countries, it may be prudent to give travelers the vaccine outside the usual North American influenza season, although availability of the vaccine can be a problem in the off-season. Prophylaxis with rimantadine or amantidine is another option if there is a poor match between the circulating influenza A strain and the current vaccine.

Pneumococcal infections are more common and more likely to be bacteremic in HIV-infected persons. Rates may be more than 100-fold higher than in an age-matched non-HIV-infected population. Thus the pneumococcal vaccine is recommended in HIV-infected persons, preferably early in the course of HIV infection. Asymptomatic HIV-infected persons with CD4 counts less than $500/mm^3$ are substantially less likely to respond to the pneumococcal capsular polysaccharide than healthy young adults, although even with advanced stages of immunosuppression, some HIV-infected persons are able to mount an antibody response. Pneumococcal infections may not be more common during travel, but penicillin-resistant strains are more prevalent in many areas of the world than they are in the United States, and any serious illness during travel can be disruptive.

Because hepatitis B and HIV share similar routes of transmission, many HIV-infected persons will already be immune to hepatitis B or be chronic carriers of hepatitis B surface antigen (HBsAg). The hepatitis B vaccine appears to be safe to use and should be given to hepatitis B-susceptible, HIV-infected persons who meet the usual criteria for the vaccine. HIV-infected persons are more likely to become chronic carriers of HBsAg if they become infected with hepatitis B virus. They also respond less well to the vaccine, with only 50% to 70% developing antibody titers that are considered protective.

Rates of invasive *H. influenzae* infections are substantially higher in HIV-infected persons than in the general population. Because many of the strains causing invasive disease are not serotype B (e.g., only 33% of strains were serotype B in one study in HIV-infected men), the conjugate vaccine directed against type B disease in common use may have limited benefit. Given that the vaccine appears to be safe, administration of the vaccine may be considered.

Vaccines for Travel to Developing Countries

A second group of vaccines listed in Table 13-4 are frequently administered before travel to developing countries. Because of the increased risk of vaccine-associated poliomyelitis in immunosuppressed persons, the enhanced inactivated parenteral polio vaccine (eIPV) should be used instead of oral live polio vaccine (OPV) in HIV-infected persons and their

Table 13-4
Immunizations for Adult HIV-Infected Travelers

Indication	Vaccine	Comments
Routine	Diphtheria-tetanus*	Booster interval 10 years
	Haemophilus influenzae b, conjugate	Optional
	Hepatitis B†	Assess antibody level following vaccine
	Influenza	Yearly
	Pneumococcal	Recommended; one booster after 5 years
Standard for travel to developing countries	Hepatitis A‡	Give minimum of 4 weeks before departure
	Immune globulin‡	Duration 3-5 months; dose dependent
	Measles or MMR§	Avoid in late stage HIV
	Polio, enhanced inactivated (eIPV)	Avoid live oral polio vaccine
	Typhoid, inactivated Vi polysaccharide	Booster interval 3 years; avoid live oral typhoid vaccine (Ty21a)
For selected destinations or circumstances	Japanese encephalitis	Assess risks and benefits; no efficacy data
	Meningococcus	No efficacy data
	Rabies	Use IM vaccine series, no efficacy data; assess antibody level following vaccination
	Yellow fever**	Do not give if CD4 counts $<200/mm^3$; booster interval 10 years
	BCG (Bacille Calmette-Guérin)	Avoid BCG

Adapted from Wilson ME, von Reyn CF, Fineberg HV: Infections in HIV-infected travelers: risks and prevention, *Ann Intern Med* 114:582, 1991.
*Recommendations assume a history of routine childhood immunizations.
†Omit if person is already immune to hepatitis B.
‡Omit if person has serologic evidence of immunity to hepatitis A.
§May be omitted if patient has serologic evidence of measles immunity.
¶Rarely indicated.
**Required by many countries in Africa and South America and by other countries for travelers who have visited or been in transit through countries where yellow fever is endemic.

household contacts. The inactivated Vi polysaccharide typhoid vaccine should also be used in preference to the oral typhoid vaccine (Ty21a), although no cases of progressive infection with this attenuated strain of *Salmonella typhi* have been reported. Travelers who lack immunity to hepatitis A should be given one of the inactivated hepatitis A vaccines, ideally at least 4 weeks before departure. Immune globulin is a safe alternative for persons who do not have time to receive the vaccine. The commercially available serologic tests for hepatitis A antibody assess whether a person is immune because of past infection but are not sufficiently sensitive to pick up vaccine-induced antibodies. Hence, routine serologic testing after hepatitis A vaccination is not recommended.

Recommendations about the measles vaccine in HIV-infected persons differ from advice about other live vaccines. This live vaccine is recommended for HIV-infected persons, unless they have severe immunosuppression. A case of fatal giant cell pneumonitis associated with measles vaccine virus has been reported in a young man with late-stage AIDS. The following observations underlie the current recommendation: (1) Measles infection in HIV-infected persons can be atypical, severe, and sometimes fatal; (2) measles vaccine has generally been safe (with exception noted previously), although most of the experience in HIV infection has been in young children; (3) treatment modalities for measles are limited; (4) measles is highly contagious and exposure is often inapparent; and (5) risk of exposure is greater during travel to many developing countries than it is in the United States. The measles cases in the United States now are imported or related to imported cases. The current recommendation is for two doses of measles vaccine (the first dose usually given at age 12 to 15 months with a second dose in childhood). Some adults who never experienced natural infection because of measles vaccination in infancy have not received a second vaccine dose, and may be candidates for the second dose before travel. It may be worthwhile to assess measles antibody status in HIV-infected persons even if born before 1957, if they have no history of natural measles.

Special Vaccines for Specific Destinations or Activities

Other vaccines listed in Table 13-4 are recommended only for specific destinations or special circumstances. The traditional inactivated cholera vaccine is safe, but it is no longer available in the United States. HIV-infected persons are probably at increased risk for cholera because gastric acid is an important barrier to infection. Newer vaccines are not yet available. Education about the need for rehydration for severe diarrhea and the availability of oral rehydration salts is important for all travelers.

Rabies vaccine should be given to HIV-infected persons who meet the usual criteria for the vaccine. The more immunogenic intramuscular route and dose (1 ml) should be used (instead of 0.1 ml dose via intradermal route) because it offers a greater potential for efficacy. For persons at high risk of exposure, it may be prudent to measure antibodies to assess if the usual three-dose series has provided protective levels of antibodies.

The yellow fever vaccine often poses the most difficult dilemma because infection with yellow fever may be lethal and effective treatment is unavailable, the vaccine contains live virus, and proof of vaccination is required for entry into many countries. There are three main options for an HIV-infected person who plans to travel to yellow fever endemic countries. Transmission of yellow fever is focal in endemic areas and many travelers to countries requiring yellow fever vaccine are at no risk of infection. A reasonable option for a person visiting an area without current yellow fever transmission is to provide a letter of waiver saying that the vaccine is contraindicated for medical reasons. Another approach is to change the itinerary to avoid countries requiring the vaccine. The third option is to give the vaccine. HIV-infected persons with CD4 counts greater than $200/mm^3$ who cannot avoid exposure to the yellow fever virus should be offered the vaccine. In persons with lower CD4 counts, the possible risks and benefits should be considered on an individual basis. For HIV-infected persons who receive the vaccine and who will be at moderate or high risk of exposure, it may be prudent to assess levels of neutralizing antibodies after vaccination (consult state health department or Centers for Disease and Control, Fort Collins, CO, at 970-221-6400). Whether or not the vaccine is given, the traveler should be given explicit instructions in ways to avoid mosquito bites. Insect control maneuvers can help to prevent many infections in addition to malaria and yellow fever. Use of permethrin sprayed on clothing may be a useful adjunct to other approaches to preventing bites.

Chemoprophylaxis for Traveler's Diarrhea

All HIV-infected persons should be given advice, and preferably written materials, describing ways to avoid risky food and beverages. Those traveling to developing countries should be given a prescription for antimicrobial agents, either to be taken as prophylaxis or to be used as empiric therapy in the event of acute diarrheal illness (see Chapters 6 and 26). Because HIV-infected persons have a higher risk for diarrhea than other travelers, the threshold for recommending prophylactic antibiotics may be lower. This issue should be discussed and individual preferences considered. Some considerations in the decision to use prophylaxis versus early empiric therapy include destination and duration of stay, available medical facilities at the destination, allergies, and other concurrent medications. If the traveler is already taking sulfamethoxazole/trimethoprim for *Pneumocystis* prophylaxis, a different agent should be chosen for early self-treatment of diarrhea. A quinolone, such as norfloxacin or ciprofloxacin, is a reasonable choice.

Antimalarial Prophylaxis

Antimalarial agents and advice about personal protective measures to prevent mosquito bites should be given to HIV-infected travelers, as to others. Many HIV-infected persons are allergic to sulfonamides, so use of sulfadoxine/pyrimethamine (Fansidar), which contains a long-acting sulfonamide, as presumptive therapy may not be an option. Mefloquine is currently a first-line drug recommended for most chloroquine-resistant malarious areas. Because of the high frequency of underlying neurologic problems in HIV-infected persons, it is important to review any history of seizures or current signs or symptoms of CNS disease before prescribing this agent. Atovaquone/proguanil (Malarone) is another first-line drug for malaria chemoprophylaxis that may be considered if the HIV-infected traveler is not already on atovaquone.

HIV-UNINFECTED TRAVELER

Routes of HIV Transmission in Other Countries

Routes of transmission of HIV infection are the same throughout the world, yet risks may exist that may catch travelers unaware. Too often in the United States, HIV is perceived as an infection spread primarily through homosexual activities and intravenous drug use. Some generally informed persons believe that if they avoid those activities, they are at no risk. However, sexual contacts with new partners, including heterosexual relations, are the most common means of exposure to HIV during travel. The pretravel evaluation is an opportunity to give explicit advice and education about the risks of casual sex. In addition to sexual contacts, other possible sources of exposure to HIV during travel, especially in developing countries, include parenteral exposures (needles used for injections of medications, acupuncture, tattoos, ear piercing, body piercing, injection drug use, invasive medical procedures) and blood and blood products. In many countries with limited resources, blood is not routinely screened for HIV infection. In a 1993–1994 survey of blood transfusion practices in 12 countries in Central and South American only 9 countries screened donors for HIV.

Avoiding HIV Infection During Travel

The pretravel visit should include education about how to avoid HIV infection and should begin with the assumption that the traveler may have casual sex during the trip. For example, a study in 1991 and 1992 found 18.6% of travelers reported a new sexual partner on their most recent trip, and 5.7% acquired a sexually transmitted infection. Strategies to reduce risk include avoiding sex. Those who plan to (or think they might) have sex with a new partner should be advised to pack latex condoms, since ones of good quality are not readily available in many countries. Anyone anticipating the need for injections (or planning prolonged stay in remote areas) should consider taking sterile needles and syringes, accompanied by a letter on an official letterhead explaining that the needles are for medical purposes only. Invasive procedures (including dental work) should be limited to those absolutely required. Medical facilities should be chosen carefully. Persons planning a long stay should identify a reliable medical facility soon after arrival, before a medical crisis arises.

Medical students, humanitarian volunteers, and other health care workers who may have intimate contact with local residents should gather information before departure about rates of infection in the area where they will be working and availability of protective measures, screening tests, and drugs to treat HIV. Health care personnel should be counseled about potential risks and ways to reduce them. In some instances, health care workers may want to take with them supplies of disposable gloves, protective eyewear, and a course of drugs that could be used for postexposure treatment. In countries where antiviral drugs have had limited use, rates of zidovudine resistance may be low, but in places where standard antiviral drug regimens have been used extensively to treat HIV-infected persons, emergence of drug-resistant viral strains may render the commonly used post exposure prophylaxis drug protocols ineffective for that purpose.

Although the emphasis is given to prevention of infections during travel (Table 13-5), the greatest threat to health and well-being in many countries comes from injury, especially motor vehicle accidents. Injury is the event most likely to lead to emergency blood transfusion, with the attendant risk of infection by HIV or other blood-borne pathogens. Although injury may seem unavoidable, in fact, some simple maneuvers can reduce the risk of some kinds of injury. Travelers have some control over choice of car, use of seat belts, time of day for travel, use of two-wheeled vehicles, sobriety

Table 13-5
Strategies to Reduce Risk for HIV Infection During Travel

Avoid sex with new partners
Use condoms, if having sex
Take sterile needles and syringes
Avoid invasive procedures (unless urgently needed), tattoos, ear and body piercing
Choose medical facilities carefully
Avoid injury, motor vehicle accidents

and wakefulness during driving, and level of attentiveness during driving. Mention of motor vehicle-related risks during the pretravel session can reinforce the need to take extra precautions.

REFERENCES

Angel JB et al: Vaccine-associated measles pneumonitis in an adult with AIDS, *Ann Intern Med* 129:104, 1998.

Chariyalertsak S et al: Case-control study of risk factors for *Penicillium marneffei* infection in human immunodeficiency virus-infected patients in northern Thailand, *Clin Infect Dis* 24:1080, 1997.

Colebunders R et al: Incidence of malaria and efficacy of oral quinine in patients recently infected with human immunodeficiency virus in Kinshasa, Zaire, *J Infect* 21:167, 1990.

Fleming AF: Opportunistic infections in AIDS in developed and developing countries, *Trans R Soc Trop Med Hyg* 84(suppl 1):1, 1990.

Fuller JD et al: Influenza vaccination of human immunodeficiency virus (HIV)-infected adults: impact on plasma levels of HIV type 1 RNA and determinants of antibody response, *Clin Infect Dis* 28:541, 1999.

Gamester CF, Tilzey AJ, Banatvala JE: Medical students' risk of infection with blood-borne viruses at home and abroad: questionnaire survey, *BMJ* 318:158, 1999.

Godofsky EW et al: Sinusitis in HIV-infected patients: a clinical and radiographic review, *Am J Med* 93:163, 1992.

Gotuzzo E et al: Association between the acquired immunodeficiency syndrome and infection with *Salmonella typhi* or *Salmonella paratyphi* in an endemic typhoid area, *Arch Intern Med* 151:381, 1991.

Goujon C et al: Good tolerance and efficacy of yellow fever vaccine among carriers of human immunodeficiency, *J Travel Med* 2:145, 1995.

Hawkes S et al: Risk behaviour and HIV prevalence in international travelers, *AIDS* 8:247, 1994.

Hess G et al: Immunogenicity and safety of an inactivated hepatitis A vaccine in anti-HIV positive and negative homosexual med, *J Med Virol* 46:40, 1995.

Kaplan JE, Masur H, Holmes K: USPHS/IDSA guidelines for the prevention of opportunistic infections in persons infected with human immunodeficiency virus: an overview, *Clin Infect Dis* 21(suppl)S12, 1995.

Kaul DR, Cinti SK, Carver PL, Kazanjian PH: HIV protease inhibitors: advances in therapy and adverse reactions, including metabolic complications, *Pharmacotherapy* 19(3):281, 1999.

Kemper CA, Linett A, Kane C, Deresinski SC: Frequency of travel of adults infected with HIV, *J Travel Med* 2:85, 1995.

Lopez-Velez R et al: Clinicoepidemiologic characteristics, prognostic factors, and survival analysis of patients coinfected with human immunodeficiency virus and *Leishmania* in an area of Madrid, Spain, *Am J Trop Med Hyg* 58:436, 1998.

Rhoads JL et al: Safety and immunogenicity of multiple conventional immunizations administered during early HIV infection, *J Acquir Immune Defic Syndr* 4:724, 1991.

Stanley SK et al: Effect of immunization with a common recall antigen on viral expression in patients infected with human immunodeficiency virus type 1, *N Engl J Med* 334:1222, 1996.

Taburet A-M, Singlas E: Drug interactions with antiviral drugs, *Clin Pharmacokinet* 30:385, 1996.

U.S. Department of State. Human immunodeficiency virus testing requirements for entry into foreign countries. Updated annually. For copy, send self-addressed stamped envelope to: Bureau of Consular Affairs, CA/PA, Room 5807, Department of State, Washington, DC, 20520. Can also access information from the web site: http://travel.state.gov

Wilson ME: *A world guide to infections: diseases, distribution, diagnosis,* New York, 1991, Oxford University Press.

Wilson ME, von Reyn CF, Fineberg HV: Infections in HIV-infected travelers: risks and prevention, *Ann Intern Med* 114:582, 1991.

Zurlo JJ et al: Sinusitis in HIV-1 infection, *Am J Med* 93:157, 1992.

CHAPTER 14

Travel with Chronic Medical Conditions

Mari C. Sullivan and Elaine C. Jong

It is important for the traveler with chronic medical conditions to consider factors such as access to medical care, the possible increased demands for aerobic exercise, changes in diet, availability of medical supplies, and the effects of altitude on illnesses when planning a trip to a foreign destination; thus advance planning is essential for persons in this category of travelers. Another factor that could make a significant difference in the success of a journey is being able to travel with a companion. The traveling companion need not be medically oriented but could provide invaluable help in getting professional assistance should an urgent medical need arise.

There are many remote areas of the world where medical care may be hours or days away from a traveler stricken by illness or complications of a preexisting condition. If an individual with a chronic disease is very stressed by the thought of remote travel and lack of access to care, it may be justified to counsel that traveler to adjust his or her itinerary to one that includes the availability of adequate medical care. The traveler with chronic medical conditions has to consider whether the anticipated benefits of the planned travel experience are worth accepting the potential health risks associated with a given itinerary.

Air travel can be stressful because of the noise, turbulence, crowding, limited seating space, and psychological factors (fear of flying). In addition, air travel may present high-altitude barometric and oxygen stresses, as well as rapidly transport the traveler across many time zones, necessitating special changes in the timing of medications. Travel by land or sea routes may be less stressful for people with medical conditions, but still requires advance planning. Regardless of mode of transportation, if special medical equipment must be taken along (wheelchairs, portable oxygen tanks, dialysis equipment and fluids, oversize or excess baggage for supplies, etc.), travelers should contact the medical departments of major airline, railroad, or cruise ship companies for specific information and guidance before confirming reservations.

CHRONIC OBSTRUCTIVE PULMONARY DISEASE AND OTHER LUNG DISEASES

The effects of exercise, exposure to cold, altitude, and extreme heat can be significant stressors for the traveler with underlying lung disease. The presence of environmental allergens and pollution in various cities of the world, such as Beijing, Mexico City, and Kathmandu, to name a few, are additional significant considerations.

Modern jet aircraft can pressurize passenger cabins to sea level up to a cruising altitude of 22,500 ft. Higher cruise altitudes between 30,300 and 40,000 ft are generally used by commercial aircraft for longer trips, with a cabin pressure simulating an altitude between 5000 ft (as in Denver) and 8000 ft (as in Mexico City). Healthy passengers can tolerate this moderate change in altitude, but patients with chronic obstructive pulmonary disease (COPD) may have increased hypoxemia owing not only to diminished oxygen pressure, but also to impaired hypoxic ventilatory drive, decreased cardiac reserve, and mechanical limitations. An example of the last is restricted lung expansion resulting from abdominal distention from trapped gases in the bowel expanding at the higher altitudes. Apple juice is a major cause of intestinal gas; carbonated drinks are not. Keeping this in mind, the choice of beverages used to maintain hydration during air travel is important. The relatively low humidity inside the passenger cabin (10% to 12%) may cause difficulty for patients with thick pulmonary secretions or tracheostomies, so adequate individual hydration must be maintained while avoiding beverages that cause excessive intestinal gas, diuresis, or sedation.

In general, overeating, alcoholic beverages, sedatives, and cigarette smoking should be avoided by patients with respiratory conditions during air travel and once at destination. Although American air carriers have made smoking illegal on all flights, this may not be true of international carriers. In foreign countries, travelers may find that there are no anti-smoking policies in place. It is important that travelers who are concerned about environmental exposure to tobacco smoke be aware that smoking by others could present a problem in restaurants, hotels, banks, conference rooms, and other public places of business, as well as on buses and other modes of public transportation. Thus the prevalence of smoking among the residents of the areas to be visited and the existence of smoke-free environments may influence the choice of itinerary for this group of travelers.

Table 14-1 presents some pulmonary contraindications to air travel. However, these contraindications are general and certain individuals with chronic lung disease who fall into one of these categories may be able to travel on the advice of their personal physicians. Most experts recommend supplemental oxygen during air travel for people with a baseline Po_2 of 70 mm Hg or less at sea level. Table 14-2 shows the drop in the arterial Po_2 going from sea level to an altitude of 8000 ft in healthy young adults and in a group of patients with COPD. Dillard and colleagues have proposed a formula that used the preflight Pao_2 and FEV1 on the ground *(G)* for a given patient to predict the Pao_2 at cruising altitude *(Alt)*:

$$Pao_2\ Alt = 0.453\ (Pao_2\ G) + 0.386\ (\text{FEV1 \% predicted}) + 2.440$$

They recommend that if the predicted Pao_2 at altitude is 40 to 55 mm Hg, the patient is likely to require supplemental oxygen during a long flight (6 hours) on commercial aircraft.

Supplemental Oxygen

Supplemental oxygen supplies can be arranged on most airlines (with at least 48 hours notice) by a signed letter or prescription from the patient's physician (see Chapter 2). This must state the desired flow rate, type of mask, and whether the oxygen is to be used intermittently or continu-

Table 14-1
Respiratory Contraindications to Air Travel*

Conditions Adversely Affected by Hypoxia
Active bronchospasm
Cyanosis
Dyspnea at rest or during exercise
Pneumonia or acute upper respiratory tract infection
Pulmonary hypertension with or without cor pulmonale
Severe anemia (hemoglobin level 7.5 gm/dl) or sickling hemoglobinopathies
Unstable coexisting cardiac disorders, such as arrhythmias, angina pectoris, and recent myocardial infarction (within 3 to 4 weeks)

Conditions Adversely Affected by Pressure Changes
Thoracic surgery in the preceding 3 weeks
Noncommunicating lung cysts
Otitis media, sinusitis, or recent middle ear surgery
Pneumothorax or pneumomediastinum

Inadequate Pulmonary Function (As Evidenced By One or More of the Following)
Diffusing capacity less than 50% of predicted
Hypercapnia ($Paco_2$ >50 mm Hg)
Hypoxemia while breathing room air (Pao_2 <50 mm Hg)
Maximum voluntary ventilation less than 40 L/min
Vital capacity less than 50% of predicted

Other Contraindications
Contagious diseases, including active tuberculosis

From Gong H Jr: Advising COPD patients about commercial air travel, *J Repir Dis* 11:484-499, 1990.
*These contraindications are relative, since patients may significantly improve with appropriate therapy and supplemental oxygen.

ously. Most of the time, there is an extra charge for this service. Some airlines such as Cathay Pacific, Air Canada, Air Malta, and Virgin Atlantic will provide this service at no charge or minimal charges, whereas other carriers such as Alitalia charge the cost of the airfare for in-flight oxygen.

Special arrangements have to be made with oxygen distributors at each airport for supplies of oxygen needed on the ground during layovers and airport transfers to connecting flights, and even for the final destination if it is more than 5000 ft above sea level. Travelers with moderate to severe COPD who are already hypoxic at ambient conditions at home should not plan trips to high altitudes. The risk for high altitude pulmonary edema is significant in these individuals.

The traveling companion should be instructed that visual impairment, fatigue, headache, sleepiness, dizziness, personality changes, impaired memory or judgment, and incoordination may be signs of oxygen deficiency and that medical assistance may be needed.

Travelers with Asthma

In 1998 the CDC estimated that 17,299,000 people have asthma in the United States alone. A review by Gern and Busse shows that patients with underlying asthma are much more likely to have significant complications

Table 14-2
Decline in Blood Oxygen Tension with Increase in Altitude in Tow Patient Groups

Group	Pa_{O_2} sea level	Pa_{O_2} 5500 ft	Pa_{O_2} 8000 ft*
Healthy young adults	98 mm Hg	68 mm Hg	60-63 mm Hg
Patients with COPD	72.4 mm Hg	—	47.7 mm Hg†

From Dillard TA, Berg BW, Rajagopol KR, et al: Hypoxia during air travel in patients with chronic obstructive pulmonary disease, *Ann Intern Med* 111:362-367, 1989.
*A given cruising altitude of 35,000 ft above sea level will result in a cabin altitude varying from 5000 to 8000 ft among different aircraft models according to pressurization schedules.
†After 45 minutes' steady-state hypobaric exposure, equivalent to 8000 ft above sea level.

from exposure to rhinovirus and influenza virus infections than those without asthma. Respiratory infections are among the common ailments of travelers with personal stress, air travel, contact with strangers, and environmental contamination contributing to the risk of exposure. Thus it is important for the traveler with asthma and other chronic respiratory conditions to have annual immunization with the flu vaccine, to be up to date on all other recommended vaccines (including pneumococcal vaccine), and to optimize health status before departure.

Travelers with asthma should carry with them an adequate supply of medications. Medications should be hand-carried and not placed in checked baggage during travel. Asthma is a problem worldwide, and while it is best for patients to use medications acquired at home, traveling patients should be informed in case of lost or missing supplies that certain common medications may be available under different brand names but similar formation when abroad. For example, *albuterol* may be available as *salbutamol* in other countries.

In addition to the chemical air pollution in many cities of the world, molds and pollens may present new or unidentified triggers for exacerbations of asthma. Travelers may visit regions of the world where dust mites and cockroaches are prevalent, and exposure to byproducts of these could pose increased risks for triggering asthma attacks. Travelers with any remote history of asthma or reactive airway disease should be warned that travel to a new place could trigger asthma even if they have been asymptomatic for years.

Travelers with asthma should have a peak flow meter and know how to use this device for self-assessment of subtle exacerbations of their condition while traveling. Specific instructions on when and how to self-treat an exacerbation should be given. Depending on the travel itinerary and circumstances, the traveling patient should include short-acting bronchodilator multidose inhalers (MDIs), a course of oral prednisone, one or more oral antibiotics (e.g., azithromycin, levofloxacin, amoxicillin plus clavulinate, second- or third- generation cephalosporin, etc.) against common respiratory pathogens, oral medications against viral influenza (amantidine, rimantidine, zanamivir, etc.), and extra steroid MDIs in their travel medicine kit (Chapter 1).

Patients with asthma traveling to colder environments should be instructed to wear hats with a facemask to rewarm inhaled air, and appropriate clothing. Patients should be instructed to wear a respirator capable of filtering chemical pollutants if planning travel to cities of the world where air pollution is a significant problem.

Unlike patients with COPD, patients with asthma generally do well at altitude. Some theories for this are that they are less exposed to allergens and other etiologic factors responsible for triggering asthma exacerbations. In addition, patients with asthma may be more sensitive to declines in their respiratory function, and may spontaneously limit or decrease their activity levels as this occurs. This may have a protective effect when trekking to altitude and in other types of travel.

CARDIOVASCULAR DISEASE

The decrease in arterial PO_2 at cruising altitudes of commercial aircraft was discussed previously. In patients with cardiopulmonary disease, the hypoxemia that develops may produce symptoms during prolonged commercial air flights. Supplemental oxygen should be considered and arrangements made in advance.

Patients should be sure to carry their prescribed medications in their hand-held carry-on baggage, as well as copies of recent medical records (electrocardiogram, vital signs, list of diagnoses, list of prescription medication and doses, and name and telephone number of their personal physician or cardiologist). Salty foods, carbonated beverages, immoderate consumption of alcoholic beverages, and fatty or spicy foods should be avoided during flight. Carrying along healthy snack food from home is a good precaution against unsuitable airline food. Passengers should get up and walk around the aircraft cabin periodically and/or flex and extend their lower extremities while seated at least once an hour to decrease venous stasis and pooling.

A study of medical emergencies among commercial air travelers by Cummins and Schubach, examined cases where emergency medical technicians were called to the airport; the majority of emergencies among air travelers happened on the ground within the air terminal. Only 25% experienced their problem during flight; the most common medical problems were abdominal pain, chest pain, shortness of breath, syncope, and seizures. Although the rate of medical emergencies for inbound passengers was low (1 of every 39,600 inbound passengers), the authors suggested that given the volume of passengers involved, a large number of people can be anticipated to experience medical problems requiring emergency assistance during air travel or in the hours immediately before or after. Five cardiac arrests occurred among the 754 travelers who experienced emergencies in the 1-year survey: one of these cardiac arrests took place on board an aircraft (on the ground before take-off), one on the ground at the concourse gate minutes after deplaning, and three in travelers who had deplaned and were at the baggage claims area.

Given the physical and emotional stress on passengers in air terminals, as they rush to cover relatively long distances on foot to make connecting flights or to retrieve their bags in the baggage claim area, several commonsense tips for air travelers could be given:

1. Allow plenty of time for travel to the airport, airport parking, standing in line at the ticket counter to check in, and passage through security checks to get to the departure gate.

2. Request an aisle seat, at the time the ticket is booked, for increased mobility and leg room (although the aisle seat places a passenger at increased risk of injuries from baggage falling out of overhead bins, should the aircraft experience severe turbulence, compared with a window seat).
3. Request special in-flight meals (low salt, vegetarian, etc.) in advance, at the time the ticket is booked.
4. Request assistance by wheelchair or airport motor cart for transport within the airport terminal if there are problems with ambulation, exercise tolerance, or any other disabilities.
5. Pack lightly, and utilize luggage with wheels or a baggage cart for transport of carry-on bags within the terminal.
6. Wear comfortable clothing in layers that can be added for warmth, or removed for cooling, and wear comfortable "broken-in" low-heeled walking shoes for travel.

Patients with unstable angina, uncontrolled congestive heart failure, and/or uncontrolled cardiac dysrhythmias should defer travel until these conditions have been stable for 3 months. Patient with recent myocardial infarction may travel if stable after 4 to 6 weeks. It has been suggested that patients with a recent myocardial infarction (MI) or coronary artery bypass graft are safe to travel to altitude as long as they remain well for 3 months following their surgery or MI. Patients should not fly for at least 3 weeks after heart, lung, or gastrointestinal surgery. Patients with recent cerebral infarct (stroke) may travel by air after 2 to 6 weeks.

Patients with a history of cardiac disease may want to consider purchasing evacuation insurance to ensure that if they are traveling to a remote country, they can be evacuated out. They should review the policy to ensure that they will be covered for preexisting conditions, and should determine if the level of evacuation will meet their needs. Some of these companies will provide a fully equipped and staffed air ambulance (fixed-wing or helicopter) to evacuate a cardiac case to the nearest regional medical center that could provide a level of care similar to the standard of care available in the patient's home country. Other companies will evacuate a patient to the nearest in-country medical center, where the care may or may not approximate prevailing Western standards. Sometimes, the outcome of the evacuation is determined by weather, environment, availability of aircraft and fuel, and political factors.

Cardiac Pacemaker

Travelers with implanted cardiac pacemakers should have a thorough cardiac evaluation before extended overseas travel. The model and lot number of the pacemaker, as well as a copy of the patient's ECG with and without the pacemaker activated, should be carried on the trip along with the other important documents (passport, immunization booklet, traveler's health history; see Chapter 1). Identification of potential medical resources along the planned itinerary is advised, since not all type of medical facilities stock replacement batteries, pacemaker units, and electrodes.

Travel within the continental United States is usually without problems, since many pacemaker patients can have their units checked via electronic telephone diagnostic programs. Unfortunately, these types of calls are not relayed by international satellite communications, so a pacemaker checkup overseas would involve consulting a knowledgeable local medical doctor. A pacemaker identification code form is available from local branches of the American Heart Association.

DIABETES MELLITUS

Patients traveling with diabetes need to consider how to adapt their treatment programs to unfamiliar foods, irregular schedules, and varying amounts of exercise. Good planning and advance preparation are key in avoiding stress and problems arising as a result of traveling with diabetes. It is important to make plane and hotel reservations in advance and to allow reasonable time between connecting flights. Organize assistance ahead of time if the connection time will be a problem. Schedule necessary travel immunizations several weeks before travel. In addition to the usual travel vaccines, patients with diabetes should be encouraged to receive an annual flu shot, as well as the pneumococcal polysaccharide vaccine.

Table 14-3 lists supplies and medications that patients with diabetes need to assemble before departure. The America Diabetes Association is an excellent additional source of information for the traveler with diabetes. They publish "The Diabetes Travel Guide" ($14.95), which includes information about diabetes supplies and a guide to insulin manufactured in the United States and abroad. Insulin manufactured in the United States is sold as U-100 strength but it can be sold as U-40 or U-80 overseas. This guide helps to address these concerns, as well as other issues.

The management of diabetes is usually based on a 24-hour medication schedule. When traveling north or south, no adjustments in the 24-hour schedule are needed. Traveling westward results in a longer day, and traveling eastward results in a shorter day. When five or fewer time zones are crossed, no change is required in the usual insulin routine. However, when six or more time zones are crossed, adjustment in the usual schedule is advisable.

Table 14-3
Checklist of Supplies for Insulin-Dependent Patients

Insulin sufficient to last the entire trip plus at least one extra week
Disposable U-100 syringes and needles to last entire trip plus one week
At least one bottle of Humalog (Lispro) insulin
Reagent strips and lancets for blood glucose testing
Portable blood glucose monitor with extra batteries
Ketone-detecting urine test strips (for use during illness)
Glucose tablets
Glucagon emergency kit
Snacks; Power Bars, peanut butter crackers, fruit juice, to take on board
Diabetes identification tag or (MedicAlert) bracelet
Billfold card detailing insulin dose and doctor's name and telephone number
Signed statement from personal physician on letterhead stationary documenting medical diagnosis and necessity for carrying supply of insulin, syringes, and needles for diabetic treatment
Prescription from personal physician detailing insulin dose, in case supplies from home are lost, damaged, or stolen.
All oral medications including antibiotics, antiemetic and antidiarrheal agents, as well as essential OTC medications.

Adapted from Diabetes Day-by-Day #29 On the Go? Alexandria, VA, The American Diabetes Association.

The timing for oral diabetic medication is not as critical as that for insulin. People taking pills for their diabetes should simply take their medicine at the prescribed time, using local time. Patients wearing an insulin pump (CSII therapy) may have to make some minor adjustments in their basal insulin rates as they travel and upon arrival. It is important to carry a letter from the physician explaining this device and the fact that it is attached by tubing and a subcutaneous needle to the person wearing the pump. Most airport security personnel in major international airports are familiar with insulin pumps, but the traveler may find that he or she is asked to remove the pump.

Frequent blood sugar monitoring is essential for safety. In addition to the typical measurements before breakfast, lunch, and dinner, travelers should check blood glucose levels about every 6 hours whenever their daily routine is disrupted. Even individuals who are normally lax about home glucose monitoring should test at least four times per day while traveling. Most significant problems associated with fluctuations in blood sugars can be avoided by frequent checking of blood sugars. It is essential that the traveler with diabetes have an adequate supply of the proper blood glucose (BG) strips for his or her particular meter, and that they have batteries and even a back-up meter to use should they have a problem with their meter.

Diabetes and High Altitude

It is important to note that meters are not accurate at altitude and that there have been a number of reported deaths from diabetic ketoacidosis (DKA) in patients with diabetes traveling to high altitude. This could, in part, be a result of people depending on meter readings that were reading too low. Carrying urine ketone dipstick tests (Ketostix) will allow the patient to detect early ketoacidosis and to evacuate to a lower altitude if it is present.

Traveling East Across Six or More Time Zones

There are a number of references dealing with the adjustment of insulin doses during travel through multiple east-to-west or west-to-east time zones. There have been some recent studies that demonstrate that straightforward and simple advice with regard to insulin management while traveling is preferred to elaborate protocols to alter insulin dosages. Some of the suggestions in a study by Gill and Redmond were that the patient be advised to check BGs frequently during the flight, carry quick-acting carbohydrate source in the hand luggage, and avoid airline "diabetic meals" which are not standardized.

Patients planning a long trip across many time zones may be greatly benefited by switching from *regular insulin* to one of the recombinant insulin analogs *Humalog* (Lispro) or Novalog (insulin aspart). These agents have a rapid onset of action and can be taken with a meal, unlike regular insulin that must be injected at least 30 minutes before a meal to avoid postprandial hypoglycemia. Another significant advantage of analog/recombinant insulin is that it remains in the body for a maximum of 2 to 4 hours, thereby decreasing the likelihood of between-meal hypoglycemia.

Another advantage is that the Humalog or Novalog cartridges, when used with an insulin pen injection device, make administration of insulin extremely easy. A very popular version of an insulin pen, which can be carried in a shirt pocket or a handbag, is made by Novo Nordisk Pharmaceuticals. The desired dose of insulin, which is housed in the cartridge, is dialed into the device, and is delivered with a 30-gauge ½-inch needle at the end of the pen. Although the Humalog pen cartridges are made by Eli Lilly, they are compatible with other pen systems such as the Novo Nordisk product.

The use of Humalog or Novalog insulin would give the traveler the flexibility of cutting back their basal insulin (NPH or UltraLente) dose by 10%, and using a small dose of Humalog to correct any resulting hyperglycemia. The exact doses need to be individualized. If the patient with diabetes is interested in changing to this type of regimen, he or she should do so at least a month or two ahead of time to allow adequate time to adjust insulin regimens before travel.

One approach to east-to-west travel across time zones is described in the following: Individuals who normally take insulin once daily before breakfast should take the usual dose at the usual time on the day of departure (Table 14-4). The first morning at destination, just before breakfast (local time), two thirds of the usual morning dose of insulin is taken, since fewer than 24 hours will have elapsed since the previous morning's insulin injection. This reduced dose is designed to prevent hypoglycemia early in the day, particularly under circumstances that may involve extra activity or disruption of meal schedules.

To protect against an elevation in blood glucose as a result of the reduced morning dose, blood glucose should be tested before dinner that evening, that is, about 10 hours after the morning insulin dose. If the blood glucose is greater than 240 mg/dl, the patient should take the remaining one third of the usual insulin dose that was omitted that morning. The

Table 14-4
Insulin Adjustment When Traveling East Across Multiple Time Zones*

	Day of departure	First morning at destination	10 Hr after morning dose	Second day at destination
Single-dose schedule	Usual Dose	Two-thirds usual dose	Test blood glucose Remaining one-third of morning dose if blood sugar over 240	Usual dose
Two-dose schedule	Usual morning and evening doses	Two-thirds usual morning dose	Test blood glucose Usual evening dose plus remaining one-third of morning dose if blood sugar over 240	Usual two doses

Adapted from Benson E, Metz R: Management of diabetic during intercontinental travel, *Bull Mason Clin* 38:145-151, Winter, 1984-1985.
*People initially traveling east will use westbound schedule on return journeys (see Table 14-5).

usual insulin dose is then resumed beginning the morning of the second day at the destination.

People who customarily take two insulin injections daily also administer only two thirds of their usual morning dose of insulin the first morning at the destination (Table 14-4). That evening, if a before-dinner blood test for glucose shows 240 mg/dl or less, they simply take their usual evening dose of insulin. However, if the blood sugar is greater than 240 mg/dl, they should add to their evening dose the one third of the morning dose that was omitted.

Traveling West Across Six or More Time Zones

On the day of departure, the usual dose of insulin is taken before breakfast (Table 14-5). In flight, meals are eaten at the times provided for other passengers. It is advisable to check blood glucose before meals or at 6-hour intervals during the flight. About 18 hours after the morning insulin injection, whether still in flight or at the destination, the blood glucose should be tested. If the blood glucose is 240 mg/dl or less, the individual may safely wait until the first morning at destination to take the usual insulin dose at the usual time (local time), even though more than 24 hours will have elapsed. However, if the blood glucose level is greater than 240 mg/dl, a supplemental dose of insulin equal to one third of the usual morning dose should be taken, followed by a meal or snack. For example, if the usual morning does is 30 U of NPH plus 12 U of regular insulin, then the supplemental dose is 10 U of NPH plus 4 U of regular. The next morning (local time), the usual insulin dose is taken.

Patients who normally take insulin on a twice-daily schedule should leave their wristwatches unadjusted during the flight. At about the time of the evening meal at the point of departure (i.e., about 10 to 12 hours after the morning dose of insulin), the usual second dose is taken, followed by a meal or snack (see Table 14-5). From that time on, travelers on this dosage schedule follow the same plan as those who take one injection

Table 14-5
Insulin Adjustment When Traveling West Across Multiple Time Zones*

	Day of departure	18 Hr after morning dose	First morning at destination
Single-dose schedule	Usual dose	One-third usual dose followed by meal or snack if blood sugar over 240	Usual dose
Two-dose schedule	Usual morning and evening doses	One-third usual morning dose followed by meal or snack if blood sugar over 240	Usual two doses

Adapted from Benson E, Metz R: Management of diabetic during intercontinental travel, *Bull Mason Clin* 38:145-151, Winter, 1984-1985.
*People initially traveling west will use eastbound schedule on return journey (see Table 14-4).

daily. Thus, at about 18 hours after the first dose of insulin and 6 hours after the second, the blood is tested, and an extra dose of insulin equal to one third of the morning dose is taken if the blood glucose is more than 240 mg/dl.

Regardless of the method used to adjust insulin dosages while traveling, it is essential that the person on insulin therapy understand how to recognize and treat hypoglycemia, how to monitor and interpret blood glucose results, and how to adjust insulin for a decrease or increase in the amount of carbohydrate present in the meal. A visit to a Certified Diabetes Educator (CDE) or an endocrinologist with a special interest in diabetes prior to travel can be invaluable. These professionals can suggest individualized programs of insulin management to address changes in time zones, exercise levels and illnesses while traveling.

Prevention of Hypoglycemia

Travel usually involves a drastic departure from daily routines. Meals may be delayed or unavailable. Physical activity is often greatly increased. These factors increase the risk of hypoglycemia. The principle of eating extra food when engaged in extra activity becomes especially important when traveling. Suitable snacks, such as crackers, dried fruits, or nuts, should be carried for use if meals are delayed or to supplement meals if necessary. Concentrated commercially available food bars such as "Power Bars" suit this purpose very well.

Persons with diabetes should receive instruction from their diabetes care provider on recognition and treatment of hypoglycemia. A person with hypoglycemia may feel weak, drowsy, dizzy, or confused. Paleness, headache, trembling, sweating, rapid heartbeat, and a cold, clammy feeling are also signs of low blood sugar. Sugar cubes or other sources of rapidly absorbed sugar should also be available in case hypoglycemic symptoms develop. Commercially available products to treat hypoglycemia are highly recommended. These products have a measured amount of concentrated carbohydrate content and are very stable.

Traveling companions should be advised of the early signs of hypoglycemia and should understand the importance of administering sugar-containing drinks if the person becomes glassy-eyed, grows confused or irritable, or is noted to be sweating inappropriately. If the person is too confused to swallow, food or fluid should not be administered. Instead, glucagon should be administered by injection.

Anyone using insulin as part of his or her diabetes treatment should travel with a glucagon emergency kit. Traveling companions should be briefed on proper use of the glucagon emergency kit. If the patient on insulin is traveling with a tour group, then the tour group leader or the person assigned to deal with medical problems for the group should be briefed on the use of glucagon, and should be familiar with the kit and where the traveling patient is carrying it.

The traveler with diabetes who becomes stuporous or unconscious needs skilled medical care as soon as possible. However, one should NOT delay the administration of glucagon while attempting to obtain skilled medical care. Giving glucagon to a person with diabetes who does not need it may cause a significant rise in their blood sugar, but this can be corrected relatively simply. Delaying glucagon administration in a diabetic person with severe hypoglycemia could result in severe medical complications. Glucagon can be administered by injection, even if the person of concern is stuporous or seizing. Any route of administration is reasonable, intramuscularly (IM) or subcutaneously (SC) in an emergency situation. Once glucagon is administered, if the person regains full consciousness and is able to take food orally, a carbohydrate-protein snack should be given.

Names of English-speaking physicians overseas can be obtained from a number of sources listed in the Appendix.

ARTIFICIAL HIP JOINTS AND OTHER ORTHOPEDIC HARDWARE

The metal components in artificial hip replacements and metal pins used for internal fixation of bone fractures may trigger the electromagnetic security alarms at airport passenger check-in stations. A traveler with an implanted orthopedic device or hardware should carry a signed letter from his or her personal physician on letterhead stationery stating that such a condition exists. This may avoid lengthy explanations and delays in departure.

REFERENCES

ANA Commission on Emergency Medical Services: Medical aspects of transportation aboard commercial aircraft, *JAMA* 247:1007, 1982.

Benson E, Metz R: Management of diabetes during intercontinental travel, *Bull Mason Clin* 38:145, Winter 1984-1985.

Cottrell JJ: Altitude exposures during aircraft flight: flying higher, *Chest* 92:81, 1988.

Cummins RO, Schubach JA: Frequency and types of medical emergencies among commercial air travelers, *JAMA* 264:1295, 1989.

Cummins RO: High-altitude flights and risk of cardiac stress, *JAMA* 260:3668, 1988.

Dillard TA, Berg BW, Rajagopol KR, et al: Hypoxemi during air travel in patients with chronic obstructive pulmonary disease, *Ann Intern Med* 111:362, 1989.

Gern JE, Busse WW: Relationship of viral infections to wheezing illnesses and asthma, *Nature Rev Immunnol* 2:132, 2002.

Gill GV, Redmond S: Insulin treatment, time-zones and air travel: a survey of current advice from British diabetic clinics, *Diabt Med* 10:744, 1993.

Gong H Jr: Advising COPD patients about commercial air travel, *J Respir Dis* 5:20, 1984.

Gong H Jr: Advising patients with pulmonary diseases on air travel, *Ann Intern Med* 111:349, 1989.

Gong H Jr: Air travel and oxygen therapy in cardiopulmonary patients, *Chest* 101: 1104, 1992.

Mitka M: Why the rise in asthma? New insight, few answers, *JAMA* 281:2171, 1999.

Peacock A: ABC of oxygen, *BMJ* 317:1063, 1998.

Poundstone W: Air travel and supplemental oxygen. Friendly skies for respiratory patients? *Respir Ther* 12:79, 1983.

Quinn S: Diabetes and diet. We are still learning, *Med Clin North Am* 77:773, 1993.

Sane T, Kovisto VA, Nikkanen P, et al: Adjustment of insulin doses of diabetic patients during long distance flights, *BMJ* 301:5211, 1990.

Schwartz JS, Bencowitz HZ, Moser KM: Air travel hypoxemia with chronic obstructive lung disease, *Ann Intern Med* 100:473, 1984.

Wick RL Jr: High-altitude flights and risk of cardiac disease (letter), *JAMA* 261: 2504, 1989.

CHAPTER 15

The Business Expatriate

William H. Shoff, Amy J. Behrman, and Suzanne M. Sheperd

Anyone living in a foreign country is an expatriate including executives, government employees, humanitarian aid workers, laborers, long-term travelers, managers, military personnel, missionaries, professionals, students, teachers, and persons visiting friends and relatives for extended periods. This chapter addresses the travel medicine issues of business expatriates (BE) alone and in conjunction with their family, although many of the concerns of other types of expatriates will be addressed by inference.

In the past, the world of the BE was one of numerous markets in many countries, connected in various ways but not immediately responsive to each other. That world has changed dramatically. Witness the Thai bhat debacle (December 8, 1997) and the ensuing domino effect involving Russia (August 17, 1998), Brazil, and other countries (fall, 1998), and the giant hedge fund Long Term Capital Management and others (fall, 1998). This series of events demonstrated the impact of globalization. First, there was the world with its many markets. Now, there is only one market, the world.

Multinational corporations number more than 35,000 with 150,000 affiliate corporations demonstrating that the BE market is huge. Executives, professionals, and specially trained workers are being sent to foreign countries to live, teach, train, and work for weeks to years. The cost of moving and establishing a BE with or without family varies from less than $250,000 to more than $500,000. It is essential to the operations of the corporations involved that their workers and their workers' families be happy, healthy, safe, and secure in order to be productive. The direct and indirect monetary costs to repatriate a business expatriate and family members owing to illness, injury or death can exceed $600,000. With the independent costs of expatriation and repatriation both high therefore, the cost of failure of the expatriate assignment is also high.

Currently, about 5% to 7% of BEs do not complete their assignments because of compromised happiness, health, safety, security, or any combination of these. The risks to the BE and family members are numerous, and they increase in frequency the longer the duration of stay, as do their risks for encountering all the problems experienced by the native population. In addition, expatriates are more vulnerable for two reasons: first, they have not developed any tolerance or immunity to local diseases; second, they are living in an unfamiliar environment. At any moment these risks can escalate further because of indiscretion. An example of a specific risk is a motor vehicle crash, which poses a significantly greater chance for death outside the United States (0 to 5.4 times greater in Europe and 2.5 to 40 times greater in the rest of the world) *(www.asirt.org)*.

An example of a broadly-based factor that may affect risk is the cultural divide. Cultural issues intervene every minute of every day and take on more weight than the hackneyed expression "culture shock" implies. One does not settle into business as usual "a few weeks after the shock wears off." Table 15-1 lists some issues that expatriates must keep in mind while preparing to live and work in another culture. The risks the BE and family members will encounter is magnified by any combination of the following factors:

- Inadequate pretravel preparation
- Foregoing recommended preventive measures
- Lack of a local social support network
- Lessening of behavioral inhibitions
- Chronic illness

The ability of an individual to adjust to a foreign assignment has been shown to be related to the following:

- Social support
- Strong internal locus of control
- Good self-esteem
- Sense of coherence

The BE and family members are truly strangers in a strange land. Inadequate preparation and insufficient vigilance by the them may lead to compromise in their well-being and effectiveness, with far-reaching consequences to them, the corporation, or both.

Planning and managing the expatriate experience involves professionals in several disciplines: human resources, occupational medicine, primary care medicine, security, and travel medicine. Other professional services are added as appropriate. For maximum benefit, these professionals should interface with each other or should interface with a common professional, usually the occupational physician, who coordinates the collected efforts. The focus in this chapter is on the role of travel medicine.

Pretravel preparation relative to health, safety, and security begins months before departure. If the assignment is for 6 months or less, it is recommended that the initial consultation take place 3 months before departure. If the assignment is longer than 6 months, it is recommended that the initial consultation take place 6 months before departure. Table 15-2 lists the tasks of pretravel preparation.

Formulation of a complete medical problem list confronts three potential issues:

- It identifies problems that may be too complicated to be managed in the assigned country because of frequency of exacerbation or lack of proper resources.
- If any psychiatric, drug, or alcohol problem(s) is identified, it raises the question of whether the person is stable enough to handle the rigors and uncertainties of the expatriate assignment.
- It avoids the improper assertion later by the BE and/or accompanying family member(s) that a given problem arose secondary to the assignment.

The role of the travel health specialist is defined as follows:

- Review the traveler's medical history including immunizations.
- Educate the traveler to risks, prevention strategies, accessing appropriate medical care, and chronic disease management.

Text continued on p. 250

Table 15-1
Expatriate Cultural Issues

Issue	Comments
Family/couple counseling	Assess impact of move on all family members. All members of family should be involved in decision-making process relative to moving and establishing a new home in the assigned country (AC). Preferred counselor should have background in family systems and experience with expatriates.
Preassignment visit to AC	If assignment is longer than 12 months, it is advisable to visit AC before beginning the assignment, particularly, if a spouse and children are included.
Learn local manners and business protocols	Cross-cultural complexities ensure problems at all levels of interaction. Routine gestures, manners, or business practices in one culture may be an insult or embarrassment in another culture. (See references: Adams JW, Axtel RE, Morrison T, et al.)
Study the dominant language(s)	Language barriers consistently block communication. The target language is that spoke by employers, government officials, health care professionals, and co-workers. Idioms vary from region to region. Word meanings sometimes change from place to place, even with similar spellings.
History	What historical relationship is there between the assigned country, the culture of origin of the BE and family, and the country in which the BE and family currently live?
Myths and stereotypes	What myths and stereotypes are operating in the assigned country?
Expatriate expectations	What are they relative to health care, child care, education, entertainment, housing, shopping?
Policy and procedure	What are policies, procedures, and practices of government, health care industry, and employer's industry?
Culture	What are the cultural norms relative to age, race, ethnicity, gender, religion, dress, etc?
Rights	What are the rights of individuals, families, the community, and workers?
Readiness to change	What is the culture's receptivity to change? What is the individual's ability to effect change?
Commercial sex	What is the role of commercial sex workers in the assigned country?
Resources for the newly arrived expatriate	Other successful expatriates, expatriate managers, native employees

Table 15-2
Expatriate Medical Checklist

Comprehensive Medical Evaluation (Primary Care Practitioner)

- Generate complete health problem list
- Complete history and physical examination
- Status of all active medical/surgical illnesses
- Significant past medical illnesses not included above
- Surgical procedures not included above
- Adverse drug reactions
  - Allergic
  - Nonallergic
- Hospitalizations not included above
- Current medications

Baseline Studies: Obtain Copies 1 to 2 Months before Departure

- Lab studies: CBC, electrolytes, BUN/creatinine, lipid panel, liver function tests, thyroid panel, fasting blood sugar
- Imaging studies: chest x-ray study for anyone >age 30 yr, mammogram as indicated
- ECG: age >35
- Exercise stress test: age >40 yr
- Pap smear as indicated
- PPD skin test (tuberculosis status)
- Hepatitis B immunization status: immunize or verify antibodies
- Hepatitis C status
- HIV status
- RPR status
- Blood type and Rh factor
- Sigmoidoscopy (flexible)/colonoscopy (as indicated): age >50 yr
- Other studies as indicated (e.g., PSA)

Studies Pertinent to the Management of any Chronic Condition: Obtain Recent Copy

- Discuss guidelines for prescription and nonprescription health products
- Adequate supply to last months (at least)
- May not be available in assigned country (AC)
- Keep in original containers to avoid legal complications
- Purchasing brands versus generics in AC
  - One study of generic chloroquine and selected antibacterials from Nigeria and Thailand revealed that 36.5% of the samples were substandard relative to pharmocopoeial limits (Shakoor, 1997).

Consultations (Nontravel Medicine)

- Specialists managing chronic conditions: obtain letter updating status
- Dental
  - Allow time for corrective measures (months)
  - Fillings may need replacement
  - Peridontal disease may need treatment
  - Dental hardware
    - Evaluate and replace as necessary
    - Carry extra set, particularly if appearance is important part of job
  - Dental care in AC may not meet the standards of Western medicine

Continued

Table 15-2
Expatriate Medical Checklist—cont'd

Eye (Other than Above)
- All persons: obtain two pair of sunglasses that provide 100% UV protection
- Lens wearers
- Comprehensive evaluation (intraocular pressure, acuity, fundus, etc.)
- Carry at least one extra set of lenses
- Carry copy of lens prescription
- Age >50 and no eye complaint: comprehensive evaluation

Hearing (Comprehensive Evaluation)
- Hearing impaired
- Occupational sound exposure
- Age >50 and no hearing complaint

Travel Medicine Consultation
- Vaccine preventable diseases
  - Update routine child and adult immunizations: selected comments follow
    - Hepatitis B
      - All unimmunized persons be immunized
      - Exposure risks: sexual transmission, dirty needles/instruments (medical and nonmedical, e.g., tattoos), and transfusions
    - Influenza: Most recent vaccine
    - Measles: All persons receive a 2-dose series since 1980 or verify immunity with positive titer
      - Significant measles vaccine quality control issues existed before 1980 (Hill, 1989).
      - Assumption that most persons borne before 1956 have immunity to measles is challenged by the observation that during the measles resurgence in the late 1980s, 28% of health care workers who contracted measles were borne before 1956 (Guide to Adult Imm, ACP, 1994)
    - Pneumococcus: 23-valent vaccine for all adults
      - Multidrug resistant pneumococci are increasing worldwide (Wenzel, 2000)
      - One recent study demonstrates cost-effectiveness of immunizing young adults (Pepper, 2000).
    - Tetanus-diphtheria
    - Varivax
  - Update travel-related immunizations: recommended for all developing countries except where noted)
    - Hepatitis A: Many travel health specialists administer it to children 1 year or older
    - Hepatitis E: All women of childbearing age, if vaccine available
      - Mortality in pregnant women up to 20% when infected during third trimester
      - Consider immunizing men and children (morbidity similar to hepatitis A)
      - Japanese encephalitis: when AC is an endemic country
      - Meningococcal vaccine (quadrivalent: A, C, Y, W-135)
        - When AC is in African meningitis belt
        - Check for recent meningococcal activity in other ACs
        - When traveling to the Haj
  - Rabies
  - Typhoid
  - Other vaccines might be indicated under special circumstances, depending on availability.
    - Anthrax
    - Cholera: the new vaccines
    - Tick-borne encephalitis

Table 15-2
Expatriate Medical Checklist—cont'd

Insurance: Minimally Recommended Coverage per Individual
Health: $100,000
Evacuation: Unlimited

Potential Illness/Injury Risks

- Accidents, particularly motor vehicle
- Altitude
- Blood-borne pathogens
  - Groups at risk: health care workers, injured persons, any other person with percutaneous/mucous membrane exposures to bodily fluids
  - Organisms: HIV, hepatitis B, hepatitis C, rabies, Ebola, other hemorrhagic fevers
  - Consider dispensing post-exposure kits for HIV exposure (occupation and non-occupational) to persons at high risk.
- Drinking water: know how to judge when water is safe and how to make it safe
- Envenomations (nonmarine): insects, snakes, other
- Food
  - >400 million metric tons of food crosses international borders each year.
  - Contaminated food may have a local or international source.
  - Hands should be thoroughly washed with soap and running safe water before handling any food. No-added water soaps for hand washing are becoming more widely available.
  - Raw or inadequately prepared foods are the source of food-borne diseases
    - ~1.5 billion episodes of infectious diarrhea occur worldwide each year in children <5 years of age leading to >3 million deaths.
    - Organisms are killed by heat (70° C/158° F to all parts of the foodstuff) or cold (−20° C _ 7 days or −35° C _ 15 hours).
    - After cooking, food held and served at 60° C/140° F is considered safe.
    - Fresh vegetables should be thoroughly rinsed with safe water and then soaked in an iodine wash (commercially available in many developing countries).
    - Two studies indicate that although the rate of diarrheal illness in expatriates may decrease to some degree over time, it is a persisting problem (Herwaldt, 2000; Shlim, 1999).
  - Mycotoxins: No international guideline has been set for safe levels of these toxins
  - Aflatoxins (carcinogenic and immunosuppressive) in corn and peanuts under humid tropical conditions.
    - Ochratoxin A in wheat and other grains in temperate conditions
    - Patulin in bruised fruit, particularly apples.
  - Seafood toxins: stable to heat and cold.
  - Pesticide residues not monitored in developing countries.
- Insect-borne diseases
- Pollution:
  - Exposure will be much larger in developing because of limited regulation.
  - Sources
    - Air: domestic coal use (Asia, Eastern Europe), power generation stations, cars.
    - Ground: garbage, industrial wastes, pesticides, toxic chemicals.
- Scuba diving: barotrauma, decompression sickness, gas embolism
- Sexually transmitted diseases
- Soil: several parasites enter the body via skin penetration
- Swimming or other aquatic exposure (fresh or salt water)
- Infectious diseases
- Aquatic envenomations

Continued

Table 15-2
Expatriate Medical Checklist—cont'd

Females of Child-Bearing Age
Review potential for an unexpected pregnancy.
Review potential for rape.

Safety and Security Risks: Four Areas of Planning (Savage, 2001)
Advance intelligence: information about known risks can be obtained from several sources.
- U.S. Department of State for travel advisory at http://travel.state.gov
- Regional Security Officer at U.S. Embassy in AC (name and phone number can be obtained from (202-647-4000) to learn about current security risks.
- Private security companies: Air Security International, Control Risk Group
  - Parvus International/Armour (see Bibliography: Private security companies).
  - iJET Travel Intelligence (see Bibliography)
- Important documents file: place in home/office before departure for use in time of crisis
  - Passport photocopy and extra passport photos
  - Health
    - Medical problem list, eye lens prescription, pertinent tests results
    - Photocopy of health insurance card
    - Photocopy of travel health insurance policy
    - Photocopy of International Certificate of Vaccination
    - Photocopy of other important legal documents, such as power of attorney
- Prepare a plan in the event that adversity occurs.
- Carry duplicates of important documents in case originals are lost or stolen while traveling.

CBC, Complete blood count; *BUN,* blood urea nitrogen; *LFT,* liver function test; *FBS,* fasting blood sugar; *ECG,* electrocardiogram; *HIV,* human immunodeficiency virus; *PPD,* purified protein derivative; *RPR,* rapid plasma reagin; *PSA,* prostate-specific antigen.

- ▼ Administer travel-related vaccines.
- ▼ Provide relevant prescriptions and possibly travel health products.
- ▼ Suggest appropriate referrals.
- ▼ Coordinate with primary care physicians, occupational medicine professionals, and other professionals as needed.

Although many safety and security concerns are dealt with by the corporation's security department, the travel medicine consultant should not assume that these issues have been adequately covered; therefore take the opportunity to reemphasize this important subject. In addition, many travelers are not aware of the increased risks involved in developing countries, having traveled mostly in developed countries. Corporations have a strategic interest in addressing the items on the pretravel checklist because of the enormous costs of investment and the desire to avoid failure, whenever possible.

Even though the information discussed in this chapter is promoted by many travel health and occupational health professionals, there is evidence that far too many BE and their families are not properly prepared when they reach their assignment or do not follow recommendations. In a survey of corporate travelers (226 responding) from one multinational corporation, the following was reported: 51% were provided health kits; 50% or more did not follow simple food precautions; 43% who went to malarious areas were compliant with antimalarial prophylaxis; 35% developed diarrhea; 29% developed respiratory illnesses; and 12% sought medical care for their problems.

In a study assessing attitudes and practices regarding preventing malaria (4990 expatriates), the following was reported: the use of prophylactic medications against malaria decreased over time from 69.2% (year 1) to 34.5% (year 10); 17.5% used pyrimethamine alone (ineffective) for malaria prophylaxis; and 7.5% used bed nets.

Fegan reported a reluctance of expatriates (106 surveyed) to take long-term malaria chemoprophylaxis. In a Dutch study assessing hepatitis B vaccination status (864 expatriates), the following was reported: 37% were vaccinated in 1991 compared with 14% in 1987 to 1989; 5% in both groups were positive for hepatitis B markers suggesting that high-risk groups were not being reached with the increased vaccination rate; 65% young females with low-risk behavior were vaccinated, but only 20% older males with high-risk behavior were vaccinated.

Relying on occupational medicine staff of corporations to convince potential BEs that the principles of prevention outlined in this chapter are important has been often ineffective because of individual resistance and noncompliance for any number of reasons, in the experience of the authors cited in dealing with several multinational corporations. Corporations must develop and enforce policies relative to placement and management of the expatriate experience that embodies these principles. It is a strategic move that will pay excellent dividends for the corporation, the individual employees involved, and their families.

The expatriate experience is not complete until BE and his or her family return home and become assimilated back into the corporate community and society. This transition is often difficult. Two thirds of returning executives and one fourth of returning managers leave the parent company within a year of return at a considerable financial cost to the company (approximately $1 million per executive). In addition, family members endure reverse culture shock. To minimize this loss, businesses should have a program to assess and prepare the returning BE for a new role in the parent company. It is advisable for the BE and family members to seek personal/family counseling as soon as possible after returning. A screening medical evaluation of the asymptomatic expatriates is sometimes recommended to detect latent travel-associated parasitic infections. Libman reported that stool examination coupled with serologic testing had a sensitivity of 89% for detecting asymptomatic schistosomiasis, filariasis, and strongyloidiasis in returning expatriates. A coordinated professional effort to manage the return of the BE and family members is as important to the success of that effort as it was when they departed for the assignment in the new country.

REFERENCES

Abueva JE: Management: return of the native executive; many repatriations fail, at huge cost to companies, *New York Times,* May 17, 2000.

Adams JW: *U.S. Expatriate handbook: guide to living & working abroad,* West Virginia University College of Business & Economics, 1998. *www.wvu.edu/~colbe*

American College of Physicians and Infectious Diseases Society of America: *Guide for adult immunization,* ed 3, Philadelphia, 1994, ACP.

Anderzen I, Arnetz BB: Psychophysiological reactions to international adjustment. Results from a controlled, longitudinal study, *Psychother Psychosomat* 68:67, 1999.

Association for Safe International Travel (www.asirt.org).

Axtel RE: *Do's and taboos around the world,* ed 3, New York, 2000, Wiley.

Bunn W: Vaccine and international health programs for employees traveling and living abroad, *J Trav Med,* 8 (Suppl 1):S20, 2001.

Emmett EA: What is the strategic value of occupational and environmental medicine? *J Occup Environ Med* 38:1124, 1996.

Eono P, Polaert C, Louis JP: [Malaria in expatriates in Abidjan] [French], *Medecine Tropicale* 59:358, 1999.

Expatriate web sites: www.globalassignment.com, www.expatexchange.com, www.expatforum.com, www.overseasdigest.com, www.odci.gov/cia/publications/factbook/index.HTML.

Fegan D, Glennon J: Malaria prophylaxis in long-term expatriate mineworkers in Ghana, *Occup Med* 43:135, 1993.

Fleming LE, Bennett MF, Rao N: Culture and health. In Herzstein JA et al, editors: *International occupational and environmental medicine,* St Louis, 1998, Mosby.

Friedman TL: *The lexus and the olive tree,* New York, 2000, Anchor Books.

Goettsch W et al: Broader vaccination of expatriates against HBV infection: do we reach those at highest risk? *Int J Epidemiol* 28:1161, 1999.

Hill DR, Pearson RD: Measles prophylaxis for international travel, *Ann Intern Med* 111:699, 1989.

iJET Travel Intelligence *(www.ijet.com).*

Kemmerer TP et al: Health problems of corporate travelers: risk factors and management, *J Trav Med* 5:184, 1998.

Libman MD, MacLear JD, Gyorkos TW: Screening for schistosomiasis, filariasis, and strongyloidiasis among expatriates returning from the tropics, *Clin Infect Dis* 17:353, 1993.

Morrison T, Wayne CA, Borden GA: *Kiss, bow, or shake hands: how to do business in sixty countries,* Holbrook, Mass, 1994, Adams Media Corporation.

Motarjemi Y et al: Food safety. In Herzstein JA et al editors: *International occupational and environmental medicine,* St Louis, 1998, Mosby.

Oatman RL: *The art of executive protection,* Baltimore, 1997, Noble House.

Pepper PV, Owens DK: Cost-effectiveness of the pneumococcal vaccine in the United States Navy and Marine Corps, *Clin Infect Dis* 30:157, 2000.

Private security company websites: Air Security International *(www.airsecurity.com),* Control Risk Group *(www.control-risk.com),* Kroll Information Services *(www.kinsonline.com),* U.S. Department of State Patterns of Global Terrorism *(www.state.gov/s/ct/ris/pgtrpt/2000).*

Savage PV: Threats of security during international travel. In Steffen R, DuPont HI: *Textbook of travel medicine and health,* ed 2, Hamilton, Ontario, 2001, B.C. Decker.

Savage PV: *The safe travel book,* San Francisco, 1999, Lexington Books.

Shakoor O, Taylor RB, Behrens RH: Assessment of the incidence of substandard drugs in developing countries, *Trop Med Int Health* 2:839, 1997.

Shlim DR, Valk TH: Expatriates and long-term travelers. In DuPont HL, Steffen R, editors: *Textbook of travel medicine,* ed 2, Hamilton, Ontario, 2000, B.C. Decker.

Shlim DR et al: Persistent high risk of diarrhea among foreigners in Nepal during the first 2 years of residence, *Clin Infect Dis* 29:613, 1999.

Siciliano RL: *The safety minute: 01,* Boston, 1996, Safety Zone Press.

Stewart L, Leggat PA: Culture shock and travelers, *J Trav Med* 5(2):84, 1998.

Wenzel RP, Edmond MB: Managing antibiotic resistance, *N Engl J Med* 343:1961, 2000.

CHAPTER 16

Health Screening in Immigrants, Refugees, and Internationally Adopted Orphans

Thomas R. Hawn and Elaine C. Jong

Health screening of immigrants, refugees, and internationally adopted orphans includes identifying and treating problems based on the prevalence of risk factors and diseases among populations of varying socioeconomic, cultural, and geographic backgrounds. Problems in communication owing to foreign language, political fears, and different cultural concepts of health may contribute to inaccurate assessments of illness in these patients. Health screening recommendations need to be individualized for cultural and geographic backgrounds. In addition to a standard well-patient checkup, several issues need to be considered (Table 16-1). Immigrants may have difficulties related to malnutrition, trauma, human rights abuses, family dislocation, and cultural adaptation. Several infectious problems that may be prevalent include tuberculosis, hepatitis B, human immunodeficiency virus (HIV) infection, syphilis, and parasitic diseases. A multidisciplinary approach may help to identify problems, mobilize resources for support, and promote effective cross-cultural communication. An overview of the components involved in health screening of immigrants and refugees is described in this chapter.

UNITED STATES ENTRANCE REQUIREMENTS

The United States Public Health Service (USPHS) has health-related entrance requirements defined under the Immigration and Nationality Act of 1990. Health screening examinations are required for permanent residency but not for asylum status or temporary residency. Individuals can be excluded from the United States on health-related grounds if they have a specific "communicable disease of public health significance," a physical or mental disorder that is a threat to the welfare of others, or an addiction to drugs. Class A conditions of public health significance are grounds for exclusion and include infectious tuberculosis (active disease, sputum smear-positive), human immunodeficiency virus (HIV) positive serology, untreated lepromatous leprosy (Hansen's disease), and untreated sexually transmitted diseases (syphilis, gonorrhea, chancroid, granuloma inguinale, and lymphogranuloma venereum). Class B conditions are not grounds for exclusion but must be reported to consular authorities. Class B conditions include inactive or treated tuberculosis, treated sexually transmitted diseases, tuberculoid leprosy, and treated lepromatous leprosy.

Screening requirements for tuberculosis include skin testing of all applicants over age 2 years. If the purified protein derivative (PPD) reaction

Table 16-1
Screening Considerations in Immigrants and Refugees

Health area	Screening considerations
History	Trauma, family status, cultural adaptation, nutritional status
Examination	Routine, including skin and dental examination
Immunizations	Routine
Infectious Diseases	
Tuberculosis	Tuberculin skin test ± chest radiograph
Hepatitis B	Hepatitis serology
HIV, syphilis	HIV serology and RPR as indicated
Malaria and extraintestinal parasites	Blood smear or specific serologic studies
Intestinal parasites	Stool microscopy for ova and parasites
Other	CBC and differential including eosinophils

HIV, Human immunodeficiency virus; *RPR,* rapid plasma reagin; *CBC,* complete blood count.

is greater than 5 mm of induration, then a chest radiograph must be obtained. An evaluation is then made to determine if applicants have active-infectious (Class A, smear positive), active-noninfectious (Class B1, smear negative), inactive (Class B2 or B3), or latent disease (normal chest radiograph). Individuals who are Class A must be treated until their sputum smears are negative before they immigrate. All applicants who are 15 years or older must have serologic testing for HIV and syphilis. In addition, a physical examination must be performed to look for evidence of sexually transmitted diseases and Hansen's disease. Besides mandatory screening for the Class A and B conditions, applicants must be up-to-date on immunizations for diphtheria, tetanus, pertussis, measles, mumps, rubella, polio, *Haemophilus influenzae* b, hepatitis B, varicella, pneumococcus, and influenza. The Division of Quarantine can also detain individuals with acute illnesses including cholera, diphtheria, plague, suspected smallpox, yellow fever, and viral hemorrhagic fever.

ROUTINE HEALTH CARE

Health screening of immigrants and refugees should begin with a standard well-patient check-up. Routine immunizations should be documented and brought up to date. In this category are tetanus, diphtheria, polio, measles, mumps, rubella, and hepatitis B. In patients less than 7 years old, pertussis and *H. influenzae* b vaccines are also advised. Recent developments in Centers of Disease Control and Prevention policies include the recommendation of varicella virus and conjugated pneumococcal vaccines for children. Recommended immunization schedules are outlined in Table 11-2 and discussed in detail with travel vaccines in Chapters 4 and 11.

TUBERCULOSIS

Although skin tests and chest x-ray studies are used to qualify immigrants, refugees, and orphans for entry into the United States, tuberculosis remains a common problem within these populations. From 1986 to 1997,

Table 16-2
Tuberculosis Incidence in Countries of Origin

Area	Smear positive (rate)†	All forms (rate)*
Sub-Saharan Africa	103	229
East and South Asia	79	174
North Africa and West Asia	54	120
South America	54	120
Central America and Caribbean	54	120
Total	77	171
United States, 1997		8
Harlem, New York, 1989		169

From Centers for Disease Control and Prevention: Tuberculosis in developing countries. *MMWR* 39:561, 1990; Centers for Disease Control and Prevention: Summary of notifiable diseases, United States, *MMWR* 46:1, 1998; Barnes PF, Barrows SA: Tuberculosis in the 1990s, *Ann Intern Med* 119:400, 1993.
*Per 100,000 population.

the number of tuberculosis cases among foreign-born people rose from 4925 to 7702, which corresponded to 22% and 39% of the national total, respectively. The incidence of tuberculosis infections among immigrants and refugees tends to reflect the rates present in the countries of origin. Table 16-2 shows the rate per 100,000 population for developing countries. Individuals with infectious tuberculosis who are on treatment with negative sputum smears can immigrate and require follow-up care in the United States. Some individuals with advanced pulmonary tuberculosis will be identified clinically months after arrival in the United States. In retrospect, such patients may not match the x-ray study submitted in his or her name to the immigration authorities. In addition, extrapulmonary tuberculosis needs to be considered and may be missed by conventional screening methods. Chapter 22 discusses tuberculosis in travelers and foreign-born people. The sections on patient compliance with therapeutic regimens and drug resistance are of special significance in this population. Tuberculosis control programs are essential for assisting with completion of therapy of those with active disease, contact tracing, screening, and provision of preventive therapy for appropriate individuals.

HEPATITIS B STATUS

Asymptomatic carriage of hepatitis B virus infection has a prevalence of up to 20% in some areas of the world (Table 16-3). Adoptive families of foreign orphans who are hepatitis B surface antigen-positive (HBSAg) should consider receiving the hepatitis B vaccine before the arrival of the new family member (Chapter 4). Sponsors and close social contacts of immigrants and refugees should also consider the vaccine if they do not already have immunity. Chapter 19 discusses viral hepatitis and the various blood tests used to identify infectivity and immunity with regard to hepatitis B. Foreign-born pregnant women who are asymptomatic carriers of hepatitis B should be identified, so that vertical transmission of the infection from mother to baby can be interrupted by giving hepatitis B

Table 16-3
Hepatitis B Virus Carriage in Refugee Populations

Country of origin	No. tested	No. positive	%	(95% CI)*
Southeast Asia				
Laos (Hmong)	8879	1374	15.5	(14.7-16.2)
Cambodia	4748	724	15.2	(14.2-16.3)
Thailand†	233	33	14.2	(10.1-19.5)
Vietnam	10,561	1460	13.8	(13.2-14.5)
Laos (other)	4238	494	11.7	(10.7-12.7)
Africa/Mideast/Asia				
Iraq	23	3	13.0	(3.4-34.7)‡
Ethiopia	944	89	9.4	(7.7-11.5)
Angola	14	1	7.1	(0.4-35.8)‡
Afghanistan	418	17	4.1	(2.5-6.6)
Iran	293	7	2.4	(1.1-5.1)
Eastern Europe				
Bulgaria	38	2	5.3	(0.9-19.1)
Romania	754	31	4.1	(2.9-5.9)
Poland	903	16	1.8	(1.1-2.9)
Former Union of Soviet Socialist Republics	4504	66	1.5	(1.1-1.9)
Former Czechoslovakia	168	2	1.2	(0.2-4.7)
Hungary	94	1	1.1	(0.1-6.6)

From Centers for Disease Control and Prevention: Screening for hepatitis B virus infection among refugees arriving in the United States, 1979-1991, *MMWR* 40:784, 1991.
*Confidence interval, calculated by the quadratic method.
†Includes only children born in Thailand whose mothers were Cambodian refugees.
‡The measured prevalence of HBsAg has not been reported to exceed 20% in any known population.

immune globulin (HBIG) and the hepatitis B vaccine to the baby shortly after birth (Chapters 4, 11, and 19).

HIV

Immigrants to the United States come from countries with a wide range of incidence of infection with HIV. If the visa application is for temporary or asylum status, HIV testing is not mandatory. For those applying for permanent residence, testing is required. This policy has been controversial, since HIV is not transmitted casually and does not pose an infectious risk to the general public. If the HIV status of an individual is unknown, evaluation for risk factors can guide decisions to screen with serologic studies.

SYPHILIS

Immigrants and refugees who have a positive syphilis serology test are usually required to receive treatment before entry into the United States. Prevalence rates in two surveys of refugees were 2% and 7.5%, respectively. Syphilis diagnosis, management, and treatment are covered in greater detail in Chapter 38. Judging an adequate response to treatment depends on the stage of disease and on the pretreatment Venereal Disease Research Laboratory (VDRL) titer. Most patients with an initial episode of primary syphilis revert to a nonreactive VDRL or RPR test status within 1 year after conventional benzathine penicillin G treatment; patients in the secondary stage who are treated usually revert within 2 years.

MALARIA AND OTHER EXTRAINTESTINAL PARASITES

Recurrent malaria in individuals from areas where *Plasmodia* species are endemic may not present with signs and symptoms that are clinically distinguishable from more commonly seen causes of febrile illness in the United States. In addition, such patients may self-diagnose malaria at the beginning of a fever, treat themselves with leftover medications brought with them, and present to health care providers when the acute attack is over and the parasitemia has cleared. A high index of suspicion must be used in the evaluation of any foreign-born person presenting with a history of recurrent fevers. A laboratory diagnosis should be sought (Chapter 17). If the diagnosis of malaria cannot be made from blood smears, but the patient's risk for infection is high based on geographic exposure and history of previous attacks, a presumptive course of therapy to eradicate latent hepatic malaria caused by *Plasmodium vivax* and *P. ovale* can be considered (Chapters 5 and 17). The elimination of recurrent malaria (by presumptive treatment) from the differential diagnosis of fever in the foreign-born patient may simplify the workup of further febrile episodes.

Infection with the lung fluke *Paragonimus* should be considered in patients with pulmonary findings mimicking tuberculosis who remain ill despite adequate treatment for tuberculosis (Chapters 22 and 43). *Strongyloides* infection in patients of foreign origin can present as a puzzling cause of hypereosinophilia in the presence of normal stool examinations or as vague complaints of abdominal discomfort without significant hypereosinophilia. *Strongyloides* causes pneumonia and disseminated infections in patients of foreign origin who become immunocompromised (Chapters 40 and 44).

Cysticercosis is a disseminated infection with larvae from the pork tapeworm *Taenia solium.* It can present as an asymptomatic, inactive old infection with "rice grain" calcifications noted in the subcutaneous tissues and muscles on screening roentgenograms taken for other purposes, or as active disease causing seizures and focal neurologic deficits. Such patients have neurocysticercosis and may have ring-enhancing cystic lesions on computed tomography scan studies (Chapter 41).

Amoebic abscesses and echinococcal cysts may remain silent for many years until focal and systemic symptoms result from the expanding space-occupying lesions. Accidental rupture of a silent echinococcal cyst may cause acute anaphylactic shock in the infected patient. Diagnosis and treatment of these infections are covered in Chapters 26 and 41.

INTESTINAL PARASITES

Protozoan parasites such as *Giardia lamblia* and *Entamoeba histolytica* can present as asymptomatic infections. Young children with asymptomatic infections pose a significant infectious risk to others in their environment because of unsanitary hygiene habits and close contact with other children and adults in the home and in daycare settings. Chapter 26 discusses diagnosis and treatment.

Infections with multiple helminths are common in refugee populations. Worm burdens and the mix of species present will depend on the patient's previous geographic exposure. With the exception of *Strongyloides* and *Enterobius* (pinworm), the common intestinal helminths are not directly transmissible from person to person.

Liver fluke infections (*Clonorchis sinensis* and *Opisthorchis* spp.) may persist asymptomatically for decades after departure of the human host from an endemic area and be detected later as a cause of ascending cholangitis and biliary obstruction. Such infections should be identified and treated in people from Southeast Asia, Hong Kong, People's Republic of China, Korea, and the eastern part of the former Soviet Union (Chapter 43).

Schistosomiasis is caused by species of long-lived human blood flukes and can be found in immigrants and refugees from Africa, South America, Puerto Rico, the Middle East, and Southeast Asia (Table 16-4). Light infections are usually asymptomatic, but schistosomiasis should be considered in the medical evaluation of eosinophilia, hepatosplenomegaly, colonic dysfunction, or hematuria in people originating from endemic areas (Chapter 43).

Screening asymptomatic individuals for intestinal infections with stool microscopy may help to identify parasites with potential long-term health consequences. Some of these disease risks include developmental delay in children (*Trichuriasis trichuria, Ascaris lumbricoides,* hookworm, and possibly *G. lamblia*), cirrhosis (*Schistosoma* spp.), bladder cancer (*Schistosoma haematobium*), cholangiocarcinoma and cholangitis (*C. sinensis* and *Opisthorchis* spp.), central nervous system infections (*T. solium, Paragonimus* spp., and *Schistosoma* spp.), vitamin B_{12} deficiency (*Diphyllobothrium latum*), and liver abscesses (*E. histolytica and Echinococcus granulosa*). The optimal screening approach to asymptomatic individuals is not well defined. The sensitivity of one stool study for detecting parasites can be quite limited depending on the organism. Whereas *A. lumbricoides* and *T. trichuria* are generally easy to detect, *S. stercoralis, Schistosoma* spp., *C. sinensis,* and *Opisthorchis* spp. are often not identified by conventional techniques. The risk of infection with various helminths depends on the patient's native country and living conditions. Owing to the expense and limited sensitivity of stool studies, empiric treatment of all asymptomatic immigrant children is probably reasonable because of the risk of developmental delay. Treatment could include mebendazole or albendazole for hookworm, *T. trichuria* and *A. lumbricoides*. For adults, the optimal screening strategy is not clear. A recent cost-effectiveness study concluded that presumptive treatment of all immigrants (regardless of age or immunosuppressed status) with albendazole (400 mg/day for 5 days) would save both lives and money. Universal screening with treatment of patients with positive stool studies was also found to decrease mortality but to be less cost effective than presumptive treatment of everyone.

SKIN LESIONS

Early lesions of leprosy are unimpressive compared with the disfiguring changes associated with severe advanced leprosy. Clinicians need a high index of suspicion when an erythematous or hypopigmented, macular, anesthetic skin lesion is encountered in a patient from a tropical area. Early diagnosis and treatment control the disease in the patient (Chapter 35). Other less common skin conditions sometimes found in immigrants

Table 16-4
Prevalence (%) of Pathogenic Intestinal Parasites in Refugees and Immigrants

Country **Year** **Author** **Number**	Southeast Asia 1981 Borchardt et al. 6241	Southeast Asia 1988 Molina et al. 2520	Central America 1990 Salas et al. 125	Central America 1983 Sarfaty et al. 96	China 1973 Seah 400	Ethiopia 1987 Parenti et al. 239
G. lamblia	11	11	22	16	4	12
E. histolytica	1	0.5	4	2	1	2
T. trichuria	16	2	27	23	6	4
Hookworm	26	15	5	1	2	4
S. stercoralis	5	4		1	1	2
A. lumbricoides	30	1	16	18	3	4
Schistosoma spp.						4
C. sinensis or *O. viverrini*	8	2			16	
Taenia spp.	0.5					0.5

include cutaneous larva migrans (Chapter 30), myiasis (Chapter 31), cercarial dermatitis (Chapter 30), and cutaneous leishmaniasis (Chapter 34).

MATERNAL AND CHILD HEALTH

Women and children have unique challenges on arrival in a new country. The physical, mental, and cultural hurdles that children encounter are magnified owing to their vulnerability and need to navigate many developmental milestones. Whereas an adult may have no serious deficits from an infection with *T. trichuria,* a child may suffer impairments in cognitive and physical development. Other potential problems that occur on immigration include dietary adjustments, dental disease, and compromised nutrition and immunity as a result of decreased rates of breastfeeding. Newly arrived refugees may be prone to malnutrition because of dietary deficits sustained during long stays in refugee camps or long journeys of escape to final receiving countries. Table 16-5 shows that a significant number of refugee children less than 5 years old had moderate to severe malnutrition. Even after arrival in "the land of plenty," some ethnic groups may continue to have patterns of poor nutrition because they cannot find familiar food items, and food coupons may not cover the right ingredients. Children and teenagers may become "junk food" addicts because they are too embarrassed to take ethnic foods to school. Language difficulties can exacerbate these problems. In the 1990 U.S. census, 28% of immigrant households with school-aged children were identified as "linguistically isolated" (those in which no one over the age of 14 spoke English). Infectious problems are often more problematic for children than adults.

Pregnant women may also have difficulty meeting nutritional requirements. They may not find traditional sources of protein and calcium, and milk may not be an adequate substitute owing to the common problem of

Table 16-5
Malnutrition Rates in Refugee Children < 5 Years of Age

Country and camp (date)	<80% weight-for-height
Ethiopia (May 1989)	
Hartisheik (n = 1350)	23%
Malawi (June 1988)	
Nsanje (n = 575)	6%
Thailand (November 1979)	
Sakeo	18%
Khao-I-Dang	5%
Somalia (May 1980)	
Sabacad	35%
Amalow	24%
Malke Hiday	26%
Sudan (January 1985)	
Wad Sherife	52%
Wad Kowli	32%

From Centers for Disease Control and Prevention: Nutritional Status of Somali Refugees-Eastern Ethiopia, September 1988-May 1989, *MMWR* 38:455, 1989.

lactose intolerance. They are also at increased risk for vitamin deficiencies, which can have detrimental impact on their children in utero. Diseases from vitamin deficiencies include neural tube defects (folate), anemia (iron), beriberi (thiamine), xerophthalmia, and blindness (vitamin A).

The vulnerability of children is further heightened by declines in breastfeeding rates on emigration. Advantages of breastfeeding over formula feeding include health, nutritional, immunologic, developmental, and economic benefits. While breastfeeding rates are nearly 100% in many countries from which people emigrate, the drop in rates on moving to the United States is discouraging. One study found that rates of exclusively breast-fed infants at 5 months declined from 85% in native countries to 14% in the United States. Several factors contributed to this problem including economic pressures, marketing practices including the temporary availability of free formula, lack of support, and the social stigma against breastfeeding. Given the compelling advantages of breastfeeding, supportive resources need to be enlisted shortly after immigration to enable mothers to continue breastfeeding.

CULTURAL CONSIDERATIONS AND ADAPTATION

The cultural background of immigrants intricately influences their health care experience. The effectiveness of clinicians in their interactions and interventions with immigrants is affected by their knowledge and awareness of the cultural systems of their patients. Standard Western approaches to problems may misidentify problems. For example, the apparently simple task of communicating the health consequences and infectious risks of hepatitis B among Khmer immigrants highlights the enormous complexity of translating concepts of illness between cultures. The literal translation of hepatitis B as "liver disease" *(rauk tlaam)* was a meaningless term to 82% of surveyed immigrants. In fact, a number of patients identified a benign rash as the predominant association with liver disease. In contrast, when liver disease was described as a symptom complex (such as yellow illness or *khan leoung*), respondents more readily recognized the serious consequences associated with hepatitis B infection. The motivation to change behavior and seek health care is not conveyed with the literal translation. This communication barrier reflects a difference in concepts of illness with the pathophysiologic, organ-based approach of Western medicine contrasted with the symptom-based approach of the Cambodians. Without acknowledgement of this difference, clinicians will have difficulty communicating biomedical information to their patients.

To more effectively communicate culturally meaningful information, clinicians need to be educated about and incorporate the different concepts of health and illness of their patients. This can be achieved partially by working closely with culturally adept interpreters and community leaders who can convey the complexity and subtleties of these concepts. Extra time invested in asking patients about their view of their health problem or proposed treatment may provide clues for successful intervention. Issues such as compliance with prescribed medications are affected by these concepts. In one survey of Cambodian patients, 67% of respondents reported noncompliance with their medications. Causes of noncompliance included misunderstanding the intent of the medication, side effects, concern about the influence of the medication on "internal strength," and cultural ideas about pharmacokinetics. Western medicine was often viewed as too "strong" and used cautiously, especially when a patient was ill or had decreased "internal strength." Individuals would often lower the dose of the medication to adjust for this problem. Immigrants may also take medications prescribed by ethnic healers, which may contain substances whose effect may confuse the clinical or therapeutic evaluation by unknowing Western physicians. Without awareness of such cultural aspects of compliance, therapeutic interventions become useless and sometimes dangerous.

Psychosocial adjustments may be among the most challenging problems for the cross-cultural health care provider. The sense of punctuality for appointments in industrialized countries may be contrary to less pressured concepts of time in other cultures. Adverse effects from prescribed medications may not be voluntarily reported for fear of displeasing the physician. The gender of the health care provider may greatly influence which health problems are discussed during the patient's clinic visit. Finally, evaluation of mental health in populations of foreign patients presents a dilemma, as it may be culturally unacceptable for some patients to admit to having mental illness. Furthermore, in some cultures the concept of the existence of mental illness is significantly different from Western approaches. The pressures of geographic translocation, learning English, finding a job, and worrying about money may be expressed as somatic complaints. The health care provider may order expensive diagnostic tests that are unnecessary.

With the complexity and diversity of different cultural concepts of health and illness, it is challenging for the clinician to provide meaningful and effective care for foreign patients. If health care providers begin with an openness to the nuances of the culture and experiences of their patients, it may help them to devise more effective communication strategies and therapeutic interventions. The Western biomedical explanation of disease processes may not be appropriate for some patients. Explanations for a patient's illness or complaints may have to be interpreted in culturally understandable terms for a healing transaction to take place. In addition to listening to the patient's concept of his or her illness, the medical practitioner is best guided by medically trained personnel from the ethnic group under consideration or by people with expertise in cross-cultural medicine.

REFERENCES

American Academy of Pediatrics: Breastfeeding and the use of human milk, *Pediatrics* 100:1035, 1997.

American Academy of Pediatrics: Health care for children of immigrant families, *Pediatrics* 100:153, 1997.

Barnes PF, Barrows SA: Tuberculosis in the 1990s, *Ann Intern Med* 119:400, 1993.

Berger JT: Culture and ethnicity in clinical care, *Arch Intern Med* 158:2085, 1998.

Borchardt KA et al: Intestinal parasites in Southeast Asian refugees, *West J Med* 135:93, 1981.

From Centers for Disease Control and Prevention: Nutritional Status of Somali Refugees-Eastern Ethiopia, September 1988-May 1989, *MMWR* 38:455, 1989.

Centers for Disease Control and Prevention: Tuberculosis in developing countries, *MMWR* 39:561, 1990.

Centers for Disease Control and Prevention: Screening for hepatitis B virus infection among refugees arriving in the United States, 1979-1991, *MMWR* 40:784, 1991.

Centers for Disease Control and Prevention: Famine-affected, refugee, and displaced populations: recommendations for public health issues, *MMWR* 41(No. RR-13):1, 1992.

Centers for Disease Control and Prevention: Summary of notifiable diseases, United States. *MMWR* 46:1, 1998.

Centers for Disease Control and Prevention: Recommendations for prevention and control of tuberculosis among foreign-born persons, *MMWR* 47 (RR16):1, 1998.
Centers for Disease Control and Prevention: Notice to readers: recommended childhood immunization schedule—United States, 1999, *MMWR* 48:8, 1999.
Committee on Maternal, Adolescent, and Child Health: Medical care for indigent and culturally displaced obstetrical patients and their newborns, *JAMA* 245:1159, 1981.
Dashefsky B, Teele D: Infectious disease problems in Indochinese refugees, *Pediatr Ann* 12:232, 1983.
Erickson V, Hoang GN: Health problems among Indochinese refugees, *Am J Public Health* 70:1003, 1980.
Forrester JE et al: Randomised trial of albendazole and pyrantel in symptomless trichuriasis in children, *Lancet* 352:1103, 1998.
Gavagan T, Brodyaga L: Medical care for immigrants and refugees, *Am Fam Physician* 57:1061, 1998.
Ghaemi-Ahmadi S: Attitudes toward breast-feeding and infant feeding among Iranian, Afghan, and Southeast Asian immigrant women in the United States: implications for health and nutrition education, *J Am Dietet Assoc* 92:354, 1992.
Gostin LO et al: Screening immigrants and international travelers for the human immunodeficiency virus, *N Engl J Med* 322:1743, 1990.
Hostetter MK et al: Medical evaluation of internationally adopted children, *N Engl J Med* 325:479, 1991.
Jackson JC et al: Hepatitis B among the Khmer: issues of translation and concepts of illness, *J Gen Intern Med* 12:292, 1997.
Johnson RJ et al: Paragonimiasis: diagnosis and the use of praziquantel in treatment, *Rev Infect Dis* 7:200, 1985.
Molina CD, Molina MM, Molina JM: Intestinal parasites in Southeast Asian refugees two years after immigration, *West J Med* 149:422, 1988.
Muennig P et al: The cost effectiveness of strategies for the treatment of intestinal parasites in immigrants, *N Engl J Med* 340:773, 1999.
Nelson KR, Bui H, Sarnet JH: Screening in special immigrant populations: a "case study" of recent Vietnamese immigrants, *Am J Med* 102:435, 1997.
Nutman TB et al: Eosinophilia in Southeast Asian refugees: evaluation at a referral center, *J Infect Dis* 155:309, 1987.
Parenti DM et al: Health status of Ethiopian refugees in the United States, *Am J Public Health* 77:1542, 1987.
Parrish RA: Intestinal parasites in Southeast Asian refugee children, *West J Med* 143:47, 1985.
Popkin BM, Bilsborrow RE, Akin JS: Breast-feeding patterns in low-income countries, *Science* 218:1088, 1982.
Rust GS: Health status of migrant farmworkers: a literature review and commentary, *Am J Public Health* 80:1213, 1990.
Salas SD, Heifetz R, Barrett-Connor E: Intestinal parasites in Central American immigrants in the United States, *Arch Intern Med* 150:1514, 1990.
Sarfaty M, Rosenberg Z, Siegel J: Intestinal parasites in immigrant children from Central America, *West J Med* 139:329, 1983.
Seah SKK: Intestinal parasites in Chinese immigrants in a Canadian city, *J Trop Med Hyg* 76:291, 1973.
Shimada J et al: "Strong medicine": Cambodian views of medicine and medical compliance, *J Gen Intern Med* 10:369, 1995.
Tong MJ et al: A comparative study of hepatitis B viral markers in the family members of Asian and non-Asian patients with hepatitis B surface antigen-positive hepatocellular carcinoma and with chronic hepatitis B infection, *J Infect Dis* 140:506, 1979.
US Department of Health and Human Services: *Technical instructions for medical examination of aliens,* Atlanta, 1991, Centers for Disease Control and Prevention.
Verner E et al: Diagnostic and therapeutic approach to Ethiopian immigrants seropositive for syphilis, *Isr J Med Sci* 24:151, 1988.
Wilson ME: *A world guide to infections: disease, distribution, diagnosis,* New York, 1991, Oxford University Press.

SECTION III

FEVER

CHAPTER 17

Malaria Diagnosis and Treatment

Matthew J. Thompson, Nicholas J. White,
and Elaine C. Jong

GENERAL CONSIDERATIONS

Physicians and other health care practitioners working in temperate malaria-free areas and countries may be unfamiliar with the various clinical presentations of this disease, which can mimic influenza or even a gastrointestinal illness (see later discussion). However, undiagnosed and untreated malaria can, in some cases, rapidly progress to a fatal outcome. For this reason, a diagnosis of malaria should be considered in any ill person with a fever if an appropriate travel history can be obtained. In general, patients at risk for malaria will come from one of the following groups:

1. Immigrants and refugees.
2. Travelers, even if the stay in an endemic area was limited to a few hours (includes missionaries, Peace Corps and other volunteer groups, professional and technical workers).
3. Military personnel with foreign assignments.
4. Recipients of blood transfusions.
5. Infants of immigrant or refugee mothers (congenital infections).
6. Intravenous drug users (parenteral transmission).
7. People living in nonendemic areas where undiagnosed imported infections may occur (proximity to international airports, military bases, refugee resettlements, and so forth).

ETIOLOGY

Malaria is a protozoan parasite infection spread from person to person in endemic areas by female mosquitoes of the genus *Anopheles.* Four species of malaria regularly cause disease in humans.

- *Plasmodium vivax*—worldwide distribution, most common in Asia, South America, Oceania, India
- *Plasmodium falciparum*—worldwide distribution; untreated infections can rapidly progress to severe illness and death
- *Plasmodium oval*—worldwide distribution; relatively uncommon outside of Africa
- *Plasmodium malariae*—much less common than *Plasmodium vivax* or *Plasmodium falciparum;* worldwide distribution; asymptomatic low-level erythrocytic infections persisting for years are possible.

PRESENTATION

Epidemiology

Malaria is endemic in most tropical areas of the world, but the risk may vary from season to season and also even within some regions. Malaria may be less of a risk in urban compared with rural areas within a given area or country. It is difficult to generalize about transmission of malaria, since this can vary enormously even within areas as small as a few square miles. In sub-Saharan Africa, transmission is often intense, and most imported cases of malaria in travelers originate from this continent.

Chloroquine-resistant *P. falciparum* has spread from Southeast Asia and South America and is now found throughout sub-Saharan Africa and most parts of the Indian subcontinent and Oceania. There are few areas, such as Central America, where chloroquine can be relied on to treat falciparum malaria. Resistance to sulfadoxine-pyrimethamine (Fansidar) is also widespread.

A list of countries with details of areas within countries where malaria is endemic can be found in *Health Information for International Travel,* a biennial manual prepared by the Centers for Disease Control and Prevention (CDC). This publication is written for health care practitioners and may be less useful for the lay traveler. Copies of this booklet may be obtained from the U.S. Government Printing Office or the Foundation for Public Health. Updated advice from the CDC specifically for travelers is also available online (see Appendix).

The malarious areas, especially those where chloroquine-resistant *P. falciparum* malaria is a risk, may change between the publication dates of *Health Information for International Travel.* Reports from the field by way of returned travelers, foreign press releases, and other sources should be confirmed with published postings from the CDC Malaria Branch online, in the *MMWR,* or in other media (see Appendix). For general information, a world map showing where malaria and chloroquine-resistant *P. falciparum* malaria are usually a concern is given in Fig. 17-1.

PATHOGENESIS

Natural Life Cycle

After inoculation of the malaria parasites (sporozoites) during feeding by a female anopheline mosquito, there is an asymptomatic incubation period that usually lasts between 1 and 3 weeks but can be as long as a year (with *P. vivax*). The sporozoites invade the liver parenchymal cells and then replicate during the incubation period (preerythrocytic schizogony). Eventually, the cells rupture and parasite forms (merozoites) are released into the bloodstream, where red blood cells are rapidly infected (erythrocytic stage) (see Fig. 5-3).

1. The merozoites mature in infected red cells. It is the blood stage infection that causes the symptoms and signs of malaria. There is no extravascular pathogenic process. The early red cell infective stages are called *ring trophozoites* and may resemble signet rings or the headphones of a stereo headset.
2. Most merozoites eventually develop in red cells through a stage of asexual division into a *schizont,* or ball of new merozoites. During this process, the erythrocyte's hemoglobin is consumed and eventually the cell bursts to liberate new merozoites that invade new red cells and amplify the infection.
3. After several cycles of asexual reproduction, a proportion of merozoites will develop into sexual forms of the parasite. A single male or female *gametocyte* is formed. These await ingestion by another feeding anopheline

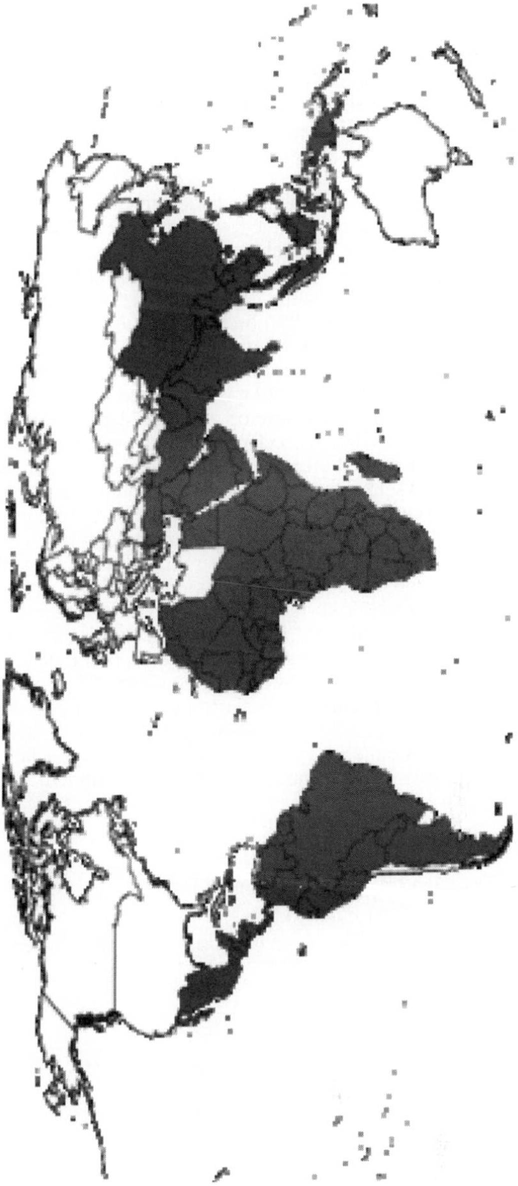

Fig. 17-1 Malaria endemic countries, 2000. Countries with malaria risk are shaded. (From Centers for Disease Control and Prevention, www.ncid.cdc.gov/travel/yb/utils/ybdynamic.asp. Accessed 08/28/02.)

mosquito before fusing in the mosquito's midgut, invading and developing in the wall of the gut, and then emigrating to the mosquito's salivary gland to complete the cycle.

Blood-Borne Malaria

The merozoites released by parasitized red cells can infect only other red cells, thus causing autoinfections and blood-borne infections, including *transfusion-associated* and *congenital malaria.*

Clinical Correlates

What may be considered the incubation period in malaria infections is complicated by the fact that each of the four human species has a variable incubation period, that is, the interval between infection with sporozoites and the onset of clinical illness with fever. *P. falciparum* has the shortest incubation period (8 days or more, average 13 days) with somewhat longer incubation periods generally observed for the other species. See Table 17-1 for data on the interval between date of return and onset of illness among imported malaria cases in U.S. travelers reported to the CDC.

The erythrocytic stage of the infection is associated with spiking fevers and chills, which may eventually develop a 48- to 72-hour periodicity in prolonged primary attacks or in secondary attacks of malaria. Although the various malarias were named after the fever intervals (i.e., tertian, quartan), this periodicity is seldom seen nowadays. Fever and illness are caused by the release of proinflammatory cytokines (particularly tumor necrosis factor) and other inflammatory mediators. The pathology of severe falciparum malaria is associated with the sequestration of red cells containing mature forms of the parasite in the microvasculature of vital organs.

Although the fever and other systemic signs and symptoms may be severe with *P. vivax, P. ovale,* and *P. malariae* infections, clinical attacks are rarely fatal, even if undiagnosed and untreated. Appropriate drug treatment will abort the clinical attack by destroying the erythrocytic stages of the malarial parasites. In contrast, malaria caused by a *P. falciparum* infection may progress rapidly to parasitize a large number of erythrocytes, with severe systemic consequences of multiple organ failure and death unless appropriate drug treatment is promptly instituted.

Table 17-1
Malaria in Returning Travelers to the United States

Interval	P. vivax no. (%)	P. falcip. no. (%)	P. malariae no. (%)
<0*	20 (3.4)	46 (10.4)	1 (2.6)
0-29	124 (21.3)	344 (77.7)	18 (47.4)
30-89	134 (23)	35 (7)	8 (21)
90-179	132 (22.7)	10 (2.2)	9 (23.7)
180-364	146 (25.1)	7 (1.6)	2 (5.3)
≥365	26 (4.5)	1 (0.2)	2 (5.3)
Total	582 (100)	443 (100)	38 (100)

From CDC: Imported malaria cases, by species and interval between date of onset: U.S. 1997, *MMWR* 50(SS-01):25, 2001.

P. falciparum infections are potentially lethal for several reasons:

1. Each schizont (the mature form of the intraerythrocytic parasite) liberates up to 32 merozoites when it ruptures. This gives the parasite an enormous growth potential.

2. Although it prefers younger erythrocytes, *P. falciparum* causing severe malaria parasitizes circulating red cells of all ages (in contrast to *P. vivax,* which tends to infect young cells only, and *P. malariae,* which has a predilection for older cells).

3. Erythrocytes containing mature forms of *P. falciparum* become rigid and nondeformable and tend to stick to normal red cells (rosetting) and to the endothelium of capillaries and postcapillary venules (cytoadherence). The resulting sequestration results from the interaction between antigenically variant parasite-derived adhesive proteins expressed on the surface of infected erythrocytes and specific receptors on the vascular endothelium. The subsequent interference with microcirculatory flow and regional metabolism is most evident in the brain but also occurs in the other vital organs. Cytoadherence and sequestration do not occur with the other three human species. Sequestration accounts for the frequently observed discrepancy between the peripheral parasite count and disease severity (i.e., patients can be very ill, and sometimes die, with relatively low peripheral blood parasite counts or parasitemias) and also explains the relative rarity with which mature trophozoites and schizonts are seen in the peripheral blood in falciparum malaria.

Immunity to Malaria

The immune response to malaria infections is inefficient, and frequent repeated attacks are required to induce protective immunity, which is rapidly lost if the individual leaves the endemic area. Acquired immunity is specific for both the species of malaria and the particular strain(s) causing the infection. The development of immunity to *P. falciparum* is gained at the expense of a high mortality in children living in areas of heavy transmission (e.g., West Africa). For this reason, severe malaria is a disease of childhood in these areas, and adults who have gained protective immunity have little or no symptoms despite malarial infection. Malaria is estimated to kill between 1 and 2 million people each year, mostly children. Symptomless parasitemias are common in the adult age group. In contrast, nonimmune travelers of all ages coming from areas without malaria (e.g., the United States) to endemic areas are vulnerable to developing severe and potentially fatal infections.

CLINICAL FEATURES

The symptoms and signs of malaria are notoriously nonspecific. The disease commonly presents as a flulike syndrome with headaches, chills, myalgias, and erratic fever. The classic periodic fever patterns that gave the infections their names (i.e., tertian, quartan) are not usually seen unless the infection is allowed to go untreated. Malaria may also present as febrile convulsions in children, may be mistaken for infectious hepatitis when jaundice is prominent or pneumonia when there is "respiratory distress" secondary to lactic acidosis, may present as coma (cerebral malaria), and on occasion may be confused with enteric infections with fever, vomiting, abdominal pain, and occasionally diarrhea. The physician should have a low threshold of suspicion in any returned traveler and should always request thick and thin blood smears or one of the other diagnostic tests if fever is present. Splenomegaly and mild anemia are relatively common in all the acute malarias, but evidence of serious organ dysfunction is virtually confined to falciparum malaria. Serious infections usually start with several days of fever and nonspecific symptoms.

Cerebral Malaria

Strictly defined, this is a coma in a patient with falciparum malaria, although any alteration in the level of consciousness should be treated similarly. It results from the sequestration of parasitized erythrocytes in the capillaries and venules of the brain, with secondary toxic and metabolic consequences. In most areas, cerebral malaria is the most frequent manifestation of severe disease, especially in children. Clinically, cerebral malaria can present with either focal or generalized neurologic features; convulsions occur, particularly in children, and contribute to coma. It must be distinguished from other causes of fever and altered consciousness (most important, bacterial, or viral meningoencephalitis).

Acute Renal Failure

Severe malaria is an important cause of acute renal failure in adults living in areas of low or unstable malaria transmission. This results from acute tubular necrosis. Some patients given oxidant antimalarial drugs may develop brisk hemolysis and hemoglobinuric renal failure ("blackwater"). This is particularly associated with the administration of primaquine to patients with glucose-6-phosphate dehydrogenase (G6PD) deficiency and with the use of quinine in severe infections.

Acute Pulmonary Edema

This is a grave manifestation of severe malaria, carrying a high mortality. It is clinically similar to the adult respiratory distress syndrome. Occasionally acute pulmonary edema also develops in *P. vivax* malaria.

Hypoglycemia

Glucose levels fall in severe malaria infections as a result of increased metabolic demands by the host and parasites, and decreased gluconeogenesis. Hypoglycemia develops in 8% of adults, 30% of children, and 50% of women in late pregnancy with severe malaria. It is usually accompanied by lactic acidosis. Quinine stimulates pancreatic insulin secretion and is an important cause of hypoglycemia especially in pregnant women.

Anemia

The hematocrit falls rapidly in severe malaria because of the accelerated clearance of both parasitized and unparasitized erthrocytes. The anemia is compounded by bone marrow dyserythropoiesis. Thrombocytopenia (circa 100,000/μl) is usual in all symptomatic malaria. Lower platelet counts may occur in severe malaria.

Bacterial Infections

Patients with severe malarial infections are particularly vulnerable to bacterial infections, such as aspiration pneumonia and spontaneous septicemia with gram-negative bacteria (particularly *Salmonellae*).

Prognosis

A variety of clinical, biochemical and hematologic features indicate a poor prognosis in severe malaria (Table 17-2).

Table 17-2
Features Indicating a Poor Prognosis in Severe Malaria

Clinical Features
Impaired consciousness
Repeated convulsions (3 in 24 hours)
Respiratory distress
Substantial bleeding
Shock
Biochemical Features
Renal impairment (serum creatinine >3 mg/dl [>264 μmol/L])
Acidosis (plasma bicarbonate <15 μmol/L)
Jaundice (serum total bilirubin >2.5 mg/dl [>43 μmol/L])
Hyperlactatemia (venous lactate >45 mg/dl [>5 μmol/L])
Hypoglycemia (blood glucose <40 mg/dl [<2.2 μmol/L])
Elevated aminotransferase levels (>3 times normal)
Hematologic Features
Parasitemia (>500,000 parasites/mm^3, or >10,000 mature trophozoites and schizonts/mm^3)
5% of neutrophils contain malaria pigment

Adapted from White NJ: The treatment of malaria, *N Engl J Med* 335:800, 1996.

Chronic Malaria

Chronic malaria refers to repeated infections. It is a major cause of chronic anemia and ill health in the rural tropics. Splenomegaly is also a reflection of repeated malaria attacks in children in endemic areas. Splenic rupture occasionally occurs as a complication of *P. vivax* infection in adults. Splenomegaly and hypersplenism are sometimes seen in adults in endemic areas; this appears to reflect an exaggerated immune response to repeated infection and will respond clinically to antimalarial prophylaxis. Nephrotic syndrome may develop in children repeatedly infected with *P. malariae* (quartan nephropathy).

LABORATORY STUDIES

The diagnosis of malaria is made by the identification of malaria parasites on the peripheral blood smear. Preparation of thick and thin smears should be a "reflex" response for any febrile patient living in or returning from a malarious area (Table 17-3). Although Giemsa stains (pH 7.2) of the blood smear are ideal for determining speciation of the parasite, the modified Wright's stain used for the routine processing of blood smears in clinical hematology laboratories is adequate.

For practical purposes, it is not essential to identify immediately the species of malaria parasite other than to distinguish *P. falciparum* from the remaining three species. If a parasitologist or other expert is not available to interpret the blood smear at the time the diagnosis must be made, three clues may help in the detection of a *P. falciparum* infection:

1. Species of malaria other than *P. falciparum* rarely achieve a level of parasitemia of more than 2%.

Table 17-3
Preparation of Blood Smears for Diagnosis of Malaria

Thin Smears
Thin smears for evaluation of the blood for malarial parasites are made the same way that routine blood smears for hematologic evaluation are made. A small drop of blood is placed at one end of a clean glass microscopic slide. A second slide is held at a 45-degree angle to the first slide, contacting the drop of blood, and spreading it out in a thin smear as the second slide is pushed along the surface of the first slide to the opposite end. After air-drying, the slide is fixed in anhydrous methanol and stained in a standard manner with reverse Field, Wright, or Giemsa stains.

Thick Smears
A thick smear for detection of malarial parasites in the blood when the parasitemia is low is made by placing one large drop of blood on a clean glass microscopic slide and using the corner of a second slide to spread the blood around to create a spot about the size of a dime. After air-drying, the slide *is not fixed* but stained directly with an aqueous stain (Wright or Giemsa stain). Exposure of the thick smear to an aqueous stain without prior fixation causes the red cells to rupture and enables the microscopist to see parasite forms in the thick layer of organic material on the slide.

2. Unlike *P. vivax* or *P. ovale,* Schuffner's dots are not seen in the red cell cytoplasm. *P. vivax*-infected red cells are usually enlarged (young cells).
3. Blue-purple "banana forms" within or outside the red cells represent the male and female gametocytes of *P. falciparum.* These forms are approximately the length of the red cell diameter and are so distinctive that they can be seen at the 400× magnification used for scanning the slide. Although the distinctive banana forms are helpful diagnostic clues, they may not be seen in early fulminant infections. Development of these sexual forms (gametocytes) may take 10 days or more in the course of a patent erythrocytic episode.

In the context of severe malaria, the microscopist should count the number of parasitized red cells (per 1000 red cells), comment on the predominant stage of parasite development (if >20% of parasites contain visible pigment, the prognosis is worse), and count the number of neutrophils containing phagocytosed parasite pigment (>5% also indicates a poor prognosis).

Fluorescent Stains

More recent techniques have used the fluorochrome acridine orange to stain parasite nuclei for detection by fluorescence microscopy. The quantitative buffy coat (or QBC) malaria test (Becton Dickinson, Franklin Lakes, NJ) uses blood collected in acridine orange and anticoagulant-coated capillary tubes for examination under a fluorescence microscope. Despite some low-technology centrifuge and microscope adaptations, this kit is still relatively expensive for many settings. A more recent modification of the same technique uses a conventional microscope fitted with a special filter to examine thick and thin films stained with acridine orange. Although both techniques are rapid, show equivalent or superior sensitivity (particularly at low parasitemias) to conventional staining, and allow limited species determination, the newer method is less expensive and allows better determination of parasite density.

Table 17-4
Rapid Antigen Tests for Detection of Malaria

Assay	*Plasmodium* species identified	Parasite antigen(s) detected
OptiMAL (Flow Inc., Portland Oregon)	*P. falciparum*, Other species*	pLDH isoenzymes
ICT Malaria P.f/P.v (AMRAD ICT, Sydney, NSW, Australia)	*P. falciparum*, Other species	HRP-2† and pan-malarial antigen‡
PATH Falciparum Malaria IC Strip (Quorum Diagnostics, Vancouver, Canada)	*P. falciparum*	HRP-2
Parasight-F test (Becton Dickinson Tropical Diagnostics, Sparks, Md)	*P. falciparum*	HRP-2
ICT Malaria P.f test (AMRAD ICT, Sydney, NSW, Australia)	*P. falciparum*	HRP-2

* *pLDH*, parasite Lactate dehydrogenase, isoenzyme specific to *P. falciparum* and *P. vivax*.
† HRP-2, Histidine-rich protein 2, specific to *P. falciparum*.
‡ Pan-specific antigen expressed by *P. falciparum, P. vivax*, and probably *P. ovale*.

Serology

Measurement of malaria antibodies in the blood is not useful in acute diagnosis, although serology is sometimes used as an adjunct to comprehensive evaluation of returned travelers with subacute febrile illness. Malaria serology is available in the United States from the CDC through state health departments.

Rapid Antigen Assays

Several immunochromatographic strip assays have been developed to detect malarial antigens in finger-stick blood samples using test strips or cards impregnated with specific antibodies (Table 17-4). These are based on detection of *P. falciparum* histidine-rich protein 2 (HRP-2) or parasite lactate dehydrogenase isoenzymes. Several newer assays also have a genus-specific antibody allowing distinction of *Plasmodium falciparum* from the other three less serious malaria species. These assays require minimal technical training and instrumentation, allowing use in rural settings or places without facilities for microscopy. In addition, their sensitivity and specificity are similar to conventional stained slides. This rapidly evolving technology may facilitate more accurate diagnosis and treatment among travelers to remote areas. Final Food and Drug Administration approval for these tests is still pending. Potential disadvantages include the cost of the test kits themselves and the inability to determine parasite load or full speciation.

TREATMENT

Acute Therapy

Most patients can be treated with oral medications. Parenteral treatment should be reserved for vomiting patients or those who are seriously ill.

Table 17-5
Treatment of Uncomplicated Malaria

Malaria	Drug regimens adult dose	Pediatric dose
Chloroquine sensitive*	Chloroquine phosphate 10 mg base/kg followed by *either* 5 mg/kg at 12, 24, and 36 hr later, *or* 10 mg base/kg at 24 hr and 5 mg/kg at 48 hr later (total dose 25 mg base/kg)	Same as adult dose
Chloroquine resistant	Pyrimethamine 25 mg + sulfadoxine 500 mg (Fansidar) tablets-take 3 tablets in a single dose (or one of other regimens listed under multidrug resistant falciparum malaria)	Pyrimethamine + sulfadoxine (Fansidar)† 1 mg + 20 mg/kg in a single dose (<1 yr = ¼ tablet; 1-3 yr = ½ tablet; 4-8 yr = 1 tablet; 9-14 yr = 2 tablets). Aim at no less than 1.25mg/kg of pyrimethamine
Multi-drug resistant (chloroquine resistant, Fansidar resistant, etc.)	Mefloquine‡ (Lariam) 25 mg base/kg; the dose should be split (i.e., 15 mg/kg, followed by 10 mg/kg 8 to 24 hr later)	Same as adult dose regimen (25 mg base/kg) adjusted for weight§
	Artemether-lumefantrine‖ (Riamet, Co-Artem) 1.5 mg + 9 mg/kg usual adult dose 4 tablets at 0, 8, 24, 36, 48 and 60 hours Taken with food if possible	Usual individual doses at same times: 25-35 kg; 3 tabs, 15-25 kg 2 tabs, <15 kg 1 tab. Taken with food if possible
	Or; halofantrine (Halfan)¶ 8 mg base/kg as a single dose, repeated at 6 and 12 hr later	Halofantrine 2% suspension 8 mg base/kg as a single dose, repeated at 6 and 12 hr later
	Quinine sulfate 10 mg salt/kg three times daily for 7 days + *either* tetracycline 4 mg/kg four times daily for 7 days *or* doxycycline 3 mg/kg once daily for 7 days *or* clindamycin 10 mg/kg twice daily for 3-7 days	Same as adult dose regimen, adjusted for weight#

Patients with a diagnosis of *P. falciparum* malaria should not go home unaccompanied, since deterioration can occur after treatment has started. It is always best to administer the first dose of antimalarial drug(s) as soon as the diagnosis is made and observe the patient for 1 hour. If vomiting occurs within 30 minutes, the full dose is given again (usually after metoclopramide, 10 mg PO, IM, or IV); if vomiting occurs between 30 and 60 minutes, half the dose is readministered (with the exception of atovaquone/proguanil, see later discussion). If parenteral therapy must be used, a changeover to oral therapy should be made as soon as the patient is alert and able to swallow. Table 17-5 presents the regimens commonly

Table 17-5
Treatment of Uncomplicated Malaria—cont'd

Malaria	Drug regimens adult dose	Pediatric dose
	Or; Atovaquone 250 mg + proguanil 100 mg (Malarone) 4 tablets single dose daily for 3 days.** Taken with food if possible	Atovaquone 250 mg + proguanil 100 mg (Malarone) tablets: 11-20 kg = 1 tablet daily for 3 days; 21-30 kg = 2 tablets as a single dose daily for 3 days; 31-40 kg = 3 tablets as a single dose daily for 3 days; >40 kg same as adult. Taken with food if possible

Adapted from White NJ: The treatment of malaria, *N Engl J Med* 335:800, 1996, and Newton P, White NJ: Malaria: new developments in treatment and prevention, *Annu Rev Med* 50:179, 1999.

**P. vivax* and *P. ovale* malaria patients should be treated with primaquine 0.25 mg base/kg/day (0.33-0.5 mg base/kg/day in Oceania and SouthEast Asia) for 14 days after the last dose of chloroquine, provided that the patient is not G6PD-deficient, pregnant, or newborn (see Chapter 5).

†Pyrimethamine-sulfadoxine (Fansidar) is contraindicated in infants less than 2 months old, and should not be given to pregnant women in the third trimester.

‡When available artesunate or artemether 4mg/kg/day should also be given for 3 days, and the mefloquine started on day 2 of the combination regimen. If mefloquine is not available, give same total dose of artesunate (10 to 12 mg/kg) over 7 days (see text).

§Mefloquine can be used for children weighing less than 15 kg with dose calculated based on weight, although this usage is not FDA-approved (see Luxemburger C et al: Mefloquine in infants and young children, *Ann Trop Paediatr* 16:281, 1996).

‖Artemether and artesunate compounds are not available in the United States.

¶Halofantrine prolongs atrioventricular and ventricular repolarisation, and should not be used in patients with preexisting cardiac conduction abnormalities, long QTc intervals or within 1 month of receiving mefloquine. It should also not be taken with fatty foods, or with drugs which prolong the QTc interval (such as quinine, quinidine, chloroquine, tricyclic antidepressants, neuroleptic drugs, terfenadine, astemizole).

#Tetracycline or doxycycline should not be given to children 8 years of age or younger, or to pregnant women.

**Atovaquone-proguanil (Malarone) daily dose can be split and given twice per day.

used for treatment of uncomplicated malaria. Other regimens are given for field or special situations. (Table 17-6).

Chloroquine-resistant falciparum malaria is now present in most areas of the tropics (see Fig. 5-1). If one is in doubt and the patient is seriously ill, one should assume that the malaria is chloroquine resistant. Recommended treatments are given in Table 17-5. The clinical status of the patient and the level of parasitemia should be followed frequently until the parasitemia has cleared and the individual is improved clinically. Patients with severe malaria require intensive-care nursing and monitoring. If the clinical status does not improve despite appropriate supportive measures

Table 17-6
Treatment of Severe Malaria in Patients Unable to Take Oral Medication

Precautions:
To avoid fatal hypotension, *never* give chloroquine, quinine, or quinidine by intravenous bolus injection. If the patient remains severely ill, the dose of quinine or quinidine should be reduced on the third day of treatment by one third to one half. Oral treatment should replace parenteral treatment as soon as the patient can take oral drugs reliably. Quinine and quinidine may induce hyperinsulinemic hypoglycemia.

Chloroquine-Resistant Malaria
Well-staffed and well-equipped hospital
*Quinine dihydrochloride**: give initial dose of *either* 7 mg salt/kg by rate-controlled IV infusion in 5% dextrose over 30 min followed by 10 mg/kg over 4 hr, *or* an initial dose of 20 mg salt/kg IV in 5% dextrose or 0.9% saline over 4 hr; *then* give maintenance dose of 10 mg salt/kg (maximum dose 1800 mg/day) infused over 2-4 hr q8h (resistant areas) or q12h (sensitive areas), until the patient can take oral drugs.
or
Quinidine gluconate[†]: give initial dose of 10 mg base/kg (maximum dose 600 mg) in 0.9% saline by rate-controlled IV infusion over 1-2 hr; followed by maintenance dose of 0.02 mg base/kg/min with cardiac monitoring, until the patient is able to take oral drugs.
or
Artemether[‡] give initial dose of 3.2 mg/kg by IM injection followed by 1.6 mg/kg daily for 5 to 7 days.
or
Artesunate[§] give initial dose of 2.4 mg/kg by IV bolus injection followed by 1.2 mg/kg at 12 and 24 hr, then daily.

Rural health facility
Quinine dihydrochloride[†]: 20 mg salt/kg by IM injection to the anterior thigh (split the initial dose between the two thighs) followed by 10 mg/kg q8hr (resistant areas) or q12h (sensitive areas), until the patient can take oral drugs.
or
Artemether[‡]: give initial dose of 3.2 mg/kg by IM injection followed by 1.6 mg/kg q24h.
or
Artesunate[§]: give initial dose of 2.4 mg/kg by IV bolus injection or IM followed by 1.2 mg/kg after 12 hr, then 1.2 mg/kg q24h

Definite Chloroquine-Sensitive Malaria
Well-staffed and well-equipped hospital
Chloroquine: 10 mg base/kg by rate-controlled IV infusion over 8 hr, followed by 15 mg/kg over 24 hr.

Rural health facility
Chloroquine: 3.5 mg base/kg by IM or SQ injection q6h until the patient can take oral drugs; or, 2.5 mg base/kg IM or SQ q4h until the patient can take oral drugs.

Adapted from White NJ: The treatment of malaria, *N Engl J Med* 335:800, 1996; Newton P, White NJ: Malaria: new developments in treatment and prevention, *Annu Rev Med* 50:179, 1999.
*Quinine dihydrochloride for parenteral use is no longer available in the United States.
[†]The regimen currently recommended by the CDC for treatment of severe malaria is a lower dose; 10 mg salt/kg initially which corresponds to 6.2 mg/kg base followed by 0.02 mg salt/kg/min (0.012 mg base/kg/min). This may lead to underdosing. Quinidine is much more cardiotoxic than quinine. The electrocardiogram must be monitored continuously, and the infusion stopped if the QT_c interval is prolonged by more than 25%. Saline should be infused if hypotension develops.
[‡]Artemether is not available in the United States.
[§]Artesunate is not available in the United States.

Table 17-7
Types of Resistance Seen in Malaria

RI: Disappearance of parasites on blood films, clinical recovery, recrudescence weeks later (within 28 days of last treatment dose).
RII: Reduction in parasitemia (>75% fall in 48 hours) and clinical symptoms, but parasitemia does not clear within 7 days.
RIII: No response to therapy (assessed at 48 hours) (i.e., parasitemia does not fall by ≥75%).

and the fall in the percentage of infected red cells on the peripheral smear is less than 75% by the third day (i.e., >48 hours) of treatment, drug resistance must be considered (Table 17-7).

Chloroquine-Resistant Falciparum Malaria

It must be emphasized that resistance is a relative phenomenon. Many patients from areas of chloroquine-resistant malaria will have some response to chloroquine (with low or intermediate levels of resistance), but the infection will tend to come back again (recrudesce). High-grade chloroquine resistance is found in some parts of South America, Indochina, Papua New Guinea, and Africa. Advice for departing travelers should be based on the most up-to-date information (see Chapter 5).

Sulfadoxine/Pyrimethamine (Fansidar)-Resistant Falciparum Malaria

Strains of falciparum malaria resistant to sulfadoxine/pyrimethamine (Fansidar) are now widespread in Asia and South America, and resistance is increasing in sub-Saharan Africa. In such instances, treatment options include quinine plus tetracycline or clindamycin, atovaquone/proguanil, mefloquine (with artesunate if available), or artemether-lumefantrine (Table 17-5).

Mefloquine-Resistant Falciparum Malaria

Highly mefloquine-resistant *P. falciparum* parasites are found on the eastern and western borders of Thailand, and adjacent parts of Democratic Kampuchea (Cambodia) and Myanmar (Burma), respectively, and southern Vietnam, but not been conclusively documented elsewhere.

Qinghaosu

Qinghaosu (artemisinin) and its derivatives (artemether, artesunate, dihydroartemisinin) developed in the People's Republic of China, appear to be the most rapidly effective of all antimalarials. They are active against all malaria species and hold particular promise for the treatment of severe malaria. They are extremely well tolerated by adults and children. There is increasing acceptance that antimalarial treatment should be with a combination of an artemisinin derivative (artesunate, artemether, dihydroartemisinin) and a drug with a slower rate of elimination to increase efficacy, reduce transmission of the infection, and to provide mutual protection from drug resistance. Unfortunately, these compounds are not available for clinical use in the United States at present but are widely available in tropical countries.

Atovaquone/Proguanil (Malarone)

Atovaquone, an antibiotic that has been used in the treatment of *Pneumocystis carinii* pneumonia, is marketed for use as an antimalarial in a fixed dose combination with proguanil (Malarone). Atovaquone/proguanil is licensed in the United States for the treatment and prevention of chloroquine-resistant *P. falciparum* (CRPF) malaria. Atovaquone/proguanil is available as an adult tablet (250 mg/100 mg) and as a pediatric tablet containing one fourth the adult tablet (62.5 mg/25 mg). Pediatric doses are based on body weight (Table 17-5). The combination tablet should be taken within 45 minutes of eating or drinking a milky drink to enhance absorption. In the event of vomiting within 60 minutes after dosing, the dose should be repeated. Metoclopramide may reduce the bioavailability of atovaquone and should be used only if other antiemetics are not available. Tetracycline and rifampin also interact with atovaquone and reduce levels by approximately 40% to 50%.

Halofantrine

Halofantrine (Halfan) is an antimalarial drug available in some countries. This drug is active against multidrug resistant malaria, but it prolongs atrioventricular and ventricular repolarization and has been associated with sudden death. It is contraindicated in patients with preexisting cardiac conduction abnormalities, long QTc intervals, or within 1 month of receiving mefloquine. It should also not be taken with fatty foods, which markedly increase its absorption, or with drugs which prolong the QTc interval (e.g., quinine, quinidine and quinidine-like antiarrhythmics, chloroquine, tricyclic antidepressants, neuroleptic drugs, terfenadine, astemizole).

Chloroquine-Resistant Vivax Malaria

P. vivax is intrinsically resistant to Fansidar, so chloroquine is the drug of choice for diagnosed cases. Chloroquine resistance in *P. vivax* has been reported from parts of Papua New Guinea, Sumatra, Irian Jaya, the Solomon Islands, Vanuatu, and recently from Myanmar (Burma) and India, although in general *P. vivax* remains chloroquine sensitive in Southeast Asia and Southern Asia.

In areas of chloroquine-resistant vivax malaria, quinine sulfate (plus or minus doxycycline) may be used for treatment. In addition, atovaquone/proguanil, mefloquine, artemether-lumefantrine (Riamet, Co-artem), and halofantrine (Halfan) have excellent efficacy in treating all four species of malaria, including uncomplicated multidrug resistant falciparum malaria, and could be used depending on availability. Clinically relevant drug resistance has not been reported in *P. ovale* or *P. malariae.*

Management of Severe Malaria

Severe falciparum malaria is a serious disease with high mortality that requires intensive care nursing and the advice of a specialist. There is the same urgency to treat this condition with adequate doses of parenteral antimalarials since there is to treat septicemia with antibacterials. Cerebral malaria has a treated mortality of 20%. All comatose patients should have a *lumbar puncture* to exclude meningitis.

Intravenous antimalarials (Table 17-6) should be given by slow constant-rate infusion as soon as possible after admission. Chloroquine should be given only if the patient *definitely* contracted malaria in an area of known sensitivity. Otherwise, in the United States the patient should be given intravenous quinidine. Elsewhere, quinine, artemether (intramuscular) or artesunate are available and should be used, since they are safer and equally effective.

Careful *hemodynamic monitoring* and attention to fluid balance are critical. After rehydration, the central venous pressure and pulmonary capillary wedge pressures should be maintained as low as is compatible with adequate cardiac output and urine flow.

Hemofiltration should be instituted if the blood urea nitrogen and creatinine continue to rise despite adequate rehydration, or if metabolic acidosis, hyperkalemia, or hypervolemic pulmonary edema with oliguria develop. Renal function typically returns slowly to normal after several days or weeks.

The *blood glucose* should be checked regularly (4 hourly), particularly in cerebral malaria patients. Intravenous maintenance fluids should include 5% to 10% glucose.

Sudden unexplained deterioration in a patient with severe falciparum malaria should be assumed to be *hypoglycemia* or *supervening bacterial septicemia.* Empirical treatment with glucose and broad-spectrum antimicrobials is justified after blood glucose and cultures have been taken.

Convulsions are common and should be treated promptly with intravenous benzodiazepines. The role of prophylactic anticonvulsants is uncertain.

In certain severe cases of falciparum malaria, the patient's clinical status will not respond adequately to appropriate drug therapy, and an *exchange blood transfusion* may be a valuable adjunct to drug therapy to replace the rigid erythrocytes that develop in severe malaria with more deformable donor cells. This should be considered de novo if the patient is seriously ill provided adequate facilities are available. Such cases should be discussed with a local tropical medicine consultant or with the CDC malaria consultant, who is available for emergency telephone consultation 24 hours a day (see Appendix).

The use of steroids or heparin is contraindicated as adjunctive treatment of cerebral and other severe forms of falciparum malaria.

Treatment in Rural Areas

Where severe malaria occurs in endemic areas, facilities for intensive care are not usually available. Where intravenous infusions cannot be maintained safely, the parenteral antimalarials can all be given by deep intramuscular injection to the anterior thigh. Absorption is adequate even in the most seriously ill patient (see Table 17-6). Where injections cannot be given, rectal, oral or nasogastric administration is better than nothing at all.

Radical Cure

In cases of *P. vivax* or *P. ovale* malaria, when the person is not returning shortly to an endemic malarious area, "radical cure" therapy with primaquine phosphate (see Table 17-5) is initiated at the time of the last dose of chloroquine. This is done to eradicate latent malarial parasites in the liver (exoerythrocytic stage) and thus prevent future malarial attacks (see Chapter 5). Although there is little evidence of true *P. vivax* resistance to primaquine, strains acquired in Indonesia and Oceania require higher doses of primaquine to achieve radical cure.

Prevention of Malaria

Mosquito vector control measures (e.g., control of breeding sites, bed nets impregnated with residual pyrethroid insecticides) and timely diagnosis coupled with appropriate drug treatment of acute attacks may be the only attainable goals for indigenous people living in malarious areas, where transmission of the disease regularly occurs and where local economics cannot support a widespread control program. Several different malaria vaccine candidates have undergone field trials, including those directed against the preerythrocytic stages and the blood stages, as well as those that block the transmission of infection. The success of such vaccines has been limited by the parasites' ability to vary key antigenic structures; future candidate vaccines will have to use a variety of novel approaches to target complex antigenic structures on multiple parasite stages of development.

For travelers going from nonendemic to endemic areas, the chances of developing malaria can be reduced by simple measures to avoid being bitten by mosquitoes (e.g., insect repellents, use of insecticide treated mosquito netting, not going outdoors at dawn and dusk). Prevention of acute malarial attacks during and following travel can usually be achieved by chemoprophylaxis.

See Chapter 5 for detailed information on chemoprophylaxis for malaria.

SPECIAL THERAPEUTIC CONSIDERATIONS

Malaria During Pregnancy

Falciparum malaria in nonimmune pregnant women carries a high fetal and maternal mortality. The placenta is a site of preferential sequestration of infected red cells. This acts as an enormous reservoir of developing parasites and interferes with uteroplacental function. In endemic areas, the main adverse effect of any malaria in pregnancy is a reduction in birth weight; the primigravida is at greatest risk. Chemoprophylaxis is therefore justified in pregnancy, even in subjects who live permanently in malarious areas.

Travelers who are pregnant should seriously consider the risks and benefits of prophylaxis to themselves and their babies. Although the safety of chloroquine and mefloquine appears acceptable in such circumstances, rigorous safety data is lacking. Proguanil (Paludrine), like chloroquine, has a long history of use as a prophylactic agent in pregnancy without apparent complications. The fixed drug combination of atovaquone/proguanil (Malarone) has not yet been fully evaluated in pregnancy. If pregnant women do travel to malarious areas, they must take effective prophylaxis, since the risks of malaria far outweigh the potential adverse effects of prophylaxis (see Chapters 5 and 12).

Treatment of malarial infections in pregnant women should be exactly the same as the treatment of other patients, with the caveat that since complications are more likely to arise, treatment should be started in the hospital, if possible. There is no convincing evidence that treatment with quinine, quinidine, chloroquine, or artemisinin derivatives adversely affects pregnancy. Many practitioners avoid the use of mefloquine in pregnancy, especially in the first trimester. Fansidar could be used in the first two trimesters for chloroquine-resistant falciparum infections, but should be avoided near term to reduce the risk of neonatal jaundice. The use of primaquine, doxycycline, or tetracycline is contraindicated in pregnancy.

Quinine sulfate plus clindamycin probably represents the safest therapy for chloroquine and multidrug resistant falciparum malaria during pregnancy. Hypoglycemia is particularly common in pregnant women receiving quinine. Fetal monitoring is essential (if available), as fetal distress is extremely common in malaria (often unsuspected) and urgent delivery may be necessary to save the baby.

Malaria in Infancy

After protection from maternal antibody wanes, the young child in endemic areas becomes increasingly vulnerable to malaria. The initial attacks of falciparum malaria are often severe and sometimes fatal. Convulsions are common, and sudden death may occur. Children are less likely than adults to develop acute renal failure, acute pulmonary edema, or jaundice; but they are more likely to develop seizures, lactic acidosis, hypoglycemia, and severe anemia. Approximately 10% of children surviving cerebral malaria will have a residual neurologic deficit (usually hemiplegia). In 50% of cases this resolves, and in 25% there is improvement, but 25% do not recover. More subtle residual deficits may be more common. Where hospital facilities for intensive care are available, children with severe malaria should be admitted and treated with parenteral antimalarials (see Table 17-6). A lumbar puncture should be performed on all comatose children irrespective of the blood smear results to exclude other potentially treatable infections.

Children with uncomplicated infections who are not vomiting may be treated with oral medication (see Table 17-5).

In practice in the rural tropics, it may not be possible to give intravenous infusions to severely ill or vomiting children. In this case, chloroquine (parenteral form) may be administered by subcutaneous or intramuscular injection and quinine, artemether, or artesunate (parenteral forms) by intramuscular injection or suppository. Quinine, quinidine, or chloroquine should never be administered by intravenous injection, only by infusion (see Table 17-6).

Management of children, like that of adults, should concentrate on lowering the temperature, carefully monitoring fluid balance, giving prompt "first-aid," treating seizures, and administering antimalarial drugs. Even in otherwise uncomplicated falciparum malaria, seizures are common and should be treated appropriately; the role of prophylactic anticonvulsants, however, is still uncertain.

COMMONLY ENCOUNTERED PRACTICAL PROBLEMS

1. Misdiagnosis
   - A. False-positive blood smear:
     1. Platelets, dirt, or accumulations of stain are misinterpreted as being malaria parasites.
   - B. False-negative blood smear:
     1. Inexperienced observers (thick films can be difficult to read).
     2. Incorrect stain, buffer, pH, and so forth.
     3. Failure to examine at least 20 fields.
   - C. Immune individual with asymptomatic parasitemia (usually African) has coexistent bacterial or viral infection.
   - D. Physicians convinced patient could not have malaria because "he took all the pills."
   - E. Incorrect diagnosis: jaundice thought to be viral hepatitis, prominent abdominal symptoms ascribed to enteric infections.
2. Failure to appreciate seriousness of infection:
   - A. For example, a returned traveler with fever who is told he has influenza and to return in 3 days if not better (i.e., failure to *think* of malaria).

B. *P. falciparum* misdiagnosed as one of the other three species, or "mixed" infection (i.e., *P. falciparum* plus another species) is missed.
C. Failure to admit to hospital those patients with *P. falciparum* and high parasitemia (>2%), those who are obtunded, confused or aggressive, those who are jaundiced, young children, or pregnant women.
D. Failure to count parasitemia; terms such as *heavy infection* or *many parasites* are too imprecise.
E. *False* conclusion that because the parasitemia is low, the infection is not severe; the message from (D) and (E) is that a low parasitemia can still mean severe disease, whereas a high one usually does mean a severe infection.

3. Therapeutic dilemmas (always seek expert advice):
   A. Patient has uncomplicated falciparum malaria from a chloroquine-resistant area, but no quinine or mefloquine is available:
      1. If from pyrimethamine-sulfadoxine (Fansidar) sensitive area, give this in treatment doses.
      2. If from Fansidar-resistant area, give an artemisinin derivative, atovaquone/proguanil (Malarone) or quinidine (Table 17-5).
   B. Patient has high fever and is vomiting, but there are no parenteral drugs:
      1. Give acetaminophen suppository, try tepid sponging, fanning, and cooling blankets and try again with oral medication or suppository formulation when temperature is down (while waiting for intravenous drugs or transferring the patient).
   C. Patient is seriously ill but there are no facilities for intravenous infusion:
      1. Give intramuscular artesunate, artemether, quinine dihydrochloride or quinidine (Table 17-5). If no previous treatment, give a loading dose.
   D. Patient develops severe hemolytic anemia and "blackwater" (i.e., black urine) while receiving parenteral quinine or quinidine:
      1. Continue the drugs and transfuse as necessary; if acute renal failure develops, consider hemodialysis.
   E. Patient with severe falciparum malaria suddenly deteriorates:
      1. Check blood glucose; if patient is hypoglycemic, correct with parenteral dextrose.
      2. Draw blood cultures and treat with empirical broad-spectrum antimicrobials.
      3. Check arterial blood gases and pH. Measure arterial lactate-correct pH if <7.2.
      4. If patient is tachypneic, consider metabolic acidosis, pulmonary edema, or pneumonia.
4. Recheck of parasite counts on blood slide indicates poor response to the antimalarial drug regimen:
   A. Ensure compliance with treatment, and consider decreased absorption resulting from acute illness, vomiting, or IM injections.
   B. Gametocytes (sexual stages) of *P. falciparum* (banana forms) on the peripheral blood smear may persist despite definitive antimalarial drug treatment, because commonly used drug regimens do not eliminate the gametocytes of *P. falciparum*.

C. Consider possibility of resistance and changing to a different antimalarial. If resistance (or recrudescence) occur:
   1. Chloroquine failure: change to sulfadoxine/pyrimethamine (Fansidar), except in Southeast Asia or South America, and repeat primaquine therapy for *P. vivax* or *P. ovale* infections (Table 17-5)
   2. Sulfadoxine/pyrimethamine (Fansidar) failure: change to atovaquone/proguanil (Malarone), mefloquine (plus artesunate if available), artemether-lumefantrine (Riamet, Co-Artem), or one of the quinine/quinidine-antibiotic combinations.
   3. Mefloquine failure: change to atovaquone/proguanil (Malarone), artesunate plus tetracycline or doxycycline or clindamycin or mefloquine, or artemether-lumefantrine (Riamet, Co-Artem).

REFERENCES

Collins WE, Jeffery GM: Primaquine resistance in Plasmodium vivax, *Am J Trop Med Hyg* 55:243, 1996.

Cooke AH et al: Comparison of a parasite lactate dehydrogenase-based immunochromatographic antigen detection assay (OptiMAL) with microscopy for the detection of malaria parasites in human blood samples, *Am J Trop Med Hyg* 60:173, 1999.

Craig MH, Sharp BL: Comparative evaluation of four techniques for the diagnosis of *Plasmodium falciparum* infections, *Trans R Soc Trop Med Hyg* 91:279, 1997.

Hien TT, White NJ: Qinghaosu, *Lancet* 341:603, 1993.

Kawamoto F: Rapid diagnosis of malaria by fluorescence microscopy with light microscope and interference filter, *Lancet* 337:200, 1991.

Kwiatkowski D, Marsh K: Development of a malaria vaccine, *Lancet* 350:1696, 1997.

Looareesuwan S et al: Malarone (atovaquone and proguanil hydrochloride): a review of its clinical development for treatment of malaria, *Am J Trop Med Hyg* 60:533, 1999.

Looareesuwan S et al: Quinine and severe falciparum malaria in late pregnancy, *Lancet* 1:4, 1985.

Luxemburger C et al: Mefloquine in infants and young children, *Ann Trop Paediatr* 16:281, 1996.

Miller KD, Greenberg AF, Campbell CC: Treatment of severe malaria in the United States with a continuous infusion of quinidine gluconate and exchange transfusion, *N Engl J Med* 329:65, 1989.

Newton P, White NJ: Malaria: new developments in treatment and prevention, *Annu Rev Med* 50:179, 1999.

Nosten F et al: Cardiac effects of antimalarial treatment with halofantrine, *Lancet* 341:1054, 1993.

Phillips RE et al: Intravenous quinidine for the treatment of severe malaria: clinical and pharmacokinetic studies, *N Engl J Med* 312:1273, 1985.

Silamut K, White NJ: Relation of the stage of parasite development in the peripheral blood to prognosis in severe falciparum malaria, *Trans R Soc Trop Med Hyg* 87:436, 1993.

The Medical Letter: Drugs for parasitic infections. March, 2000, pp 1-12.

Trang TTM et al: Acute renal failure in patients with severe falciparum malaria, *Clin Infect Dis* 15:874, 1992.

Wardlaw SC, Levine RA: Quantitative buffy coat analysis, a new laboratory tool functioning as a screening complete blood count, *JAMA* 249:617, 1983.

White NJ: Drug resistance in malaria, *Br Med Bull* 54:703, 1998.

White NJ: The treatment of malaria, *N Engl J Med* 335:800, 1996.

White NJ: Why is it that antimalarial drug treatments do not always work? *Ann Trop Med Parasitol* 92:449, 1998.

World Health Organization: Severe and complicated malaria, *Trans R Soc Trop Med Hyg* 84 (suppl 2):1, 1990.
Mills CD, Burgess DC, Taylor HJ, Kain KC: Evaluation of a rapid and inexpensive dipstick assay for the diagnosis of *Plasmodium falciparum* malaria, *Bull World Health Organ* 77:553, 1999.
Pieroni P et al: Comparison of the ParaSight-F test and the ICT Malaria Pf test with the polymerase chain reaction for the diagnosis of *Plasmodium falciparum* malaria in travelers, *Trans R Soc Trop Med Hyg* 92:166, 1998.
Palmer CJ et al: Evaluation of the OptiMAL test for rapid diagnosis of *Plasmodium vivax* and *Plasmodium falciparum* malaria, *J Clin Microbiol* 36:203, 1998.
Tjitra E et al: Field evaluation of the ICT malaria P.f/P.v immunochromatographic test for detection of *Plasmodium falciparum* and *Plasmodium vivax* in patients with a presumptive clinical diagnosis of malaria in eastern Indonesia, *J Clin Microbiol* 37:2412, 1999.

CHAPTER 18

Travel-Acquired Illnesses Associated with Fever

W. Conrad Liles and Wesley C. Van Voorhis

The evaluation of fever in travelers poses a diagnostic challenge to clinicians for many reasons. First, there are many possible etiologies, some of which are geographically localized and are, thus, unfamiliar (Table 18-1). Diagnosis may be delayed owing to lack of familiarity with routes of infection or clinical presentations of these geographically limited illnesses. Fever in travelers may be caused by infections that are potentially fatal if not recognized and treated expediently (Table 18-2). Furthermore, some infectious diseases that cause fever in travelers are highly communicable (Table 18-3). These infections represent a considerable public health danger, and some have been associated with fatal nosocomial transmission. However, the most common febrile illnesses in travelers are self-limited and remain undiagnosed, such as viral upper respiratory infections and gastrointestinal infections (see Table 18-1). Thus the challenge facing the clinician in the evaluation of fever in travelers is the detection of serious treatable or communicable infections while not submitting the majority of travelers with benign, self-limited causes of fever to expensive or invasive diagnostic evaluations. To succeed, the clinician must know as much as possible about the epidemiology, distribution, mode of transmission, and clinical characteristics of the etiologies of fever in travelers. In this chapter, diseases that cause fever in travelers are discussed, but many of the specific etiologies of fever are covered in detail in other chapters.

EPIDEMIOLOGY

Studies of fever in travelers have been impaired by the highly mobile nature of travelers and by the fact that they seek help abroad or fail to present to physicians at all. Perhaps the best studies of fever in travelers have been retrospective surveys. In these studies, returning travelers from the tropics were asked to fill out a questionnaire after short-term travel. Because these surveys were conducted relatively soon after the return from travel, infections developing longer than 6 months after travel (Table 18-4) may not have been detected. The incidence of "high fever over several days" in short-term (<3 weeks) travelers in the survey by Steffen et al. was 1.9%. Of the prolonged fevers reported, 39% occurred only while the traveler was abroad, 37% occurred both abroad and at home, and 24% occurred at home only. Prolonged fever was significantly associated with longer stays (>4 weeks) in the tropics.

Table 18-1
Relative Risk of Travelers Contracting Infectious Diseases in Developing Countries

High risk	Moderate risk	Low risk	Very low risk
Escherichia coli enteritis	Shigellosis	Amebiasis	Anisakiasis
Upper respiratory infection		Ascariasis	Anthrax
Viral gastroenteritis		Chancroid	Chagas' disease
Campylobacteriosis		Cholera	Chikungunya
Chlamydia		Enterobiasis	Clonorchiasis
Dengue		Hepatitis B	Congo-Crimean hemorrhagic fever
Epstein-Barr virus		HIV	Diphtheria
Giardiasis		Leptospirosis	Ebola-Marburg hemorrhagic fever
Gonorrhea		Lyme disease	Echinococcosis
Hepatitis A		Malaria (with prophylaxis)	Filariasis
Herpes simplex		Rubella	Gnathostomiasis
Malaria (without prophylaxis)		Rubeola	Lassa fever
Salmonellosis		Schistosomiasis	Legionellosis
		Strongyloidiasis	Lymphogranuloma venereum
		Syphilis	Melioidosis
		Trichuriasis	Paragonimiasis
		Tropical sprue	Pinta
		Tuberculosis	Plague
		Typhoid fever	Polio
			Psittacosis
			Q fever
			Rabies
			Relapsing fever
			Rickettsial spotted fevers
			Toxocariasis
			Trichinosis
			Trypanosomiasis
			Tularemia
			Typhus
			Yaws
			Yellow fever

Most causes of febrile illnesses were undiagnosed in these surveys. In general, sophisticated and uniform analyses of the causes of fevers were not completed. Thus it is impossible to comment on the incidence of infections that are commonly self-limited febrile syndromes in travelers but require specific tests to detect (e.g., serologic studies to diagnose dengue virus infections). Among the most common causes of fevers were infectious diarrhea and acute respiratory tract infections (Table 18-1). Hepatitis was the next most common vaccine-preventable cause of fevers, with malaria in travelers not taking chemoprophylaxis trailing behind. Enteric fever (i.e., typhoid or paratyphoid fever) is an example of a rarer cause of fever. Many of the other severe and/or contagious infections that can be acquired in the tropics are likely rare in travelers, although the frequencies of these infections vary among surveys.

Table 18-2
Selected Potentially Fatal Febrile Tropical Infections with Established Treatments

Infection	Treatment
Viruses	
Congo-Crimean hemorrhagic fever	Ribavirin
Lassa fever	Ribavirin
Bacteria	
Anthrax	Penicillin
Bartonellosis	Penicillin, tetracycline, chloramphenicol, or streptomycin
Brazilian purpuric fever	Ampicillin or chloramphenicol
Brucellosis	Tetracycline plus aminoglycoside, TMP-SMX or rifampin
Leptospirosis	Penicillin or ampicillin
Melioidosis	Ceftazidime
Plague	Streptomycin or tetracycline
Rickettsial spotted fevers	Tetracycline or chloramphenicol
Tuberculosis	Isoniazid, rifampin, ethambutol, plus pyrazinamide
Tularemia	Streptomycin or gentamicin
Typhoid fever	Ciprofloxacin
Typhus	Tetracycline or chloramphenicol
Parasites	
Amebiasis (liver abscess)	Metronidazole
African trypanosomiasis	Suramin or pentamidine; melarsoprol or difluoromethylornithine for CNS infection
Malaria	Quinine or quinidine, plus tetracycline (or doxycycline)
Schistosomiasis	Praziquantel (consider corticosteroids)
Visceral leishmaniasis	Stibogluconate sodium or pentamidine

TMP-SMX, Trimethoprim-sulfamethoxazole; *CNS*, central nervous system.

MEDICAL HISTORY

The medical history, including pretravel preparation and the details of activities and exposures during travel, is of paramount importance in identifying the differential diagnosis of fever in travelers.

Vaccinations and Prophylaxis

As a first step, it is important to establish the vaccination status of a patient. Vaccinations are not 100% effective, but efficacy ranges from the near-complete, 10-year protection provided by yellow fever vaccine to the approximate 50% efficacious 6-month protection provided by the parenteral cholera vaccine. The efficacy of the current hepatitis A and hepatitis B vaccine series is greater than 90%, and that of the oral typhoid vaccine series is 70% to 90%. When a dose of oral polio vaccine is repeated in adult life as recommended, vaccine efficacy approaches

Table 18-3
Selected Tropical Diseases with Documented Potential for Nosocomial Transmission

Argentine hemorrhagic fever (Junin)
Bolivian hemorrhagic fever (Machupo)
Congo-Crimean hemorrhagic fever
Ebola virus disease
Lassa fever
Marburg virus disease
Meningococcal infection
Plague
Rubella
Rubeola
Tuberculosis
Varicella

Table 18-4
Selected Febrile Illnesses of Travelers Classified by Incubation Period and Typical Clinical Course

Short Incubation(<28 days)		Long Incubation(>28 days)	
Acute course	**Prolonged or relapsing course**	**Acute course**	**Prolonged or relapsing course**
Arbovirus infection	Brucellosis	African trypanosomiasis	African trypanosomiasis
Bacterial dysentery	Epstein-Barr virus	Amebiasis	Amebiasis
Childhood viruses	Q fever	Hepatitis B and C	American trypanosomiasis
Dengue	Relapsing fever	Malaria	Brucellosis
Hepatitis A, E	Schistosomiasis	Rabies	Filariasis
Influenza	Typhoid fever		Leishmaniasis
Leptospirosis			Melioidosis
Malaria			Paragonimiasis
Plague			Schistosomiasis
Rickettsial spotted fevers			Strongyloidiasis
Rubella			Tuberculosis
Rubeola			
Tularemia			
Typhus			
Yellow fever			

Adapted in part from Salata RA, Olds RG: Infectious diseases in travelers and immigrants. In Warren KS, Mahmoud AAF, editors: *Tropical and geographic medicine,* ed 2, New York, 1990, McGraw-Hill.

90% to 100%. Thus a documented history of recent vaccination administered appropriately renders the diagnosis of yellow fever, hepatitis A, hepatitis B, polio, or typhoid fever unlikely. Similarly, administration of immune globulin within 3 months of exposure makes hepatitis A highly unlikely.

A history of compliance with prophylaxis for malaria or diarrhea is helpful, although one should bear in mind that prophylaxis for malaria is not 100% effective (see Chapters 5 and 17). It is also important to inquire as to previous diagnostic tests and treatment, some of which may have occurred while traveling.

Exposures

It is important to learn the details of itinerary, duration, and style of travel, as well as the particular characteristics of a given trip to ascertain the risk of serious disease presenting as fever. The travel itinerary is important because many diseases are limited in their geographic distribution (see Tables 18-6, 18-8, 18-10, 18-11, and 18-12). In addition to geographic exposure, there appears to be a significant association between length of travel and serious illness. Indeed, the pathogens and clinical presentations of infection can vary significantly between short-term travelers and immigrants exposed to similar conditions in the same geographic area.

For example, fever secondary to filariasis is uncommon in short-term travelers to endemic areas, but is a more frequent cause of fever in immigrants from areas of active transmission, or in individuals who previously resided in such areas. The reason for this difference is that clinical disease is dependent on parasite reproduction within the human host, and both male and female larval forms must be in close proximity within the skin to mate, a circumstance that may require thousands of mosquito bites. Schistosomiasis may present as Katayama fever (acute schistosomiasis) among travelers, but this syndrome is rarely observed in natives of endemic areas. In contrast, immigrants may present with symptoms of chronic schistosomiasis, such as abdominal discomfort, ascites, and splenomegaly, which are almost never observed in travelers. Age at time of exposure, underlying health, genetic factors, and intensity and duration of parasite exposure probably all contribute to these observations. American trypanosomiasis (Chagas' disease) is rare in short-term travelers because of lack of exposure to the vector, the reduviid bug, which commonly lives in thatched roofs and cracks in the walls of mud huts. However, Chagas' disease is recognized increasingly in the United States among immigrants from Latin America.

Travel style can be associated with an increased risk of serious illness, especially if an individual resided with natives or participated in an "adventure tour," as opposed to staying in urban, first-class hotels. Younger age and being a student are also associated with increased risk of becoming ill while traveling.

The various exposures encountered by the traveler are clues that can narrow the differential diagnosis (Table 18-5). It is important to inquire specifically about insect bites, animal contact, sexual contact, injections, transfusions, caring for ill individuals (see Table 18-3), and ingestion of unpurified water, unpeeled raw fruits, raw vegetables, raw or undercooked meat/seafood, or unpasteurized dairy products. One should inquire about bathing or swimming in fresh water in areas where schistosomiasis is prevalent; cercariae penetrate the skin in fresh water, thereby establishing the infection. Given that travelers may be reluctant to volunteer information regarding sexual contact abroad, a complete sexual history is always important.

Some groups of patients, such as Peace Corps volunteers, missionaries, and military personnel, may present with diseases seen in both travelers and immigrants, presumably reflecting a significantly more intense and prolonged exposure to infectious agents.

Table 18-5
Exposures Suggesting Specific Infections

Animal Contact
Anthrax
Babesiosis
Brucellosis
Capnocytophaga canimorsus
Hantavirus
Lassa fever
Leptospirosis
Plague
Psittacosis
Q fever
Rabies
Rat-bite fever
Toxoplasmosis
Viral hemorrhagic fevers
All tick-borne diseases

Ticks, Fleas, Lice, Mites
Babesiosis
Colorado tick fever
Congo-Crimean hemorrhagic fever
Ehrlichiosis
Kyasanur Forest disease
Lyme disease
Murine typhus
Omsk hemorrhagic fever
Plague
Q fever
Relapsing fever
Rickettsialpox
Rickettsial spotted fevers
Scrub typhus
Tick-borne encephalitis
Tularemia
Typhus

Transfusions or Injections
Babesiosis
Bartonellosis
Chagas' disease
Hepatitis B and C
HIV
HTLV-I
Leishmaniasis
Malaria
Q fever
Toxoplasmosis

Raw/Uncooked Meat/Seafood
Cholera
Hepatitis A
Toxoplasmosis
Trichinosis
Vibrio parahaemolyticus, V. vulnificus
Viral gastroenteritis

Sexual Contact
Chlamydia (PID)
Gonorrhea (PID and disseminated infection)
Hepatitis B (and possibly C)
Herpes simplex
HIV
HTLV-I
Syphilis

Mosquitoes
Bancroftian filariasis
Alphavirus diseases
- Chikungunya
- Eastern equine encephalitis
- Mayaro fever
- O'nyong-nyong
- Ross River
- Sindbis
- Venezuelan equine encephalitis
- Western equine encephalitis

Flavivirus diseases
- Dengue
- Japanese encephalitis
- St. Louis encephalitis
- Yellow fever
- Others

Bunyavirus diseases
- La Crosse
- Oropouche
- Tahyna
- Rift Valley fever

Fresh Water (or Unpeeled Fruits/Vegetables)
Amebiasis
Campylobacter enteritis
Dracunculiasis
Hepatitis A and E
Leptospirosis
Salmonellosis (Typhoid fever)
Schistosomiasis
Shigellosis
Viral gastroenteritis

Ingestion of Unpasteurized Milk
Brucellosis
Listeriosis
Q fever
Salmonellosis
Tuberculosis

HIV, Human immunodeficiency virus; *HTLV,* human T-cell lymphotrophic virus type 1; *PID,* pelvic inflammatory disease.

Clinical Characteristics

Incubation Period

Knowledge of the apparent incubation period of illness in a specific case can narrow the diagnostic possibilities (Table 18-4). Likewise, it is important to establish the onset of fever in relation to exposures. Certain diseases may present very long after the period of exposure, such as amebic abscess, malaria (especially if due to *Plasmodium vivax, P. ovale,* or *P. malariae*), echinococcosis, and filariasis. It is also helpful to note whether the course of illness has been acute or chronic as outlined in Table 18-4. This table is helpful as a guide, but many of the chronic illnesses listed, such as American and African trypanosomiasis, may present as acute febrile syndromes during primary infection.

Fever Patterns

Fever patterns, although potentially helpful, may not be as characteristic of certain diseases in short-term travelers as they are in immigrants. Fevers of primary malaria rarely exhibit the intermittent pattern of tertian or quartan fevers (every 2 or 3 days, respectively) characteristically experienced by partially immune individuals. "Saddle-back fever," which refers to the phenomenon in which fever lysis is followed within several days by the resumption of high fevers, is found in 60% of cases of dengue fever, but can also be seen in relapsing fever resulting from *Borrelia* species or with *P. malariae* (quartan malaria) infection. Continuous fever with temperature/pulse dissociation is often present in enteric (typhoid or paratyphoid) fever and typhus, but is also common in arboviral infections. Remittent fevers, in which the body temperature fluctuates more than 2° C (3.6° F) but does not completely return to normal, can occur in pulmonary tuberculosis, but may also be seen with bacterial sepsis and bacterial abscesses.

Specific Symptoms

Specific symptoms may be helpful in the diagnostic analysis. Severe myalgias, although characteristic of many febrile illnesses, are extremely severe in arboviral infections such as chikungunya and dengue. Chills, though present in many febrile syndromes, are especially prominent in malaria, bacterial infections or sepsis, and dengue. Spontaneous bleeding suggests the possibility of infection with one of the hemorrhagic viruses (e.g., Lassa fever, yellow fever, dengue hemorrhagic fever), but is also reported with various bacterial and rickettsial diseases (Table 18-6). The bleeding diathesis may range from slightly increased capillary fragility leading to easy bruising typical of mild dengue, to severe epistaxis, gastrointestinal bleeding, and possible spontaneous central nervous system hemorrhage seen with severe hemorrhagic viral diseases, such as Lassa fever.

Diarrhea associated with fever is typically caused by *Campylobacter* species, enterohemorrhagic and enteroinvasive *Escherichia coli* strains, *Salmonella* species, *Shigella* species, *Entamoeba histolytica,* and intestinal viruses, but occasionally may be present in infections with other gastrointestinal pathogens such as hookworm, and rarely with *Giardia lamblia* (Chapters 25, 26, and 40). However, it is important to remember that many systemic illnesses can present with diarrhea. For example, diarrhea and/or nausea and vomiting were reported in 43% of cases of malaria in one series.

Respiratory symptoms suggest viral upper respiratory infections but may be manifestations of tuberculosis, bacterial pneumonia, Q fever,

Table 18-6
Important Tropical Infections Associated with Spontaneous Bleeding

Infection	Geographic distribution
Viruses	
Argentine hemorrhagic fever (Junin)	South America
Bolivian hemorrhagic fever (Machupo)	South America
Chikungunya	Africa, Asia
Crimean-Congo hemorrhagic fever	Africa, Asia, and eastern Europe
Dengue	Tropical regions of Africa, South America, Central America and the Caribbean, Asia, and Oceania
Ebola virus	Africa
Hantaan virus (Hemorrhagic fever with renal syndrome)	Asia, Africa, Oceania, the Americas, Europe
Kyasanur Forest disease	India
Lassa fever	Africa
Marburg virus	Africa
Omsk hemorrhagic fever	Asia (the former USSR)
Rift Valley fever	Africa
Yellow fever	Africa, South and Central America
Bacteria	
Brazilian purpuric fever	South America
Leptospirosis	Widespread
Meningococcal infection	Widespread
Melioidosis	Asia, Oceania, Africa, and focal spots in the Americas
Plague	Asia, Africa, Europe, and the Americas
Rocky Mountain spotted fever	North and South America
Typhus	Widespread
Vibrio vulnificus	Widespread in coastal regions

Adapted in part from Wilson ME: *A world guide to infections: diseases, distribution, diagnosis,* New York, 1991, Oxford University Press.

melioidosis, or the pulmonary migration phase of helminths such as *Ascaris lumbricoides* and *Strongyloides stercoralis.* The finding of hepatosplenomegaly suggests malaria, hepatic amebiasis, acute schistosomiasis (Katayama fever), disseminated leishmaniasis, Epstein-Barr virus infection, or enteric fever, among other infectious diseases (Table 18-7). The presence of lymphadenopathy should alert the clinician to the possibility of Epstein-Barr virus, human immunodeficiency virus (HIV), acute schistosomiasis, plague, typhoid, tularemia, trypanosomiasis, and other possible pathogens (Table 18-7). During the evaluation of such a patient, one should bear in mind that neoplastic and collagen vascular diseases may also induce a syndrome of lymphadenopathy and fever.

Meningismus, confusion, and other signs of central nervous system dysfunction may be caused by a variety of viral, parasitic, and bacterial agents (Table 18-8). Because many of these pathogens are restricted to certain ecologic niches, the likelihood of infection with a given pathogen can often be estimated from the patient's geographic itinerary, season of

Table 18-7
Selected Febrile Illnesses Causing Organomegaly and/or Lymphadenopathy*

	Hepatomegaly	Splenomegaly	Generalized adenopathy	Localized adenopathy
Viruses				
Cytomegalovirus	+/−	+	+/−	+/−
Dengue	+/−	+/−	+	−
Epstein-Barr virus	+/−	++	++	+
Hepatitis A and B	++	+/−	+/−	−
HIV	+/−	+/−	++	+
HTLV-I	++	++	++	+/−
Bacteria				
Anthrax	−	−	−	+
Brucellosis	+	++	+	+/−
Ehrlichiosis	+	+	−	−
Endocarditis	−	+	+/−	−
Enteric fever	++	++	+/−	−
Leptospirosis	+/−	+	+	−
Melioidosis	+/−	+/−	+	+
Plague	+	+	−	++
Q fever	++	++	−	−
Relapsing fever	++	++	+/−	+/−
Spotted fevers	+	+	+/−	+/−
Tuberculosis	+/−	+/−	+/−	++
Tularemia	+/−	+/−	+/−	++
Typhus	+/−	++	+/−	−
Parasites				
Acute schistosomiasis	++	++	++	+/−
African trypanosomiasis	+/−	+	++	+
Amebiasis (hepatic)	++	+/−	−	−
Babesiosis	++	++	+/−	+/−
Fascioliasis	++	+/−	−	−
Filariasis	−	−	+	++
Malaria	++	+	−	−
Toxocariasis visceral larva migrans)	++	+/−	−	−
Toxoplasmosis	+/−	+/−	+	+
Visceral leishmaniasis	++	++	+	++

HIV, Human immunodeficiency virus; *HTLV*, human T-cell lymphotrophic virus type 1.
*Approximate frequency of physical finding in specified infection: ++, common; +, frequent; +/−, infrequent; −, rare/absent.

Table 18-8
Important Tropical Infections Causing Meningitis and Encephalitis

Infection	Geographic distribution
Viruses	
California group encephalitis	Americas, Asia
Chikungunya	Africa, Asia
Crimean-Congo hemorrhagic fever	Africa, Asia, Europe
Japanese encephalitis	Asia, Oceania
Kyasanur Forest disease	Asia (India)
Lymphocytic choriomeningitis	Widespread
Murray Valley encephalitis	Oceania (Australia)
Omsk hemorrhagic fever	Europe (former USSR)
Oropouche	South America
Poliomyelitis	Africa, Asia
Rabies	Africa, Americas, Asia, Europe
Rift Valley fever	Africa
Tick-borne encephalitis	Asia, Europe
Venezuelan equine encephalitis	Americas
West Nile fever	Africa, Asia, Europe, Oceania
Bacteria	
Bartonellosis	South America (Andes)
Brucellosis	Widespread
Leptospirosis	Widespread
Listeriosis	Widespread
Lyme disease	Widespread (especially America and Europe)
Meningococcal infection	Widespread (especially sub-Saharan Africa, Northern India, and Nepal)
Rickettsioses	Widespread
Salmonellosis	Widespread
Syphilis	Widespread
Tuberculosis	Widespread
Fungi	
Blastomycosis	Africa, Americas, Asia, Europe
Coccidioidomycosis	Americas
Cryptococcosis	Widespread
Histoplasmosis	Widespread
Sporotrichosis	Widespread
Protozoa	
African trypanosomiasis	Africa
Malaria	Widespread
Primary amebic meningoencephalitis	Widespread
Toxoplasmosis	Widespread
Helminths	
Cysticercosis *(Taenia solium)*	Widespread
Eosinophilic meningitis *(Angiostrongylus cantonensis)*	Asia, Oceania, Africa, Americas
Gnathostomiasis	Asia, Oceania, Africa, Americas
Paragonimiasis	Africa, Asia, South America
Strongyloidiasis (in immunocompromised hosts)	Widespread
Toxocariasis	Widespread
Trichinosis	Widespread

Adapted in part from Wilson ME: *A world guide to infections: diseases, distribution, diagnosis,* New York, 1991, Oxford University Press.

travel, and exposure history. For example, Japanese B encephalitis virus is limited to the Far East, is a disease of summer in temperate climates, and is transmitted by mosquitoes. Spinal cord disease associated with fever can result from schistosomiasis, human T-cell lymphotrophic virus type 1 (HTLV-1) infection, or polio virus infection. Eosinophilic meningitis caused by the nematode *Angiostrongylus cantonensis* occurs widely in the humid tropics, especially in Oceania and Southeast Asia. Infection of the central nervous system by either *Gnathostoma spinigerum* or *Taenia solium* (i.e., neurocysticercosis) may also produce an eosinophilic cerebrospinal fluid pleocytosis (see Chapter 44).

Cutaneous manifestations of disease are common, but seldom specific (Table 18-9). The erythema chronicum migrans of Lyme disease and rose spots in typhoid fever are examples of unique, specific rashes. Nonetheless, cutaneous manifestations can serve to refine a differential diagnosis considerably. As an example, an eschar at the site of inoculation is typical of typhus, Boutonneuse fever, and anthrax. Cutaneous ulcers are seen in leishmaniasis, tropical phagedenic ulcer, Buruli ulcer *(Mycobacterium ulcerans),* cutaneous amebiasis, insect bites, syphilis, yaws, tuberculosis, and leprosy. When evaluating a patient who has received previous treatment, it is important to recall that rash and fever can be caused by reactions to drugs, such as sulfa drugs, antimalarials, and other antibiotics. Rickettsial diseases are frequently associated with rash, but the absence of rash may be misleading and does not exclude the possibility of rickettsial disease (see Table 18-13).

INFECTIOUS DISEASES IN THE TRAVELER WITH FEVER

Selected infectious diseases that should be considered in the traveler with fever are discussed in this section, with the goal of providing an overview. References to other chapters in this book are given as appropriate; however, the reader is encouraged to consult, when possible, standard textbooks on infectious diseases and tropical medicine (see Appendix), and to contact the Centers for Disease Control and Prevention (CDC) for current and detailed information on the diagnosis and treatment of exotic diseases. The experts at the CDC can provide 24-hour emergency medical consultation by telephone to health care providers dealing with a very ill patient; the telephone numbers are given on the inside covers of this book.

Malaria

Fever in a traveler from a malarious area should be evaluated carefully with multiple blood smears for malaria. Malaria was diagnosed in 61% of recent travelers to Africa hospitalized in London with fever, but was present in only 8% of Swiss travelers to Africa and Asia with high fevers over several days (overall incidence: 97 per 100,000). Although malaria is discussed in greater detail in Chapter 17, a few points are worth repeating here. *Plasmodium falciparum* infection can be life threatening when associated with high parasitemia, blackwater fever, cerebral malaria, or adult respiratory distress syndrome. *P. falciparum* is the species associated most often with drug resistance, such that one cannot exclude the diagnosis even when the patient received “adequate” malaria prophylaxis (Chapter 5). Drug resistance is now widespread, and compliance with prophylaxis does not provide absolute protection from malaria infection. In a study by Greenberg et al., 94% of fatal *P. falciparum* infections occurred within 2 weeks of exposure, and more than 80% of these infections

Table 18-9
Selected Infections Characteristically Associated with Fever and Cutaneous Signs

Infection	Typical skin manifestations/rash
Viruses	
Dengue	Diffuse scarlatiniform or macular rash; occasional petechiae or ecchymoses
Ebola/Marburg viruses	Maculopapular rash on trunk
Herpes simplex virus	Vesicles
HIV (acute)	Morbilliform rash
Rubella	Maculopapular rash
Rubeola	Maculopapular rash
Varicella	Vesicles or pustules
Viral hemorrhagic fevers	Petechiae, ecchymoses
Yellow fever, hepatitis viruses	Jaundice
Bacteria	
Anthrax	Eschar
Bartonellosis	Erythematous papules and nodules
Leptospirosis	Possible pretibial maculopapular rash
Lyme disease	Large, annular erythematous macule(s)
Meningococcal infection	Petechiae and purpura-may involve palms/soles
Rickettsial spotted fevers	Diffuse macular or maculopapular rash-may involve palms/soles; possible petechiae and eschar at primary inoculation site
Scarlet fever	Diffuse maculopapular rash
Scrub typhus	Eschar; diffuse macular or maculopapular rash
Syphilis (secondary)	Papular rash, possibly involving palms/soles
Tularemia	Ulcerated papule at inoculation site
Typhoid fever	Rose-colored papules on trunk ("rose spots")
Typhus	Diffuse macular or maculopapular rash; occasional petechiae
Parasites	
Acute schistosomiasis (Katayama fever)	Urticaria
African trypanosomiasis	Chancre, followed by generalized erythematous rash; possible erythema nodosum
American trypanosomiasis	Erythematous nodule at inoculation site; may be associated with periorbital edema
Leishmaniasis	Ulcers, nodules
Onchocerciasis	Subcutaneous nodule(s), dermatitis
Strongyloidiasis	Cutaneous larva currens (erythematous, serpiginous subcutaneous papules, often perirectal, associated with pruritus)

were acquired in sub-Saharan Africa. Clinical manifestations of *P. vivax* and *P. ovale* infections can develop up to 5 years after exposure. The diagnosis of malaria in immune individuals or individuals who have received prophylaxis or partial treatment may be complicated by low parasitemia. Multiple blood smears or, occasionally, serologies may be helpful in difficult cases (Chapter 17).

Typhoid and Paratyphoid Fever (Enteric Fevers)

Enteric fever is caused by *Salmonella typhi* or *S. paratyphi*. Persistently rising fever, relative bradycardia, rose spots, and normal leukocyte counts are all clues to the diagnosis; however, some or all of these characteristics are not present in many cases. The organism can be cultured from the blood in more than 80% of patients during the first week of illness, and from bone marrow aspirated from the iliac crest in more than 90% of documented cases, providing that no antimicrobial drugs have been administered before obtaining the culture. The organism can be cultured from the stool during the incubation period occasionally, and in one third to two thirds of patients during the second through fourth weeks of illness. Serology may be helpful if the patient has not been immunized with typhoid vaccine.

Neither the oral nor the parenteral vaccines provide complete immunity (Chapter 4). In immunized populations, however, a higher percentage of individuals with enteric fever will have disease caused by *S. paratyphi*, although disease caused by *S. typhi* still occurs. In the series reported by Ryan et al., 62% of documented cases of typhoid in the United States were imported. Students were more likely to have imported typhoid than any other occupational group. The mean age of the patients with imported typhoid was 29 years; 59% were U.S. citizens. The countries where the highest proportion of imported typhoid was acquired were Mexico (39%) and India (14%). The highest incidence rates for contracting typhoid were reported for travel to Peru (173 per million travelers), India (118 per million), Pakistan (105 per million), Chile (58 per million), and Haiti (42 per million). Resistance to antimicrobials has been reported for *S. typhi* isolates in many countries, although fluoroquinolones are usually effective (Chapter 25).

Arboviral Diseases

Arboviral diseases are caused by arthropod-borne viruses; most are zoonoses. More than 400 arboviruses, classified into many families and genera, have been described (Table 18-10). Arboviral diseases are present throughout the tropics; however, some arboviruses, such as O'nyong-nyong, Mayaro, Ross River, Oropouche, and Rift Valley fever viruses, are limited in geographic distribution (Table 18-10). Diagnosis usually depends on clinical suspicion and serologic confirmation, the latter generally requiring acute and convalescent serum samples.

The arboviral diseases can generally be divided into four syndromes based on clinical presentation: (1) undifferentiated fever, (2) dengue fever, (3) hemorrhagic fever, and (4) encephalitis. The syndrome of undifferentiated fever (e.g., Oropouche, Mayaro, and sand fly fever) is generally characterized by one or more of the following: fever, headache, myalgias, pharyngitis, coryza, nausea, vomiting, and diarrhea. The dengue fever syndrome (dengue, chikungunya, O'nyong-nyong, Sindbis, West Nile, Ross River viruses) is characterized by fever, rash, and leukopenia. The syndrome of hemorrhagic fevers (Lassa fever, Ebola, Marburg, Congo-Crimean, Argentine, Bolivian, dengue, yellow fever viruses) ranges from mild petechiae to severe purpura and bleeding diathesis. Signs and symptoms of central nervous system dysfunction predominate in the encephalitis syndrome.

Dengue Fever

Dengue is the most widespread arbovirus, with a worldwide distribution throughout the tropics, and it is frequently encountered in travelers return-

Table 18-10
Epidemiology of Important Arboviruses*

Family (Genus) virus	Human disease	Distribution	Vector
Togaviridae (Alphavirus)			
Mayaro	Fever, arthritis, rash	South America	Mosquito
Ross River	Arthritis, rash, sometimes fever	Australia, S. Pacific	Mosquito
Chikungunya	Fever, arthritis, hemorrhagic fever	Africa, Asia, Philippines	Mosquito
Eastern encephalitis	Fever, encephalitis	Americas	Mosquito
Western encephalitis	Fever, encephalitis	Americas	Mosquito
Venezuelan encephalitis	Fever, sometimes encephalitis	Americas	Mosquito
Flaviviridae (Flavivirus)			
Dengue (4 types)	Fever, rash, hemorrhagic fever	Worldwide (tropics)	Mosquito
Yellow fever	Fever, hemorrhagic fever	Tropical Americas, Africa	Mosquito
St. Louis encephalitis	Encephalitis, hepatitis (rare)	Americas	Mosquito
Japanese encephalitis	Encephalitis	Asia, Pacific	Mosquito
West Nile	Fever, rash, hepatitis, encephalitis	Asia, Europe, Africa	Mosquito
Kyasanur Forest	Hemorrhagic fever, meningoencephalitis	India	Tick
Omsk hemorrhagic fever	Hemorrhagic fever	Former Soviet Union	Tick
Tick-borne encephalitis	Encephalitis	Europe, Asia	Tick
Bunyaviridae (Bunyavirus)			
La Crosse encephalitis	Encephalitis	North America	Mosquito
Oropouche	Fever	Brazil, Panama	Midge

Bunyaviridae (Phlebovirus)			
Sand fly fever viruses	Fever	Asia, Africa, tropical Americas	Sand fly, mosquito
Rift Valley fever	Fever, hemorrhagic fever, encephalitis, retinitis	Africa	Mosquito
Bunyaviridae (Nairovirus)			
Crimean-Congo hemorrhagic fever	Hemorrhagic fever	Asia, Europe, Africa	Tick
Bunyaviridae (Hantavirus)			
Hantaan	Hemorrhagic fever, renal syndrome	Asia	Rodent-borne
Puumala	Hemorrhagic fever, renal syndrome	Europe	Rodent-borne
Sin Nombre	Hantavirus pulmonary syndrome	Western United States	Rodent-borne
Arenaviridae (Arenavirus)			
Junin	Hemorrhagic fever	Argentina	Rodent-borne
Machupo	Hemorrhagic fever	Bolivia	Rodent-borne
Lassa fever	Hemorrhagic fever	West Africa	Rodent-borne
Reoviridae (Orbivirus)			
Colorado tick fever	Fever	Western United States	Tick
Filoviridae (Filovirus)			
Marburg	Hemorrhagic fever	Africa	Unknown
Ebola	Hemorrhagic fever	Africa	Unknown

Adapted from Shope RE. In Wyngaarden JB, Smith LH, Bennett JC, editors: *Cecil's textbook of medicine*, ed 19, Philadelphia, 1992, WB Saunders.
*Some of the viruses listed are not transmitted by arthropods and thus are not arboviruses.

ing from the tropics. Dengue virus is a single-stranded RNA flavivirus transmitted by the day-biting urban mosquito, *Aedes aegypti,* or the jungle mosquito, *A. albopictus.* Four serotypes, 1, 2, 3, and 4, are recognized. Infection with one serotype results in immunity to that particular serotype; however, after a short period of cross-protection, individuals are susceptible to infection with another serotype.

Clinical infection ranges from a mild febrile syndrome to dengue hemorrhagic fever (DHF). Grade 1 DHF is defined by a platelet count less than $100{,}000/mm^3$ and evidence of hemoconcentration (hematocrit increase $>20\%$). Grade 2 DHF is manifested by spontaneous bleeding, and grades 3 and 4 DHF are marked by circulatory failure and profound shock that are referred to as the dengue shock syndrome.

The incubation period of dengue is 5 to 8 days. A viral prodrome of nausea and vomiting is common, followed by high fever for a mean of 5 days; the fever often lyses abruptly. Myalgias are particularly prominent, giving rise to the common name of "breakbone fever." Headache (especially retroorbital), lymphadenopathy (frequently cervical), and/or rash (scarlatiniform, maculopapular, or petechial) frequently develop. The rash may occur late during the course of illness, and fever may reappear after several days. (Note: this "saddle back" fever pattern is present in about 60% of cases.)

Increasing evidence suggests that previous infection with one serotype of virus may predispose an individual to more severe disease on infection with another serotype. This immune enhancement of viral pathogenesis is thought to result from immunoglobulin-mediated dengue virus uptake into macrophages, where growth is favored. Thus the hemorrhagic fever/shock syndrome, which is most common in indigenous children, is unlikely to occur in a traveler who has not been previously infected with dengue. Prolonged convalescent periods, characterized by extreme fatigue often persisting for months, have been noted by many travelers who have acquired dengue fever.

Yellow Fever

In the Americas, yellow fever is transmitted by *Haemagogus* mosquitoes in the jungle environment and *A. aegypti* in urban settings. In Africa, transmission to humans occurs via *Aedes* spp. In both urban and rural environments, only 50 to 200 cases of yellow fever per year have been reported recently from the tropical Americas. All recent cases of American yellow fever were acquired in the jungle environment, but sporadic urban transmission still occurs in large outbreaks in Africa. Although *A. aegypti* is ubiquitous in the Far East, yellow fever virus transmission has never been reported from this region. The reason is unclear, but either the lack of virus importation into the region or possible immune cross-resistance induced by endemic dengue immunity may be responsible. The spectrum of clinical disease ranges from a dengue feverlike illness to a severe hemorrhagic illness associated with hepatic and renal failure. The disease is almost 100% preventable by vaccination with live attenuated 17D-strain vaccine (Chapter 4).

Chikungunya

Chikungunya virus infection has been noted in a number of travelers from Southeast Asia and Africa. This disease presents in a fashion similar to dengue fever. Myalgias and arthralgias are particularly severe with chikungunya.

Hemorrhagic Syndromes

Viruses causing hemorrhagic syndromes, such as Lassa fever virus, Ebola virus, Marburg virus, and Machupo virus, have been associated with life-threatening infections that can be spread nosocomially (Table 18-11). Patients who are suspected of having one of these viruses should be placed in respiratory isolation. Laboratory work should be kept to a necessary minimum and the laboratory alerted to the possibility of contagious virus in patient specimens. The CDC and the state health department should be contacted immediately.

An arthropod vector has not been identified for many of these viruses, such as Lassa fever, which is transmitted via contact with rodent reservoirs in rural West Africa or contact with humans known to be infected with Lassa fever virus. Early symptoms include fever, malaise, weakness, and myalgias. A few days later, cough, pharyngitis, chest, and epigastric pain develop. Vomiting and diarrhea occur by about day 5, associated with fever of 39° C to 40° C. By the sixth day, respiratory distress, cardiac instability, hepatic and renal failure, and hemorrhagic phenomena begin to appear. Lassa fever can be diagnosed by either the isolation of virus or the demonstration of a fourfold increase in antibody titer. Early treatment with ribavirin may improve outcome with Lassa fever virus, Hantaan virus, and other hemorrhagic viruses with the exception of Ebola, yellow fever, and dengue viruses. Other viruses of importance are listed in Table 18-11.

Rickettsial Diseases

Rickettsial diseases are acute, usually self-limited febrile illnesses caused by obligate intracellular gram-negative bacteria of the family Rickettsiaceae. Rickettsial diseases can be divided into five major groups: typhus, scrub typhus, spotted fevers, Q fever, and trench fever. All are transmitted by ticks, fleas, lice, or mites, except for Q fever, which is usually acquired by inhalation of aerosolized organisms. Rickettsiaceae are widely distributed throughout the world (Table 18-12).

The spectrum of illness ranges widely and includes subclinical infection. Incubation periods for the various diseases vary widely, on the order of 2 to 30 days (Table 18-13). Clinical illness is generally characterized by an abrupt onset of fever, chills, and sweats, frequently associated with rash, headache, conjunctivitis, pharyngitis, epistaxis, myalgias, arthralgias, and hepatosplenomegaly. An eschar often develops at the site of the bite of the mite or tick in scrub typhus and the spotted fever group. Vasculitis underlies the typical pathologic manifestations of rickettsial disease. Complications are rare, but include encephalitis, renal failure, and shock.

Most rickettsial disease reported in the United States is acquired domestically (e.g., Rocky Mountain spotted fever). Tick typhus (Mediterranean spotted fever, boutonneuse fever, South-African tick typhus, among others) appears to be the most common rickettsial disease of travelers, accounting for 67 of 76 cases of rickettsial disease reported to the CDC from 1976 through 1986. Tick typhus is endemic to areas in southern Europe, Africa, and the Middle East, although most cases were reported in travelers to Africa. Murine typhus and scrub typhus were the other rickettsial diseases diagnosed in travelers and reported to the CDC.

Diagnosis of rickettsial disease generally depends on clinical suspicion (often mandating empiric antibiotic therapy), the Weil-Felix reaction (Rickettsiaceae share antigens with *Proteus mirabilis* strains), and specific

Text continued on p. 308

Table 18-11
Epidemiology and Clinical Characteristics of Viral Hemorrhagic Fevers

Disease	Clinical syndrome	Geographic distribution	Vector
Yellow fever	Ranges from mild febrile illnesses to severe hepatitis and renal failure (with albuminuria); biphasic course of illness may be noted	Tropical South America and sub-Saharan Africa	*Aedes aegypti* mosquito *Haemagogus* mosquito (urban Americas)
Dengue	Classic dengue-fever, severe myalgias, and morbilliform rash Dengue hemorrhagic fever-shock and DIC	Tropical and subtropical regions of the Americas, Africa, Asia, and Australia	*Aedes aegypti* mosquito
Lassa fever	Fever, severe headache, lumbar pain, chest pain, and thrombocytopenia; possible encephalitis, pneumonitis, and myocarditis	Sub-Saharan Africa	None (high potential for person-to-person transmission)
Argentine hemorrhagic fever (Junin virus)	Insidious onset of fever, myalgia, headache, conjunctivitis, epigastric pain, nausea, and vomiting; possible shock	Argentina (especially Buenos Aires province)	None
Bolivian hemorrhagic fever (Machupo virus)	Similar to Argentine hemorrhagic fever	Bolivia (department of Beni)	None
Marburg virus	Abrupt onset of fever, headache, conjunctivitis, myalgia, nausea, and vomiting; severe hemorrhagic complications and shock are common	Laboratory outbreaks involved with handling infected monkey tissues/cells	None (high potential for person-to-person transmission)
Ebola virus	Similar to Marburg virus	Isolated outbreaks in Zaire and Sudan	None (high potential for person-to-person transmission)
Crimean-Congo hemorrhagic fever	Abrupt onset of fever, headache, arthralgia, myalgia, conjunctivitis, and abdominal pain; purpura and ecchymoses are common	Africa, Middle East, eastern Europe	*Hyalomma* species (ticks) (potential for nosocomial transmission)
Hemorrhagic fever with renal syndrome (Hantavirus)	Abrupt onset of fever, headache, lethargy, abdominal pain associated with oliguria and acute renal failure; petechiae are common[†]	Balkans, former Soviet Union, Korea, and China	None

DIC, Disseminated intravascular coagulopathy.

Table 18-12
Epidemiology of Rickettsial Diseases

Disease	Organism	Natural cycle		Usual mode of transmission to humans	Common occupational or environmental association	Geographic distribution
Typhus Group						
Murine typhus	*Rickettsia mooseri (R. typhi)*	Flea	Rodents	Infected flea feces into broken skin or aerosol to mucous membrane	Rat-infected premises (shops, warehouses, grain elevators)	Scattered foci, worldwide
Epidemic typhus	*R. prowazekii*	Body louse	Human	Infected feces or crushed louse into broken skin, or aerosol to mucous membranes	Louse-infected human population with louse transfer	Worldwide
Brill-Zinsser disease	*R. prowazekii*	Recrudescence months to years after primary attack of louse-borne typhus			Unknown, stress	Worldwide
Spotted Feber Group (Selected Examples)						
Rocky Mountain spotted fever	*R. rickettsii*	Ixodid ticks	Ticks/small mammals	Tick bite, mechanical transfer to mucous membranes, ?airborne	Tick-infested terrain, houses, dogs	Western hemisphere
Ehrlichiosis	*Ehrlichia canis*	Ticks	Dogs	Tick bite	Tick-infested areas	At least 12 states in United States, primarily southern states
Boutonneuse fever	*R. conorii*	Ixodid ticks	Ticks/rodents, dogs	Tick bite	Tick-infested terrain, houses, dogs	Mediterranean littoral, Africa, Indian subcontinent

Continued

Table 18-12
Epidemiology of Rickettsial Diseases—cont'd

Disease	Organism	Natural cycle		Usual mode of transmission to humans	Common occupational or environmental association	Geographic distribution
Rickettsialpox	*R. akari*	Mouse mite	Mite/mice	Mouse mite bite	Unique mouse- and mite-infested premises (incinerators)	United States, former Soviet Union, Korea, Central Africa
Others						
Q fever	*Coxiella burnetii*	Ticks	Ticks/mammals	Inhalation of dried airborne infective material; tick bite	Domestic animals or products, dairies, lambing pens, slaughterhouses	Worldwide
Scrub typhus (tsutsugamushi disease)	*R. tsutsugamushi* (multiple serotypes)	Chiggers (harvest mites)	Chigger/rodents	Chigger bite	Chigger-infested terrain; secondary scrub, grass airfields, golf courses	Asia, Australia, New Guinea, Pacific Islands
Trench fever	*Rochalimaea quintana*	Body louse	Humans	Infected feces or crushed louse into broken skin; aerosol to mucous membranes	Lousy human population with louse transfer	Africa, Mexico, South America, Eastern Europe

Adapted from Hornick Rb. In Wyngaarden JB, Smith LH, Bennett JC, editors: *Cecil's textbook of medicine,* ed 19, Philadelphia, 1992, WB Saunders.

Table 18-13
Clinical Features of Important Rickettsial Diseases

Disease	Usual Incubation Period in Days (Range)	Eschar	Onset, Day of Disease	Rash: Distribution	Rash: Type	Usual Duration of Disease in Days[*] (Range)	Usual Severity[†]	Fever after Chemotherapy (Hours)
Typhus Group								
Murine typhus	12 (8-16)	None	5-7	Trunk → extremities	Macular, maculopapular	12 (8-16)	Moderate	48-72
Epidemic typhus	12 (10-14)	None	5-7	Trunk → extremities	Macular, maculopapular, petechial	14 (10-18)	Severe	48-72
Brill-Zinsser disease	—	None		Trunk → extremities	Macular	7-11	Relatively mild	48-72
Spotted Fever Group (Selected Examples)								
Rocky Mountain spotted fever	7 (3-12)	None	3-5	Extremities → trunk, face	Macular, maculo-papular, petechial	16 (10-20)	Severe	72
Ehrlichiosis	7-21	None	Rare?	Unknown	Petechial	7 (3-19)	Mild	72
Boutonneuse fever	5-7	Often present	3-4	Trunk, extremities, face, palms, soles	Macular, maculo-papular, petechial	10 (7-14)	Moderate	—
Rickettsialpox	?9-17	Often present	1-3	Trunk → face, extremities	Papulovesicular	7 (3-11)	Relatively mild	—
Others								
Q fever	10-19	None		None		(2-21)	Relatively mild[‡]	48 (sometimes slow)
Scrub typhus (tsutsugamushi disease)	1-12 (9-18)	Often present	4-6	Trunk → extremities	Macular, maculopapular	14 (10-20)	Mild to severe	24-36

Adapted from Hornick RB: In Wyngaarden JB, Smith LH, Bennett JC (eds): *Cecil textbook of medicine,* ed 19, Philadelphia, 1992, WB Saunders.
*Untreated disease.
[†]Severity can vary greatly.
[‡]Occasionally, subacute infections occur (e.g., hepatitis, endocarditis).

serologies. Therapy consists of tetracycline (2 g/day), doxycycline (200 mg/day), or chloramphenicol (1.5 to 2 g/day), generally for 3 to 4 days after defervescence and a minimum of 1 week total therapy. Recent evidence suggests that the quinolone antibiotics may be acceptable alternatives for the therapy of rickettsial spotted fevers other than Rocky Mountain spotted fever.

Helminths

Schistosomiasis (bilharziasis)

Schistosomiasis is caused by a fluke and transmitted by freshwater exposure in endemic regions. Katayama fever, or acute schistosomiasis, develops 2 to 10 weeks after exposure. This serum sickness-like illness is believed to represent a reaction against antigen-antibody complexes formed as a result of egg deposition. This syndrome is most severe in *Schistosoma japonicum* infections, in which egg production is greatest. Characteristic clinical manifestations include fevers, chills, sweating, headache, cough, lymphadenopathy, hepatosplenomegaly, and eosinophilia. Although death has been reported in *S. japonicum* infections, most patients with Katayama fever experience a self-limited illness that is commonly undiagnosed. Travelers appear to be more likely to develop this syndrome than natives. Serologic studies are helpful in the diagnosis. Recommended treatment involves administration of praziquantel and corticosteroids (see Chapter 43).

Filariasis

The filariasis syndromes associated with fever include onchocerciasis (river blindness), lymphatic filariasis (lymphangitis, often complicated by bacterial superinfection), and nocturnal fever with or without pulmonary symptoms resulting from circulating microfilariae. Eosinophilia is common in patients with filariasis. The diagnosis is usually established by the demonstration of microfilariae in skin snips (onchocerciasis) or in blood. (Note: in lymphatic filariasis, the microfilariae often circulate nocturnally.) Serologic study may be helpful when the disease is suspected (see Chapter 42).

Strongyloidiasis

Strongyloidiasis, usually acquired when larvae in contaminated soil penetrate the skin, rarely causes a febrile illness in travelers. However, immunocompromised hosts can develop a life-threatening hyperinfection syndrome, frequently complicated by significant disseminated strongyloidiasis outside of the gastrointestinal tract (see Chapters 40 and 44).

Trichinosis

Trichinosis, usually associated with eosinophilia, muscle pain, and fever, can be acquired by travelers who ingest undercooked meat (see Chapter 44).

Paragonimiasis

Paragonimiasis is an illness caused by a lung fluke that induces a febrile response either during its migration to the lungs or by its obstruction or destruction of lung parenchyma. Hemoptysis can occur, thereby mimicking pulmonary tuberculosis. The disease is acquired by ingestion of raw freshwater crustaceans or plants in Asia, South America, and Africa. Diagnosis can be established by examination of the sputum and stool for ova. Serologic studies are available (see Chapter 43).

Echinococcosis

The echinococcus usually causes hydatid cyst disease involving the lungs or liver. Fever is usually absent unless the cyst(s) becomes secondarily infected (see Chapter 41).

Protozoa

Amebiasis

E. histolytica is usually acquired by ingesting cysts in contaminated water or food, but may be transmitted sexually. Both amebic dysentery and amebic liver abscess may cause fever. Amebic liver abscess is associated with right upper quadrant discomfort, hepatomegaly, an elevated right hemidiaphragm, and high serologic reactivity to *E. histolytica* antigens. Often, *E. histolytica* cannot be identified in the stool at the time of presentation of amebic abscess. Treatment is with metronidazole plus another agent to clear luminal cysts, such as iodoquinol (see Chapter 26).

Chagas' Disease

Chagas' disease (American trypanosomiasis), caused by infection with *T. cruzi,* is typically acquired by dwelling in mud or thatched-roof housing via the bite of the reduviid bug. It is also transmitted frequently by blood transfusion in endemic countries and occasionally in the United States. After an incubation period of 1 to 2 weeks, *T. cruzi* causes a febrile illness during the acute stage of infection that persists for 2 to 4 weeks. The illness is accompanied by local swelling at the site of inoculation of trypanosomes, lymphadenopathy, hepatosplenomegaly, and influenza-like symptoms. Trypanosomes may be seen during the acute stage of infection in peripheral blood by blood smear or in biopsy specimens obtained from the site of inoculation. Serology studies may be helpful. Treatment during the acute stage of infection with benznidazole or nifurtimox may be beneficial in attenuating the progression to chronic Chagas' disease. This disease is rare among travelers (see Chapter 23).

African Trypanosomiasis

African trypanosomiasis (infection with *Trypanosoma brucei gambiense* or *T. brucei rhodesiense*) causes a febrile syndrome due to circulating trypanosomes. The disease is transmitted by the bite of the tsetse fly in Africa. Occasionally, a chancre can be seen at the site of inoculation during acute infection. Lymphadenopathy is common, particularly in the posterior cervical chain. Later, the trypanosomes invade the central nervous system, and lumbar puncture must be performed to determine which treatment regimen should be administered. If disease has progressed to the central nervous system, treatment with arsenicals or difluoromethylornithine is recommended. Otherwise, treatment with suramin is preferred. African trypanosomiasis is uncommon among travelers (see Chapter 24).

Visceral Leishmaniasis

Visceral leishmaniasis, or kala-azar as it is called in advanced stages, is characterized by hepatosplenomegaly, severe wasting, and fevers. *Leishmania* spp. are transmitted by the bite of the sandfly. The kala-azar syndrome is usually caused by *L. donovani.* Visceral leishmaniasis is extremely uncommon among travelers. *L. tropica* was reported to cause a febrile syndrome in U.S. soldiers stationed in the Persian Gulf. This clinical syndrome, while not as severe as kala-azar, was associated with fevers and leishmanial forms in bone marrow biopsy specimens obtained from affected soldiers. Treatment with pentavalent antimonials led to apparent cure.

Toxoplasmosis

Toxoplasmosis, which can cause an acute febrile syndrome, may be acquired by travelers via the consumption of undercooked meat. Transmission may occur in unexpected places, such as France, where infection with *Toxoplasma gondii* is much more common because of the popular ingestion of uncooked meat.

Bacteria

Tuberculosis

Tuberculosis is an uncommon disease among short-term travelers (Table 18-1). Travelers at increased risk are those going abroad to perform medical service and in travelers residing abroad for prolonged lengths of time. Occasionally, tuberculosis (TB) transmission has been reported among air travelers as the result of relatively poor air turnover on airlines and the presence of a passenger with active pulmonary TB. Statistics are not available for the average traveler, but purified protein derivative (PPD) conversion occurred at a rate of 3% to 4% in infantryman stationed in Vietnam, whereas the rate is less than 1% per year for those stationed in the United States. Health care workers, missionaries, teachers, and others who anticipate close daily contact with resident populations in countries where the incidence of tuberculosis is high should receive the PPD skin test before travel to establish a baseline status and following travel (see Chapter 22).

Meningococcal Meningitis

Meningococcal infection occurs sporadically in travelers to endemic areas (sub-Saharan Africa and Nepal) and in epidemics during times of crowding. An example of the latter is the reported high incidence of meningococcal disease and carriage after pilgrimage to Mecca. Purpuric lesions and signs of meningismus are helpful diagnostic clues, but individuals may present with only fever and respiratory symptoms. Diagnosis is established by culture of blood and cerebrospinal fluid, and treatment with parenteral penicillin or chloramphenicol is usually effective. Contacts of documented cases should receive prophylaxis with rifampin or ciprofloxacin. Travelers going to areas of known meningococcal transmission should receive the meningococcal vaccine before departure (see Chapter 4).

Leptospirosis

Leptospirosis is acquired by contact with water contaminated by animal urine containing the responsible spirochetes and is common in the tropics and subtropics (Chapter 20). This disease may be contracted by abattoir workers, swimmers, and campers. Clinical illness ranges from relatively mild disease to fulminant hepatic failure (Weil's disease). Definitive diagnosis is based on either serologic studies or the demonstration of leptospires in specimens of clinical fluids.

Brucellosis

Brucellosis is usually transmitted by unpasteurized dairy products, but may be encountered in abattoirs. Illness ranges from an indolent febrile syndrome to fulminant endocarditis.

Plague

Plague is reported to be epidemic in humans in certain regions of Vietnam and is endemic in rodent populations in the southwestern United States and other areas of the world. Larger outbreaks can occur, as in India in 1994. Plague causes a clinical syndrome of painful regional lymphadenitis associated with necrotizing pneumonia and septicemia. Prophylactic tetracycline may be given to travelers at risk (see Chapter 4), since the plague vaccine is not widely available.

Melioidosis

Melioidosis, caused by *Pseudomonas pseudomallei*, produces a tuberculosis-like illness or septicemia. The disease is particularly prevalent in Southeast Asia, where it is especially common in rice paddy workers. Many Vietnam veterans have serologic evidence of past infection with *P. pseudomallei*. Like tuberculosis, the bacteria may remain dormant for many years before reactivating and causing illness.

Relapsing Fever

Relapsing fever (caused by *Borrelia* species) is a worldwide tick-borne endemic disease, but louse-borne human-human transmission still occurs in highlands of Ethiopia, Sudan, Somalia, Chad, Bolivia, and Peru. Diagnosis depends on the demonstration of extracellular spirochetes by blood smear and Giemsa staining.

Bartonellosis

Bartonellosis is transmitted by sandflies in river valleys with elevations between 2000 and 8000 ft in Peru, Ecuador, and Colombia. This infection can lead to acute hemolysis (i.e., Oroya fever), in which organisms adherent to erythrocytes may be detected on pathologic stains, or chronic skin disease (i.e., verruga peruana, lesions that may be sessile, miliary, nodular, pedunculated, or confluent, and may be as large as 1 to 2 cm).

Anthrax

Anthrax generally has been associated with exposure to infected animals, contaminated animal hides, and wool. Because *Bacillus anthracis* spores can survive for prolonged periods, contaminated hides or wool remain infectious, and may rarely be responsible for disease transmission in the United States. Anthrax is sometimes associated with a local eschar, where bacteria proliferate and invade the bloodstream. Travelers purchasing souvenirs or articles of clothing made with contaminated animal hides or wool are a group at theoretical risk for the acquisition of anthrax; hunters are another potential group at risk.

Sexually Transmitted Diseases

Gonorrhea, syphilis, chlamydia, herpes simplex, and chancroid are all sexually transmitted diseases that may give rise to fevers (see Chapters 33 to 39).

Viruses

Respiratory and Enteric Viruses

Common respiratory and enteric viruses are the most common causes of fever in travelers, accounting for over 50% of cases of febrile illness in travelers in most series.

Hepatitis

Hepatitis viruses are a relatively common cause of fever in travelers (100 to 200 per 100,000 travelers); prodromal symptoms associated with fever may precede frank icterus. Hepatitis A occurs most frequently, but more than 90% of cases could be prevented by pretravel immunization with hepatitis A vaccine. Hepatitis B and C may occur in health care workers, individuals with a history of sexual contact abroad, and patients who receive blood transfusions (see Chapter 19). Hepatitis E has been serologically confirmed in a few returned travelers; it undoubtedly occurs more often.

Human Immunodeficiency Virus (HIV)

Acute HIV infection, resulting from sexual activity, blood transfusion, and intravenous drug use, has been reported among returned travelers (see Chapters 13 and 36).

Infectious Mononucleosis

Acute infection with Epstein-Barr virus (EBV) may occur in susceptible travelers; especially in the 15- to 30-year-old age group. Hepatosplenomegaly, lymphadenopathy, heterophile antibodies, and the presence of atypical lymphocytes on the blood smear are helpful clues. Specific EBV serologies are useful to establish the diagnosis of acute infection. Cytomegalovirus (CMV) infections may cause an infectious mononucleosis-like illness in travelers and may be diagnosed by CMV serologies.

Measles

Rubeola (measles) remains an important cause of morbidity and mortality in developing countries and poses a substantial risk to travelers who have not received adequate immunization. Furthermore, the syndrome of atypical measles may result from exposure to wild virus in individuals who may have received killed virus vaccine (used in the United States before 1963). Complications include progressive pneumonitis (especially in pregnant or immunocompromised patients), pulmonary bacterial superinfection, and encephalitis.

APPROACH TO THE TRAVELER WITH FEVER

A thorough but directed evaluation, bearing in mind that most fevers are self-limited, is warranted for the traveler presenting with fever. A careful history covering pretravel prophylaxis, itinerary, travel "style," exposures, apparent incubation period, fever pattern, symptoms, previous treatment, and diagnostic studies is essential. Laboratory tests to consider in the diagnostic evaluation include blood smears for malaria (and Borrelia, trypanosomes, Babesia, etc.), complete blood count and white cell differential, absolute eosinophil count, serum electrolytes, blood urea nitrogen and creatinine, glucose, bilirubin, hepatic transaminases, urinalysis, chest x-ray study, PPD skin test, hepatitis serologies, and bacterial cultures of blood, urine, and stool. In many instances, it is prudent to obtain and save an acute serum sample for future comparative serologic studies. Suspected cases of viral hemorrhagic fevers, severe malaria, and enteric fever should be immediately hospitalized. Travel in a rural African environment is a significant risk factor for exposure to viral hemorrhagic fevers, although other hemorrhagic viruses including those causing dengue fever, Hantaan, yellow fever, and Crimean-Congo hemorrhagic fever have a more cosmopolitan distribution in widely scattered parts of the world

(Table 18-6). All cases of suspected viral hemorrhagic fevers should be reported immediately to both the local health department and the CDC.

The clinically stable patient with travel-related fever in whom the initial history, physical examination, and screening laboratory studies are unremarkable may be observed. The patient should be instructed to keep a temperature record and return in 2 to 3 days if fever fails to resolve, or sooner if symptoms worsen. Because the majority of travel-related febrile illnesses represent common self-limited viral syndromes, most fevers will resolve spontaneously. If fever persists, however, repeat malarial smears and blood cultures may be warranted. Directed serologic studies to detect diseases compatible with the patient's history and physical examination should be considered. Imaging studies (e.g., abdominal computed tomography or ultrasound) and biopsies (e.g., bone marrow, liver, lymph nodes) may be indicated. Hospitalization may be justified to expedite the workup in certain circumstances. During the evaluation of perplexing cases of apparent travel-related illness, the clinician should bear in mind that noninfectious disorders, such as occult malignancies, systemic lupus erythematosus, and temporal arteritis may present with fever.

Presumptive empiric therapy directed against a likely pathogen may be justified, especially when adequate diagnostic studies are not readily available or a patient is clinically deteriorating. Examples include oral quinine or intravenous quinidine for suspected infection with *P. falciparum,* chloramphenicol or quinolones for suspected enteric fever, and ribavirin for suspected Lassa fever (Table 18-2). Early initiation of appropriate therapy may significantly reduce morbidity and potential mortality from these serious febrile illnesses of travelers.

REFERENCES

Abramowicz M, editor: Drugs for parasitic infections, *Med Lett* 40:1, 1998.

Centers for Disease Control and Prevention: *Health information for international travel,* Washington DC, 2001-2002 (revised annually), Government Printing Office.

Cowley RG: Implications of the Vietnam war for tuberculosis in the United States, *Arch Environ Health* 21:479, 1970.

Ericsson CD, Patterson TF, DuPont HL: Clinical presentation as a guide to therapy for travelers' diarrhea, *Am J Med* 294:91, 1987.

Fallon RJ et al: Assessment of antimicrobial treatment of acute typhoid and paratyphoid fever, *J Infect* 16:129, 1988.

Frame JD: Clinical features of Lassa fever in Liberia, *Rev Infect Dis* 11(suppl 4):783, 1989.

Gear JH: Clinical aspects of African hemorrhagic fevers, *Rev Infect Dis* 11(suppl 4):777, 1989.

Greenberg AE, Lobel HO: Mortality from *Plasmodium falciparum* malaria in travelers from the United States, 1959-1987, *Ann Intern Med* 113:326, 1990.

Gubler DJ: Dengue and dengue hemorrhagic fever, *Clin Microbiol Rev* 11:480, 1998.

Gust ID, Purcell RH: Report of a workshop: waterborne non-A non-B hepatitis, *J Infect Dis* 156:630, 1987.

Harris RL: Boutonneuse fever in American travelers, *J Infect Dis* 153:126, 1986.

Huggins JW: Prospects for treatment of viral hemorrhagic fevers with ribavirin, a broad-spectrum antiviral drug, *Rev Infect Dis* 11(suppl 4):750, 1989.

Istre GR et al: Acute schistosomiasis among Americans rafting the Omo river, Ethiopia, *JAMA* 251:508, 1984.

Kain KC, Keystone JS: Malaria in travelers. Epidemiology, disease, and prevention, *Infect Dis Clin North Am* 12:267, 1998.

Kendrick MA: Study of illness among Americans returning from international travel, July 11-August 24, 1971 (preliminary data), *J Infect Dis* 126:684, 1972.

Levy MJ, Herrera JL, DiPalma JA: Immune globulin and vaccine therapy to prevent hepatitis A infection, *Am J Med* 105:416, 1998.

Liles WC, Van Voorhis WC: Fever in Travelers to Tropical Countries. In Root RK, Waldvogel F, Corey L, Stamm WE, editors: *Clinical infectious diseases—a practical approach,* New York, 1999, Oxford University Press.

Maddison SE: Serodiagnosis of parasitic diseases, *Clin Microbiol Rev* 4:457, 1991.

McDonald JC, MacLean JD, McDade JE: Imported rickettsial disease: clinical and epidemiologic features, *Am J Med* 85:799, 1988.

Moore PS et al: Group A meningococcal carriage in travelers returning from Saudi Arabia, *JAMA* 260:2686, 1988.

Panisko DM, Keystone JS: Treatment of Malaria-1990, *Drugs* 39:160, 1990.

Piessens WF, Partano R: Host-vector-parasite relationships in human filariasis, *Semin Infect Dis* 74:542, 1980.

Raoult D et al: Mediterranean spotted fever: clinical, laboratory and epidemiological features of 199 cases, *Am J Trop Med Hyg* 35:845, 1986.

Raoult D, Drancourt M: Antimicrobial therapy of rickettsial diseases, *Antimicrob Agents Chemother* 35:2457, 1991.

Revak DM et al: Brucellosis contracted during foreign travel, *Postgrad Med* 85:101, 1989.

Rigau-Perez JG, Gubler DJ, Vorndam AV, Clark GG: Dengue: a literature review and case study of travelers from the United States, 1986-1994, *J Travel Med* 4:65, 1997.

Rigau-Perez JG et al: Dengue and haemmorhagic fever, *Lancet* 352:971, 1998.

Ryan CA, Hargrett-Bean NT, Blake PA: *Salmonella typhi* infections in the United States, 1975-1984: increasing role of foreign travel, *Rev Infect Dis* 11:1, 1989.

Salata RA, Olds RG: Infectious diseases in travelers and immigrants. In Warren KS, Mahmoud AAF, editors: *Tropical and geographic medicine,* ed 2, New York, 1990, McGraw-Hill.

Schwartz E et al: The effect of oral and parenteral typhoid vaccination on the rate of infection with *Salmonella typhi* and *Salmonella paratyphi* A among foreigners in Nepal, *Arch Intern Med* 150:349, 1990.

Steffen R et al: Health problems after travel to developing countries, *J Infect Dis* 156:84, 1987.

Strickland GT: Fever in travelers. In Strickland GT, editor: *Hunter's tropical medicine,* ed 7, Philadelphia, 1991, WB Saunders.

Tilzey AJ, Webster M, Banavala JE: Patients with suspected Lassa fever in London during 1984: problems in their management, *BMJ* 291:1554, 1985.

Wilson ME: *A world guide to infections: diseases, distribution, diagnosis,* New York, 1991, Oxford University Press.

CHAPTER 19

Viral Hepatitis in Travelers and Immigrants

Russell McMullen and Elaine C. Jong

The various forms of viral hepatitis are ubiquitous and constitute a particular concern for travelers and immigrants, and the physicians responsible for their health care. As the list of viral agents known to cause liver inflammation has lengthened, so has the list of serologic studies available that allow for more precise diagnosis; however, this increase requires more knowledge and understanding for correct analysis and application of clinical information in the increasingly complex field of hepatology. Complicating the diagnosis of acute liver inflammation, a number of other infections that may be acquired while traveling can mimic the symptoms of classic viral hepatitis, as can untoward effects of a number of medications and other potential hepatotoxins.

Beyond recognition and diagnosis of acute or chronic liver infection, the physician treating travelers must understand the principles of prophylaxis for viral hepatitis and also know those areas where particular types of hepatitis are endemic; consideration must also be given to the purpose of the travel being undertaken, as well as the likelihood of intimate contact between the individual traveler and native people.

In addition to advising and treating travelers from one's home country, the physician treating immigrants must also be particularly aware of the epidemiology of the various forms of viral hepatitis, the existence of carrier states, and the differential diagnosis of hepatitis in the immigrant population.

Physicians must also take special considerations into account when dealing with the problem of chronic hepatitis B in mothers, a situation quite prevalent in the immigrant population. Maternal-fetal transmission of this viral disease, and the long-term sequelae, can be prevented with appropriate diagnosis and treatment.

EPIDEMIOLOGY AND ETIOLOGY

The physician treating both travelers and immigrants must be familiar with several different viral agents responsible for hepatitis: the *hepatitis A virus* (HAV); the *hepatitis B virus* (HBV); *hepatitis C virus* (HCV), of which there appear to be at least two different serotypes; *hepatitis D virus* (HDV), formerly known as the *delta agent;* and the *hepatitis E virus* (HEV), formerly known as *enterically transmitted non-A, non-B hepatitis.* The epidemiology of these individual infections will be considered below (Table 19-1). In addition, there is evidence to suggest that other

Table 19-1
Characteristics of Viral Hepatitis

Type	Incubation period	Transmission	Area of high prevalence	Age preference	Fatality rate	Chronicity
A	2-6 weeks Mean: 26 days	Fecal-oral Contaminated food and water	Worldwide greatest in tropics and developing world	Children Young adults	$<$0.5%	No
B	2-6 months Mean: 12 weeks	Maternal-fetal Sexual drug use Skin to skin Blood products	China Southeast Asia/ Oceania Sub-Saharan Africa Middle East Amazon Basin Balkans	All ages, but especially neonates, children, young adults	1%-3%	Neonates 85% Children 25%; young adults 5-10%
C	6-12 weeks Mean: 8 weeks	Drug use Blood products Sexual (?) Idiopathic	Worldwide greatest in Middle East, West Africa, China, Japan	Adults Neonates	Rare (more common if hepatitis B is present?)	$>$50%
D	3-6 weeks following superinfection	Drug use Sexual (Same as hepatitis B)	Southern Italy Middle East North Africa West Africa Amazon Basin	Adults (All ages?)	Co-infection 2%-10% Superinfection 5%-20%	Co-infection 5% Superinfection 80%
E	2-9 weeks Mean: 6 weeks	Contaminated water Fecal-oral	Similar to hepatitis A Especially: India, Pakistan, Nepal, Southeast Asia, Middle East	Young adults Children	$<$1% In pregnancy 10%-20%	No

*From McMullen R: Hepatitis and international travel. In Bia F, editor: *The travel medicine advisor,* Atlanta, 1993, American Health Consultants.

types of viral hepatitis also exist; although they have not yet been characterized, the field is likely to become more crowded with recognized viral hepatopathogens.

Hepatitis A

The HAV is a 27-nm RNA virus. Transmission of hepatitis A is almost exclusively via the *fecal-oral route,* although parenteral transmission may occasionally occur. The virus is found throughout the world, but from the standpoint of the traveler, inadequate sewage facilities and contaminated water in developing nations are often responsible for transmission, as is person-to-person transmission, particularly because of poor personal hygiene by food handlers. Consumption of contaminated food (e.g., shellfish, as well as any ready-to-eat food handled by an infected person) may also put the traveler at risk. As an indication of the difference in risk in developed versus nondeveloped countries, serologic evidence of prior hepatitis A infection was present in 2.3% of young Scandinavian soldiers, was found in 20% to 30% of middle-aged, middle-class New Yorkers, but has been found in almost 100% of Southeast Asian populations. There is epidemiologic evidence that this changes as developing countries undergo modernization: only 50% of young urban Thais are seropositive, and the major 1988 hepatitis A outbreak in China indicates a large pool of susceptible young adults.

Hepatitis B

The agent of hepatitis B is a 42-nm DNA virus. The intact virion, also known as the Dane particle, consists of identifiable subviral fragments, including the hepatitis B surface antigen (HBsAg), a core antigen (HBcAg), a DNA polymerase molecule, and the "e" antigen (HBeAg). Circulating HBsAg is the prime marker of active infection, whereas HBeAg is an indicator of high infectivity. Identifiable groups at risk of contracting hepatitis B include persons receiving contaminated blood products (a low risk in the United States, where banked blood is screened for HBsAg), organ transplant recipients, health care workers having frequent contact with blood products, hemodialysis patients, homosexual males with multiple sexual partners, and sexual and household contacts of HBsAg-positive carriers. Of most concern to the traveler is the risk of exposure through sexual or close personal contact with carriers in the native population. Other travelers at risk include those who seek cut-rate medical or dental care in countries where hepatitis B is endemic, or those who receive unexpected emergency care in suboptimal situations.

The risk of transmission of hepatitis B during travel reflects the prevalence of the disease worldwide (Fig. 19-1). In the United States, there is evidence of past hepatitis B infection in 10% of the population, but the HBsAg-positive carrier rate is less than 1%. The same percentages hold for northern European countries, but areas of North Africa, sub-Saharan Africa, Oceania, and much of East Asia have much higher rates of infection. Evidence for previous infection may be present in up to 70% to 80% of the population, and the underlying carrier rates range from 5% to 15%. An estimated 170 million persons worldwide are chronic carriers of HBV.

One reason for the high rate of infection and carrier state is the phenomenon of peripartum maternal-fetal vertical transmission. As many as 30% to 50% of the women who are HBsAg carriers, or who are acutely infected in the third trimester, will transmit the infection to their offspring unless specific prophylactic measures are taken at the time of

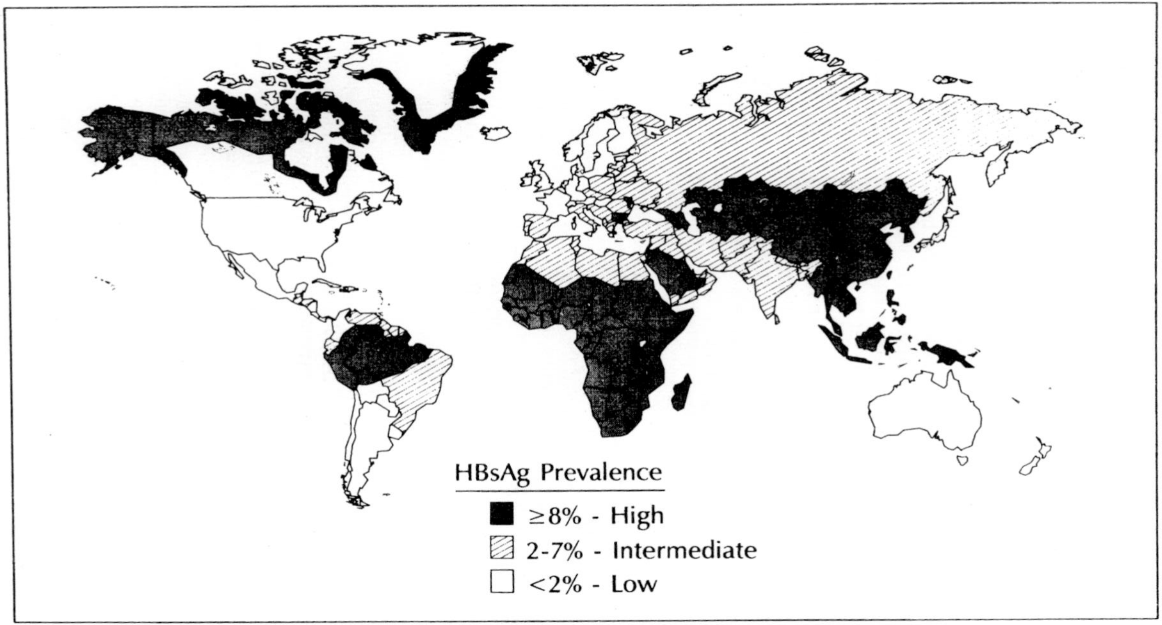

Fig. 19-1 Geographic distribution of hepatitis B prevalence. (From Health Information for International Travel 1993, Atlanta, 1993, Centers for Disease Control.)

birth. Infants whose mothers are HBsAg-positive and also HBeAg-positive have an 85% to 95% of becoming infected unless treated immediately after birth. Immigrants from areas with high rates of HBV infection require screening, in particular pregnant females, who require careful management if positive. Household contacts and sexual contacts of HBV carriers should be screened and offered prophylaxis with hepatitis B vaccine when appropriate (Chapters 4 and 16).

Hepatitis C

A viral agent causing what was previously referred to as non-A, non-B hepatitis (NANBH) has been identified serologically and named hepatitis C. HCV became the most common cause of transfusion-associated hepatitis in the United States after screening for HBsAg decreased the percentage of posttransfusion hepatitis resulting from hepatitis B to 10%. Older studies suggested that as many as 3% to 7% of units of what would now be regarded as high-risk blood products were capable of transmission of NANBH, and rates of infection from 5% to 15% in patients receiving 1 to 5 units of blood were documented. The risk of posttransfusion hepatitis resulting from what is now known to be hepatitis C initially decreased when blood was screened for surrogate markers for NANBH (using the liver enzyme alanine aminotransferase [ALT] and the core antibody to hepatitis B); it has now undergone about a 10-fold decrease with routine screening of donor blood for antibody to hepatitis C.

Transmission of HCV also occurs with parenteral drug abuse and most of the other mechanisms by which HBV is spread. Although data from some studies have been contradictory, there appears to be a mildly increased incidence of infection in homosexual males and in long-term heterosexual partners of infected individuals: inoculation of body fluids containing virus through mucosal lesions is presumed to be the mechanism of spread. The likelihood of transmission to health care workers after needlestick or other parenteral exposure to blood or body fluids appears to be significant, and correlated to the viral load of the source patient. Rates of transmission from 1% to 10% have been reported for HCV, in contrast to 5% to 30% for HBV.

The worldwide epidemiology of HCV is still being defined. Unfortunately, a large proportion of infections with HCV, both in the United States and abroad, have no clear reason for transmission established, and therefore there is no good way to counsel travelers regarding avoidance of transmission risk. It has been established that some countries have a particularly high prevalence of anti-HCV antibody. Included in this are certain sub-Saharan African nations, Egypt and parts of the Arabian Peninsula, Thailand, and Japan. A second serotype of HCV appears to be common in Japan; it has a shorter incubation period than that seen in the strain predominant in the United States.

Hepatitis D

Hepatitis D (formerly the "delta agent") is a defective virus that is dependent on the genetic mechanism of the HBV for replication. Active hepatitis D is found only in patients who are positive for HBsAg, and anti-hepatitis D antibody has been found only in the sera of active HBsAg carriers or those with serologic evidence of past infection. Hepatitis D is most prevalent in southern Italy and North Africa, but increased rates are also seen in the middle East and sub-Saharan Africa. Epidemics have also occurred in the Amazon Basin. Risk factors for the transmission of the virus appear to be much the same as for HBV. In the United States, hepatitis D is found almost exclusively in drug abusers with concomitant hepatitis B infection or in HBV carriers with a history of many transfusions. The mortality rate in acute HBV infection appears to be greater when hepatitis D coinfection is present, but not as high as when hepatitis D superinfection of a chronic hepatitis B carrier occurs.

Hepatitis E

What had previously been called enterically transmitted non-A, non-B hepatitis is now known as hepatitis E. HEV has been demonstrated in stool using immune electron microscopy, and although the virus has been found to resemble HAV in terms of both transmission and epidemiology, it is serologically unrelated.

HEV has been the source of several large epidemics in India, Nepal, and Burma, usually in association with flooding or other problems with the water supply. Well-studied outbreaks have occurred in African refugee camps and in two villages in Mexico; the latter have been the only documented major outbreaks in North America. With the advent of serologic testing, evidence for frequent sporadic transmission of endemic infection has been documented in a number of countries, including Egypt, Hong Kong, and nations in sub-Saharan Africa; most symptomatic cases seem to occur in young adults or older children. The very few cases in the United States have been imported by recent travelers from abroad, primarily Mexico and India; secondary transmission has not been documented.

In general, hepatitis E is clinically similar to hepatitis A; however, the mortality in some outbreaks has been higher than that seen with hepatitis A, perhaps owing to malnutrition and concomitant disease among the victims. A mortality rate of 10% to 20% among women late in pregnancy has been a consistent finding in epidemics. Administration of immune globulin derived from pooled serum banks in nonendemic regions for hepatitis E appear to offer no protection against infection.

CLINICAL SYNDROMES

Uncomplicated infections with the different viral agents have both similarities and differences, but can be divided into the prodromal, icteric, and convalescent phases. Some hepatitis infections result in either fulminant or chronic hepatitis, both of which can lead to complications, including death.

Prodrome

The incubation period for hepatitis A is 2 to 6 weeks, with a mean of 3.7 weeks, and the onset of the disease is typically rather rapid. The incubation times for hepatitis B (2 to 6 months; mean 11.8 weeks) and hepatitis C (6 to 12 weeks; mean 7.8 weeks) are longer, and the onset is generally more indolent. The incubation periods for hepatitis D and E are not so well defined, but for HDV appears to range from 3 to 6 weeks, and for HEV to range from 2 to 9 weeks (with a mean of 6 weeks).

Beyond the differing incubation periods and the rapidity of onset of symptoms, the prodrome in the different types of infections may be remarkably similar. Fatigue and malaise are often the initial symptoms, followed by gastrointestinal symptoms including anorexia, nausea, and occasional diarrhea. A low-grade fever may also be present. Right upper quadrant tenderness is almost universally found, and hepatomegaly is detectable in a majority of cases.

Arthralgia and an urticarial rash are seen about 10% of the time as part of the prodrome of hepatitis B. They are thought to be due to the formation of hepatitis B antigen-antibody immune complexes. This is seen rarely in HAV infection and may occur occasionally in hepatitis C.

Patients with hepatitis A are infectious for approximately 2 weeks before the onset of clinical disease, during which time they are shedding viral particles in their stool. Shedding declines with the onset of jaundice, and the patient is noninfectious 1 to 2 weeks after clinical disease develops. There is no carrier state. By contrast, patients with HBV infection may have low levels of HBsAg detectable within 1 to 2 weeks after inoculation and theoretically may be infectious; a smaller inoculum will delay the appearance of HBsAg in serum. The timing for infectivity with HCV is not known.

Icteric Phase

Most cases of all three major types of hepatitis remain subclinical. In the case of hepatitis A, this is because worldwide most infections occur in children, who seldom become very ill; adults are much more likely to become jaundiced. An estimated 10% to 20% of HBV and 30% of HCV infections result in jaundice. Patients may first notice darkening of the urine, then the appearance of scleral or palatine icterus, and, finally, frank jaundice. Pruritus may become prominent. As this stage, symptoms of hepatitis A begin to improve, and infectivity clears as HAV disappears from the stool. However, symptoms of hepatitis B and hepatitis C may persist after the onset of jaundice, and infectivity remains.

Convalescent Phase

Gradual return to well-being is the rule in all types of hepatitis that do not become fulminant or progress to a chronic carrier state. In all, 90% of cases of hepatitis A are characterized by return of liver function tests to normal within 12 weeks; the balance takes somewhat longer, but no carrier state develops. In contrast, the resolution of infection in hepatitis B typically takes 6 to 20 weeks, and the marker of cure is disappearance of HBsAg and appearance of antibody to it (anti-HBs); 5% to 10% of adult patients become chronic carriers of HBsAg. Hepatitis C symptoms may resolve quickly or may follow a smoldering course; the latter is highly associated with development of a chronic carrier state.

Fulminant Hepatitis

Development of fulminant hepatitis is the most feared complication of acute hepatitis infection. An overwhelming infection, it results in massive hepatic necrosis, extreme initial elevation of bilirubin, and persistently abnormal bilirubin despite a return of hepatic enzymes to normal. Hepatic encephalopathy occurs owing to the extreme liver dysfunction. Fulminant hepatitis occurs in only a small number of cases of acute hepatitis but is more common in hepatitis B (1% to 3%) than in hepatitis A (0.5% to 1.0%). The role of HCV in fulminant hepatitis remains controversial; although it may be a cofactor in some cases, most evidence suggests it is rarely, if ever, the sole cause. Regardless of viral etiology, the prognosis in cases of infectious fulminant hepatitis is grim. Without liver transplantation, the mortality rate is 60% to 90%. The mortality rate for fulminant hepatitis B is much higher if hepatitis D coinfection is present, and the rate in hepatitis D superinfection of chronic hepatitis B is particularly high.

Carrier States

A chronic carrier state does not occur after hepatitis A or hepatitis E, as far as is known, but can be seen after either HBV, HCV, or HDV infection. In all 5% to 10% of people in the United States infected with HBV become carriers of the virus. The rate is higher (15% to 20%) in geographic areas with high endemic rates of disease; the carrier state is more likely after maternal-fetal transmission. The most dreaded complication of the HBV carrier state is hepatocellular carcinoma, which is 300 times more likely to develop in carriers. The chronic carrier state can also develop with HCV and, in fact, is probably more common than in HBV infection. Chronic HCV infection appears to be independently associated with hepatocellular carcinoma, and there is some evidence that chronic HCV infection may increase the likelihood of hepatocellular carcinoma in HBV carriers.

Chronic Hepatitis

Hepatitis B and hepatitis C can result in either chronic persistent or chronic active hepatitis, although the percentage of cases in which this occurs remains unclear. In chronic persistent hepatitis, the inflammation remains confined to the portal area and there is no progression to significant fibrosis or cirrhosis. In contrast, chronic active hepatitis involves greater distribution of inflammation, with bridging necrosis between the portal areas; eventually fibrosis develops. Cirrhosis and hepatic failure represent long-term potential complications of chronic active hepatitis.

DIFFERENTIAL DIAGNOSIS

Before the diagnosis of a specific viral hepatitis can be made, several other potential sources of hepatocellular injury must be considered. Particular attention should be paid to diseases endemic to areas from which travelers or immigrants have come, but other less exotic causes of jaundice must be considered (Table 19-2).

Viral Diseases

Yellow fever: Yellow fever should be considered in any jaundiced patient who has been traveling in the endemic areas of South America or West and Central Africa. However, the incubation period of the severe, icteric form of yellow fever is 3 to 6 days, and the diagnosis can be effectively excluded if the patient departed from an endemic area more than a week previously. Also, the onset is quite abrupt, with marked systemic symptoms, rather than the often more insidious onset typical of viral hepatitis.

Epstein-Barr Virus: The syndrome of mononucleosis can include hepatic enzyme abnormalities, although they are typically low grade. Jaundice can be seen with more severe inflammation.

Cytomegalovirus: A syndrome similar to that of mononucleosis can also be seen in this infection.

Herpes simplex: Disseminated infection can result in hepatic necrosis, but this complication is generally seen only in immunocompromised patients.

Coxsackievirus: Severe infections can result in hepatitis.

Nonviral Infections

Typhoid: Diffuse hepatic involvement in typhoid may result in frank jaundice. Acute cholecystitis, with resultant biliary stasis, may also develop in the first stage of typhoid. The same risk factors that predispose a traveler to hepatitis A predispose to typhoid.

Table 19-2
Historical Clues in Diagnosis of Hepatitis

Recent travel history
Ethnic background and birthplace (especially Asian, Oceanic, or North African; or close exposure to these individuals)
Sexual orientation and patterns of contact
Known exposure to an infectious agent causing hepatitis (including health care workers with high-risk exposure)
Immunizations against hepatitis
Past or current medical conditions
Previous hepatitis, including type (if known); other liver disease
History of, or symptoms suggestive of, biliary tract disease
Transfusions or administration of blood products
Hemodialysis
History of organ transplantation
History of recent surgery (benign postoperative jaundice?)
History of frequent previous jaundice (Gilbert's syndrome?)
Current pregnancy (third trimester: consider cholestatic jaundice of pregnancy or acute fatty liver of pregnancy)
Drug history
Illicit drug usage (especially parenteral)
Prescription medications (include oral contraceptives)
Over-the-counter medications (include vitamins)
Toxin exposure
Alcohol usage
Occupational exposure
Mushroom ingestion

Malaria: Hepatomegaly and jaundice occasionally occur, most commonly in severe falciparum malaria.

Liver abscess: Both bacterial and amoebic liver abscess may cause focal hepatomegaly and tenderness. Amoebic liver abscess is particularly a risk in travelers to developing tropical countries.

Q Fever: Hepatomegaly and jaundice may be prominent symptoms. Exposure to cows, goats, or sheep when the animals are giving birth is a major risk factor for the disease, but exposure to the animal hides of these species can also result in transmission.

Secondary syphilis: Alkaline phosphatase will be markedly elevated if liver inflammation is associated with secondary syphilis.

Leptospirosis: Liver dysfunction may occur in the "immune" secondary phase of the disease.

Toxoplasmosis: The infection usually results in only mild liver function abnormalities in immunocompetent individuals.

Helminthic Infestations

Ascariasis: Hepatosplenomegaly may be seen when a patient is first infected, and biliary tract obstruction is a late complication that may occur in immigrants or returning longtime travelers.

Schistosomiasis: Marked systemic illness accompanied by hepatomegaly can be seen in acute illness due to *Schistosoma mansoni* or *Schistosoma japonicum.*

Flukes: A number of other flukes may cause infections that ultimately result in biliary tract obstruction. These include *Clonorchis sinensis,* the *Opisthorchis* species, and *Fasciola hepatica* (which may cause a picture of acute liver disease during the invasive phase).

Toxic Hepatitis

Many toxins, including prescription medications, over-the-counter medications, fat-soluble vitamins and niacin, alcohol, industrial agents, and toxin of the mushroom *Amanita phalloides,* can cause hepatitis. A detailed drug history should be taken in any jaundiced patient.

Biliary Tract Disease

Cholecystitis or obstructive biliary tract disease should be in the differential diagnosis if the diagnosis of hepatitis is considered.

Gilbert's Syndrome

This benign defect in hepatic glucuronyl transferase activity can cause increased bilirubin in fasting or mildly ill patients. The increase is virtually all unconjugated (indirect) bilirubin.

Pregnancy

In the third trimester of pregnancy, two syndromes can be seen. Cholestatic jaundice of pregnancy is a benign condition without significant hepatic damage, but acute fatty liver results in marked hepatocellular damage and has a high mortality rate.

DIAGNOSIS

Diagnosis of hepatitis is generally dependent on demonstration of abnormal liver function and evidence of liver cell inflammation. Screening laboratory tests usually confirm that hepatitis is present, although values may be normal in those with chronic hepatitis and those who are carriers.

The transaminases, alanine aminotransferase (ALT) and aspartate aminotransferase, are the prime markers for hepatocellular injury. They will usually be quite elevated in acute hepatitis, with values as high as several thousand international units. In chronic hepatitis, they may be normal or just mildly elevated until an acute exacerbation of the disease occurs, at which point they may rise dramatically. Decreasing levels of the transaminases will generally parallel the resolution of acute liver inflammation, although normalization following fulminant hepatitis may be an ominous indicator of massive hepatocellular death.

Abnormalities in the serum bilirubin level directly reflect the functional abnormality in hepatitis. The level will generally mirror the degree of enzyme elevation. An exception to this can occur when massive cell death has occurred. The transaminases can be deceptively normal while the bilirubin remains quite high, reflecting the poor functional capability of the little remaining parenchymal tissue. In a mildly ill or otherwise normal patient who is jaundiced, fractionation of bilirubin to determine the proportion that is unconjugated (indirect) may be useful to establish the diagnosis of Gilbert's syndrome rather than hepatitis.

Unfortunately, although these general screening tests may be of benefit in detecting that the patient's liver is diseased, they are of little benefit in identifying which type of hepatitis the patient may have. To identify type, more specific laboratory tests are necessary.

Hepatitis A

For the diagnosis of hepatitis A, there is an assay for antibody to the HAV (anti-HAV). In the acute disease, the anti-HAV will be of immunoglobulin class IgM, whereas within 6 months of resolution of the infection, the anti-HAV will all be IgG. If the IgM fraction is identified in the serum of the acutely jaundiced patient, a presumptive diagnosis of acute hepatitis A is made (Fig. 19-2).

The presence of IgG antibody is believed to confer immunity to reinfection and it will generally be present for life after infection. Antibody levels decline after immunization with hepatitis A vaccine, so booster doses will ultimately be recommended.

Hepatitis B

Diagnosis of hepatitis B infections is much more complex (Figs. 19-3 to 19-5). A number of serologic tests aid in the diagnosis. Results reflect the presence of the viral components or the immune system's response to them during the various stages of the disease. Early in the course of the acute infection, the HBsAg can be detected, often before there are any clinical signs of infection. As long as this is found in the serum, the patient remains infectious, and if it remains present 20 weeks after the onset of jaundice, the patient is presumed to be a carrier.

Disappearance of the HBsAg from the blood is followed, after a period of several weeks, by the development of the anti-HBs antibody, which is a marker for resolution of the infection. The patient is not infectious and is considered cured. This is also the only hepatitis B serology that should be positive in the patient who has been successfully vaccinated.

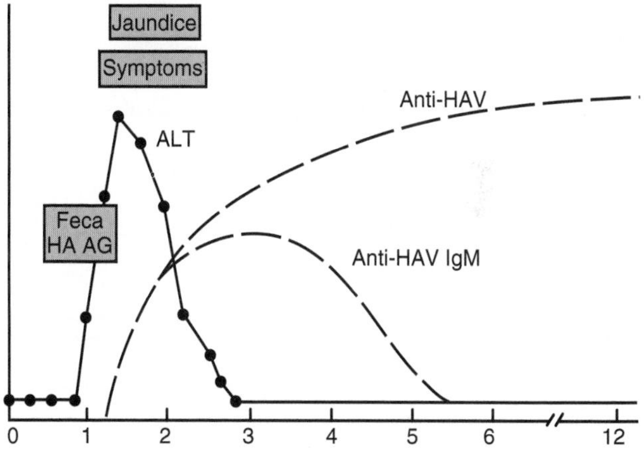

Fig. 19-2 The clinical, serologic, and biochemical course of typical type A hepatitis. *HA Ag,* Hepatitis A antigen; *ALT,* alanine aminotransferase; *anti-HAV,* antibody to hepatitis A virus. (From Hoofnagle JH: *Perspectives on viral hepatitis,* vol 2, Chicago, 1981, Abbott Laboratories.)

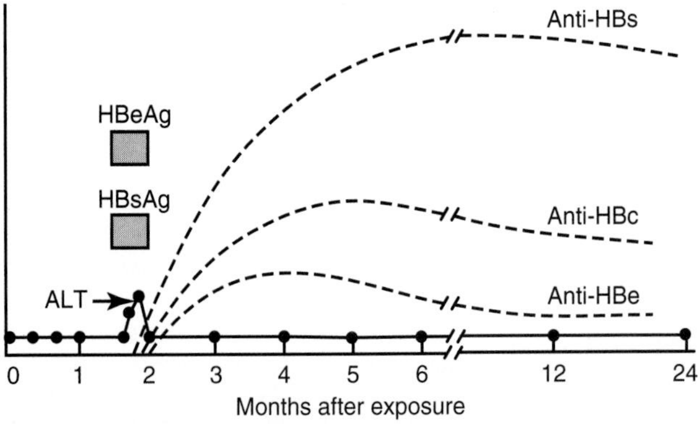

Fig. 19-3 The clinical, serologic, and biochemical course of a subclinical asymptomatic hepatitis B virus infection. (From Hoofnagle JH: *Perspectives on viral hepatitis,* vol 2, Chicago, 1981, Abbott Laboratories.)

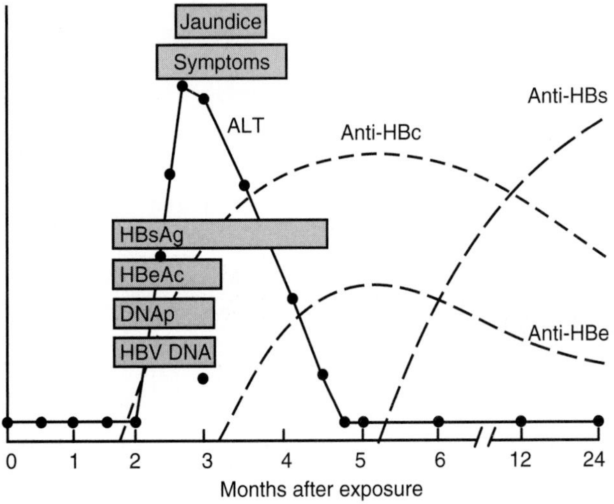

Fig. 19-4 The clinical, serologic, and biochemical course of typical acute type B hepatitis. *ALT,* Alanine aminotransferase; *HBsAg,* hepatitis B surface antigen; *HBeAg,* hepatitis B e antigen; *DNA-p,* serum hepatitis B virus DNA polymerase activity; *HBV-DNA,* serum hepatitis B virus DNA; *Anti-HBs,* antibody to HBsAg; *Anti-Hbe,* antibody to HBeAg; *Anti-HBc,* antibody to hepatitis B core antigen. (From Hoofnagle JH: *Perspectives on viral hepatitis,* vol 2, Chicago, 1981, Abbott Laboratories.)

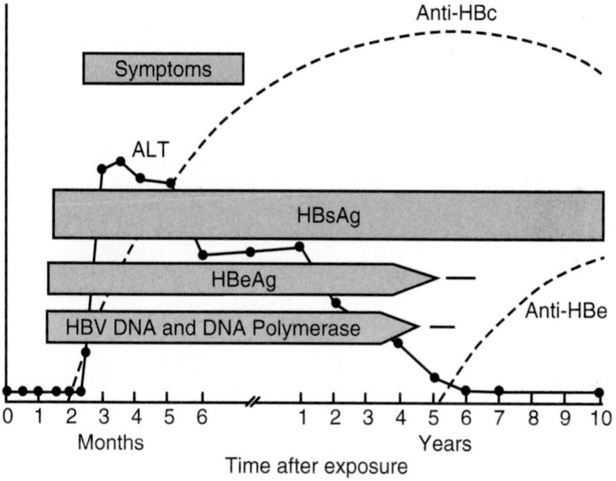

Fig. 19-5 The clinical, serologic, and biochemical course of a chronic type B hepatitis infection. (From Hoofnagle JH: *Perspectives on viral hepatitis,* vol 2, Chicago, 1981, Abbott Laboratories.)

Subsequent to the development of HBsAg, but before anti-HBs appears, antibody to the core of HBV develops (anti-HBc). This generally occurs at about the time of the onset of clinical illness, but it may be the only marker of HBV present if HBsAg has disappeared and anti-HBs has not yet appeared (the "core window"). An assay for IgM can determine if the anti-HBc present is due to acute or remote infection.

Another marker for hepatitis B infection is the HBeAg, or "e" antigen. This viral component is part of the nucleus and circulates freely during the acute infection. It is indicative of a high degree of infectiousness; presence of HBeAg more than 10 weeks beyond the symptomatic period indicates that the patient will probably become a chronic carrier (25% to 50% of carriers are positive). By contrast, if the patient develops anti-HBe, it is a sign of probable resolution of infection (Table 19-3).

Hepatitis C

Diagnosis of hepatitis C has been made possible by development of assays for HCV markers. The first-generation enzyme-linked immunosorbent assay (ELISA) test did not become positive until a mean of 15 weeks after onset of clinical illness and thus proved of little benefit in diagnosis of acute hepatitis C, but it did result in a significant decrease in the incidence of transfusion-associated hepatitis in the United States by identifying chronic carriers of HCV. Second-generation ELISA tests are more sensitive and specific, generally becoming positive earlier in the course of infection, sometimes at the time symptoms first become apparent. The radioimmunoblot assay is used as a confirmatory test for positive hepatitis C ELISA screens.

Table 19-3
Interpretation of Hepatitis B Serologic Tests

			Serologic Test
HBsAg	**Anti-HBs**	**Anti-HBc**	**Suggested diagnoses and follow-up**
+	–	–	Early hepatitis B infection: probably preclinical or early clinical illness HBeAg/anti-HBe testing possibly indicated: If –/– ("e window") or –/+: resolution likely If +/–: still highly infectious Needs follow-up testing until anti-HBs is positive (i.e., acute infection has resolved)
+	–	+	Diagnostic of either of the following: (1) Acute HBV infection: has not developed anti-HBs yet. Consider "e" antigen testing as outlined previously. Needs follow-up until anti-HBs positive. Anti-HBc IgM distinguishes 1 from 2 (2) Chronic HBV carrier. Consider hepatitis A, hepatitis C, or hepatitis D superinfection as diagnosis if acute hepatitis present. Consider other virus or toxin
+	+	+	Acute hepatitis B Atypical pattern; usually HBsAg is gone by the time anti-HBs appears; should resolve, since antibody is present
–	+	+	Remote hepatitis B infection Recovery is indicated by positive anti-HBs Consider hepatitis A, hepatitis C, other virus, or other cause if acute hepatitis present
–	–	+	One of the following: (1) Remote HBV infection: anti-HBs now at undetectable level. If HBeAg is negative, assume remote infection and consider HAV, HCV, other virus, or other cause if acute hepatitis present (2) Immediate past HBV infection: the "core window" after HBsAg disappears but before anti-HBs appears. A positive test for HBeAg suggests this diagnosis: While the patient is still infectious (positive HbeAg), the infection is in the process of resolution, since HBsAg has disappeared. Follow-up is needed to be sure anti-HBs becomes positive. The immunoglobulin class of anti-HBc may distinguish 1 from 2 (3) Low-level carrier state: HBsAg is too low to measure. If acute infection is present, consider HAV, HCV, or other virus, or other cause
–	+	–	Either of the following: (1) Remote HBV infection: anti-HBc now too low to detect (2) Past immunization with hepatitis B vaccine: the vaccine contains low levels of HBsAg only. If acute infection is present, consider HAV, HCV, other virus, or other cause of hepatitis
–	–	–	No evidence of HBV infection Consider HAV, HCV, other virus, or other cause if hepatitis present

An assay for presence of hepatitis C RNA in serum and plasma that uses the polymerase chain reaction (PCR) is the most sensitive test yet developed and is positive early in infection, making it potentially the most useful test for diagnosis of acute infection and for confirming ongoing chronic infection with low-level viremia. The HCV RNA bDNA assay is used for quantitative assay of HCV in patients, including those with an extremely high viral load, and is calibrated to international units established by the World Health Association. Despite the increased sensitivity of the newer HCV RNA bDNA assay currently available, a negative result does not ensure that a patient is virus negative. The more sensitive qualitative PCR should be performed to rule out the possibility of low-level viremia.

Hepatitis D

An antibody assay exists for hepatitis D, but it is often only transiently positive at the time of acute infection; it does remain persistently positive in chronic carriers of the infection. An IgM assay will be positive in acute infections and can differentiate acute from chronic disease. Hepatitis D should be considered in cases of fulminant hepatitis, or if a patient who is a known hepatitis B carrier suffers an acute exacerbation.

Hepatitis E

Serologic tests for hepatitis E that use ELISA technology have been developed and used in studies to screen for both prevalence and incidence in countries where this disease is endemic. The tests are not currently commercially available in the United States, but serologic confirmation of cases can be obtained through the Hepatitis Branch of the Centers for Disease and Prevention.

Epstein-Barr Virus and Cytomegalovirus

The other viral infections that are most commonly considered in the differential diagnosis of hepatitis, which are EBV and CMV, can be ruled out by using acute and convalescent antibody titers. The Monospot test may be useful for the diagnosis of mononucleosis resulting from EBV, but it is frequently negative early in the course of the illness and may remain so.

HBV Infection in Pregnancy

As a general policy, immigrants to this country from areas where hepatitis B is endemic should be screened for HBsAg, but the screening process becomes extremely important in pregnant women. The influx of refugees from Southeast Asia and other areas where hepatitis B is endemic has made this even more critical (Chapter 16).

The cause for concern is the risk of maternal-fetal transmission. Up to 90% of infants born to HBeAg-positive mothers will themselves become chronic carriers, with the risk of long-term complications and death and also the risk of passing the infection on to their offspring. High-dose (0.5 ml) hepatitis B immune globulin (HBIG) given at birth has been shown to decrease the immediate infection rate by 80%. When the passive immunity granted by HBIG disappears, significant risk of infection via maternal-fetal contact returns, so it is recommended that infants at risk receive the first of their three hepatitis B vaccinations at birth. This combination of HBIG and hepatitis B vaccine has been shown to be 90% effective in preventing infection in children born to mothers who are HBV carriers (see Chapters 11 and 12).

TREATMENT

There is no specific treatment for acute viral hepatitis. Hospitalization is indicated for those people who are unable to care for themselves or who are unable to eat. The other indication for hospitalization is hepatic failure, which requires intensive support and careful laboratory monitoring.

Diet was formerly a matter of great concern in treating hepatitis, but the feeling now is that a general diet with relatively high carbohydrate and low fat content is tolerated best. Activity level is also generally recommended to be as tolerated by the patient. People will usually respond more positively to being as active as possible rather than confined to bed until liver function results approach normal.

Medications in acute hepatitis represent a difficult issue. In general, it is wise to avoid all medications, if possible, but especially any medications that are known to be hepatotoxic. Alcohol, even in modest quantities, should be avoided in the immediate period of infection, although it is probably not necessary to prescribe it for 12 months (as some urge) in the absence of evidence of severe liver disease.

Prothrombin time is a functional assay of the liver's ability to synthesize coagulation factors. Vitamin K may be indicated in modest doses if it appears that acute liver infection is interfering with normal factor production.

Interferon given intramuscularly has been used with mild success in treatment of chronic hepatitis C; 25% of patients treated have persistent normalization of transaminase levels, although the long-term significance is unclear. The effects of interferon alpha for treatment of chronic hepatitis B have been variable and unpredictable. Newer antiviral agents, such as lamivudine, are being tested in combination chemotherapeutic regimens.

PREVENTION

Hepatitis A can be prevented in travelers through the administration of immune globulin (IG), which passively immunizes the patient with anti-HAV obtained from large plasma pools. IG recipients receive protection against infection with hepatitis A virus immediately after administration from the transfer of preformed antibodies contained in the product. Recommendations are that short-term travelers receive 0.02 ml/kg (2 ml for an adult) of IG, and those contemplating stays of 3 months or longer should receive 0.06 ml/kg (5 ml for an adult). In those staying for prolonged periods, additional doses of IG are necessary every 5 months. Studies suggest that protective efficacy in preventing seroconversion is about 85% and that over a year about 1 in 500 people relying on IG prophylaxis will develop icteric hepatitis.

Although theoretically it is better to avoid giving IG and live virus vaccines together, in practice, no difficulty has been seen with oral polio or yellow fever vaccine, both of which are live (there is no concern with inactivated vaccines). However, the *immune responses to the components of the measles, mumps, and rubella vaccine (MMR) are inhibited by IG.* Thus, it is imperative that MMR or the individual components not be given for 3 months after or during the 2 weeks before administering IG.

Travelers who are at risk for hepatitis A may opt for prophylaxis with one of the inactivated hepatitis A virus vaccines currently available. The inactivated vaccines have a rate of seroconversion of greater than 95% 1 month after immunization, but a booster dose 6 to 12 months after the initial dose is recommended to ensure long-lasting high levels of immunity (see Chapter 4). Because a dose of IG sufficient to give protection for up to 3 months is less expensive than hepatitis A vaccine, one-time travelers may be tempted to opt for IG as a measure of economy. They should understand that the efficacy of IG appears to be considerably less. Again, because of the price of hepatitis A vaccine, it may be cost effective to perform HAV antibody screening in travelers who are likely to have been previously infected. Examples of people who should be considered for testing include those with a history of jaundice, natives or long-term residents of areas where hepatitis A is endemic, or those born before the close of World War II, when sanitary conditions were not as carefully maintained.

Reasonable precautions should be exercised in eating and sanitation habits, even in those persons who opt for IG or hepatitis A vaccine. These should include drinking hot, carbonated, or canned or bottled beverages; eating hot, well-cooked food and particularly avoiding raw or poorly cooked seafood; and avoiding unpeeled fruits and uncooked vegetables, which may be fertilized with "night soil." These measures will help with prevention of infections in general.

Prophylaxis for hepatitis B is indicated for travelers depending on risk of exposure. Examples of those who require prophylaxis include health care workers, those who anticipate receiving medical care in endemic regions, and those who expect to have sexual or other intimate contact with natives in countries where hepatitis B is endemic. Long-term travelers (more than 6 months) to endemic areas should receive prophylaxis as well, regardless of anticipated activities. If protection against hepatitis A and hepatitis B are needed by a traveler, the recently released hepatitis A plus hepatitis B combination vaccine may be used (see Chapter 4). HBIG is not indicated for preexposure prophylaxis in travelers. It is expensive and the benefits over IG are small and transient. Immigrants who are household or sexual contacts of persons found to be HBsAg-positive should receive the hepatitis B vaccine if not immune.

There are no firm data that indicate IG is protective against hepatitis C if given before exposure. IG manufactured in the United States does not contain antibody against HEV. There is some evidence that IG manufactured where hepatitis E is endemic does not confer good protection either.

Immunity to hepatitis D is conferred with immunity to hepatitis B. Vaccine for hepatitis B should be given to those at risk. HBV carriers can only avoid risky exposures for HDV.

REFERENCES

Aach RD et al: Hepatitis C virus infections in post-transfusion hepatitis, *N Engl J Med* 25:1325, 1991.

Centers for Disease Control: Enterically transmitted non-A non-B hepatitis-East Africa, *MMWR* 36:241, 1987.

Centers for Disease Control: Enterically transmitted non-A non-B hepatitis-Mexico, *MMWR* 36:597, 1987.

Centers for Disease Control: Hepatitis B virus: a comprehensive strategy for eliminating transmission in the United States through universal childhood vaccination: recommendations of the Immunization Practices Advisory Committee (ACIP), *MMWR* 40:1, 1991.

Centers for Disease Control: Protection against viral hepatitis: recommendations of the Immunization Practices Advisory Committee (ACIP), *MMWR* 39(RR-2): 1, 1990.

Centers for Disease Control and Prevention: Hepatitis E among U.S. travelers, 1989-1992, *MMWR* 42:1, 1993.

Davis GL: Update on the management of chronic hepatitis B, *Rev Gastroenterol Disord* 2:106, 2002.

Davis GL et al: Treatment of chronic hepatitis C with recombinant interferon alfa: a multicenter randomized, controlled trial, *N Engl J Med* 321:1501, 1989.

Everhart JE et al: Risk for non-A, non-B (type C) hepatitis through sexual or household contact with chronic carriers, *Ann Intern Med* 112:544, 1990.
Halliday ML et al: An epidemic of hepatitis A attributable to the ingestion of raw clams in Shanghai, China, *J Infect Dis* 164:852, 1991.
Hoofnagle JH: Type D (delta) hepatitis, *JAMA* 261:1321, 1989.
Lange WR, Frame JD: High incidence of viral hepatitis among American missionaries in Africa, *Am J Trop Med Hyg* 43:527, 1990.
Lewin S, Walters T, Locarnini S: Hepatitis B treatment: rational combination chemotherapy on viral kinetic and animal model studies, *Antiviral Res* 55:381, 2002.
Lok ASF et al: Seroepidemiologic survey of hepatitis E in Hong Kong by recombinant-based enzyme immunoassays, *Lancet* 340:1205, 1992.
McMullen R: Hepatitis and international travel. In Bia F, editor: *The travel medicine advisor,* Atlanta, 1993, American Health Consultants.
McMullen R, Jong EC: Incidence of antibody to hepatitis A among employees of a multinational corporation: implications for immunoglobulin prophylaxis. In Steffen R, editors: *Travel medicine,* Berlin, 1989, Springer-Verlag.
Pierce PF, Cappello M, Bernard KW: Subclinical infection with hepatitis A in Peace Corps volunteers following immune globulin prophylaxis, *Am J Trop Med Hyg* 42:465, 1990.
Steffen R et al: Health problems after travel to developing countries, *J Infect Dis* 156:84, 1987.
Winokur PL, Stapleton JT: Immunoglobulin prophylaxis for hepatitis A, *Clin Infect Dis* 14:580, 1992.
World Health Organization: The First International Standard for HCV RNA Quantification, *Vox Sang* 76:149, 1999.

CHAPTER 20

Leptospirosis

Vernon E. Ansdell

Leptospirosis is the most common zoonosis worldwide. It occurs in all areas except polar regions and is particularly common in the tropics and subtropics. Typical cases present abruptly with high fever and chills, intense headache, severe myalgias, and conjunctival suffusion. Many cases have a nonspecific presentation, however, and are often misdiagnosed. Adventurous travelers, especially to tropical and subtropical regions, are at increased risk of leptospirosis and should be identified and counseled appropriately before departure. The diagnosis of leptospirosis is fraught with problems. A combined approach using culture (blood, urine, cerebrospinal fluid) plus serology (acute and convalescent sera) is recommended to optimize the diagnostic yield. Antibiotic treatment should be started as soon as the diagnosis is suspected, after acute diagnostic specimens are obtained, to maximize benefit.

ETIOLOGY

Leptospirosis is caused by an aerobic, tightly coiled, highly motile spirochete with hooked ends measuring 0.1 μm in diameter and from 6 to 20 μm in length. Because the organism is slender and highly motile, it is capable of passing through membrane filters 0.2 μm in diameter. The organism survives best in moist, warm conditions (optimal temperature 28° C to 30° C) in a slightly alkaline environment (optimal pH 7.2 to 7.4). The genus *Leptospira* includes two species: *L. interrogans,* which is pathogenic, and *L. biflexa,* which is saprophytic and nonpathogenic. *L. interrogans* is divided into 23 serogroups and over 200 serovars, most of which can cause infections in humans. Serovars from common serogroups that cause infection in humans include icterohaemorrhagiae, canicola, hardjo, hebdomadis, grippotyphosa, pomona, australis and ballum.

EPIDEMIOLOGY

Leptospirosis occurs worldwide except in polar regions. Human infection may be epidemic, sporadic, or endemic. Leptospirosis is most common in warm, moist, tropical and subtropical regions, especially areas that have heavy rainfall and neutral or alkaline soil. Infection is often seen in agricultural areas with large numbers of livestock or rodents, or in areas with large wildlife populations. It is most common in the rainy season in the tropics and in the summer and fall in temperate climates, probably reflecting the increased opportunity for exposure to contaminated freshwater.

Leptospirosis is a zoonosis with many wild and domestic animal reservoirs including rats, mice, mongooses, pigs, dogs and cattle. The cycle of transmission is shown in Fig. 20-1. After infection, animals often harbor leptospires in the kidneys. The organism multiplies and may be shed in the urine for months or years. Infected animals are often asymptomatic.

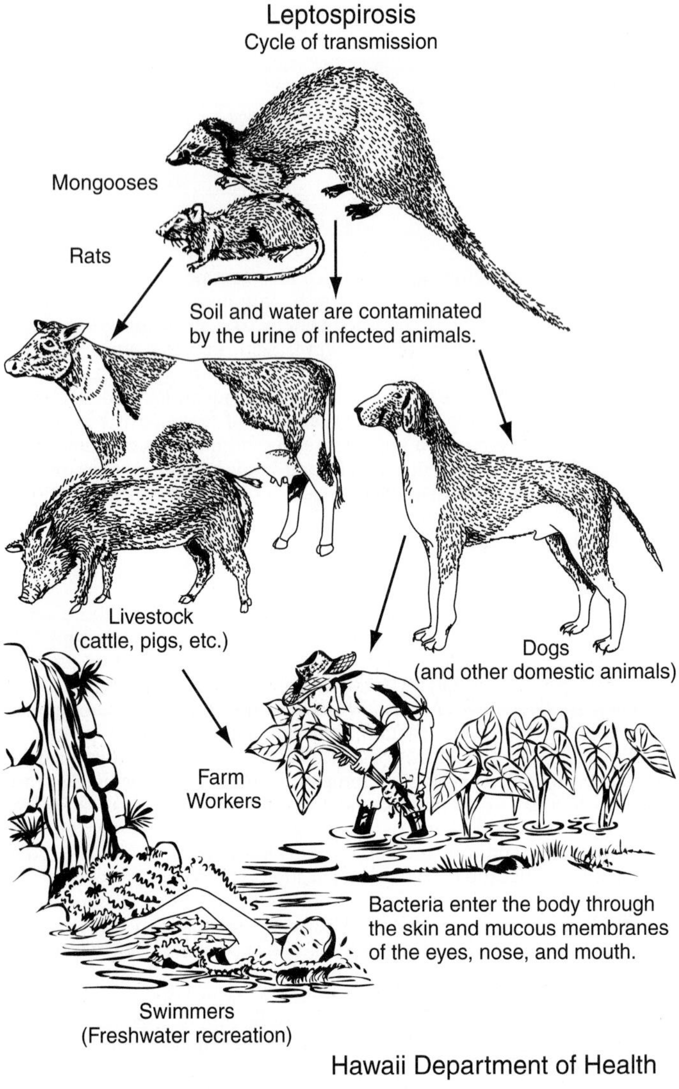

Fig. 20-1 Cycle of transmission of Leptospirosis from animal to man.

Leptospira proliferate in fresh water, damp soil, vegetation, and mud. Humans become infected by exposure to infected animal urine either by direct contact or as the result of indirect exposure through contaminated water or moist soil. Indirect contact is the commonest source of infection and may occur via contaminated mud or fresh water in rivers, lakes, and streams. It occurs in a wide variety of occupational (e.g., rice or sugarcane farmers, sewage workers, miners) and recreational (e.g., rafting, hiking, swimming, fishing, gardening) situations. Direct contact with contaminated urine and tissues of infected animals may occur in hunters, dairy or cattle farmers, abattoir workers, or veterinarians. Infection is acquired through damaged skin (e.g., cuts and abrasions) or via exposed mucous membranes of the nose, mouth, and eyes. Very rarely, infection may be the result of laboratory accidents, animal bites (contaminated with urine), blood transfusions, organ transplants, ingestion of breast milk, sexual intercourse, or congenital transmission.

High antibody prevalence rates have been reported from many tropical and subtropical countries. Examples include Belize, 37%; Tahiti, 30%; Thailand, 27%; and Vietnam, 23%. Average annual incidence rates in tropical and subtropical countries are also high, for example, Tahiti, 20 per 100,000 and Barbados, 123 per 100,000. In contrast, the average annual incidence rate in the United States is 0.02 per 100,000. Typically, at least half the cases of leptospirosis diagnosed in the United States are from Hawaii, and average annual incidence rates on the island of Kauai may be as high as 24 per 100,000. Leptospirosis is most common on the Hawaiian islands that have the most rainfall (Kauai and Hawaii Island), especially in the windward (wetter) areas of those islands. Historically an occupational disease of sugarcane workers in Hawaii, leptospirosis has become increasingly recognized as a recreational disease in recent years.

Some serovars appear to be associated with particular animals. Examples include icterohaemorrhagiae (rats), canicola (dogs), pomona (swine), autumnalis (rats, raccoons), hardjo (cattle) and bratislava (swine, badgers).

It has been noted that outbreaks of leptospirosis often occur after periods of heavy rainfall and flooding. It is thought that rain washes the organism from the river banks into surface waters, while at the same time flooding results in increased human contact with water and forces infected animals into closer contact with humans. A major outbreak occurred after widespread flooding in Nicaragua in 1995 and was responsible for more than 2000 cases and more than 40 deaths. An outbreak in white water rafters in Costa Rica in 1996 was also linked to heavy rainfall. In 1998 the largest outbreak in recorded U.S. history involved a group of triathletes who had swum in a lake after heavy rainfall in Illinois. More than 60 cases were reported in this outbreak. A further example of the association of leptospirosis with flooding was in late 1998, in the aftermath of Hurricane Mitch, when outbreaks of leptospirosis were reported from various countries in Central America including Honduras, Guatemala, and Nicaragua.

Recently there have been several reports of leptospirosis in travelers; nevertheless, the infection continues to be underrecognized in this group. With the increased popularity of recreational and wilderness activities in travelers, there is an increased risk of leptospirosis, particularly in tropical and subtropical regions. Travel medicine specialists should make special efforts to identify and counsel travelers at risk of leptospirosis. This is particularly important in travelers to areas that have experienced recent flooding because they may be at increased risk of infection. In certain situations prophylactic antibiotics may be indicated. It is also important to consider the diagnosis of leptospirosis in a returned traveler who presents with appropriate exposure history and relevant clinical features. Clinicians who see returned travelers need to have a high index of suspicion for leptospirosis, particularly bearing in mind the potentially long incubation period of up to 30 days. Prompt diagnosis is particularly important because appropriate antibiotic treatment needs to be started early to maximize its benefit.

CLINICAL MANIFESTATIONS

The incubation period is usually 7 to 14 days but may range from 2 to 30 days. More than 90% of cases are relatively mild and self-limited. The remaining cases may be severe, often associated with jaundice, potentially life threatening and sometimes referred to as Weil's syndrome (named after Adolf Weil, who was the first to describe the severe form of leptospirosis in 1892). Totally asymptomatic cases are probably rare.

The illness may be biphasic. The first or leptospiremic phase typically lasts 3 to 7 days and represents the period when organisms are present in the blood. The second (leptospiruric) or immune phase, may be clinically silent or last for 1 month or longer. It coincides with the formation of circulating immunoglobulin M (IgM) antibodies. In the commoner, milder (anicteric) form of leptospirosis, there may be a clinically apparent, symptom-free interval of 1 to 3 days between the first and second phases (Fig. 20-2).

ANICTERIC LEPTOSPIROSIS

Leptospirosis has protean manifestations. Classic presentation is with fever, headache, myalgias, and conjunctional suffusion. Typically, the onset is abrupt with high fever (often greater than 39° C), chills, and a severe

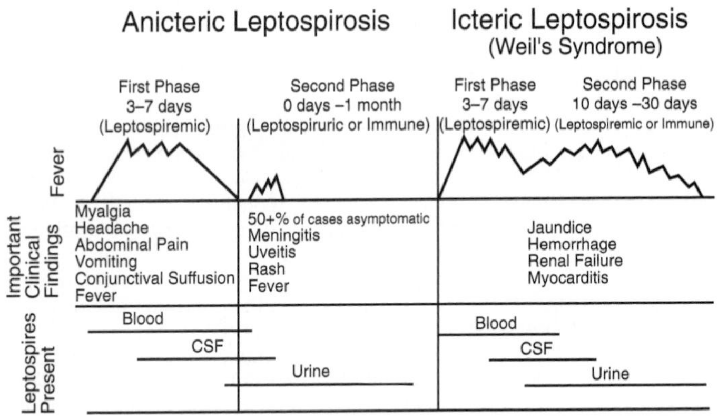

Fig. 20-2 The clinical course of leptospirosis: anicteric and icteric disease. *CSF*, Cerebrospinal fluid. (Adapted from Feigin RD, Anderson DC: Leptospirosis. In Feigin RD, Cherry JD, editors: *Textbook of pediatric infectious diseases*, ed 4, vol 2, Philadelphia, 1998, WB Saunders.)

frontal headache. Patients may report that this is the worst headache they have ever experienced. Muscle pain and tenderness are common and typically involve the muscles of the calves, thighs, and lower back. Conjunctival suffusion* (not conjunctivitis) is virtually pathognomonic of leptospirosis when observed. It usually appears on the third or fourth day of illness and is probably common, although it may be mild and easily overlooked if not sought diligently. Large studies have shown a prevalence of anywhere from 8% to 100%. Subconjunctival hemorrhages are often present.

Gastrointestinal symptoms may include abdominal pain, nausea, vomiting, and diarrhea. Pulmonary involvement occurs in 20% to 70% of cases. Respiratory symptoms may include cough, sometimes with hemoptysis, dyspnea, chest pain, and sore throat. Rashes are present in 10% to 30% of patients during the first week of illness, but typically last only 1 to 2 days. They may be erythematous, macular, maculopapular, urticarial, petechial, or purpuric.

There may be a symptom-free period of 1 to 3 days followed by the second (leptospiruric) or immune phase. This is often clinically inapparent. The hallmark of this phase is aseptic meningitis and symptoms include headaches, neck stiffness, nausea, vomiting, and photophobia. There may be a low-grade temperature. Rashes may also be present during this phase. Inflammation of the anterior uveal tract has been reported in 2% to 10% of patients. It presents clinically as iritis, iridocyclitis, or chorioretinitis several weeks or months after the initial illness. It is usually bilateral and may run a prolonged or recurrent course. Rarely, long-term neuropsychiatric changes such as headaches, inability to concentrate, mood swings, depression, and psychosis have been reported after infection.

SEVERE (ICTERIC) LEPTOSPIROSIS (WEIL'S DISEASE)

Approximately 10% of patients with leptospirosis develop a severe, potentially life-threatening form of the disease. The onset of illness is indistinguishable from the milder form of leptospirosis. After 4 to 9 days, however, there is progression to a severe illness characterized by complications such as jaundice, renal failure, hemorrhage, and cardiopulmonary insufficiency or failure. Jaundice usually appears between the fifth and ninth days of illness and may last for several weeks. It may be marked but liver failure is rare because severe hepatocellular damage is unusual. Tender hepatomegaly is common and splenomegaly may occur. Renal involvement is common and may be evident within 3 to 4 days of onset. Several factors may be involved in the pathogenesis of renal insufficiency including hypovolemia, hypotension, and acute tubular necrosis. Oliguric or nonoliguric renal failure usually occurs during the second week of illness. Peritoneal or hemodialysis may be required, although many cases can be managed without dialysis. Hemorrhage appears to be the result of severe vasculitis with endothelial damage resulting in capillary injury. Hemorrhagic manifestations include petechiae, purpura, bleeding gums, epistaxis, hemoptysis, gastrointestinal hemorrhage, and, rarely, subarachnoid or adrenal hemorrhage. Cardiac involvement may result in myocarditis or pericarditis, and there may be arrhythmias such as atrial fibrillation, atrial flutter, and a variety of conduction disturbances. Congestive heart failure may occur and evidence of myocarditis is often present in fatal cases. Pulmonary involvement may be prominent in severe lep-

*Dilation of conjunctival vessels without inflammation.

tospirosis. It may manifest as pulmonary hemorrhage, pneumonic consolidation, pleural effusions, or adult respiratory distress syndrome (ARDS). Epidemics of leptospirosis with severe, sometimes fatal, pulmonary hemorrhage have been reported from Korea, China, Brazil, and Nicaragua. No single serovar was isolated in these cases. Typically, jaundice was rare or absent in these cases distinguishing them from classic Weil's syndrome and emphasizing that jaundice is not necessarily present in severe leptospirosis.

Overall mortality for leptospirosis is probably less than 1%. In severe leptospirosis, the mortality rate is about 5% to 10%, but may be higher in developing countries where facilities for dialysis and intensive care are often not readily available. Mortality is higher in elderly patients or if there is serious underlying disease. Leptospirosis in pregnancy may be responsible for spontaneous abortion, particularly if infection occurs early in pregnancy. Congenital infection is probably rare.

DIFFERENTIAL DIAGNOSIS

Clinical manifestations of leptospirosis are variable and often nonspecific. Clinicians should have a high index of suspicion to avoid misdiagnosis. There may be diagnostic clues or "red flags" that should alert clinicians to the possibility of leptospirosis (Table 20-1). There is often a broad differential diagnosis, particularly in a traveler who has recently returned from the tropics (Table 20-2). For example, leptospirosis may present as an unexplained febrile illness, pharyngitis, aseptic meningitis, or hemorrhagic fever; or it may mimic infections such as dengue fever, malaria, viral hepatitis, or typhus.

DIAGNOSIS

Culture

Cultures should be obtained whenever possible because they may detect cases that would be missed by serology alone. Blood and, where appropriate, cerebrospinal fluid (CSF) should be cultured during the first 7 to 10 days of illness, before administration of antibiotics. Urine should be cultured during the second week of illness and for up to 30 days after onset (Fig. 20-2). Tissue specimens and dialysis fluid can also be cultured in appropriate situations. Cultures should be inoculated as soon as possible using special media (e.g., Fletcher semisolid or Tween 80-albumin

Table 20-1
Diagnostic Red Flags

- History of contact with freshwater or mud
- History of contact with animals
- History of skin cuts or abrasions
- Abrupt onset of severe headache
- Severe myalgias (calves, thighs, lumbar area)
- Conjunctival suffusion
- Fever and new onset atrial fibrillation
- Jaundice with relatively mild transaminase elevation
- Fever, jaundice, and thrombocytopenia
- Hepatitis and neutrophil leukocytosis
- Fever and elevated creatine kinase levels
- Fever and elevated amylase levels

[EMJH]). Blood that cannot be inoculated immediately should be heparinized. If there is any delay in inoculating urine, it should be alkalinized using bovine serum albumin. It is important to emphasize that cultures may take anywhere from 1 to 6 weeks to become positive.

Immunodiagnosis

IgM antibodies appear as early as 4 days after the onset of symptoms but are usually not demonstrable until the second week. They usually peak by the third or fourth week. The appearance of serum antibodies may be suppressed or delayed by antibiotics or corticosteroids. The current reference standard is the microscopic agglutination test (MAT), a labor- and skill-intensive test available only in specialized reference laboratories worldwide. Paired sera drawn 14 to 28 days apart should be obtained. Serologic diagnosis is usually based on demonstrating a fourfold rise or single MAT titer of at least 1 in 200. To make the diagnosis of leptospirosis it is particularly important to obtain convalescent serum because the acute serum is often negative for antibodies. Even paired sera may fail to detect infection in up to 10% of patients with culture-positive leptospirosis. Unfortunately, serovars present in the tropics may not be represented in the serovar pool, so that sera from patients with leptospirosis from tropical areas may test negative, emphasizing the importance of obtaining cultures whenever possible.

Rapid screening serologic tests that are sometimes used include enzyme-linked immunosorbent assay (ELISA), dot-ELISA, indirect hemagglutination, IgM dipstick, latex agglutination, and indirect fluorescent antibody. These alternative tests tend to have variable sensitivities and specificities depending on the location of the test and the case definition used.

Polymerase chain reaction offers the attractive possibility of rapid, early diagnosis. Unfortunately the test is not routinely available and remains unproven as a reliable means of diagnosis.

LABORATORY AND RADIOLOGIC FINDINGS

The total white blood cell count is variable but is usually elevated in severe disease. A neutrophil (polymorph) leukocytosis is common, in con-

Table 20-2
Differential Diagnosis

- Influenza
- Streptococcal pharyngitis
- Viral hepatitis
- Aseptic meningitis
- Legionnaires' disease
- Brucellosis
- Toxoplasmosis
- Hanta virus
- Dengue fever
- Malaria
- Typhoid fever
- Rickettsial diseases (e.g., typhus, Q fever)
- Hemorrhagic fevers
- Relapsing fever

trast to viral hepatitis. A mild to moderate thrombocytopenia (platelet counts 50,000 to 120,000/mm^3) is common and may occur in up to 50% of cases. Platelet counts of less than 50,000/mm^3 are less common but may be seen in severe disease. Prothrombin time may be prolonged in severe leptospirosis, but can be corrected with vitamin K. Erythrocyte sedimentation rate is commonly elevated and is often greater than 50 mm/hr.

Liver function abnormalities include elevated bilirubin (up to 20 mg/dL or higher) but with relatively mild increase in alkaline phosphatase and transaminase levels. Elevated serum amylase has been reported in 47% to 80% of cases, but in only a few of these cases did patients have any evidence of pancreatitis. Creatine kinase levels are elevated in more than half the patients during the first week of illness. This may help to differentiate leptospirosis from viral hepatitis.

Urinalysis is abnormal in at least 70% of cases, although the abnormalities may be slight and transient, particularly in mild cases. Abnormalities may include proteinuria, hyaline or granular casts, pyuria, and hematuria.

CSF obtained during the second (immune) phase of illness shows features of an aseptic meningitis. The CSF cell count is usually less than 500/mm^3. Polymorphonuclear leukocytes predominate early in the illness, but mononuclear cells increase later. CSF protein may be elevated (up to 300 mg/dL), but CSF glucose is usually normal.

Chest x-ray study abnormalities have been noted in 23% to 67% of patients. Abnormalities develop 3 to 9 days after the onset of illness. X-ray studies may be abnormal despite normal clinical examination. Abnormalities include small nodular densities; large confluent areas of consolidation; and diffuse, ill-defined, ground-glass densities. These abnormalities are usually bilateral, nonlobar, and predominantly peripheral.

TREATMENT

Antibiotic treatment should be started as soon as the diagnosis of leptospirosis is suspected because antimicrobial agents are most effective if initiated during the first 4 days of illness. Early antibiotic treatment has been shown to reduce the duration and severity of illness. There is evidence of some benefit, however, even if treatment with intravenous penicillin is started relatively late in the course of severe illness. Antibiotics should be continued for 7 to 10 days. The organism is sensitive to a wide range of antibiotics. Penicillin, ampicillin, amoxicillin, or doxycycline is often recommended. Erythromycin, third-generation cephalosporins such as ceftriaxone and cefotaxime, and some fluoroquinolones also appear to be effective. The organism may be resistant to chloramphenicol, vancomycin, aminoglycosides, and first-generation cephalosporins.

In the early stages of infection, it is usually impossible to be certain of the diagnosis of leptospirosis. Hence, antibiotic coverage needs to be broad enough to include other possible diagnoses. Supportive care, if necessary in an intensive care unit, is also important and meticulous attention to fluid and electrolyte balance is essential. Peritoneal dialysis or hemodialysis has helped to reduce the mortality from leptospirosis because, in the past, renal failure was an important cause of death. Jarisch-Herxheimer reactions have been reported after treatment of leptospirosis with penicillin, but they appear to be less common than with other spirochetal infections. Steroids have not yet been proved to be of any benefit.

PREVENTION

Travelers at risk of leptospirosis should be identified and counseled appropriately before departure. Recommendations for prevention include avoiding potentially contaminated fresh water, damp soil, or mud whenever possible; wearing protective waterproof clothing; and covering cuts and abrasions with waterproof dressings. Submersion in potentially contaminated freshwater should be avoided, since the organism can enter via the mucous membranes of the eyes, nose, and mouth. Drinking water may be contaminated with leptospires and should be purified by boiling or treating with iodine or chlorine. Filtration may not be adequate because the organism is slender and highly motile and can pass through membrane filters up to 0.2 μm in diameter.

Travelers to areas that have recently experienced flooding may be at increased risk of infection and should be especially careful. In very high-risk situations they may be candidates for prophylactic antibiotics.

A killed whole cell vaccine is available for immunization of high-risk humans in China, Japan, Vietnam, Israel, and certain European countries. However, safety and efficacy in humans remain uncertain. In addition, it is important to emphasize that the vaccines are serovar specific and even if an inexpensive, safe, and effective vaccine were available, it would have limited value for travelers. Animal vaccines are effective and widely available but offer only short-term, serovar-specific protection. Previous infection provides protection only against the infecting serovar. Therefore second infections are possible in high-risk individuals with recurrent exposure to infection (e.g., rice farmers).

Chemoprophylaxis using doxycycline, 200 mg once a week beginning before the first exposure and ending after the last exposure, was effective in preventing leptospirosis in U.S. military personnel in Panama. Short-term, high-risk travelers may be suitable candidates for chemoprophylaxis. Doxycycline, 100 mg once a day, for prevention of malaria probably also protects against leptospirosis. Travelers at risk of both malaria and leptospirosis may be particularly appropriate candidates for doxycycline chemoprophylaxis rather than alternative antimalarials such as mefloquine (Larium) or atovaquone and proguanil (Malarone).

REFERENCES

Ansdell VE, Sasaki DM: Leptospirosis in Hawaii: important implications for the adventurous traveler in the tropics. Third Conference on International Travel Medicine, Paris, France, 1993.

Antony SJ: Leptospirosis: an emerging pathogen in travel medicine. A review of its clinical manifestations and management, *J Travel Med* 3:113, 1996.

Berman SJ et al: Sporadic anicteric leptospirosis in South Vietnam, *Ann Intern Med* 19:167, 1973.

CDC: Update: outbreak of acute febrile illness among athletes participating in Eco-Challenge—Sabah 2000—Borneo, Malaysia, 2000, *MMWR* 50:21, 2001.

CDC: Outbreak of leptospirosis among white-water rafters—Costa Rica 1996, *MMWR* 46:577, 1997.

Edwards CN, Everard COR: Hyperamylasemia and pancreatitis in leptospirosis, *Am J Gastroenterol* 86:1665, 1991.

Faine S, Bolin C, Perolat P: *Leptospira and leptospirosis,* Melbourne, 1999, MedSci.

Farr RW: Leptospirosis, *Clin Infect Dis* 21:1, 1995.

Ferguson IR: Leptospirosis update, *BMJ* 302:128, 1991.

Heron LG et al: Leptospirosis presenting as a haemorrhagic fever in a traveler from Africa, *Med J Austral* 167:477, 1997.

Jackson LA et al: Outbreak of leptospirosis associated with swimming, *Pediatr Infect Dis J* 12:48, 1993.

Katz AR et al: Assessment of the clinical presentation and treatment of 353 cases of laboratory confirmed leptospirosis in Hawaii, 1974-1998, *CID* 33:1834, 2001.

Korman TM, Globan MS, Smythe LD: Leptospirosis in a returned traveler: isolation of a new Leptopira serovar, *Aust NZ J Med* 27:716, 1997.

Monsuez J, Kidouche R, LeGueno B, Postic D: Leptospirosis presenting as haemorrhagic fever in a visitor to Africa, *Lancet* 349:254, 1997.

Morgan J et al: Outbreak of leptospirosis among triathlon participants and community residents in Springfield, Illinois, 1998, *CID* 34:1593, 2002.

O'Neill KM, Rickman LS, Lazarus AA: Pulmonary manifestations of leptospirosis, *Rev Infect Dis* 13:705, 1991.

Sasaki DM et al: Active surveillance and risk factors for leptospirosis in Hawaii, *Am J Trop Med Hyg* 48:35, 1993.

Sehgal SC et al: Randomized controlled trial of doxycycline prophylaxis against leptospirosis in an endemic area, *Int J Antimicrob Agents* 13:249, 2000.

Takafuji ET et al: An efficacy trial of doxycycline chemoprophylaxis against leptospirosis, *N Eng J Med* 310:497, 1984.

Trevejo RT et al: Epidemic leptospirosis associated with pulmonary hemorrhage—Nicaragua, 1995, *J Infect Dis* 178:1457, 1998.

Van Crevel R, Speelman P, Grevekamp C, Terpstra WJ: Leptospirosis in travelers, *Clin Infect Dis* 19:132, 1994.

Watt G et al: Placebo-controlled trial of intravenous penicillin for severe and late leptospirosis, *Lancet* 1:433, 1988.

CHAPTER 21

Lyme Disease

David H. Spach

In 1977, Steere and co-workers reported on an epidemic of arthritis in the region of Old Lyme, Connecticut, and thus catalyzed a flurry of critical studies that soon described *Ixodes* ticks as the vector, identified the spirochete *Borrelia burgdorferi* as the causative infectious pathogen, and characterized the broad clinical manifestations of Lyme disease. Interestingly, several authors had previously described patients in Europe with clinical manifestations similar to patients with Lyme disease, and subsequently the European borreliosis was also shown to be caused by infection with *B. burgdorferi.* Currently, Lyme disease is appreciated as an important vector-borne disease that occurs worldwide. A consideration of Lyme disease is especially relevant to outdoors and adventure travelers, since the ticks that cause Lyme disease are expanding into new geographic areas.

CAUSATIVE ORGANISM

B. burgdorferi is a 0.2 by 25 μm unicellular spirochete that has a central protoplasmic cylinder surrounded by an outer envelope that contains important surface proteins. In different regions of the world, distinct *B. burgdorferi* strains exist. Investigators have analyzed specific antigenic differences to classify *B. burgdorferi* into four species: (1) *B. burgdorferi* sensu stricto, (2) *B. garinii,* (3) *B. afzelii,* and (4) *B. japonica.* In the United States, all isolates, to date, have been *B. burgdorferi* sensu stricto. In Europe, however, most isolates have been either *B. garinii* or *B. afzelii.* The distinct antigenic strains may explain some of the differences observed in the predominant clinical manifestations in persons infected with *B. burgdorferi* in the United States versus those infected in Europe.

TRANSMISSION

In the United States, *B. burgdorferi* can be potentially transmitted to humans via one of two types of *Ixodes* ticks: *I. scapularis* (formerly known as *I. dammini* and commonly referred to as the deer tick) (Fig. 21-1) and *I. pacificus* (commonly referred to as the western black-legged tick). Dennis and co-workers have published a national map showing the distribution of the *Ixodes* ticks in the United States. This map shows *I. scapularis* most concentrated in the northeastern and upper north central states and *I. pacificus* clustered in west coastal states. In Europe, *I. ricinus* serves as the primary vector for *B. burgdorferi,* whereas *I. persulcatus* is the major vector in Asia. In the former Soviet Union, *I. persulcatus* and *I. ricinus*

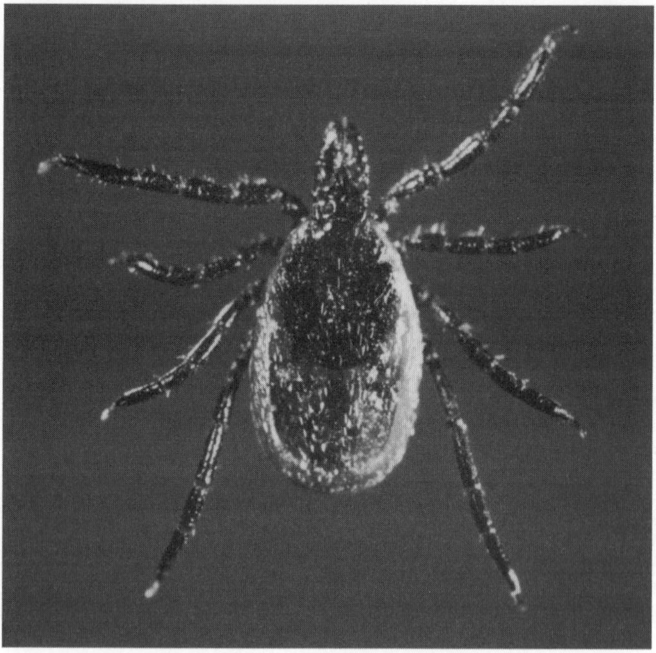

Fig. 21-1 Adult *Ixodes scapularis* female tick.

transmit both *B. burgdorferi* and tick-borne encephalitis virus during the same seasons and in the same locations.

In the northeastern and upper north central United States, the white-footed mouse, *Peromyscus leucopus,* serves as the most common reservoir for *B. burgdorferi.* The white-tailed deer also plays a major role because the adult *I. scapularis* ticks prefer to mate on these animals. In most of the western United States, the dusky-footed wood rat is the major reservoir for *B. burgdorferi,* but two species of *Ixodes* ticks, *I. neotomae* and *I. pacificus,* are involved in the life cycle of *B. burgdorferi.* In this so-called California bicycle, the *I. neotomae* ticks play the role of infecting the wood rat with *B. burgdorferi,* whereas the *I. pacificus* ticks play the role of transmitting *B. burgdorferi* to humans after acquiring *B. burgdorferi* from the wood rat reservoir.

The life cycle of these *Ixodes* ticks includes three stages, typically lasting 2 years, and requiring a blood meal at each stage to mature to the next stage. The cycle begins in the spring when the adult female tick releases her eggs, which hatch as 6-legged larvae. During the summer, the larvae take a blood meal, followed by a dormant phase in the fall. In the spring, the ticks molt and enter the second phase of their life cycle as 8-legged nymphal ticks. In the late spring or summer, the nymphal ticks take a blood meal and subsequently molt as 8-legged adults in the fall. The adults mate and the male then dies; the female, however, takes one more blood meal before she lays her eggs and dies. Although ticks at any of

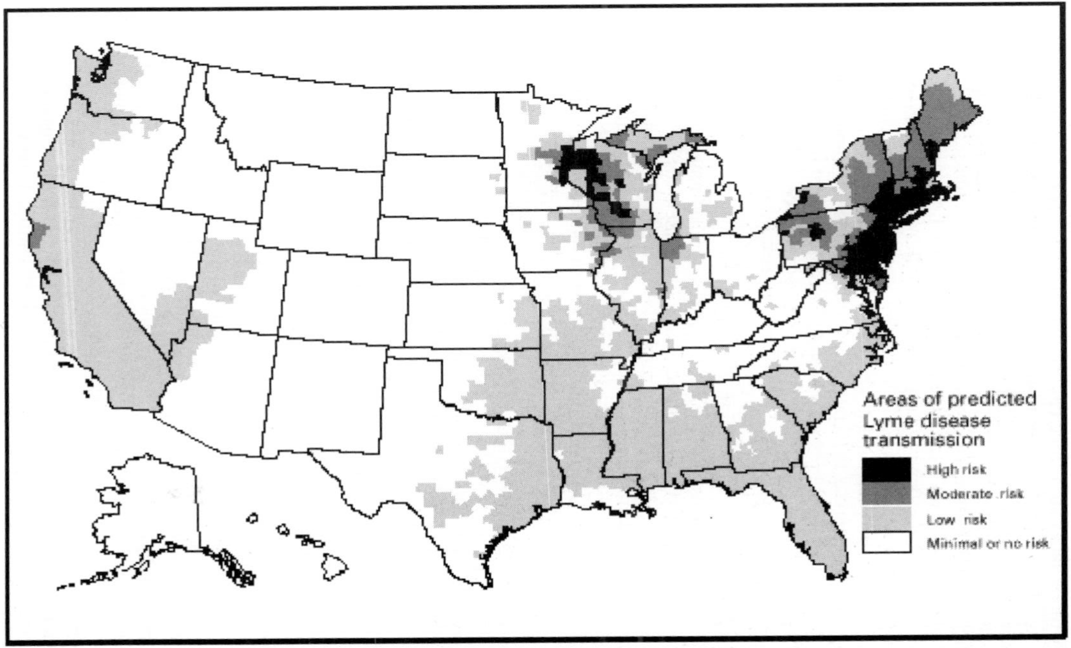

Fig. 21-2 Lyme disease cases in United States in 1996. (From Centers for Disease Control and Prevention.)

these three stages are competent vectors for *B. burgdorferi* transmission to humans, most cases of Lyme disease result from the bite of the 2 to 3 mm nymphal tick. In the United States, *Ixodes* ticks also serve as the vector for the infectious pathogens that cause babesiosis and human granulocytic ehrlichiosis. Bites from *Ixodes* ticks are generally painless, and fewer than 50% of patients with Lyme disease recall a tick bite. Animal laboratory studies show that efficient transmission of *B. burgdorferi* by *I. scapularis* requires a minimum of 36 to 48 hours of tick attachment, but human cases have apparently occurred after shorter periods of tick attachment. Nevertheless, it does appear that, in general, transmission to humans probably requires at least 8 hours of attachment. The requirement for prolonged attachment correlates with the change in *B. burgdorferi* outer surface protein OspA (noninfectious state) to OspC (infectious state).

EPIDEMIOLOGY

In 1982, after it was realized that Lyme disease had emerged as a major vector-borne disease in the United States, the Centers for Disease Control and Prevention (CDC) initiated surveillance for Lyme disease. In 1991 Lyme disease became a reportable disease, with a case defined for surveillance purposes as (1) erythema migrans rash of at least 5 cm, or (2) a positive serology result combined with at least one compatible manifestation of musculoskeletal, neurologic, or cardiovascular disease. In the last two decades, Lyme disease has become the most common vector-borne disease reported in the United States. In 1996, 16,455 cases of Lyme disease involving 45 states were reported to the CDC (Fig. 21-2). Detailed information from 1996 surveillance data found that most cases originated from the Northeast, Mid-Atlantic, and upper North central regions. Among all 1996 reported cases, 91% originated from one of eight states: Connecticut, Rhode Island, New York, New Jersey, Delaware, Pennsylvania, Maryland, and Wisconsin. The highest incidence was in Nantucket County, which reported 1247 cases of Lyme disease per 100,000 persons. No reported cases originated from Alaska, Arizona, Colorado, Montana, or South Dakota. The highly endemic regions for Lyme disease correlate with the regions that have a high density of *Ixodes* ticks.

In the United States, most human infections with *B. burgdorferi* occur from May to August, corresponding with the most active feeding period of the *Ixodes* nymphal ticks and maximal human outdoor exposure. The timing of cases in the western United States is generally several weeks later than in the eastern United States, mainly because of the later onset of warmer weather. Lyme disease occurs in children and adults and has an approximately equal distribution among males and females.

Worldwide, the disease occurs in many areas of Europe, especially Germany, Austria, Switzerland, and France. Lyme disease has also been reported from Sweden, the former Soviet Union, China, Japan, and Australia.

CLINICAL MANIFESTATIONS

From a conceptual standpoint, Lyme disease can be categorized into three different stages: (1) early localized (onset days to weeks after infection), (2) early disseminated (days to months), and (3) late (months to years). From a practical perspective, most patients do not pass through all three phases; the manifestations of the stages can overlap, specific clinical manifestations can occur independently, and some patients develop asymptomatic infection. Clinical features of Lyme disease in the United States

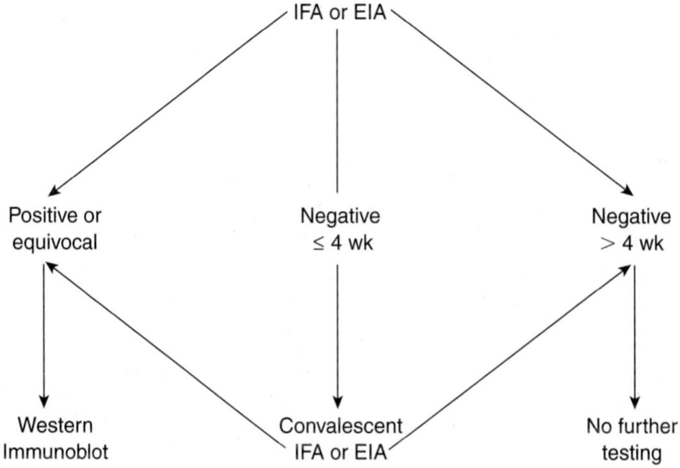

Fig. 21-3 Recommended approach for serologic testing of patients with suspected Lyme disease. (From Centers for Disease Control and Prevention.)

differ somewhat from those in Europe; erythema migrans and arthritis occur more frequently among patients in the United States, whereas neurologic and chronic skin conditions are more common in European patients.

Early Localized Infection

The most common clinical manifestation of Lyme disease in the United States is the erythematous macular rash known as erythema migrans. This lesion develops in 60% to 80% of Lyme disease cases, typically appearing at the site of the tick bite 7 to 10 days after the bite. Patients often also have concomitant mild to moderate constitutional symptoms, including low-grade fever, headache, fatigue, myalgias, and regional lymphadenopathy. The typical appearance of erythema migrans is a round or oval, well-demarcated, erythematous lesion at least 5 cm in diameter (median, 15 cm). The lesion can appear in one of several forms, including a solid lesion, a bulls-eye pattern, or as multiple rings. If untreated, the erythema migrans lesion gradually expands, typically developing partial central clearing and reaching a diameter of more than 30 cm. Erythema migrans and associated early symptoms typically persist for 3 to 4 weeks if left untreated. In some instances, patients and medical providers may confuse erythema migrans with an allergic reaction to an insect bite. An insect bite typically is painful, has its onset within 24 hours of the bite, and usually resolves within several days. Erythema migrans, on the other hand, is usually painless, has a delayed onset of typically 7 to 10 days, and will persist for weeks if not treated.

Although *B. burgdorferi* infection is initially limited to the primary cutaneous site, dissemination from the site of infection to distant sites can occur within days to a few weeks after initial inoculation. Some patients will show evidence of dissemination early in their course by developing multiple, widespread, secondary annular erythema migrans lesions; these secondary lesions are generally smaller than the initial erythema migrans lesion and can vary in number from 1 to more than 50. Years after the initial infection, patients may develop a late-stage cutaneous manifestation known as acrodermatitis chronica atrophicans; this chronic scarring skin lesion can resemble scleroderma and is considerably more common among European patients with Lyme disease than among those in the United States.

Early Disseminated Infection and Late Infection

Months after the initial infection, approximately 60% of patients with Lyme disease in the United States will develop arthralgias or arthritis. The arthritis typically consists of brief attacks of asymmetric, oligoarticular arthritis involving large joints interspersed with months of remission. Only about 10% of patients with untreated Lyme disease will develop chronic arthritis, and these patients often have the HLA-DR4 haplotype. In addition, patients with HLA-DR4 often have a poor response to antimicrobial therapy. Even with chronic Lyme arthritis, patients generally have resolution of their active flares within 5 to 6 years, and most do not develop permanent joint damage. The arthralgias also tend to involve large joints, have intermittent recurrences, and usually resolve within 5 to 6 years.

Overall, about 20% of patients with Lyme disease have some type of neurologic manifestations. Early in the course of Lyme disease, patients may develop unilateral or bilateral facial palsy. Less frequently, patients may present with a lymphocytic meningitis or meningoencephalitis within months of the initial infection. Later in the course (months to years after infection), patients may develop peripheral neuropathy that can manifest as radiculoneuritis, mononeuritis multiplex, or diffuse peripheral neuropathy. The late-appearing chronic neurologic manifestations pose special difficulty, since many of these symptoms are nonspecific and can overlap with many other diseases. The Lyme-associated chronic neurologic manifestations include subacute encephalopathy, axonal polyneuropathy, and less frequently leukoencephalopathy. Available studies suggest that subacute encephalopathy is the most common of these chronic neurologic manifestations and it is characterized by cognitive deficits and disturbances in mood and sleep. Unfortunately, patients with chronic neurologic Lyme disease may have persistence of their symptoms for several years, even longer than 10 years in some cases.

Although cardiac manifestations develop in fewer than 10% of patients with Lyme disease, they can have potentially fatal consequences. The most common cardiac abnormality is atrioventricular block, occurring in about 5% to 8% of patients with Lyme disease, typically weeks to months after the initial infection. Although some patients have required a temporary pacemaker for severe atrioventricular conduction disturbances, these abnormalities generally do not necessitate placing a permanent pacemaker if the patient receives appropriate therapy Lyme disease. Other less common cardiac manifestations include myocarditis, pericarditis, and pancarditis. Rare reports have described cases of chronic cardiomyopathy caused by *B. burgdorferi.* The prevalence of cardiac abnormalities among persons with Lyme disease who have received antibiotic therapy—typically for erythema migrans—is the same as for persons without a history of Lyme disease.

In addition to the cutaneous, joint, neurologic, and cardiac manifestations, rare reports have described involvement of just about every body site. Several lines of evidence suggest *B. burgdorferi* can be transmitted transplacentally, but adverse birth outcomes related to maternal Lyme disease appear to be rare.

DIAGNOSIS

As noted earlier, the CDC has generated a case definition for Lyme disease for surveillance purposes. This case definition, however, is not meant to be a rigid guideline for actual clinical decisions regarding who should or should not receive therapy for Lyme disease. Multiple factors play a role in the clinical decision making regarding the clinical diagnosis of Lyme disease. From a clinical perspective, a diagnosis of Lyme disease should initially be based on compatible clinical findings in a patient with a reasonable probability of previous exposure to *Ixodes* ticks; serologic testing for evidence of *B. burgdorferi* infection can then serve as an adjunct to clinical judgment. Most laboratories use the serum enzyme immunoassay (EIA) as a screening test and the serum Western immunoblot as a confirmatory test.

Recommendations for serologic testing of patients with suspected Lyme disease arose from expert groups that convened at the Second National Conference on Serologic Diagnosis of Lyme Disease in 1994; these expert groups included the CDC, the Association of State and Territorial Public Health Laboratory Directors, the Food and Drug Administration (FDA), and the National Institutes of Health. In general, these groups recommended using a two-step diagnostic process for suspected cases, with initial testing consisting of an EIA or an immunofluorescent antibody test (Fig. 21-3). If the initial test is positive or equivocal, further "confirmatory" testing should be performed using a standardized Western immunoblot because the screening tests have less than optimal specificity. If the Western immunoblot is positive, the patient is considered to have laboratory evidence of Lyme disease. Because adequate antibody responses to *B. burgdorferi* may not be generated in the first several weeks of infection, patients with a negative screening test taken less than 4 weeks after possible infection should undergo follow-up convalescent repeat testing. If, however, the patient has a negative screening test taken after 4 weeks of infection, he or she does not have laboratory evidence of Lyme disease and, in general, would not need further testing for Lyme disease because the sensitivity of the test in patients with late Lyme disease is high.

The same expert panel also generated recommendations that standardized the criteria for a positive Western immunoblot serology test. Specifically they recommended that the Western immunoblot immunoglobulin M should be considered positive if at least two of the following bands are present: 21/24 kDa (OspC), 39 kDa (BmpA), or 41 kDa (Fla). The recommended criterion for a positive Western immunoblot IgG is presence of at least five of the following 10 bands: 18 kDa, 21/24 kDa (OspC), 28 kDa, 30 kDa, 39 kDa (BmpA), 41 kDa (Fla), 45 kDa, 58 kDa (not GroEL), 66 kDa, or 93 kDa. Most commercial laboratories that perform *B. burgdorferi* Western immunoblot assays now incorporate these specific diagnostic criteria into their interpretation of the test.

Although standardization of *B. burgdorferi* Western immunoblotting now exists, several major problems still exist with serologic testing for Lyme disease. First, false-negative antibody tests are common during the initial 4 to 6 weeks of the patient's illness, a time when patients most often present with the initial erythema migrans rash. Second, antimicrobial treatment of early Lyme disease can blunt antibody responses and thus generate a false-negative test. Third, false-positives results can result from other infectious agents and other diseases including Epstein-Barr virus, oral treponemes, syphilis, relapsing fever, and rheumatoid arthritis. Fourth, test results vary significantly in different laboratories, a problem compounded by the multitude of laboratories that now perform *B. burgdorferi* serologic testing.

Other diagnostic tests, such as culture, antigen detection, polymerase chain reaction (PCR), and measurement of cell-mediated immunity to *B. burgdorferi,* are considered investigational and are not recommended for routine clinical purposes. Among these investigational techniques, PCR-based tests show the most promise, especially for patients for early-stage Lyme disease, as well those with potential false-negative antibody titers. Although several investigators have cultured *B. burgdorferi* from clinical specimens, performing cultures requires a special medium (Barbour-Stoenner-Kelly) and is neither rapid nor widely available. Some reference laboratories perform *B. burgdorferi* cerebrospinal fluid antibodies, but criteria for a positive test are not standardized.

Several studies have shown that significant problems exist with the overdiagnosis of Lyme disease. In particular, two studies found that only about one fourth of patients referred to their clinic with suspected active Lyme disease actually had active Lyme disease. One of these studies also reported that among persons referred to their clinic who had not responded to antibiotic therapy for Lyme disease, nearly 80% had not responded because the initial diagnosis of Lyme disease was not warranted.

THERAPY

Patients with early Lyme disease manifested by erythema migrans and nonspecific flu-like symptoms respond well to antimicrobial therapy administered soon after symptom onset. In general, with long delays in the initial diagnosis of Lyme disease, patients have poorer responses to antimicrobial therapy. The following treatment recommendations are based on available data from clinical trials, previously published reviews, and expert opinion (Table 21-1). The primary goals of treating patients with early-stage Lyme disease is to decrease the duration of the acute manifestations (such as erythema migrans), as well as to diminish the likelihood that later sequelae of Lyme disease will develop. More than 90% of patients with erythema migrans respond to a 14- to 21-day course of oral doxycycline or amoxicillin; some studies have supplemented amoxicillin with probenecid to enhance amoxicillin levels. In general, doxycycline should not be used to treat Lyme disease in pregnant women, lactating women, or children 8 years old or younger. Results with either cefuroxime or clarithromycin suggest similar response rates as those seen with either doxycycline or amoxicillin, and thus these two medications are considered reasonable alternatives to doxycycline or amoxicillin. Because erythromycin and azithromycin have success rates lower than doxycycline or amoxicillin, they are not recommended as first-line therapy. Treatment with doxycycline provides an advantage over amoxicillin in geographic areas where patients with Lyme disease may have concomitant babesiosis or ehrlichiosis, because doxycycline effectively treats all three of these tick-borne diseases. In one trial of patients with early-stage disseminated Lyme disease, treatment responses were similar with oral doxycycline and intravenous ceftriaxone in terms of preventing late manifestations of Lyme disease.

Table 21-1
Treatment of Lyme Disease in Adults

Manifestation	Therapy	Route	Dose	Duration
Early (Erythema migrans)	Doxycycline	PO	100 mg bid	14-21d
	Amoxicillin	PO	500 mg tid	14-21d
	Cefuroxime axetil	PO	500 mg bid	14-21d
Arthritis	Doxycycline	PO	100 mg bid	30d
	Amoxicillin	PO	500 mg tid	30d
	Ceftriaxone	IV	2 g qd	14-21d
Cardiac				
Mild (AV block with PR 0.3s)	Doxycycline	PO	100 mg bid	14-21d
Serious	Ceftriaxone	IV	2 g qd	14-21d
Neurologic				
Mild (Facial palsy)	Doxycycline	PO	100 mg bid	21-30d
	Amoxicillin	PO	500 mg tid	21-30d
Serious	Ceftriaxone	IV	2 g IV qd	14-21d

Modified from Spach DH: Ehrlichiosis, babesiosis, Rocky Mountain spotted fever, and Lyme disease. In Mandell GL, Wilfert CM: *Atlas of infectious diseases* 11:14.1, 1999.

Initial therapy of Lyme arthritis with either oral doxycycline or amoxicillin gives response rates similar to those seen with intravenous regimens. Overall response rates are in the range of 50% to 60%, but lower among those who previously received intraarticular steroids. In addition, responses are often delayed for several months. For nonresponders with well-documented Lyme arthritis, most recommend treating with either a 2- to 3-month course of oral doxycycline or a 14- to 28-day course of either intravenous ceftriaxone or intravenous cefotaxime.

Patients with early-stage neurologic Lyme disease, such as facial palsy, generally respond to oral therapy. Although the choice of drugs and duration of treatment for late neurologic Lyme disease remains controversial, most recommend using a 14- to 28-day course of intravenous therapy (ceftriaxone, cefotaxime, or penicillin). One study that compared cefotaxime with intravenous penicillin has shown better response rates with cefotaxime. Response rates with ceftriaxone and cefotaxime appear similar. From a practical perspective, the schedule of once daily intravenous ceftriaxone is significantly more convenient than giving multiple doses per day of either intravenous cefotaxime or intravenous penicillin. Overall, about 60% of patients with neurologic involvement show significant improvement in their neurologic manifestations, but, as with patients with Lyme arthritis, improvement may be delayed for several months after therapy. Studies have not been performed that would determine the responses of repeat courses of intravenous antibiotics in patients with chronic neurologic Lyme disease.

Patients with cardiac disease generally should receive intravenous therapy. Some experts recommend oral therapy for mild atrioventricular block

(PR interval less than or equal to 0.3 seconds), but others have suggested using intravenous regimens with any cardiac involvement. Regardless, patients with cardiac involvement should be observed closely and may require a temporary pacemaker.

Many patients treated for Lyme disease do not improve after therapy, and the complex reasons for poor response may include initial misdiagnosis, concomitant chronic illnesses such as fibromyalgia or depression, slowly resolving Lyme disease, permanent tissue damage caused by *B. burgdorferi,* post-Lyme autoimmune disease, persistent tissue infection with *B. burgdorferi,* and sterile inflammation caused by dead organisms. For those patients who do not respond to antibiotics and have no objective evidence of active Lyme disease, repeated courses of antibiotics have no proven benefit.

PREVENTION

The two strategies used in preventing Lyme disease include avoiding tick bites and receiving prophylactic antibiotics if a tick bite occurs. The easiest and first step in preventing Lyme disease involves decreasing the risk of receiving an *Ixodes* tick bite and minimizing the duration of a bite if it does occur. In general, specific preventive measures consist of staying in the middle of trails when walking through wooded areas, avoiding tall grass and shrubs, wearing light-colored clothing to more easily spot any tick that may crawl onto clothing, wearing long pants tucked into socks, wearing shoes or closed-toed sandals, and wearing an effective tick repellent. Frequent checks for ticks are recommended because *B. burgdorferi* is usually not transmitted to humans unless a tick has been attached for at least 8 hours. If an attached tick is found, a pair of tweezers should be used to grasp the tick close to the skin as possible, and then it should be removed by pulling perpendicular to the skin with slow steady pressure.

Prophylactic Antibiotics

Recommendations on whether to give prophylactic antibiotics to persons after an *Ixodes* tick bite has generated controversy. In general, most experts do not recommend giving prophylactic antibiotics after a tick bite, except perhaps if the bite took place in a region highly endemic for Lyme disease. The recommendations not to give prophylactic antibiotics are based on several small studies that have shown the risk of having a significant antibiotic-related adverse event is approximately the same as the person developing Lyme disease. Those against giving prophylactic antibiotics would argue to defer antibiotic treatment until the onset of clinical symptoms suggest Lyme disease. Proponents for giving antibiotics argue that prophylactic antibiotics are inexpensive and effective in preventing Lyme disease. In addition, they argue that if prophylactic antibiotics are not given, approximately 30% of patients who develop Lyme disease will not have an obvious early clinical manifestations, and these persons may subsequently develop debilitating late-stage Lyme disease. Regardless of what experts have recommended, one study performed in Maryland has shown that prophylactic antibiotics are given more than 50% of the time in actual clinical practice. Moreover, this study showed that serologic testing was performed in approximately two thirds of patients who are evaluated for prophylactic antibiotics after a tick bite. Whether or not these persons receives prophylactic antibiotics, they should receive specific information on the signs and symptoms of early Lyme disease and should promptly return for further evaluation if they develop any signs or symptoms suggestive of Lyme disease.

Lyme Disease Vaccine

Two recombinant *B. burgdorferi* OspA Lyme disease vaccines have been developed and have undergone large-scale evaluation. Both of these vaccines contain 30 μg of OspA, but differ in that the SmithKline Beecham product *(LYMErix)* contains an aluminum adjuvant, whereas the Pasteur Merieux Connaught vaccine *(ImuLyme)* does not. The *LYMErix* vaccine had received FDA approval in the United States for persons aged 15 to 70 years, but was withdrawn from the U.S. market in early 2002. These vaccines have a novel mechanism of action in that they stimulate human antibodies to OspA, and these antibodies neutralize *B. burgdorferi* in the midgut of the *Ixodes* tick while the tick takes a blood meal. Because *B. burgdorferi* within the tick changes its outer protein covering from OspA to OspC after prolonged feeding, the human OspA antibodies would not likely provide reliable protection if *B. burgdorferi* entered the human bloodstream.

Large studies in adults with these two vaccines showed that both have a protective effect of more than 75% after three doses are given. In these studies, adverse effects of the vaccine were generally limited to mild, short-term, localized reactions at the vaccine injection site. Although these vaccines appear to be effective and safe, several concerns have been generated. First, no published data exist regarding the efficacy and safety of these vaccines in children. Second, the long-term immunogenicity of the vaccine remains unknown. Third, the vaccine can confound screening EIA serologic tests because antibodies to OspA are critical in most available EIA tests. Fourth, it is theoretically possible that persons who have received the vaccine could develop a delayed immunopathogenic response based on molecular mimicry the vaccine, although there has been no indication of this in trials.

REFERENCES

Bunikis J, Barbour AG: Laboratory testing for suspected Lyme disease, *Med Clin North Am* 86:311, 2002.

Burgdorfer W et al: Lyme disease a tick-borne spirochetosis? *Science* 216:1317, 1982.

Campbell GL et al: Estimation of the incidence of Lyme disease, *Am J Epidemiol* 148:1018, 1998.

Cassatt DR et al: DbpA, but not OspA, is expressed by *Borrelia burgdorferi* during spirochetemia and is a target for protective antibodies, *Infect Immunol* 66:5379, 1998.

Centers for Disease Control and Prevention: Lyme disease 1996, *MMWR* 46:531, 1997.

Centers for Disease Control and Prevention: Recommendations for test performance and interpretation from the Second National Conference on Serologic Diagnosis of Lyme Disease, *MMWR* 44:590, 1995.

Dattwyler RJ et al: Ceftriaxone compared with doxycycline for the treatment of acute disseminated Lyme disease, *N Engl J Med* 337:289, 1997.

Dennis DT et al: Reported distribution of *Ixodes scapularis* and *Ixodes pacificus* (Acari: Ixodidae) in the United States, *J Med Entomol* 35:629, 1998.

Fix AD, Strickland T, Grant J: Tick bites and Lyme disease in an endemic setting. Problematic use of serologic testing and prophylactic antibiotic therapy, *JAMA* 279:206, 1998.

Logigian EL, Kaplan RF, Steere AC: Chronic neurologic manifestations of Lyme disease, *N Engl J Med* 323:1438, 1990.

Massarotti EM: Lyme arthritis, *Med Clin North Am* 86:297, 2002.

Piesman J et al: Duration of adult female *Ixodes dammini* attachment and transmission of *Borrelia burgdorferi,* with description of a needle aspiration isolation method, *J Infect Dis* 163:895, 1991.
Sangha O et al: Lack of cardiac manifestations among persons with previously treated Lyme disease, *Ann Intern Med* 128:346, 1998.
Schwan TG et al: Induction of an outer surface protein on *Borrelia burgdorferi* during tick feeding, *Proc Natl Acad Sci USA* 92:2909, 1995.
Sigal LH: Persistent complaints attributed to chronic Lyme disease: possible mechanisms and implications for management, *Am J Med* 96:365, 1994.
Smith RP, Schoen RT, Rahn DW, et al: Clinical characteristics and treatment outcome of early Lyme disease in patients with microbiologically confirmed erythema migrans, *Ann Intern Med* 136:421, 2002.
Steere AC et al: Lyme arthritis: an epidemic of oligoarticular arthritis in children and adults in three Connecticut communities, *Arthritis Rheum* 20:7, 1977.
Steere AC et al: Vaccination against Lyme disease with recombinant *Borrelia burgdorferi* outer-surface lipoprotein A with adjuvant, *N Engl J Med* 339:209, 1998.
Steere AC et al: The overdiagnosis of Lyme disease, *JAMA* 269:1812, 1993.
Steere AC: Lyme disease, *N Engl J Med* 345:115, 2001.

CHAPTER 22

Tuberculosis in Travelers and Immigrants

Charles M. Nolan

In many countries of the world, tuberculosis is by far the most important preventable and treatable cause of morbidity and mortality. This fact alone dictates a healthy respect for tuberculosis, and a familiarity with its manifestations, diagnosis, and management in patients born outside the United States and in persons returning from foreign travel. In addition, the worldwide epidemic of acquired immunodeficiency syndrome (AIDS), resulting from infection with the human immunodeficiency viruses (HIV), has profoundly affected the epidemiology, clinical expression, and public health significance of tuberculosis. It is incumbent on all medical practitioners to understand the mutual interactions between HIV infection and tuberculosis, and the implications of these interactions on the prevention, diagnosis, and management of tuberculosis in travelers and immigrants. It is beyond the scope of this chapter to present an exhaustive review of this subject. Rather, pertinent information will be incorporated when considerations of HIV infection affect issues covered in this chapter related to the prevention and treatment of tuberculosis in U.S. residents traveling abroad and persons immigrating to the United States from foreign countries.

The American physician who encounters tuberculosis in a patient who has traveled abroad or in one from a foreign country is not seeing a new or "exotic" disease. The basic principles that underlie the approach to all patients with tuberculosis are still applicable and should be trusted. Nevertheless, there are special considerations in the evaluation and management of tuberculosis in the context of foreign origin or travel, and the purpose of this chapter is to point out those considerations.

In digesting the material in this chapter, the reader should not attempt to focus on individual facts so much as to assimilate general principles. For example, a busy practitioner should not expect to recall the prevalence of resistance to isoniazid among *Mycobacterium tuberculosis* isolates from persons who have immigrated from Korea, or to know whether bacille Calmette-Guérin (BCG) vaccine is used on a universal scale in Ethiopia; specific information of this nature is readily available. It is important, however, to know that in many parts of the world, resistance to isoniazid is greater than in the United States; that BCG vaccination, in common usage in much of the world, affects tuberculin reactivity; and that the risk of HIV infection varies widely according to the geographic origin of the patient.

In the approach to evaluation of patients with symptoms of pulmonary disease, health care providers need to remember that tuberculosis may simulate many other diseases. All standard texts note that pneumonia, lung abscess, neoplasm, and fungal and parasitic infections may be mimicked by tuberculosis. Also, the patient who originates from, or who has traveled to, a foreign country presents an additional diagnostic challenge. For example, coccidioidomycosis is prevalent in persons from northern Mexico, as it is in the southwestern United States, and it must be considered as a cause of fibrosing, cavitary pulmonary disease in Mexican immigrants.

On the other hand, deep tissue fungal infections are rare in refugees from Southeast Asia. In this population, another chronic pleuropulmonary infection, paragonimiasis or lung fluke infection, is more often confused with tuberculosis. Paragonimiasis is endemic in Asian countries and must be suspected, particularly when the history of raw crayfish consumption is reported. The clinical illness produced by paragonimiasis may be indistinguishable from that resulting from tuberculosis, and chest x-ray findings are also similar. The diagnosis is made by locating the parasite in microscopic smears of sputum or in lung biopsy specimens. Serologic testing is available commercially or through the Centers for Disease Control and Prevention (see Appendix).

EPIDEMIOLOGY

The worldwide epidemiology of tuberculosis has been dramatically affected by the AIDS pandemic. For example, after decades of decline in the United States, tuberculosis resurged in the late 1980s because of the new risk factor, HIV infection, along with increased migration from high-prevalence countries and dismantling of the public health infrastructure for tuberculosis control. In the late 1990s, however, morbidity resulting from tuberculosis has declined, with 6 consecutive years of decreasing case numbers and rates from 1993 to 1998. The incidence of tuberculosis in the United States in 1998 was 6.8 cases per 100,000 population, the lowest ever recorded. By contrast, in sub-Saharan Africa, where one of four adults may have HIV infection, tuberculosis case rates exceed 250 per 100,000. Even higher incidences have been recorded in some Asian countries. In Cambodia and the Philippines, where at the time of this writing HIV infection is negligible, tuberculosis annual case rates exceed 300 per 100,000.

Two practical considerations arise from an understanding of tuberculosis incidence rates. First, in areas of high incidence, the disease circulates widely and the population tends to develop tuberculosis infection at an early age. Whereas among children entering school in the United States only a very small percentage have a positive tuberculin test, among Somali immigrants of comparable age, as many as 20% may have tuberculosis infection. When it is considered that the early childhood and pubertal years are times of increased risk for reactivation of tuberculosis, it follows that for children who have immigrated from areas of the world with a high incidence of tuberculosis, the index of suspicion for tuberculosis must be high during the evaluation of a compatible illness.

Second, it is important to understand that immigrants bring with them to their new home their previous annual risk of tuberculosis. Immigrants resettling in a new country continue, at least for a few years, to experience the annual risk of tuberculosis that exists in the country from which they departed. Thus a physician evaluating a recent refugee from Vietnam with cough and weight loss must take into account that tuberculosis is 50 times as likely to occur each year (given an incidence rate of 300 per 100,000 per year in Vietnam) as in a patient indigenous to the United States (where the incidence of tuberculosis is 7 per 100,000 per year) with similar symptoms.

Mycobacterium bovis and Nontuberculous Mycobacterial Infection

In evaluations for tuberculosis in patients who have lived or traveled abroad, *M. bovis* must be included. *M. bovis* infection is historically acquired by consumption of milk from infected cows. The organism may penetrate gastrointestinal mucosa, invade mesenteric lymphatic tissue, and then follow pathways of lymphohematogenous spread, as outlined in Fig. 22-1 for *M. tuberculosis.* Human infection with *M. bovis* has essentially been eliminated in developed countries as a result of the pasteurization of milk and tuberculosis-control programs for cattle. Even though these two control measures are generally absent in developing countries, infection caused by *M. bovis* is only rarely recognized in immigrants to the United States from these regions.

Extrapulmonary Tuberculosis

Also uncommon in patients from Asia and the Pacific Islands are extrapulmonary infections caused by mycobacteria other than *M. tuberculosis.* The importance of this fact, from a practical point of view, is that cervical adenitis in refugee or immigrant children from African or Asian countries should be presumed to be as a result of *M. tuberculosis* rather than to other mycobacteria, as would be the presumption in American children with cervical adenitis.

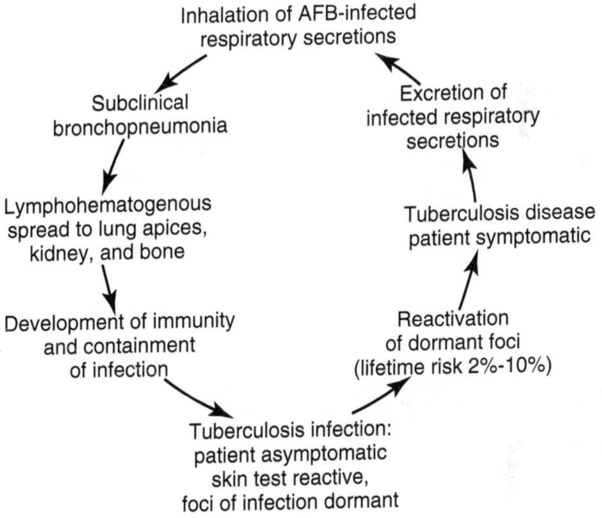

Fig. 22-1 Pathogenesis of tuberculosis.

Tuberculosis in Tourists

Despite the high incidence of tuberculosis in much of the world, American tourists to high-incidence areas are not at significant risk of exposure. The reason for this apparent paradox is that tuberculosis is not generally spread by casual personal contact. For example, careful epidemiologic studies have shown that regular contact with infectious individuals, even in an occupational setting, usually does not result in transmission of infection. The most important determinant of transmission is close ongoing contact with an infected person, such as occurs among family members.

Thus Americans visiting a high-incidence area who follow normal tourist routes for a period of no more than 2 to 3 weeks are unlikely to experience sufficient personal contact with infectious persons to acquire tuberculosis infection.

Tuberculosis in Americans with foreign travel histories is much more likely to occur in those who have traveled or lived abroad for more than several months. For instance, during the past 8 years, only a handful of cases of tuberculosis were diagnosed at the Seattle-King County Department of Public Health Tuberculosis Clinic in Americans with histories of foreign travel: a 23-year-old Peace Corps worker who had resided in Somalia for 18 months, a 40-year-old construction worker who had just returned from a 9-month tour in the Philippine Islands, a 56-year-old merchant seaman who spends at least 6 months of each year at sea and disembarking at ports in the western Pacific, a 28-year-old female medical student who spent 3 months working at a missionary hospital in India, and a 27-year-old man who had traveled for 5 months in the Indian subcontinent and Asia.

Although a number of chronic illnesses and therapies have long been known to increase the risk of reactivation of tuberculosis (see Pathogenesis), HIV infection is without historical precedence as a potential risk factor for progression of tuberculosis infection to disease. Whereas the average annual risk of tuberculosis in a skin test-positive person is approximately 1 in 1000, in an HIV-seropositive person, that annual risk may be as high as 5 in 100, a 50-fold annual increase in risk. This staggering increase is presumably due to the dysfunction in cellular immunity that is a hallmark of progressive HIV infection and AIDS.

In addition to the risk of reactivation of tuberculosis in people with HIV infection, several studies have described an increased incidence of active tuberculosis in the population group that occurs soon after initial exposure to an infectious case. This alarming phenomenon, which could have significant implications for HIV-infected travelers who may have chance, casual contact with infectious persons during travel in areas of high tuberculosis incidence, must receive urgent study.

ETIOLOGY

Tuberculosis is caused by *M. tuberculosis,* one of a family of bacterial rods characterized by the waxy component of their cell wall, mycolic acid. The designation of *M. tuberculosis* as the "acid-fast bacillus" derives from its distinguishing staining property—resistance to decolorization by acid alcohol when stained with basic fuchsin.

PATHOGENESIS

The pathogenesis of human tuberculosis is outlined in Figure 22-1. The usual mode of transmission is inhalation and implantation of respiratory secretions containing *M. tuberculosis,* the causative organism, on the respiratory bronchiole or lung alveolus, both of which lie beyond the protective mucociliary blanket of the respiratory tree. The subsequent steps in the pathogenic process that lead to tuberculosis infection generally occur without knowledge of the host. From the initial implantation site in the lungs, there may be silent lymphohematogenous spread to other organs. *Mycobacterium tuberculosis* is an obligate aerobe and thrives best when the PO_2 is 100 mm Hg or more. The organs most commonly affected by tuberculosis are those with the highest oxygen tension: the apices of the lungs, the kidneys, and the growing ends of long bones.

When the immune process stimulated by the infection becomes operative, it virtually always contains the disseminated infection. Therefore, in most patients, latent tuberculosis infection is marked only by the presence of a positive tuberculin skin test. A small proportion of infected individuals show fibrotic or fibrocalcific lesions in the upper lung fields on chest-x-ray study, presumably as a result of self-limited pulmonary disease that occurred in subclinical fashion in the past.

Most cases of active tuberculosis arise from reactivation of dormant foci of infection. All the factors that determine the small proportion of individuals whose tuberculosis infections will become reactivated are not known. However, certain conditions are known to increase the risk of reactivation: (1) recent exposure to an infectious case, or recent conversion of the tuberculin test from negative to positive, (2) silicosis, (3) diabetes mellitus, (4) diseases (e.g., HIV infection) or drug therapy (e.g., corticosteroids) associated with immunosuppression of cell-mediated immunity, and (5) conditions associated with lowered body weight, such as gastrectomy and malnutrition. Resistance to reactivation of tuberculosis also appears to be lower at certain times during the life span, particularly the first several years of life, during puberty, and in the postpartum period.

According to current knowledge, *the individual with tuberculosis infection generally is resistant to reinfection.* The major risk for tuberculosis in such individuals is that associated with reactivation of the dormant infection.

CLINICAL FEATURES

Pulmonary Tuberculosis

The onset of symptoms and signs of tuberculosis is usually gradual, over a period of weeks or months. The first symptoms are often nonspecific, consisting of fatigue, anorexia, weight loss, irregular menses, or low-grade fever. Symptoms such as these are often attributed to overwork or emotional stress. Pulmonary symptoms usually include a cough, often of imperceptible onset, which slowly progresses over weeks or months to become more frequent and finally to be associated with the production of mucoid or mucopurulent sputum. Dyspnea is uncommon.

Two symptoms that may be misleading in foreign patients are sweats and hemoptysis. These two symptoms are included among classic symptoms of pulmonary tuberculosis, but are in fact uncommon. Furthermore, it is difficult to translate these descriptive terms to other languages. Consequently, among some immigrant populations, night sweats and hemoptysis are reported so frequently as to render them virtually useless in an evaluation of tuberculosis.

Chest pain is also an uncommon symptom of tuberculosis, but, for unknown reasons, is frequently reported by refugees from Southeast Asia. When chest pain does occur, especially when there is a respiratory component, pleural effusion should be suspected.

Extrapulmonary Tuberculosis

The symptoms and signs of extrapulmonary tuberculosis generally relate specifically to the affected organ system. Lymphatic tuberculosis, which is particularly common in Asians and Africans, may involve any regional lymph nodes, but most often affects those of the neck and supraclavicular regions (scrofula). Tuberculosis of the bone and joints usually causes extreme and persistent localized pain and swelling. An exception may be Pott's disease of the spine, which can progress insidiously and become advanced before diagnosis.

Tuberculosis in Children

Tuberculosis in children from other countries, for whom English is not the primary language, is particularly difficult to diagnose. Hilar adenopathy, sufficiently extensive to cause the right middle lobe syndrome, may be entirely asymptomatic. The early stages of miliary tuberculosis may produce little in the way of specific symptoms in children, particularly when the history must be obtained through an interpreter.

Tuberculosis in Persons with HIV Infection

The onset and clinical course of symptoms of tuberculosis in persons with HIV infection may be similar to those in other patients, particularly if tuberculosis occurs, as it often does, early in the course of HIV infection as the first opportunistic infection. On the other hand, the symptoms of tuberculosis may be indistinguishable from other respiratory diseases to which HIV-infected patients are subject, such as *Pneumocystis carinii* pneumonia and bacterial pneumonia, and even those of progressive HIV infection itself. A high index of suspicion for the diagnosis must be maintained. Extrapulmonary tuberculosis, including military and meningeal tuberculosis, occurs with increased frequency in persons with HIV infection. These two forms of tuberculosis are uniformly lethal if not recognized and treated promptly. Consequently, they must be included in the differential diagnosis when persons with HIV infection experience a severe, abrupt illness with nonspecific signs, neurologic symptoms, or headache. Also, in Africa, a high proportion of patients with "slim disease," the wasting syndrome attributed to AIDS, who come to autopsy are found to have had unsuspected tuberculosis.

DIAGNOSIS

Radiographic Findings

Immunologically competent patients with pulmonary tuberculosis who have disease sufficient to cause symptoms will virtually always have an abnormal chest x-ray film. In contrast, pulmonary tuberculosis is regularly, if not frequently, encountered in HIV-infected patients even though the chest x-ray film shows only subtle, usually diffuse, changes. In immunocompetent adults, lesions resulting from tuberculosis usually occur in the apical and posterior segments of the upper lobes or in the superior segments of the lower lobes, but again this is not the rule in the patient with HIV infection. In such patients, tuberculosis is associated with a wide variety of radiographic changes, nearly all of which are also associated with hilar or mediastinal adenopathy or both; these include lobar consolidation, patchy pneumonitis, and diffuse "miliary" infiltration. Cavitation is not frequent. Indeed, it has been said, in respect to the variegated radiographic presentation of pulmonary tuberculosis in HIV-infected patients, that all such patients with respiratory symptoms must be suspected to have tuberculosis.

Hilar and mediastinal adenopathy are not commonly seen with pulmonary tuberculosis in immunologically competent adults. When noted, another diagnosis, such as lymphoma, should be considered. In children, however, active primary tuberculosis virtually always includes hilar or mediastinal adenopathy, or both. The adenopathy noted on the radiograph is usually unilateral, and in approximately half the cases is associated with parenchymal infiltration.

Skin Testing

The tuberculin skin test is a time-honored diagnostic aid in the evaluation of a patient with suspected infection, but its limitations must be understood. For example, latent tuberculosis *infection* (Fig. 22-1) is marked by a significant reaction to the tuberculin skin test, but the test is unable to differentiate patients who have *disease* due to tuberculosis from those who merely have latent infection with no disease. When used appropriately, however, the skin test can yield valuable epidemiologic information and identify individuals who may be at high risk for disease. For example, in the current case registry of active tuberculosis patients in Seattle-King County, Washington, 92% of patients have a positive tuberculin reaction.

It has recently been appreciated that the utility of the tuberculin test as a screening tool for tuberculosis infection can be enhanced if the cutoff-point between a positive and negative test varies inversely with either the risk of tuberculosis infection, or the risk of tuberculosis disease, given infection (Table 22-1). Thus the lowest cutoff-point, 5 mm, should apply to those at highest risk of infection and/or disease, such as persons with HIV infection and recently infected persons such as contacts of infectious cases and persons who have recently converted their skin test reactivity from negative to positive. The highest cutoff-point, 15 mm, should apply to those who lack all identified risk factors. The adoption of these guidelines for interpretation of the tuberculin skin test has considerably improved its utility in identifying persons most likely to be at risk of tuberculosis and to benefit from preventive therapy (see later discussions).

Culture of Tubercle Bacilli

The recovery on culture of *M. tuberculosis* is essential for the definitive diagnosis of tuberculosis. Thus the patient suspected of having mycobacterial disease according to epidemiologic information signs and symptoms, the tuberculin skin test, and the chest x-ray study should have the appropriate specimens submitted for culture. Most patients with pulmonary tuberculosis are able to produce specimens of sputum that yield *M. tuberculosis* upon culture. Sputum specimens submitted for culture should always be examined microscopically for the presence of tubercle bacilli in sputum smears using acid-fast or fluorescent antibody staining.

Many patients with pulmonary tuberculosis, particularly those with advanced symptoms and radiographic signs, and virtually all those with cavitary tuberculosis have sputum smears positive for acid-fast bacilli. Nevertheless, the absence of such a finding should not lead the clinician away from the diagnosis of tuberculosis. At least one third of patients with pulmonary tuberculosis that produce positive sputum cultures have negative sputum smears. One practical implication of the smear-negative patient with tuberculosis is that the individual should be considered to be of low infectivity for others.

Invasive procedures, such as bronchoscopy and lung biopsy, are usually not necessary to establish the diagnosis of pulmonary tuberculosis. In gen-

Table 22-1
Interpretation of Mantoux Tuberculin Test*

5 mm Induration	>10 mm Induration	>15 mm Induration
Deemed Significant in:	**Deemed Significant in:**	**Deemed Significant in:**
Persons with HIV infection IV drug users with unknown HIV status Persons with history of close contact with infectious tuberculosis Persons whose chest x-ray film shows fibrotic lesions likely to represent old, healed tuberculosis	Persons born in high-prevalence countries in Asia, Africa, and Latin America IV drug users known to he HIV seronegative Persons from low-income, medically underserved populations Residents of long-term care facilities Locally identified high-risk populations (e.g., the homeless) Persons with medical conditions reported to increase risk of tuberculosis once infection has occurred (e.g., silicosis, gastrectomy, chronic renal failure, diabetes mellitus, immunosuppressive therapy, and hematologic and other malignancies) Health care workers serving high-risk populations	Persons without risk factors listed in previous two columns

From Bernardo J: Tuberculosis: a disease of the 1990s, *Hosp Pract* 26:195,1991.
*From Centers for Disease Control and Prevention and American Thoracic Society. Test performed by intradermal injection of 0.1 ml of PPD-S, containing 5 TU, usually into forearm, with reading at 48 to 72 hours (although positive reaction may still be measurable 1 week after injection). Induration is measured *across* forearm, ignoring any erythema.

eral, several negative sputum cultures, when they have been collected and cultured appropriately, rule out the diagnosis of tuberculosis. An exception to this rule occurs in primary tuberculosis in children and in persons with HIV infection. Children with hilar and mediastinal lymphadenopathy typically have negative sputum smears, and in this instance a positive culture is not required for the diagnosis. Because of similarity in the onsets, symptoms, and radiographic appearances of several AIDS-associated respiratory diseases, including tuberculosis, it is often prudent to perform bronchoscopy to obtain additional material for smear and culture, to arrive at the correct diagnosis, and to begin appropriate therapy as rapidly as possible.

Compared with most bacteria, *M. tuberculosis* multiplies very slowly, dividing every 18 to 24 hours. Using the most modern method of culture, the isolation and identification of the causative organism require 10 to 20 days. The fact that isolation and identification are prolonged has important implications in the initial approach and the early management of patients suspected of having tuberculosis.

When extrapulmonary tuberculosis is suspected on clinical grounds, it is usually necessary to obtain tissue or other body fluids from the affected sites to establish the diagnosis. Whenever possible, tissue obtained from either open or closed biopsy should be cultured, as well as any aspirated fluid; the yield on culture will be improved. This is particularly true with pleural and lymphatic tuberculosis, in which culture of tissue gives a greater yield than culture of aspirated fluid.

TREATMENT

The goals of tuberculosis treatment are (1) to eliminate death and decrease disability resulting from tuberculosis in individual patients and (2) to interrupt and prevent transmission of the tubercle bacilli to contacts of an infectious patient. With available chemotherapeutic agents, both goals are readily achievable. However, the treatment of tuberculosis is unusual among infectious diseases in that long-term therapy, measured in months rather than days or weeks, is necessary.

The five most commonly used antituberculous drugs are described in Table 22-2. In addition to these agents, several others are available: the quinolone drugs ciprofloxacin and levofloxacin, and capreomycin, kanamycin, ethionamide, and cycloserine. However, when it is necessary to use these alternative agents in an antituberculous regimen, a chest or infectious disease specialist should be consulted. Compared with the drugs described in Table 22-2, these are less potent against *M. tuberculosis* and are difficult to administer because of potentially dangerous side effects.

It is always necessary to treat *active tuberculosis* with at least two drugs known to be potent against the infecting organism. Thus susceptibility testing of *M. tuberculosis* isolates is an essential component of optimum management of a case of active tuberculosis. Throughout the United States, susceptibility testing of tuberculosis is available free of cost through local or state health departments.

The initial empiric treatment regimen should consist of four drugs for the first 2 months: isoniazid, rifampin, pyrazinamide, and ethambutol or streptomycin. This regimen gives excellent results in pulmonary, extrapulmonary, and primary tuberculosis. The regimen can be altered as appropriate after the results of sensitivity testing on the patient's isolate are known. If drug susceptibility tests are not available, pyrazinamide may be discontinued at 8 weeks, but ethambutol or streptomycin should be continued along with isoniazid and rifampin for a total of 6 months.

Nearly all patients receiving this regimen, including those with HIV infection, will convert sputum cultures from positive to negative within 3 months of starting treatment. If a patient is still culture-positive at that time, monthly sputum cultures should be performed and the duration of total treatment should be extended to at least 3 months beyond the time of sputum conversion. The patient with persistently positive sputum cultures despite initial four-drug therapy should be suspected either of being noncompliant or of having a drug-resistant infection.

Most patients with HIV infection who contract tuberculosis respond well to routine treatment as described previously. Indeed, tuberculosis is the most treatable of all the life-threatening opportunistic infections asso-

Table 22-2
Chemotherapeutic Agents Commonly Used to Treat Tuberculosis

Drug	Daily dose	Side effects	Interactions	Remarks
Isoniazid	5-10 mg/kg up to 300 mg PO	Hepatitis, peripheral neuritis, rash, dizziness	Potentiation of phenytoin, Antabuse	Inexpensive Used in treatment of TB infection and TB disease
Rifampin	10-15 mg/kg up to 600 mg PO	Hyperbilirubinemia, fever, purpura	Inhibition of many drugs: oral contraceptives, quinidine, coumarin drugs, digoxin, oral hypoglycemics, HIV protease inhibitors, certain nonnucleoside reverse-transcriptase inhibitors	Colors urine and other body secretions orange
Ethambutol	15-25 mg/kg PO	Optic neuritis (rare at 15 mg/kg), reversible, rash		Use with caution in patients with renal disease and when eye testing is not possible
Pyrazinamide	20-25 mg/kg up to 2 g PO	Hyperuricemia, rash, hepatitis		When used for the first 2 months with isoniazid and rifampin, can shorten total duration of therapy to 6 months
Streptomycin	15-20 mg/kg up to 1 g IM	Eighth cranial nerve and renal toxicity	Potentiation of neuromuscular blocking agents	Use with caution in older patients and in those with renal disease

ciated with AIDS. Nevertheless, some authorities recommend extending the total duration of therapy for tuberculosis in such patients an additional 3 months (for a total of 9 months) because of the possibility of relapse resulting from failing immunity. In any case, treatment of tuberculosis in persons with HIV infection should be individualized, and the patient should be monitored closely throughout the course of treatment to ensure that the response has been satisfactory.

Drug Resistance

Whereas the prevalence of resistance to the five primary antituberculous drugs in Table 22-2 is less than 10% in the United States, it is higher in *M. tuberculosis* isolates from other parts of the world. Thus the prevalence of resistance to isoniazid among infecting organisms from Southeast Asian immigrants is 10% to 15%, and among Philippine immigrants it is 15% to 25%. Other areas with prevalences of isoniazid resistance greater than that in the United States are Africa, Central and South America, and countries of Asia and the Pacific Islands.

A prime factor in the development of isoniazid resistance is suspected to be uncontrolled and inappropriate use and formulation of the drug, typified by the small concentrations of isoniazid in some cough syrup preparations and the brief use of isoniazid in the treatment of nonspecific respiratory illnesses.

When applying available information on *M. tuberculosis* drug resistance to the management of the individual patient with tuberculosis, several important principles of treatment emerge:

- When there is a reasonable possibility that a patient with tuberculosis acquired the infection in a country with high isoniazid resistance rates, drug susceptibility testing is absolutely mandatory.
- Treatment before the time results of susceptibility testing are available (3 to 6 weeks from the time of presumptive diagnosis) must include at least two drugs to which the infecting organism is likely to be susceptible. For patients receiving a diagnosis of tuberculosis in the United States, regardless of national origin, the initial recommended four-drug regimen of isoniazid, rifampin, pyrazinamide, and ethambutol or streptomycin will guarantee adequate treatment while awaiting susceptibility testing in more than 95% of patients.
- When susceptibility test results indicate that the infecting organism is susceptible to isoniazid and rifampin, ethambutol can be discontinued. Pyrazinamide may be withdrawn after 2 months, and the total length of treatment should be 6 months. If the infecting organism is resistant to isoniazid, that drug should be stopped and the other three agents of the original regimen—rifampin, pyrazinamide, and ethambutol—should be continued for 6 months. In patients with isoniazid-resistant tuberculosis, the response to therapy must be monitored carefully.

In the rare instance in which resistance to two of the three agents is encountered, some prior treatment is almost certain. An unexpected sequel of the AIDS epidemic was the appearance, on the eastern U.S. seacoast, of cases of tuberculosis that were resistant to several antituberculosis drugs, including isoniazid and rifampin. This multidrug-resistant variety of tuberculosis runs a rampant, fatal course in patients with AIDS and has been documented to spread from such patients to other patients and to health care personnel in hospitals, clinics, and correctional facilities. This unfortunate offshoot of the AIDS epidemic underscored several important needs: safer hospital environments, a larger armamentarium of antituberculosis drugs, and a strong public health infrastructure to prevent and control dangerous communicable diseases.

Multidrug-resistant tuberculosis (MDR-TB) associated with HIV infection, but also occurring in patients without that diagnosis, has now been identified throughout the world. In fact, with the subsidence of HIV-associated, multidrug-resistant tuberculosis, the predominant risk factor for MDR-TB in the United States is foreign birth. During the last 8 years, all 18 MDR-TB cases diagnosed in patients evaluated at the Seattle-King County Department of Public Health TB Clinic were foreign-born. Thus physicians who practice travel medicine must remain aware of international trends of this ominous "new" variety of tuberculosis, MDR-TB. Finally, immigrants with MDR-TB are likely to have chronic infections with extensive lung damage. Treatment of tuberculosis in this setting is exceedingly difficult and has significant public health, as well as personal health, implications. Such patients should invariably be referred for consultation to a chest of infectious disease specialist.

Precautions and Contraindications

Three drugs in the antituberculosis armamentarium are safe for use in pregnancy: isoniazid, rifampin, and ethambutol. Streptomycin may have nephrotoxic effects and should be avoided in persons with renal disease. Further, ethambutol is excreted via the kidneys. Thus, if it must be used in patients with renal disease, blood levels may be needed to determine appropriate dosing. Patients with mild liver disease are usually able to tolerate a regimen of isoniazid, rifampin, and pyrazinamide. Specifically, there seems to be no added risk of liver damage from the use of antituberculous drugs in patients who are chronic asymptomatic carriers of the hepatitis B surface antigen, but the safety of antituberculosis regimens for persons with chronic hepatitis C is not known.

With the development of highly active antiretroviral therapy for patients with HIV infection, treatment of tuberculosis in persons with HIV infection has become more complicated. For example, rifampin, a mainstay of tuberculosis treatment, must be avoided in patients receiving therapy with HIV protease inhibitors and certain nonnucleoside reverse-transcriptase inhibitors, because rifampin accelerates the metabolism of those agents and lessens their antiretroviral effect. Given the increasing complexity of treatment of HIV infection, it is preferable for a clinician with training and expertise in managing both HIV infection and tuberculosis to supervise the treatment of tuberculosis in such patients.

Problems with Patient Compliance

Because of the long duration of the drug therapy that is required to cure a case of active tuberculosis, patient compliance (i.e., the ability of patients to take their medications as advised) is a major issue. When treatment is based on susceptibility testing as described earlier, failure to eradicate the infection is virtually always due to noncompliance, even in patients with HIV infection.

Although a number of tests are available to monitor compliance, most noncompliant patients are discovered by their failure to return for follow-up clinic visits. Compliance must be monitored with particular care during treatment of tubercular patients who are from other parts of the world. When the patient originates from a culture with vastly different concepts of health and illness, or when there is a language barrier so that the communication and understanding of medical advice is difficult, noncompliance is highly likely.

Patient noncompliance with prescribed antituberculosis medications has an adverse effect on both the personal and public health goals of tuberculosis treatment. Therefore it is mandatory that the practitioner who suspects noncompliance for any reason report the suspicion to the local health department and, unless there are extraordinary circumstances to consider, to refer the case for management to the appropriate public health tuberculosis clinic. Most public health tuberculosis clinics in the United States use directly observed therapy (DOT)—a concept of treatment in which every dose of medication is administered under direct observation by health services personnel—for some or all of their tuberculosis patients. Because of the key role of drug therapy in terminating the spread of tuberculosis and in preventing MDR-TB, DOT is increasingly the standard of care for tuberculosis treatment in the United States.

PREVENTION

Although medical practice has traditionally focused on curing human disease, there is currently a wide interest in disease prevention and health maintenance. In this context, medical practitioners who deal with foreign patients have both the opportunity and the responsibility to practice preventive medicine with respect to tuberculosis in that population.

Review of the pathogenesis of tuberculosis (Fig. 22-1) reveals that there are two targets for prevention of tuberculosis: (1) prevention of acquiring latent tuberculosis infection in unexposed persons and (2) in those who already have latent tuberculosis infection, progression of latent tuberculosis infection to disease. The primary way to prevent the acquisition of latent tuberculosis infection is to eliminate the excretion of tubercle bacilli from the sputum of infectious patients. This is readily done, as noted previously, by administering effective chemotherapy to persons with pulmonary tuberculosis. From a practical viewpoint, once an infectious individual is started on adequate chemotherapy, he or she ceases to spread the infection.

A second means of preventing tuberculosis infection is vaccination with BCG, a live vaccine made from an attenuated strain of *M. bovis*. BCG has been used for decades for the prevention of tuberculosis in infants and children in many parts of the world. However, because of uncertainty regarding its efficacy, it was never chosen for use in tuberculosis control programs in this country. (See Chapter 4 for additional information on BCG use in the United States.)

The second line of approach to prevention of tuberculosis—preventing disease in those with tuberculosis infection—has a place in modern private medical practice. A number of studies by the U.S. Public Health Service in the 1950s and 1960s showed that administration of isoniazid, 300 mg/day for 6 months to 1 year, had a 50% to 80% efficacy rate in preventing tuberculosis disease in persons with latent tuberculosis infection. The protective effect of isoniazid preventive therapy is believed to be lifelong.

Recent studies in HIV-infected persons have also verified that a regimen of rifampin plus pyrazinamide given for 2 months confers protection equal to that of isoniazid for persons with latent tuberculosis infection. Based on those studies, a new set of guidelines for management of persons with latent tuberculosis infection has been prepared by experts from the Centers of Disease Control and Prevention (CDC) and the American

Thoracic Society (ATS). Table 22-3 reviews the current treatment alternatives for persons with latent tuberculosis infection. According to those recent CDC/ATS guidelines, the criteria for treatment of latent tuberculosis infection have also been simplified. Treatment should be offered to such persons if:

1. They may have been recently infected with *M. tuberculosis.* Recent infection is likely in contacts of infectious cases of tuberculosis, in persons who have converted their tuberculin skin test from negative to positive within a 2-year period, in persons who have recently immigrated from parts of the world where the incidence of tuberculosis is high, and in children with a positive skin test.

2. They have medical conditions that raise the risk of progression from latent tuberculosis infection to clinical tuberculosis. Medical conditions that raise the risk of developing tuberculosis include HIV infection; treatment with immunosuppressive medications such as corticosteroids; diabetes mellitus; certain malignancies; conditions associated with low weight for height such as malnutrition, gastrectomy, and intestinal bypass surgery; and fibrotic pulmonary lesions consistent with inactive pulmonary tuberculosis.

Patients receiving preventive therapy with either isoniazid or the rifampin-pyrazinamide regimen should be seen monthly during treatment and given prescriptions for 1-month supplies of medicine at each follow-up appointment. Personal interviews for compliance checks and side effects should be performed at these monthly intervals. The most important side effect of isoniazid is hepatotoxicity. Although potentially fatal, the frequency of this side effect is very low. Every patient that starts isoniazid preventive therapy should be informed about the symptoms of hepatotoxicity and instructed to stop treatment immediately if such symptoms develop. Patients capable of following these instructions do not require laboratory monitoring of hepatocellular enzymes during isoniazid treatment.

The side effects of rifampin-pyrazinamide preventive therapy are not well defined. Pyrazinamide tends to elevate the concentration of uric

Table 22-3
Drug Regimens Recommended by the American Thoracic Society and the Centers for Disease Control and Prevention for the Treatment of Latent Tuberculosis Infection

Drug(s)	Duration	Rating
Isoniazid	9 months	Preferred
Isoniazid*	6 months	Acceptable alternative
Rifampin-pyrazinamide	2 months	Acceptable alternative
Rifampin†	4 months	Acceptable alternative

American Thoracic Society and Centers for Disease Control and Prevention: Targeted tuberculin testing and treatment of latent tuberculosis infection, *Am J Respir Crit Care Med* (in press).
*Acceptable when 9 months of isoniazid treatment is not possible to administer.
†Acceptable when pyrazinamide, started in the 2-month regimen, cannot be continued.

acid in serum and may cause arthralgias. That agent has also been associated with hepatotoxicity. It is recommended that patients receiving rifampin and pyrazinamide for 2 months should be evaluated at least clinically and with liver function testing at 2, 4, and 8 weeks for compliance with the regimen and possible side effects.

REFERENCES

Bass JB Jr et al: Treatment of tuberculosis and tuberculosis infection in adults and children. American Thoracic Society and Centers for Disease Control and Prevention, *Am J Respir Crit Care Med* 149:1359, 1994.

Centers for Disease Control and Prevention: Notice to Readers: Updated guidelines for the use of rifabutin or rifampin for the treatment and prevention of tuberculosis among HIV-infected patients taking protease inhibitors or nonnucleoside reverse transcriptase inhibitors, MMWR 49:185, 2000.

Centers for Disease Control and Prevention: Tuberculosis elimination revisited: obstacles, opportunities, and a renewed commitment. Advisory Council for the Elimination of Tuberculosis (ACET), *MMWR* 48(RR-09):1, 1999.

Centers for Disease Control and Prevention: Recommendation for prevention and control of tuberculosis among foreign-born persons: Report of the Working Group on Tuberculosis Among Foreign-Born Persons, *MMWR* 47(RR-16):1, 1998.

Centers for Disease Control and Prevention: Prevention and treatment of tuberculosis among patients infected with human immunodeficiency virus: principles of therapy and revised recommendations, *MMWR* 47(RR-20):1, 1998.

Centers for Disease Control and Prevention: The role of BCG vaccine in the prevention and control of tuberculosis in the United States: a joint statement by the Advisory Council for the Elimination of Tuberculosis and the Advisory Committee on Immunization Practices, *MMWR* 45(RR-4):1, 1996.

Dye C et al: Global burden of tuberculosis. Estimated incidence, prevalence, and mortality by country, *JAMA* 282:677, 1999.

Havlir DV, Barnes PF: Tuberculosis in patients with human immunodeficiency virus infection, *N Engl J Med* 340:367, 1999.

Nolan CM: Community-wide implementation of targeted testing and treatment of latent tuberculosis infection, *Clin Infect Dis* 29:880, 1999.

Nolan CM, Goldberg SV, Buskin SE: Hepatotoxicity associated with isoniazid preventive therapy: a 7-year survey from a public health tuberculosis clinic, *JAMA* 281:1014, 1999.

CHAPTER 23

Chagas' Disease

Martin S. Cetron and Anne C. Moore

Chagas' disease, first described in 1909 by Carlos Chagas, is endemic throughout Central and South America. The World Health Organization (WHO) and others estimate 16 to 18 million people are infected with *Trypanosoma cruzi,* the etiologic agent of this disease. *T. cruzi,* a protozoan of the order Kinetoplastida, is parasitic to insects and a wide variety of mammals. Blood-sucking reduviid bugs serve as the principal transmission vector by depositing *T. cruzi*-infected feces onto the skin. The parasite is then inoculated into dermal breaks or mucosal surfaces by inadvertent rubbing or scratching. Most transmission occurs in poor rural areas, reflecting the natural habitat of the insect vector. Two other means of transmission occur in endemic regions: transfusion of parasite-contaminated blood, which is an increasing problem with the urbanization Chagas, and congenital transmission.

Recently, there has been an increase in reports of Chagas' disease in nonendemic areas. Forty-two cases of Chagas' disease (25 of which involved classic chagasic cardiomyopathy) were reported after a retrospective review of records from 1974 through 1990 at Los Angeles County Hospital by Hagar and Rahimtoola. All patients were Latin American immigrants who acquired their infection outside the United States. Estimates by some experts suggest there may be as many as 50,000 to 100,000 people infected with *T. cruzi* now residing within the United States.

EPIDEMIOLOGY

Parasite Distribution versus Disease Distribution

T. cruzi infection of vertebrate hosts and insect vectors occurs widely throughout the Americas from 42 degrees north latitude to 46 degrees south latitude. This encompasses much of the United States (although infection is especially prominent in Florida, Texas, and Louisiana) and extends through Mexico and Central America to most of South America. Transmission to humans, on the other hand, is more restricted, occurring mainly in endemic areas in Mexico, Central America, Ecuador, Colombia, Venezuela, Guyana, Suriname, French Guiana, Brazil, Paraguay, Uruguay, Argentina, Chile, Bolivia, and Peru (Fig. 23-1). Chagas' disease represents a serious health problem in 17 countries in Latin America, threatening 25% of the population. The prevalence of infection in Latin America is estimated to be 16 to 18 million seropositive individuals; 90 million are estimated to be at risk for acquiring the infection. Clinically overt chronic

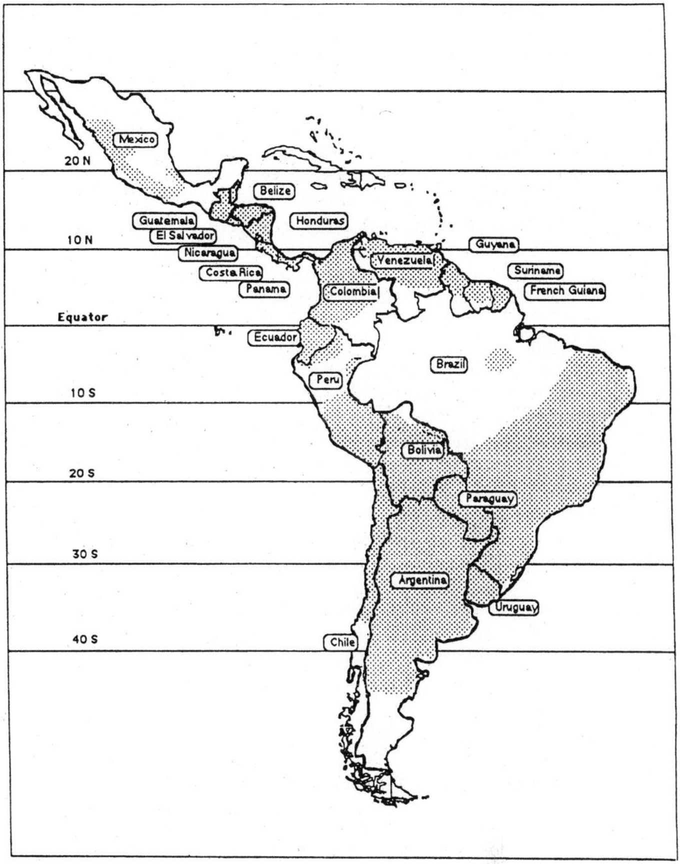

Fig. 23-1 Geographic distribution of *T. cruzi* infection. (From Epidemiology and control of African trypanosomiasis: Report of a WHO Expert Committee, *WHO Tech Rep Ser* 739:41, 1986.)

Chagas' disease occurs in approximately 20% to 30% of the infected individuals (i.e., about 5 million persons). These estimates vary widely depending on the intensity of the investigation, the geographic region involved, and the virulence of the strain of *T. cruzi.*

Vectors

T. cruzi infects many vertebrates and is transmitted by insects of the family Reduviidae, subfamily Triatominae. More than 100 triatomine species exist, each with its own feeding pattern, vertebrate host preference, and geographic/ecologic distribution. In the sylvatic cycle, the bugs prefer forested areas, but they become domesticated as a result of conversion of natural habitat to domestic uses. Most bug species prefer tropical climates with a temperature range from 24° to 30° C and relative humidity from 60% to 70%. Climatic factors account for increased transmission during the warmer months.

Triatoma infestans, T. dimidiata, Panstrongylus megistus, and *Rhodnius prolixus* are important vectors in human transmission. Colloquial names for the reduviid are commonly used (Table 23-1). In northeast Brazil, for example, they are known to locals as *barbeiros* or *bicudos*. The word *barbeiro* comes from the Portuguese word for barber, used because the bugs like to bite the exposed chin and neck. In Argentina, Uruguay, Bolivia, and Chile they are referred to as *vinchucas*. In English one hears the terms *bed bugs* or *kissing bugs,* which refer to the insect's preference for feeding at night and about the face of sleeping children.

Reservoir Hosts

T. cruzi is found in a broad range of species of sylvan mammals including monkeys, sloths, rodents, marsupials, rabbits, bats, and various carnivores. Humans can become infected by entering into the sylvatic transmission cycle of *T. cruzi,* but transmission primarily occurs because the reduviid vectors move into the domestic environment and infect peridomiciliary, then domestic animals. In endemic areas, the seroprevalence among domestic animals is high; studies have shown the following rates: 80% in dogs, 60% in cats, 19% in sheep, and 9% in goats. Guinea pigs and rabbits are often domesticated and have been shown to have a seroprevalence of 60% and 12%, respectively. Among rodents, up to 90% of mice and 60% of rats have been shown to be infected. In most cases, animals acquire their infection directly from insect bites, but in others the acquisition of infection appears to be via the food chain (e.g., cats eating infected mice).

Table 23-1
Popular Regional Names for Triatomine Bugs*

Name	Countries where used
Barbeiros, bicudos, chupanca, fincao, percevejo da parede	Brazil
Vinchucas	Argentina, Uruguay, Bolivia, Chile
Chirimacha or chinchon	Peru
Chupasangre	Ecuador
Chinche or chincha	Mexico, Colombia, Venezuela, Central America
Chinchona, chince picuda, or pik	Mexico
Chinchorro or chinchorra	Ecuador, Guatemala
Timbuck or chincha-guasu	Paraguay
Telepate	Guatemala, El Salvador
Bush chinch	Belize
Pito	Colombia
Cone nose bugs, kissing bugs, assassin bugs, Arizona tigers	United States

*Extracted from Garcia-Zapata MTA, Marsden PD: Chagas' disease, *Clin Trop Med Commun Dis* 1:558, 1986.

Transmission

Transmission by insect vector occurs in both sylvan and domestic cycles. It is the interface of these cycles, brought about by infected peridomiciliary animals such as rodents and, particularly, opossums, that leads to high rates of infection of more domestic animals, such as dogs, and eventually of humans. Triatomine vectors account for 95% of human infection. Chagas' disease tends to occur in low socioeconomic settings because of the primitive type of housing the reduviid bugs prefer. They tend first to colonize outbuildings, then move into houses built with walls of sticks and mud and covered with thatched roofs. Cracks in the walls and roofs provide the bugs with a daytime hiding place, as well as ready nighttime access to domestic animal and human hosts to obtain blood meals.

In some insectivorous animals, acquisition of the parasite is via the food chain. This has implications for transmission in countries such as Peru and Bolivia, where home-bred guinea pigs have a high prevalence of infection and serve as a reservoir of infection. It is rare, but human outbreaks following ingestion of food contaminated with infected insects or their feces have been documented.

TRANSFUSION- AND ORGAN TRANSPLANT-RELATED TRANSMISSION

Transfusion-related *T. cruzi* infection occurs because of population migration from rural to urban centers and insufficient blood bank screening programs. Between 12% and 48% of the recipients of infected blood will become infected, depending on the frequency and volume of transfusions. In Brazil the estimated number of transfusion-related infections has been as high as 20,000 per year over the last decade, although this is declining owing to increased screening of blood.

Whereas blood bank screening for antibodies to *T. cruzi* is available in several larger urban centers in Brazil (Rio de Janeiro, São Paulo, Belo Horizonte, Fortaleza, Salvador, and others), many smaller regions and poorer countries throughout Latin America (e.g., Bolivia) still lack sufficient technology and resources to ensure the safety of their blood supply. Previous strategies to sterilize blood from highly endemic areas have included the use of gentian violet. This is largely out of favor because of unacceptable staining of the skin in transfusion recipients. Increased Latin American immigration to the United States has generated concerns about the possibility of *T. cruzi* contamination of the U.S. blood supply. The issue is currently under discussion by U.S. health care authorities.

Transmission of Chagas' disease can occur through transplantation of organs from chronically infected donors. New infection in immunosuppressed transplant recipients can cause severe, sometimes fatal, acute Chagas' disease. A more common problem in reactivation of chronic Chagas' disease in immunosuppressed organ recipients. Reactivation in patients with acquired immunodeficiency syndrome has also been reported, most commonly presenting as a tumorlike lesion of the central nervous system or as an acute diffuse meningoencephalitis.

CONGENITAL TRANSMISSION

Congenital transmission is a more serious problem than previously realized, especially in highly endemic areas of Bolivia, Chile, and Brazil, where prevalence among offspring from seropositive pregnant mothers ranges from 4% to 10%. Congenital *T. cruzi* infection may be responsible for prematurity and small fetal size, although most infected newborns are asymptomatic.

It is known that parasitemia is common among infected neonates; hepatosplenomegaly, meningoencephalitis, hemorrhagic disorders, and disseminated cutaneous lesions are also well described.

Transmission by breastfeeding deserves mention because of the conflicting information previously available. Despite sporadic anecdotal reports implicating breast milk, the most recent systematic studies from Bahia (Brazil), Cordoba (Argentina), and Santa Cruz (Bolivia) do not support transmission of *T. cruzi* via colostrum. Current WHO policy explicitly states "there is no reason to restrict breast-feeding by *T. cruzi*-infected mothers."

CLINICAL FEATURES

Infection in humans is characterized by two principal stages: acute and chronic.

Acute Disease

Along with fever, patients experience local swelling at the inoculation site; this is referred to as a chagoma. If the conjunctiva or eyelid is the portal of entry, one may develop the classic unilateral periophthalmic cellulitis and palpebral edema referred to as *Romãna's sign.* This is a reliable diagnostic indicator seen in 90% of recognized acute cases. Flulike symptoms such as malaise, fever, rash, anorexia, diarrhea, and vomiting are common but nonspecific.

Acute Chagas' disease often passes undetected. It is diagnosed in only 1% to 2% of all cases, but electrocardiographic (ECG) or radiographic evidence of acute myocarditis is found in as many as 30% of acute cases if it is sought. Fulminant systemic symptoms requiring hospitalization occur only occasionally during acute Chagas' disease, but include generalized lymphadenopathy, hepatosplenomegaly, severe myocarditis, and meningoencephalitis. Disease of sufficient severity to require hospitalization carries a 5% to 10% mortality rate. The younger the patient at the time of acquisition, the more severe the acute syndrome, especially if the patient is 2 years old or less. Congenitally acquired disease carries the highest morbidity and mortality.

After the initial infection, widespread dissemination of *T. cruzi* occurs; this is followed by lifelong infection. Incubation periods of 20 to 40 days have been observed in transfusion recipients. In most instances, acute symptoms resolve within 4 to 8 weeks. The host then enters the so-called chronic stage.

Chronic Disease

Most chronically infected individuals are asymptomatic and are said to have "indeterminate" infection. In the chronic stage, infection is usually detected by demonstrating positive seroreactivity to parasite antigens in a patient who is tested because of appropriate epidemiologic risk factors. All persons with chronic infection are believed to have a low level of circulating parasitemia. Parasitemia can be detected in 20% to 50% of patients using the technique of xenodiagnosis (i.e., allowing laboratory-reared reduviids to feed on subjects' blood and monitoring the reduviids for *T. cruzi* infection). By the fourth decade of life, approximately 20% to 30% of chronically infected individuals progress to symptomatic disease.

Symptomatic chronic Chagas' disease is characterized by cardiac, gastrointestinal, and neuropathic disorders. Cardiac problems include conduction system disturbances with or without dilated cardiomyopathy. The most common digestive syndromes include megaesophagus, with symptoms similar to idiopathic achalasia, and megacolon, which causes bloating, constipation, and abdominal pain. Coexistence of cardiac and gastrointestinal symptoms does occur in the same patient. Neurologic symptoms of the central, peripheral, and autonomic nervous systems have been described in chronic Chagas' disease, but these are rare and not well studied.

Chagas' disease pathogenesis is not well understood and continues to generate controversy. Past hypotheses and debate have focused on the relative roles of the initial pathogenic insult during acute infection versus the role of autoimmune phenomena in clinical progression of disease. Several recent studies have reported low numbers of parasites in chronically infected tissue, suggesting that viable parasites and the resulting chronic inflammation may play an important role.

Table 23-2 summarizes the salient clinical features of each of the three principal manifestations of chronic infection.

Host factors alone may not entirely explain the striking regional differences in disease manifestations that occur throughout Latin America. There are areas in northern Brazil where cardiac disease is two to three times more common than intestinal disease, whereas in Argentina, Chile, and some parts of Bolivia, gastrointestinal megasyndromes predominate. These geographic differences may be due in part to differences among strains of the parasite rather than to host factors.

DIAGNOSIS

Although the clinical syndromes are fairly characteristic, diagnosis of Chagas' disease may be difficult to prove. Diagnostic approaches have involved two basic strategies: parasite detection and serologic evidence of infection. When deciding which approach to use in a given epidemiologic setting, consideration should be given to the differing sensitivities and specificities of the tests, as well as to cost and ease of performance.

Parasite Detection Methods

During the acute phase, one may culture *T. cruzi* from the blood or see circulating trypomastigote forms on direct examination of the blood. Although they can be seen on Giemsa-stained specimens either by thin or thick smear (sensitivity 60% to 70%), superior methods of detection are microscopic examination of peripheral blood buffy coat wet preparations, culture, PCR, and serodiagnosis, all of which have a detection rate of 90% to 100% in the acute phase.

Xenodiagnosis

During the chronic disease stage, parasites circulate in very low numbers, and amplification strategies are generally required to reach the threshold of detection. In endemic areas where appropriate facilities are available, xenodiagnosis has a sensitivity of 20% to 50% when serial examinations are performed. Forty nymphal-stage, laboratory-reared reduviids are divided into four small matchbox-sized containers and are allowed to simultaneously take a blood meal over 10 to 20 minutes from each of the patient's four extremities. Total blood volume consumed by the insects ranges from 4 to 20 ml. The insects' feces and intestinal contents are examined 1 to 2 months later for evidence of *T. cruzi* epimastigotes or metacyclic trypomastigotes. Although this approach is painless, the disadvantages of it are the obvious delay in diagnosis, the expense of maintaining an insect facility, and the relatively low sensitivity.

Table 23-2
Clinical Features of Chronic Chagas' Disease

Indeterminate*
Applies to at least 40% to 60% of chronically infected people
Begins 8 weeks postinfection and lasts decades, if not for life
Serologic tests for *T. cruzi* are positive
Sensitive methods of parasite detection (e.g., PCR or xenodiagnosis) demonstrate low levels of circulating *T. cruzi*
Physical examination, ECG, and chest x-ray studies are normal
Patients are asymptomatic and capable of normal activity
As much as 50% of this population may be misclassified because on careful study they show some ECG abnormalities
Patients are often unaware of infection and serve as reservoirs to maintain the parasite life cycle

Cardiac†
Most frequent symptoms are palpitations, dizziness, syncope, dyspnea, edema, and chest pain
Arrhythmias of many varieties are a hallmark of chronic chagasic heart disease
Multifocal PVCs are commonly seen early in the course
Sick sinus syndrome and sinoatrial block also occur frequently
Right bundle-branch block with left anterior hemiblock is the classic and most common conduction abnormality
Complete heart block requiring mechanical pacing is not uncommon
Sudden death is not rare and is usually due to ventricular fibrillation
Cardiomegaly is common and causes regurgitant systolic murmurs
Congestive heart failure is due to chronic inflammatory changes in the myocardium, not coronary artery disease
Apical left ventricular aneurysms are seen frequently at autopsy; they predispose patients to arterial embolization
Pancarditis is seen on histopathology

Gastrointestinal Syndromes‡
Most commonly affected segments are the esophagus and colon
Pathologic inflammatory lesions are found in Auerbach's plexus, which is responsible for the autonomic coordination of peristalsis
Esophageal dysmotility may result in progressive dilation of the lumen
Patients experience variable degrees of dysphagia and regurgitation
In the extreme form of esophageal disease, radiographic evaluation shows megaesophagus, contraction abnormalities, and distal esophageal stricture
Colonic dysmotility is manifest initially by constipation
Progressive obstipation leads to dilated megacolon, fecaloma, and severe abdominal pain
Acute volvulus may occur

---

*Disease state is labeled indeterminate because it is unclear when, or if, they will develop symptomatic Chagas' disease.
†Consider chagasic heart disease in a young patient from an endemic area (or who has a history of blood transfusion) who presents with unexplained cardiomyopathy, ECG abnormalities, or arterial emboli.
‡Consider Chagas' disease in any patient from an endemic area who presents with megaesophagus or megacolon.
PCR, Polymerase chain reaction; *ECG,* electrocardiogram; *PVCs*, premature ventricular contractions.

Blood Cultures

Centrifugation blood culture in liver infusion tryptose or brain-heart infusion medium can detect parasites in about 30% of chronically infected patients. Cultures can be repeated serially to increase yield; this is a popular procedure in endemic areas and is thought to be equivalent to xenodiagnosis in sensitivity.

Polymerase Chain Reaction

A recent strategy for indirect parasite detection is based on the amplification of *T. cruzi* DNA using the polymerase chain reaction (PCR). DNA is extracted after whole blood lysis by using various techniques; unique *T. cruzi* gene fragments are then amplified in a thermocycler. The reported detection threshold is on the order of one parasite per 20 ml blood aliquot. As of this writing, PCR has not been widely tested beyond the research setting; it is not recommended for routine diagnosis.

Serologic Detection Methods

In *T. cruzi* infection, antibodies appear during the acute phase and generally persist for life. Diagnosis of chronic Chagas' disease generally depends on antibody detection methods. The most widely used tests are immunofluorescent antibody (IFA), hemagglutination, and enzyme-linked immunosorption assay (ELISA). They use epimastigote antigens or recombinant proteins in detecting *T. cruzi* antibodies (usually IgG antibodies, except when using IFA, which can distinguish between IgG and IgM). Sensitivity for these tests in reliable laboratories with standardized reagents and careful quality-control practices should be on the order of 98%. False-positive results can occur with sera from patients with leishmaniasis (a coendemic infection in many areas of Latin America) or *T. rangeli,* an animal trypanosome nonpathogenic to humans. Because of variable test specificity, most authorities recommend performing at least two different types of serologic tests per patient. Currently, a number of laboratories are working on the development of assays based on synthetic peptides, which would have the potential for increased specificity of serologic testing.

The Parasitic Diseases Division of the Centers for Disease Control and Prevention (CDC) (404-488-7760) is available for consultation regarding the diagnosis and therapy of Chagas' disease.

TREATMENT

Antitrypanosomal Agents

Specific antitrypanosomal chemotherapy for acute Chagas' disease is strongly recommended. Therapy is most effective when initiated as early as possible after exposure; this curtails the magnitude of parasitemia and the dissemination of the organisms. Previously, most authorities did not recommend using trypanocidal agents for chronic infection because there was little evidence that treatment at this stage prevented development of cardiac or digestive symptoms. Recently, small randomized clinical trials have reported high rates of parasitologic cure in children with asymptomatic chronic *T. cruzi* infection. Although the role of parasitemia in the evolution of Chagas' disease has not been defined, and although data are needed to evaluate clinical outcomes after treatment of longstanding infection, a World Health Organization expert committee has recommended that treatment should be offered to anyone with positive serology.

Nifurtimox (Lampit) and benznidazole (Rochagan) are both active against *T. cruzi* and can effectively abolish parasitemia. Unfortunately, these trypanocidal agents carry the risk of serious toxicity; they should be used only if clearly indicated. Neither drug is currently licensed in the United States; however, nifurtimox is available from the CDC. Since 1982, nifurtimox has been released by the CDC for treatment of reactivated Chagas' disease in 24 patients with Chagas' infection. An additional five persons in the United States were treated because of exposure to *T. cruzi* in laboratory accidents. Nifurtimox has also been used to prevent reactivation of Chagas' disease in 10 cardiac or bone marrow transplant recipients. There have been no cases of acute Chagas' disease diagnosed in U.S. travelers to endemic areas.

Table 23-3 provides a summary of these medications and precautions associated with their use. Investigations of alternative therapy with fluconazole, itraconazole, or allopurinol have found only limited anti-*T. cruzi* activity in humans.

The criteria for cure in acute Chagas' disease are the elimination of parasitemia, amelioration of signs and symptoms, and, if treated early enough, reversion of serologic tests to negative within 6 to 8 months after therapy. It should be noted that parasitemia tends to wane even without treatment, and that finding parasitemia is often a function of how vigorously one looks.

Symptomatic Treatment

Therapeutic approaches are dictated by the type and severity of end-organ damage.

Patients with indeterminate-stage disease should have periodic examinations and ECGs performed.

Table 23-3
Chemotherapy for Acute Chagas' Disease

Drug	Dosage	Adverse effects
Nifurtimox	*Adults:* 10 mg/kg/day PO divided tid or qid × 60-120 days *Children:* 15-20 mg/kg/day PO divided tid or qid × 60-120 days	1. Peripheral neuritis: 30% 2. Polyneuropathy 3. Tremors and excitation 4. Insomnia 5. Anorexia and weight loss 6. Hemolysis in G6PD-deficient patients
Benznidazole (First-line drug of choice for acute disease in Brazil)	*Adults:* 5-7.5mg/kg/day PO divided bid × 60 days *Children:* 5-10 mg/kg/day PO divided bid × 60 days	1. Photosensitive rash: 50% 2. Anorexia and weight loss 3. Peripheral neuritis 4. Hematologic abnormalities 5. Secondary lymphoproliferative disorders occur in animals

Cardiac failure in Chagas' disease is managed in standard fashion with digitalis, diuretics, and angiotensin-converting enzyme inhibitors. Arrhythmias usually respond to antiarrhythmic drug therapy; use of beta-blockers should be avoided. Many patients require pacemakers for the management of high-grade atrioventricular block, but they do not work well in patients with thin-walled, dilated hearts. Anticoagulants should be considered because of the high incidence of left ventricular aneurysm and pulmonary emboli.

Megaesophagus can be managed by noninvasive dilation or by surgical intervention to remove strictured regions. Megacolon should be surgically treated by resection of the dilated segment before fecaloma or vascular complications occur. Recurrences of gastrointestinal megasyndromes that require multiple surgeries are known to occur.

PROGNOSIS

The overall prognosis of patients with chronic Chagas' disease is fairly good: 70% or more will remain in the seropositive but asymptomatic indeterminate stage. Symptomatic chronic Chagas' disease carries a variable prognosis depending on severity of end-organ damage. Heart failure, which often appears between ages 20 and 50 years, carries a 2-year mortality rate of 50%. Digestive syndromes are better tolerated, but they also account for premature mortality. In truth, it is difficult to know the morbidity and mortality directly attributable to Chagas' disease, but overall life expectancy in endemic areas is estimated to be 9 years less than in nonendemic areas.

PREVENTION

For Persons Living in Endemic Areas

Prevention strategies in endemic areas are a major priority of WHO; the Pan American Health Organization; and the Health Ministries of several Latin American countries, notably Argentina, Brazil, and Venezuela. In the absence of effective therapies and vaccines, control focuses on surveillance and vector control. Several approaches to control are used: (1) blood bank screening to eliminate transfusion-related transmission, (2) insecticide spraying to eradicate domiciliated reduviids, and (3) housing improvements using "bug-proof" construction to minimize contact between the insect vector and human hosts.

For Persons Traveling to Endemic Areas

For the traveler to Latin America, protecting oneself against *T. cruzi* infection is largely a matter of educational awareness; there are no prophylactic medications or vaccines available. Travelers should be encouraged to consult reference literature to see pictures of the reduviid bug before departure. However, as noted previously, in 20 years of CDC surveillance, there have been no cases of acute Chagas' disease in U.S. travelers to endemic areas. The following brief advice for personal protection against Chagas' disease is provided:

1. Be aware of the risk of transmission in each of the endemic areas.
2. Be familiar with the regional names and appearance of triatomine (reduviid) bugs.
3. Avoid sleeping in cracked-walled, thatched-roofed houses such as are typically found in rural villages of Latin America.
4. If sleeping in high-risk areas is unavoidable, use a hammock with a cloth-roofed mosquito net; this affords some protection against being bitten.

5. Seek local medical attention as early as possible if signs or symptoms of acute Chagas' disease occur. Do not wait until you return from your trip; antitrypanosomal therapy is most effective in the early stages of Chagas' infection.

REFERENCES

Altclas J et al: Reactivation of chronic Chagas' disease following allogeneic bone marrow transplantation and successful pre-emptive therapy with benznidazole, *Transpl Infect Dis* 1:135, 1999.

Anez N et al: Detection and significance of inapparent infection in Chagas' disease in western Venezuela, *Am J Trop Med Hyg* 65:227, 2001.

Blejer JL, Saguier MC, Salamone HJ: Antibodies to *Trypanosoma cruzi* among blood donors in Buenos Aires, Argentina, *Int J Infect Dis* 5:89, 2001.

Bocchi EA, Fiorelli A: First Guideline Group for Heart Transplantation of the Brazilian Society of Cardiololgy: the Brazilian experience with heart transplantation: a multicenter report, *J Heart Lung Transplant* 20:637, 2001.

Britto C et al: Polymerase chain reaction (PCR) as a laboratory tool for the evaluation of the parasitological cure in Chagas' disease after specific treatment, *Medicina* (B Aires) 59(Suppl 2):176, 1999.

Chagas C: Nova tripanozomiaze humana. Estudos sobre a morfolojia e o ciclo evolutivo de *Schizotrypanum cruzi* ajente etiolojico de nova entidade morbida do homen, *Mem Inst Oswaldo Cruz* 1:159, 1909.

Cohen JE, Gurtler RE: Modeling household transmission of American trypanosomiasis, *Science* 293:694, 2001.

Corti M: AIDS and Chagas' disease, *AIDS Patient Care STDS* 14:581, 2000.

Garcia-Zapata MTA, McGreevy PB, Marsden PD: American trypanosomiasis. In Strickland GT, editor: *Hunter's tropical medicine,* ed 7, Philadelphia, 1991, WB Saunders.

Grant IH et al: Transfusion-associated acute Chagas disease acquired in the United States, *Ann Intern Med* 111:849, 1989.

Hager JM, Rahimtoola SH: Chagas' heart disease in the United States, *N Engl J Med* 325:763, 1991.

Ianni BM et al: Chagas' heart disease: evolutive evaluation of electrocardiographic and chocardiographic parameters in patient with the indeterminate form, *Arq Bras Cardiol* 77:59, 2001.

Kirchhoff LV, Gam AA, Gilliam FC: American trypanosomiasis (Chagas' disease) in Central American Immigrants, *Am J Med* 82:915, 1987.

Kirchhoff LV: Is *Trypansoma cruzi* a new threat to our blood supply? *Ann Intern Med* 111:773, 1989.

Lauria-Pires L et al: Progressive chronic Chagas heart disease ten years after treatment with anti-*Trypanosoma cruzi* nitroderivatives, *Am J Trop Med Hyg* 63:111, 2000.

Moncayo-Medina A: Chagas' disease 1976-1986. In Maurice J, Pearce AM, editors: *Tropical disease research: a global partnership: Eighth Programme Report,* Geneva, 1987, WHO.

Nickerson P et al: Transfusion-associated *Trypanosoma cruzi* infection in a non-endemic area, *Ann Intern Med* 111:851, 1989.

Solari A et al: Treatment of *Trypanosoma cruzi*-infected children with nifurtimox: a 3 year follow-up by PCR, *J Antimicrob Chemother* 48:515, 2001.

CHAPTER 24

African Sleeping Sickness (Trypanosomiasis)

Carter D. Hill, Russell McMullen, and Matthew J. Thompson

The agents of African sleeping sickness are protozoa of the genus *Trypanosoma,* subgenus *Trypanozoon,* species *brucei.* Human disease is caused by two subspecies, *T. b. gambiense* and *T. b. rhodesiense,* each of which has a characteristic geographic distribution and clinical syndrome associated with it. The disease, sleeping sickness, associated with either species is a febrile illness (which may range from acute or subacute to chronic) with eventual central nervous system (CNS) involvement, progressive deterioration, and, unless treated, death.

In both types of human African trypanosomiasis (HAT), humans are a definitive host, and the intermediate hosts are species of blood-sucking tsetse flies *(Glossina).*

EPIDEMIOLOGY

Although approximately 45,000 cases of trypanosomiasis are reported each year, it is estimated that more than 450,000 carry the disease and as many as 55,000 die each year. Indeed, about 60 million of the 400 million people inhabiting sub-Saharan Africa live in areas where tsetse flies and trypanosomes are present, and thus are at risk of acquiring trypanosomiasis. HAT is responsible for considerable morbidity and poses an enormous burden to the health care and economic structures of Africa.

The two distinct forms of trypanosomiasis are known as East and West African trypanosomiasis (Fig. 24-1; Table 24-1). East African trypanosomiasis *(T. b. rhodesiense)* is found in the savanna and woodlands of eastern and central equatorial Africa. It has widespread distribution throughout these rural areas because several antelope species are major mammalian hosts and they are trypanotolerant; cattle may also be hosts, but tolerate infection poorly resulting in significant loss of livestock productivity. Humans are essentially an incidental host.

West African trypanosomiasis *(T. b. gambiense)* is found in more forested areas of Central and West Africa. Transmission occurs along rivers and lakes and is more frequent in the dry season. It tends to be an indolent illness, and relatively asymptomatic carriers perpetuate the disease cycle by providing a continued source of infectious blood meals for flies.

In addition to the endemic foci of trypanosomiasis, major epidemics of trypanosomiasis have been recognized during this century; some have claimed hundreds of thousands of victims in days before effective treatment was available. Most recently epidemics have occurred in countries

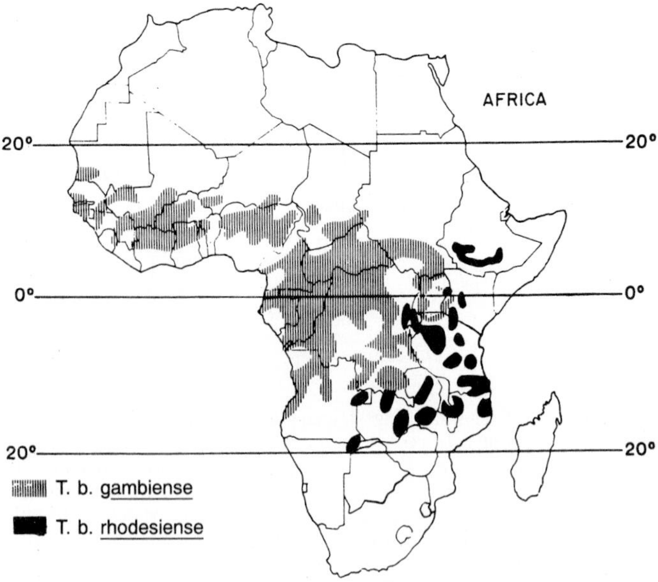

Fig. 24-1 Distribution of West African trypanosomiasis *(Trypanosoma brucei gambiense)* and East African trypanosomiasis *(Trypanosoma brucei rhodesiense).* Note that *T. b. gambiense* tends to be transmitted in forested areas along rivers, and *T. b. rhodesiense* is transmitted in separated areas of woodland and savanna. (From Strickland GT: *Hunter's tropical medicine,* ed 8, Philadelphia, 2000, WB Saunders.)

such as Uganda, Democratic Republic of Congo (formerly Zaire), Central African Republic, and Sudan; in some cases prevalence rates are higher than they have been for decades. Epidemic outbreaks may be enhanced by population movements (often owing to local unrest) that take people into areas where infected tsetse flies are present, climactic change, and possibly by alteration in virulence of the pathogens. Several recent reports have noted an apparent increase in East African trypanosomiasis in European travelers returning from East African game reserves.

Although a few studies have examined the interaction between human immunodeficiency virus (HIV) infection and trypanosomiasis, it does not appear that HIV has had much effect on the incidence of sleeping sickness; however, further studies are needed to determine the full influence these two diseases may have on each other.

HAT can be controlled. After the discovery of the causative agent and vector at the onset of the twentieth century, aggressive control measures were successful. These included culling of wildlife reservoirs, clearing of vegetation housing tsetse flies, coercion of humans into screening programs, and lastly, treating infected individuals. In recent decades, however, surveillance has diminished, fly populations have returned, wars have displaced infected individuals, and treatment attempts have been limited.

Table 24-1
Characteristics of West African and East African Trypanosomiasis

	West African	East African
Pathogen	*Trypanosoma brucei gambiense*	*Trypanosoma brucei rhodesiense*
Geographic distribution	West and Central Africa	Central, East and Southeastern Africa
Local environment	Along rivers, lakes and water holes	Savanna and cleared brush
Important hosts	Humans	Antelope, cattle, humans
Onset	Subacute to chronic	Acute to subacute
Parasitemia	Low	High
CNS invasion	Late	Early
Death in untreated illness	Months to years	2 to 9 months
Diagnosis	Lymph node aspirate CSF evaluation	Peripheral blood smear CSF evaluation
Utility of rodent inoculation for diagnosis	No	Yes
Patient population at particular risk	Rural dwellers along rivers	Tourists (on safari) Rural dwellers Rural workers (e.g., hunters, fishermen, firewood collectors, game wardens)

African trypanosomiasis is unusual in tourists because it is primarily a rural disease. A recent 30-year review identified 22 published cases (1 fatality) of imported HAT in the United States since 1967. All cases of HAT involving U.S. travelers have been of the East African trypanosomiasis, with the majority acquired on visits to game reserves. During this same time period, four cases of West African trypanosomiasis were reported; all involved African nationals who were living or studying in the United States. People who are long-term travelers or residents of endemic areas, including missionaries, rural health care workers, and Peace Corps volunteers, may be also be at increased risk for West African trypanosomiasis.

LIFE CYCLE AND TRANSMISSION

Trypomastigotes are ingested by tsetse flies during a blood meal obtained from a mammalian host (humans for West African trypanosomiasis; generally antelope or cattle, rarely humans, for East African trypanosomiasis). After multiplication and morphologic change in the fly midgut, the organisms migrate to the salivary gland; there they undergo alteration into epimastigotes, then into infective metacyclic trypomastigotes. These are inoculated back into mammalian hosts during a subsequent blood meal. The metacyclic trypomastigotes then become bloodstream trypomastigotes and multiply; large numbers are able to survive despite the host immune response because of periodic alteration of surface antigens.

PATHOGENESIS

After initial hemolymphatic dissemination, the trypanosomes eventually invade interstitial spaces and also cause an endarteritis. In this early stage of the disease, one sees involvement of the lymphatics, liver, and spleen. Pancarditis is also seen, usually with the cardiac conduction system affected, but this is more common with East African trypanosomiasis. In the later stage of the disease (which can occur within weeks in East African trypanosomiasis), the CNS is invaded; the patient develops meningoencephalitis and/or meningomyelitis and the progressive neurologic deterioration characteristic of "sleeping sickness."

The exact pathogenesis of trypanosomiasis is not well understood. It has not been proven that toxin production has a role in causing tissue damage. Some theorize that the clinical symptoms and pathologic damage are attributable to poorly understood immune mechanisms. Immune complexes associated with complement can be shown in serum and damaged tissues, and rheumatoid factor and anti-DNA antibodies are seen in serum. Perivascular infiltration is a prominent feature of the endarteritis that develops in target organs. The endarteritis plays a significant pathologic role, especially in the development of CNS disease, in which thrombosis resulting from endarteritis appears to be a major cause of deterioration.

CLINICAL FEATURES

Clinical manifestations of HAT are variable, with a large range of symptoms; it is mainly the time course that distinguishes between the East and West African illnesses. In travelers the disease is usually fulminant; therefore timely recognition and treatment are essential. A tender chancre usually develops at the site of the bite within 5 to 15 days after the bite of an infected tsetse fly, although shorter and longer periods have been reported. It tends to be more common in East African trypanosomiasis, and it seems to occur more frequently in Caucasians. The chancre is an indurated, dark red nodule that may be 2 cm or more in size; it usually heals spontaneously over several weeks.

East African Trypanosomiasis

Onset of symptoms is within hours to days after development of a chancre, although it may take longer if no chancre develops. Signs and symptoms include the following:

1. High fever, headache, and malaise occur, then subside after 2 or 3 days; these may develop a periodic pattern of recurrence. Gastrointestinal symptoms may sometimes occur.
2. Early onset of pancarditis is more common in Eastern trypanosomiasis; these patients tend to have tachycardia, whether febrile or not, and are also subject to arrhythmias and congestive failure.
3. A transient skin rash is often present. It is more commonly seen in Caucasians and is most prominent on the trunk. It consists of 5- to 10-cm erythematous patches with a clear center.
4. Edema is variably present, and usually consists of facial and periarticular swelling.
5. Lymphadenopathy is not prominent. Hepatosplenomegaly may sometimes occur.
6. Early CNS invasion occurs, followed by rapid deterioration; death may occur after a stormy 6-week course, but may take as long as 6 to 9 months.

West African Trypanosomiasis

A localized nodular lesion or chancre may develop within 5 to 10 days of the tsetse fly bite. It ulcerates and disappears over 2 to 3 weeks. In practice, this primary lesion is seldom seen. Signs and symptoms include the following:

1. Onset of symptoms is insidious and patients may be asymptomatic for many months. The hemolymphatic stage, which begins anywhere from weeks to months after infection, is characterized by high fevers; these may persist for several days, followed by periods of remission during which the patient feels relatively well. Patients may also complain of headache and malaise. Although more characteristic of East African trypanosomiasis, tachycardia may be present.
2. Lymphadenopathy is a prominent feature. Nodes are typically rubbery, discrete, and nontender, but become fibrotic with time. Posterior cervical adenopathy (Winterbottom's sign) is a classic finding. Mild hepatosplenomegaly may also be seen.
3. Generalized pruritis is common, as is facial and periarticular edema.
4. A transient skin rash is often present early in the disease.
5. Subtle neurologic signs may appear, including personality change, irritability, indifferent attitude, and deep hyperesthesia (i.e., delayed onset of intense pain when soft tissues are compressed—Kerandel's sign); these frequently predate any change in the cerebrospinal fluid (CSF).
6. Later CNS changes include aimless gaze, daytime somnolence (sometimes alternating with nighttime insomnia) and hypothermia and hyperthermia. Papilledema may be present on examination.
7. Extrapyramidal signs are also seen late in the disease and include tremor, slurred speech, ataxia, rigidity, and akinesia; many patients exhibit choreiform movements of the extremities and trunk.
8. In the final stages of the disease, progressive decreased conscious level occurs, and patients will move from indifference and difficult with arouse, will not eat spontaneously, and eventually lapses into coma.
9. The disease is invariably fatal without treatment; patients usually die of malnourishment, accidents, or intercurrent infection.

DIAGNOSIS

1. A history of travel to endemic areas is important; a high index of suspicion must be maintained when evaluating patients who have been to affected parts of Africa.
2. Definitive laboratory diagnosis depends on demonstration of trypanosomes in peripheral blood, tissue (e.g., from the chancre), lymph node aspirate, or, in late stages, CSF.
   a. Aspiration and wet prep examination of exudate from the chancre (if present) may reveal motile organisms. Giemsa stain should also be done.
   b. Examination of blood, either as a wet prep or stained preparations, frequently demonstrates trypanosomes. Giemsa-stained thick and thin smears are probably best, but standard hematology slides prepared with Wright's stain may also be diagnostic. Blood smears are more likely to be positive in the hemolymphatic stage, particularly in East African trypanosomiasis, where the level of parasitemia is usually high. Serial slides may need to be examined (much as for malaria) because parasitemia may be low and undergo daily fluctuation. If the index of suspicion is high in a patient with negative smears, other useful laboratory techniques include examination of the buffy coat of centrifuged anticoagulated whole blood, concentration using an anion-exchange column, or the Quantitative Buffy Coat (QBC) method.

c. Microscopic examination of lymph node aspirate for trypanosomes is most helpful in diagnosing West African trypanosomiasis, in which lymphadenopathy is more prominent and there are few organisms in the peripheral blood.
d. Specific trypanosomal antibody testing can be used to confirm the diagnosis, but this is not as specific or as sensitive as detection of the parasites themselves. The Parasitic Diseases Branch of the Centers for Disease Control and Prevention (CDC) (see "Quick Guide to Resources") should be consulted for availability of indirect fluorescent antibody or enzyme-linked immunosorbent assay antibody testing, trypanosome-specific DNA by polymerase chain reaction, and for guidance in diagnosis and management.
e. The card agglutination test for trypanosomiasis (CATT) is commercially available and practical for field use to detect antibodies. Although it lacks specificity it appears to be most useful in seroepidemiologic studies of *T. b. gambiense* or to identify patients requiring further diagnostic evaluation. A new rapid latex agglutination assay for antibodies to *T. b. gambiense* in serum/CSF appears to offer greater sensitivity and specificity, although confirmatory studies are needed and availability is limited.
f. Several antigen detection systems have been studied, including the trypanosomiasis card indirect agglutination test (TrypTect CIATT) with a reported sensitivity and specificity (99.3% and 99.4%, respectively) for both *T. gambiense* and *T. rhodesiense.* Again, availability is limited and further studies are needed.
g. Intraperitoneal inoculation of mice or rats with infected blood or CSF will result in parasitemia within 1 to 2 weeks; this method is very sensitive, but only for *T. b. rhodesiense,* and is rarely used (Table 24-2).
h. CSF examination must be performed on all patients. Early findings after CNS invasion include increased cells (predominantly mononuclear, may also include the morula plasma cells of Mott), increased protein levels, and small numbers of trypanosomes may also be seen on centrifuged CSF (care should be taken to avoid contamination with trypanosomes from blood during the lumbar

Table 24-2
Treatment of West African and East African Trypanosomiasis

Disease organism	Stage of disease	Drugs of choice	Alternatives
T. brucei gambiense	Early	▼ Pentamidine	▼ Surmanin ▼ Eflornithine
	Late (CNS involvement)	▼ Melarsoprol	▼ Eflornithine
T. brucei rhodesiense	Early	▼ Suramin	▼ Eflornithine
	Late (CNS involvement)	▼ Melarsoprol	▼ Eflornithine

Consult the CDC Parasitic Disease Branch for advice on treatment. These drugs may be available only through CDC Drug and Immunobiologic Service (404-639-3670/2888), and are not necessarily FDA-approved for the above indications.

puncture). Immunoglobulin M (IgM) levels are markedly increased in the CSF in later stages of CNS involvement, and the opening pressure found on lumbar puncture is often elevated.

3. Additional laboratory features of the disease are as follows:
   a. The most characteristic feature is markedly elevated serum IgM levels.
   b. The following may be seen but are more characteristic in acute illness due to *T. b. rhodesiense:*
      (1) Anemia (resulting from hemolysis, hemodilution, or disorded erythropoiesis)
      (2) Abnormal liver function
      (3) Coagulation abnormalities, including thrombocytopenia and other findings of disseminated intravascular coagulation
      (4) Leukocytosis resulting from monocytes, lymphocytes, plasma cells

DIFFERENTIAL DIAGNOSIS

With the notable exception of the chancre resulting from the tsetse fly bite, most clinical findings in African trypanosomiasis are nonspecific. Malaria should be considered, particularly in patients who present with an acute relapsing febrile illness after travel to rural East or Central Africa. Fortunately, multiple blood smears are the prime diagnostic test for both malaria and East African trypanosomiasis. Other infections that cause acute or subacute febrile illness (some of which may lead to CNS symptoms) should be considered. These include relapsing fever, typhoid, brucellosis, rickettsial and arboviral fevers, leptospirosis, acute HIV infection, mononucleosis, secondary syphilis, tuberculosis, visceral leishmaniasis, and other causes of acute to subacute meningitis. Lymphoma may also present with a similar picture. Chronic diseases that may mimic the later stages of trypanosomiasis include neurosyphilis, stage IV HIV disease (and associated CNS illnesses), CNS tumors, and severe neuropsychiatric disorders.

TREATMENT

The CDC Parasitic Disease Branch should be consulted; the staff there have considerable experience with trypanosomiasis, and most of the medications used are available only through the CDC Drug and Immunobiologic Service (404-639-3670/2888). The supply of virtually all effective agents except pentamidine has been severely limited by cutbacks in commercial production of these drugs.

The treatment regimen depends on two factors. The first factor is whether the patient has West African or East African disease. Because the two subspecies are morphologically indistinguishable, identification is usually based on the geographic locale of where the patient contracted the disease. The second factor is whether there is evidence of CNS involvement (CSF examination is mandatory even if there are no neurologic signs or symptoms). Follow-up monitoring of patients and treatment of relapses are essential, especially for patients with *T. b. rhodesiense* who should have CSF examination repeated at 3- to 6-month intervals after therapy.

Suramin (Bayer-205) is the treatment of choice for *T. b. rhodesiense* if CSF examination is normal. Severe idiosyncratic reactions occur rarely but may be more likely if the patient also has onchocerciasis; a test dose of 100 to 200 mg given intravenously is indicated for all patients. If this is tolerated, then 20 mg/kg (to a maximum of 1 g) is given on days 1, 3, 7,

14, and 21. Because suramin is not licensed in the United States, it must be obtained from the CDC Drug Service. Side effects can be severe and include fever, pruritus, skin rashes, neuropathies, hematologic changes, and, most important, nephrotoxicity. Albuminuria is common, but should be checked for before each dose; if it increases or if casts are seen, alternative drugs should be used.

Pentamidine isethionate (e.g., Pentam 300) may also be used in the absence of CNS involvement, but it is not effective against infections caused by *T. b. rhodesiense.* It is commercially available as a treatment for *Pneumocystis carinii* pneumonia, although it is labeled as investigational for treating HAT. The treatment course is 4 mg/kg a day for a total of 10 doses. The intramuscular (IM) route is recommended because intravenous administration is more likely to be associated with severe hypotension, but regardless of route, patients should be kept supine and closely monitored after each dose. Side effects also include sterile abscesses after IM use, hypoglycemia, abdominal cramping, transaminase abnormalities, nephrotoxicity, leukopenia, and thrombocytopenia.

Melarsoprol (Mel B, Melarsen oxide-BAL) is a trivalent arsenical that is effective against both *T. b. gambiense* and *T. b. rhodesiense.* It penetrates into the CSF in low but effective concentrations; hence, it has been the drug of choice when there is CNS involvement. It is also used to treat relapses after suramin or pentamidine treatment of hemolymphatic disease. Unfortunately, recent epidemics have reported treatment failure rates of up to 30%. It must be obtained through the CDC Drug Service, and their recommended treatment regimens are complicated. For minimal CNS involvement, 2 to 3.6 mg/kg/day (maximum: 200 mg/day) should be administered intravenously for 3 days. After 1 week, 3.6 mg/kg/day given intravenously should be administered for 3 days, then repeated again after 10 to 21 days. A shorter (10-day) course of 2.2 mg/kg/day given intravenously may be equally effective. Other regimens include lower initial doses, which are increased gradually to reduce the incidence of side effects, although there are not data to support the efficacy of this regimen.

Some patients experience a Jarisch-Herxheimer-like reaction after starting melarsoprol. The metabolites of the drug are toxic and may cause optic atrophy, rashes, abdominal pain, transaminase elevation, cardiotoxicity, and nephropathy. A severe reactive encephalopathy occurs in up to 10% of patients, generally in those with more advanced CNS disease. It may present as convulsions, rapidly progressing coma, or with abnormal psychiatric behaviors such as restlessness, aggression, or psychosis. Mortality with this complication is high. Patients receiving this drug should be closely observed. Concurrent administration of prednisolone may decrease the incidence of encephalopathy.

Eflornithine HCl (Ornidyl, difluoromethylornithine, DFMO) has proven more than 90% effective in trials when used for CNS disease resulting from *T. b. gambiense;* it may represent an alternative to melarsoprol, but is definitely the treatment of choice in the event of relapse after CNS treatment. It is not effective against CNS disease resulting from *T. b. rhodesiense.* The commercial viability of this drug has recently improved following a new indication of topical eflornithine for the removal of unwanted facial hair in women. Limited supplies of eflornithine are available from the WHO. In the United States, this drug is approved by the U.S. Food and Drug Administration for treatment of CNS disease resulting from *T. b. gambiense,* but is available only as an "orphan" drug (www.fda.gov/orphan; the Office of Orphan Drug Products Development). The dosage is 100 mg/kg intravenously every 6 hours for 14 days; this appears to be more effective than short (i.e., 7-day) courses. In some studies, this regimen has been followed with an additional course of 75 mg/kg/day PO every 6 hours for 21 to 30 days, although the additional benefit of this additional oral treatment is unclear. Side effects include diarrhea, vomiting, seizures (rarely), and bone marrow suppression, which is generally reversible.

Nifurtimox (Bayer 2502) is used in the acute phase of American trypanosomiasis (Chagas' disease), and may be useful against refractory cases of West African trypanosomiasis. It is available only from the CDC. The dose used has been 15 mg/kg/day orally for 30 to 60 days; 30 mg/kg/day has also been tried. Relapses are frequent and the rate of toxicity has been significant; therefore it is recommended only as a third-line treatment. Side effects include abdominal symptoms, neuropathy, and hemolysis, particularly in patients who are deficient for glucose-6-phosphate dehydrogenase.

PREVENTION

Because the risk to international travelers is relatively low, most are not counseled specifically about the risk from tsetse flies and their association with trypanosomiasis. The flies are large and capable of biting through lightweight clothing. They tend to feed during the day and appear to be attracted by bright-colored clothing and by moving vehicles. Standard insect bite prevention measures may help, including the use of DEET-containing compounds. DEET-Plus (Sawyer Products, Safety Harbor, FL) also contains R-326, a specific fly repellent reported to work for 8 hours. Clothing should extend to the wrists and ankles and should be of dull-colored heavy material, such as canvas. Screens on vehicle windows can be important. Mosquito netting can be helpful for rest periods during the day; this contrasts to malaria prevention, for which evening and nighttime protection is most important.

Areas where tsetse flies are prevalent are widely distributed, but foci are often known to native residents; it is advisable to avoid areas they designate as heavily infested. Development of land (to the exclusion of wild game) and successful production of healthy cattle are generally incompatible with tsetse infestation.

Although pentamidine or suramin have been used prophylactically against *T. b. gambiense,* chemoprophylaxis may cause side effects, development of resistant strains, and may possibly mask symptoms until CNS invasion has occurred. Given the rarity of HAT in U.S. travelers chemoprophylaxis is not recommended for short-term visitors.

A vaccine will not be available for the foreseeable future, although significant immunity occurs after Gambian sleeping sickness, suggesting that developing a vaccine is biologically plausible. At present HAT control activities in Africa rely on improved surveillance and clinical management of identified cases, reducing tsetse fly densities using odor-baited fly traps, insecticide-coated bait animals, spraying insecticides, and release of sterile insects (liberation of sterilized flies to compete with wild flies). Given the limited and costly treatments available for this disease, however, much work is needed to identify new and more effective therapeutic options.

REFERENCES

Anon: Drugs for parasitic infections, *Med Lett Drug Ther* 40:1, 1998.

Asonganyi T et al: A multi-centre evaluation of the card indirect agglutination test for trypanosomiasis (TrypTect CIATT), *Ann Trop Med Parasitol* 92(8):837, 1998.

Barrett MP: The fall and rise of sleeping sickness, *Lancet* 353:1113, 1999.

Blum J, Nkunku S, Burri C: Clinical description of encephalopathic syndromes and risk factors for their occurrence and outcomes during melarsoprol treatment of human African trypanosomiasis, *Trop Med Int Health* 6(5):390, 2001.

Bryan RT et al: African trypanosomiasis in American travelers: a 20-year review, In Steffen R et al, editors: *Travel medicine: Proceedings of the First Conference on International Travel Medicine,* Berlin, 1988, Springer-Verlag.

Burri C et al: Efficacy of new, concise schedule for melarsoprol in treatment of sleeping sickness caused by *Trypanosoma brucei gambiense:* a randomized trial, *Lancet* 355(9213):1419, 2000.

B scher P, Lejon V, Magnus E, Van Meirvenne N: Improved latex agglutination test for detection of antibodies in serum and cerebrospinal fluid of *Trypanosoma brucei gambiense* infected patients, *Acta Trop* 73(1):11, 1999.

Duggan AJ, Hutchinson MP: Sleeping sickness in Europeans: a review of 109 cases, *J Trop Med Hyg* 69:124, 1966.

Edeghere H, Olise PO, Olatunde DS: Human African trypanosomiasis (sleeping sickness): new endemic foci in Bendel State, Nigeria, *Trop Med Parasitol* 40:16, 1989.

Gear JHS, Miller GB: The clinical manifestations of Rhodesian trypanosomiasis: an account of cases contracted in the Okavango swamps of Botswana, *Am J Trop Med Hyg* 35:1146, 1986.

Haller L et al: Clinical and pathological aspects of human African trypanosomiasis (*T. b. gambiense*) with particular reference to reactive arsenical encephalopathy, *Am J Trop Med Hyg* 35:94, 1986.

Jones J: African sleeping sickness returns to UK after 4 years, *BMJ* 321:1177, 2000.

Legros D et al: Risk factors for treatment failure after melarsoprol for *Trypanosoma brucei gambiense* trypanosomiasis in Uganda, *Trans R Soc Trop Med Hyg* 93(4):439, 1999.

Maddocks S, O'Brien R: African trypanosomiasis in Australia, *N Engl J Med* 342:1254, 2000.

Meda HA et al: Human immunodeficiency virus infection and human African trypanosomiasis: a case-control study in Cote d'Ivoire, *Trans R Soc Trop Med Hyg* 89(6):693, 1995.

Milord F et al: Efficacy and toxicity of eflornithine for treatment of *Trypanosoma brucei gambiense* sleeping sickness, *Lancet* 340:652, 1992.

Moore A, Richer M: Re-emergence of epidemic sleeping sickness in southern Sudan, *Trop Med Int Health* 6(5):342, 2001.

Pepin J et al: Short-course eflornithine in Gambian trypanosomiasis: a multicentre randomized controlled trial, *Bull World Health Org* 78(11):1284, 2000.

Pepin J et al: The impact of human immunodeficiency virus infection on the epidemiology and treatment of *Trypanosoma brucei gambiense* sleeping sickness in Nioki, Zaire, *Am J Trop Med Hyg* 47(2):133, 1992.

Pepin J: Zaire (Congo): resurgence of trypanosomiasis ("patients without borders"), *Lancet* 349 (suppl III):10, 1997.

Pepin J et al: Trial of prednisolone for prevention of melarsoprol-induced encephalopathy in gambiense sleeping sickness, *Lancet* 1(8649):1246, 1989.

Quinn TC, Hill CD: African trypanosomiasis in an American hunter in East Africa, *Arch Intern Med* 143:1021, 1983.

Schofield CJ, Maudlin I: Trypanosomiasis control, *Int J Parasitol* 31:614, 2001.

Sinha A et al: African trypanosomiasis in two travelers from the United States, *Clin Infect Dis* 30(6):840, 1999.

Smith DH, Pepin J, Stich AHR: Human African trypanosomiasis: an emerging public health Crisis, *Br Med Bull* 54:341, 1998.

Stanghellini A, Josenando T: The situation of sleeping sickness in Angola: a calamity, *Trop Med Int Health* 6(5):330, 2001.

Van Nieuwenhove S et al: Sleeping sickness resurgence in the DRC: the past decade, *Trop Med Int Health* 6(5):335, 2001.
Van Voorhis WC: Therapy and prophylaxis of systemic protozoan infections, *Drugs* 40:176, 1990.
World Health Organization: Epidemiology and control of African trypanosomiasis. Report of a WHO Expert Committee. *WHO Tech Rep Ser,* No. 739. Geneva, WHO, 1986.

SECTION IV

DIARRHEA

CHAPTER 25

Approach to Diarrhea in Returned Travelers

Matthew J. Thompson and Elaine C. Jong

A common medical complaint of travelers to developing countries is that of diarrhea and gastrointestinal symptoms acquired during travel. Traveler's diarrhea (TD) is more common in younger individuals and in those of higher socioeconomic status. Perhaps this reflects a predilection for a more adventurous itinerary and an interest in foreign cuisines. It occurs more frequently in people with reduced gastric acidity and in travelers to tropical locations rather than to temperate climates; geographic destination is by far the most important determinant of attack rate.

Since the majority of cases of TD occur within the first week of travel, and since most patients travel for at least a week, the physician will seldom see a case of new-onset diarrhea in a returned traveler, unless the ingestion of contaminated food occurred on the airplane home. Thus the majority of cases of travel-acquired diarrhea seen by the physician will be *protracted* or *recurrent diarrhea.* Between 8% and 15% of patients with TD will experience symptoms for more than 1 week, and in 2% symptoms will last for 1 month or more.

HISTORY

The most important question in the investigation of TD is its duration. TD is usually a self-limited illness and lasts an average of 3.6 days. Thus there is no need for an extensive medical workup before the natural history of the case unfolds, unless the patient's general condition requires that treatment be undertaken immediately. The time of onset of the diarrhea with respect to arrival in the foreign country is important to establish, since the average incubation period of TD is 3 days.

The severity of the illness is important in the approach to the acutely ill patient with diarrhea. The average case of TD is not severe (averaging 4.6 stools per day), and systemic complaints are usually those of nausea and crampy abdominal pain. The presence of high fever, as well as blood or pus in stool specimens, suggests an invasive pathogen (e.g., *Salmonella, Shigella, Campylobacter, Escherichia coli* O157:H7, *Entamoeba histolytica*) and may help eliminate from consideration such noninvasive agents as enterotoxigenic *E. coli,* rotavirus, Norwalk agent, *Giardia lamblia,* and *Vibrio cholerae,* which tend to cause profuse watery diarrhea and cramps, without fever or bloody stools. However, blood may not be present in all patients infected with invasive organisms, and concurrent infection with more than one enteric pathogen may occur.

The complaints of "sulfur" burps, foul flatulence, and milk intolerance suggest the presence of *G. lamblia.* The recent use of antibiotics adds the diagnosis of antibiotic-associated diarrhea caused by *Clostridium difficile* to the differential.

Information on the returned traveler's efforts to self-medicate, alter diet, or diagnose and treat while abroad should be obtained. If unknown foreign medications were taken, the names, dosing schedule, and subjective response to treatment should be ascertained.

Travelers from industrialized countries are likely to carry an antiperistaltic agent such as loperamide and/or antimicrobials for empiric self-treatment of diarrhea on trips abroad (see Chapter 6). If these were used and an initial response obtained, the recurrence of symptoms may represent recrudescence of partially resistant organisms or reinfection with similar or different pathogens.

Information about possible food sources is usually not helpful, but a history of shellfish or seafood consumption may be useful. Raw and undercooked shellfish and seafood are common sources of *Vibrio parahaemolyticus,* which may present as a profuse watery diarrhea, and *Vibrio vulnificus,* which may cause fever, chills, nausea, vomiting, and abdominal pain. Hepatitis A can also be acquired in this way, and diarrhea can occasionally be among the early presenting symptoms of this infection. Norwalk agent-like particles have been isolated from shellfish, among other sources, and have been implicated in large outbreaks of gastroenteritis, including on cruise ships.

Lifestyle data should be collected (such as sexual preference in males), since tests to rule out anogenital gonococcal infection and other agents may be appropriate. A dietary history, searching for recent bulk-forming additions to the diet, and review of the patient's medicines may reveal important clues as to the etiology. Contact with an animal with diarrhea should lead one to consider *Campylobacter* and *Giardia* more seriously.

Finally, the likelihood of the patient's transmitting the diarrhea to contacts must be explored. Patients with such jobs as food handlers and institutional caregivers should be investigated regardless of the length of symptoms to make a diagnosis and initiate therapy or to delay resumption of work to avoid a potential epidemic.

CLINICAL FEATURES

The first determination to be made in the traveler with diarrhea is the need for hospitalization. The combination of orthostatic hemodynamic changes and an inability to maintain oral rehydration necessitates intravenous rehydration and possibly hospitalization. The presence of obvious toxicity or sepsis is also a clear indication for hospitalization. In cases in which significant systemic toxicity is present, blood and other body fluid cultures may be necessary, as well as early initiation of parenteral antibiotics.

The physical examination is usually of little assistance in determining the etiology of travel-acquired diarrhea but is useful to assess the general condition of the patient and to exclude other conditions that may present with diarrhea. In TD, the abdomen is usually nontender or minimally so, and the bowel tones are usually hyperactive. Focal abdominal tenderness mandates expanding the differential diagnosis to include appendicitis, biliary tract disease, peptic ulcer disease, pancreatitis, diverticulitis, and inflammatory bowel disease. Hepatic tenderness in the traveler with diarrhea may bring acute viral hepatitis or amebic liver abscess into the differential diagnosis. In elderly individuals, the rectal examination is important to rule out diarrhea around an impaction, which may ensue from previous dehydration and the use of antiperistaltic agents. Occult or gross blood in the stool supports the diagnosis of an invasive organism and impels the clinician to continue investigation if only noninvasive pathogens are identified in submitted stools (rectal hemorrhoids, peptic ulcer disease, inflammatory bowel disease, diverticulitis, malignancy and recent ingestion of rare meat as sources of blood may need to be ruled out).

LABORATORY STUDIES

The decision to do laboratory studies in the traveler with diarrhea should be based primarily on the duration of symptoms and the severity of the illness. The traveler seeking medical help who has had fewer than 5 days of diarrhea probably does not require investigation unless significant fever, abdominal pain, dehydration, or blood or mucus in the stool is present. Evaluation of travelers with protracted gastrointestinal symptoms should follow a stepwise approach to avoid unnecessary investigations and prevent important diagnoses from being overlooked.

Studies on TD show that the most commonly isolated pathogens are enterotoxigenic *E. coli, Salmonella, Shigella, Campylobacter jejuni,* and *V. parahaemolyticus.* Among travelers, viral pathogens and protozoa have been documented in 5% to 10% of diarrheal cases. Table 25-1 lists enteric pathogens that may present with diarrhea.

Patients need to be instructed on proper collection of stool samples for laboratory testing. Specimens contaminated with urine or retrieved from the toilet bowl are not satisfactory. The specimen should be caught in a specimen container, or the patient should defecate on newspaper and the mushiest portion of the stool scooped up with a clean plastic spoon and transferred to a specimen container. Alternatively, after urinating, the patient can use a large piece of plastic wrap draped like a sling and held fast between the toilet bowl and seat to catch the stool specimen. The specimen can then be transferred to a specimen container. The specimen should be submitted to the laboratory as quickly as possible, ideally within 1 to 2 hours to ensure reliability of microscopy and culture results.

If a protozoan parasite such as *E. histolytica* or *Giardia* is suspected and there is difficulty in obtaining the stool specimen promptly, the patient can be instructed to suspend a small stool sample in polyvinyl alcohol (PVA) fixative at home, to be delivered to the laboratory when convenient, or even to be mailed in (if appropriate leak-proof containers and mailers are used). Several convenient stool preservative kits are available commercially, with patient instructions in English and other languages. Alternatively, the clinical microbiology laboratory can usually furnish the PVA fixative in a small jar. Preserved stools are satisfactory for examination for intestinal protozoa and for eggs or larvae of intestinal helminths, but they cannot be used for culture of bacterial pathogens. Multiple (at least 3) specimens may need to be obtained to avoid false-negative results, since many parasites are excreted intermittently. There is some evidence that in patients who do not have frank diarrhea, a cathartic-induced (magnesium sulfate) "purged" stool specimen will enhance detection of intestinal parasites.

Laboratory investigation of diarrhea should start with *visual inspection of the stool.* Blood in the stool indicates an inflammatory process, and greasy or frothy stools imply malabsorption (which may occur in giardiasis, in a postinfectious state, or in tropical sprue).

Table 25-1
Enteric Pathogens That May Present with Diarrhea

Viruses
Norwalk agent
Rotavirus
Hepatitis A
Hepatitis E
Bacteria, Noninvasive
Enterotoxigenic *E. coli* (ETEC)
Vibrio cholerae 01
V. cholerae 0139
V. cholerae non-01
Vibrio parahaemolyticus
Clostridium perfringens type A
Clostridium difficile
Clostridium botulinum
Bacteria, Invasive
Campylobacter jejuni
Salmonella spp.
Shigella spp.
Aeromonas hydrophila
Plesiomonas shigelloides
Vibrio vulnificus (in people with liver disease)
Yersinia enterocolitica
Hemorrhagic *E. coli*, serotype 0157:H7
Clostridium perfringens type C (enteritis necroticans)
Parasites
Giardia lamblia
Entamoeba histolytica
Cryptosporidium
Cyclospora cayetanensis
Dientamoeba fragilis
Blastocystis hominis
Isospora belli
Trichinella spiralis

The search for the pathogens causing protracted diarrhea should include a stool Gram stain. This test can be of use for the rapid and accurate diagnosis of *Campylobacter* enteritis, in which the characteristic "gull wing" morphology of the organisms can allow presumptive diagnosis. The microscopic identification of white cells in the stool can be made from the Gram stain or by staining a slide of fresh diarrheal stool with methylene blue. It is important to recognize that neither the absence nor the presence of fecal white cells points toward a specific etiology. A positive test, however, may indicate the need for a continued search for an etiology if no pathogen is found during the initial evaluation.

Certain bacterial pathogens will be missed on selective media used for *Salmonella* and *Shigella,* and cultures for these microorganisms need to be specifically requested. These include *Campylobacter, Vibrio* spp., *Yersinia enterocolitica,* and *C. difficile.* Special laboratory tests are needed to identify agents such as enterotoxigenic *E. coli,* enteroinvasive *E. coli,* enteropathogenic *E. coli* (*E. coli* O157:H7), *Cryptosporidium,* and *Cyclospora* (see Chapter 26).

Serologic tests for *E. histolytica* are available at some specialty laboratories; significantly elevated antibody titers correlate well with invasive disease. Rotavirus, Norwalk agent, and hepatitis A can be diagnosed by serologic testing as well. The state health department is a good resource for finding the local or regional laboratories that perform these tests.

The complaint of flatulence and foul-smelling stools suggests giardiasis; a string test or a duodenal aspiration may be necessary to reveal the culprit (see Chapter 25). Enzyme-linked immunosorbent assay (ELISA) tests that can detect *Giardia* antigen in stool specimens are an adjunct to the standard morphologic identification of this parasite in stool specimens.

ACUTE DIARRHEA SYNDROMES

General Features

Treatment should focus on correcting dehydration and electrolyte abnormalities and maintaining adequate ongoing hydration. In some cases specific antimicrobial treatment may be appropriate, and patients may need to be observed to prevent development of complications.

Enterotoxigenic E. Coli

Travel-associated diarrhea caused by enterotoxigenic *Escherichia coli* is usually a self-limited illness, responding to the traveler's empiric self-treatment (see Chapter 6). Increasing resistance is developing to antibiotics such as trimethoprim-sulfamethoxazole in many developing countries such as Thailand; there is also sporadic resistance to quinolones and macrolides. Diarrhea caused by this agent is unlikely in the setting of prolonged gastrointestinal symptoms in the returned traveler who comes to medical attention.

SALMONELLA

Salmonella are ubiquitous gram-negative bacteria causing a range of disease in human infection: acute enterocolitis, typhoid fever, paratyphoid fever, bacteremia and septicemia, as well as focal infections (cholecystitis, meningitis, pneumonia, mycotic aortic aneurysms, osteomyelitis, and so forth). Infections may be asymptomatic, however, and asymptomatic human carriers may transmit the disease for years through unhygienic practices.

Etiology and Transmission

There are three species in the genus *Salmonella: S. typhi, S. choleraesuis,* and *S. enteritidis.* The species are further classified into serogroups and serotypes. Serogroup classification into five groups, A to E, on the basis of somatic (O) antigen identification can be done in most clinical microbiology laboratories. Serotypes are differentiated by testing for somatic (O) and flagellar (H) antigens. Although there are a large number of serotypes, 10 serotypes account for the majority of human salmonellosis diagnosed in the United States (e.g., *S. typhimurium, S. typhi*). Serotype identification is usually done at regional salmonella typing centers.

Salmonella infections are usually acquired through ingestion of contaminated food and water. Ingestion of uncooked foods, especially meat, poultry, eggs, and dairy products, is a special risk because of the high prevalence of salmonella infections in cattle and chickens. Animal reservoirs of *Salmonella* also include other fowl (turkeys, ducks), livestock (pigs, horses, sheep), dogs, cats, rodents, and reptiles (snakes, lizards, turtles). Infections can be transmitted by direct contact with these animals or their excreta. Oysters and shellfish grown in waters contaminated with sewage may transmit *Salmonella* to humans. One outbreak of salmonellosis was associated with contaminated marijuana.

Any food can be contaminated during preparation if unsanitary kitchen practices prevail with regard to cleansing of cutting boards, knives and utensils, and countertops. Food handlers with asymptomatic infections can also contaminate any food product during preparation. Although the high temperatures of cooking usually kill bacteria, certain strains of *Salmonella* are relatively heat-resistant and may survive exposure to heat that would kill other organisms. The relative resistance of salmonella to freezing, desiccation, and other environmental conditions also contributes to the transmission of infection through ice, dust, and water supplies.

Infections are dependent on the size of the inoculum dose, the vehicle of transmission, and the susceptibility of the host. An oral inoculum of 10^6 bacteria or greater, ingestion of contaminated foods high in protein and fat (ice cream, cheddar cheese, hamburger), and impaired host status (very young or very old age, diabetes, sickle cell disease, schistosomiasis) tend to promote infection. Strain-specific differences in virulence also appear to contribute to patterns of infection.

Clinical Features

Typhoid Fever

Typhoid fever is a severe and prolonged illness in humans caused by infections with *S. typhi*. The incubation period is usually 8 to 14 days and varies inversely with the size of the infectious inoculum. Untreated typhoid fever may last for several weeks and is characterized by (1) fever, headache, and abdominal tenderness early in the disease; (2) rash, prostration, and delirium during the second and third weeks of the disease; and (3) defervescence and convalescence in the fourth week of the disease. Constipation is often more common than diarrhea, especially in the early stages of the infection.

More than half the reported cases in the United States are acquired during travel or residence outside the country. The infection occurs through invasion of the gastrointestinal tract. The bacteria spread into the regional lymphatics and then into the bloodstream. The reticuloendothelial cells in the liver, spleen, bone marrow, and lymph nodes rapidly clear the early bacteremic phase, but the *S. typhi* bacteria multiply within the phagocytic cells and reenter the bloodstream and intestinal tract from intracellular sites, causing a sustained bacteremia and fecal shedding. Proliferation of reticuloendothelial cells and lymphoid tissue in the liver, spleen, mesenteric lymph nodes, and intestinal tract gives rise to complications of the disease. Common intestinal complications are bleeding and perforation.

Enteric Fever

Enteric fever is sometimes used as a synonym for typhoid fever. However, enteric fever also designates a severe systemic infection with *S. paratyphi* A, B, or C, which is often acquired during foreign travel. *Salmonella paratyphi* infection is accompanied by prostration, fever, and septicemia, but is of somewhat shorter duration than typhoid fever.

Enterocolitis

Salmonella enterocolitis can range from a mild to severe diarrheal illness with cramps, nausea, vomiting, and fever. The incubation period is usually 8 to 48 hours after exposure. The acute illness usually lasts for 1 to

2 weeks, although salmonella are shed in the feces for 4 to 6 weeks in untreated persons and up to months in some patients treated with antibiotics. Chronic enteric carriers are people who shed the same species of *Salmonella* in their feces for a year or more after the initial enterocolitis, and the species is usually *S. typhi.*

Bacteremia and Septicemia

Uncomplicated *Salmonella* enterocolitis can result in a transient bacteremia that will be detected by surveillance blood cultures. A septic presentation with spiking fevers and chills, leading to complications and even death, may be seen in patients with underlying diseases, malignancies, or altered host immunity. *Salmonella typhimurium* is the most common serotype isolated from blood.

Focal Infections

Focal infections can result from bacteremia or from contiguous spread to organs connected to the gastrointestinal tract. Focal infections have been reported in the gallbladder, appendix, peritoneum, urinary tract, bone, brain, meninges, heart, aorta, lungs, spleen, and skin. The severity of the illness and the outcome of the infection are related to the site of the infection and the nature of underlying disease or host impairment.

Laboratory Tests

Flecks of mucus in fecal specimens will show fecal leukocytes with Gram stain or Wright's stain. Stool specimens or rectal swabs should be cultured for *Salmonella* using selective isolation media, such as brilliant green, bismuth sulfite, *Salmonella-Shigella,* or xylose-lysine-deoxycholate agars. Blood and tissue specimens are cultured in the standard way.

The serologic tests are less useful for diagnosis because of problems with specificity. The serologic tests are more useful in epidemiologic investigations of outbreaks, when the antigen of a single serotype can be used to screen sera from the population under study. If the Widal test (agglutination titers of serum against *S. typhi* O and H antigens) is used to confirm the diagnosis of typhoid fever, a fourfold or greater increase in the titer in the absence of typhoid immunization is considered highly suggestive of infection. Acute and convalescent serum should be drawn 3 weeks apart. Peak serum titers usually occur during the third week of the illness.

Salmonella infection is required to be reported to the public health departments of most states.

Treatment

Antibiotic treatment may be indicated for patients with *Salmonella* enterocolitis who are severely symptomatic, or those at risk for severe infections such as neonates, elderly, immunosuppressed individuals. However, antibiotic treatment may sometimes prolong infectious carriage of *Salmonella.* Treatment should be guided by antibiotic sensitivity testing, since drug resistance to multiple antibiotics is prevalent among *Salmonella* strains. The antibiotics of choice are the quinolones or third-generation cephalosporins; newer macrolides such as azithromycin have also been used successfully (Table 25-2). High rates of resistance to ampicillin, amoxicillin, trimethoprim/sulfamethoxazole, and chloramphenicol are now present in many countries in Africa, Asia, and South America. Sporadic resistance to quinolones and third-generation cephalosporins has been reported from several developed and developing countries. Treat-

Table 25-2
Treatment for Common Bacterial Pathogens Causing Acute Diarrhea Syndromes*

Pathogen	Drug	Dosage for adults	Dosage for children
Salmonella spp.†	Ciprofloxacin	500 mg PO every 12 hours for 5 days	Not recommended for children less than 18 years old
	or Azithromycin‡	1.0 PO once then 500 mg qd for 6 days	
	or Ampicillin	0.5-1.0 gm PO or 0.5-3.0 gm IV every 6 hours for 5 days	100 mg/kg/day PO or IV in 4 divided doses for 5 days
	or Chloramphenicol	0.5-1.0 gm PO or IV every 6 hours for 5 days	50 mg/kg/day PO or IV in 4 divided doses for 5 days
	or Trimethoprim/sulfamethoxazole (Bactrim, Septra)	160/800 mg PO every 12 hours for 3 to 5 days	8/40 mg/kg/day in 2 divided doses for 3 to 5 days
Shigella spp.	Ciprofloxacin	500 mg PO every 12 hours for 5 days 1 gm PO once may be adequate	Not recommended for children less than 18 years old
	or Trimethoprim/sulfamethoxazole (Bactrim, Septra)	160/800 mg PO every 12 hours for 3 to 5 days	8/40 mg/kg/day in 2 divided doses for 3 to 5 days
	or Azithromycin‡	500 mg qd for PO once, then 250 mg qd for 4 days	
	or Tetracycline	2.5 g PO in a single dose	Not recommended for children less than 8 years old
	or Ampicillin	0.5-1.0 g PO or 0.5-3.0 g IV every 6 hours for 5 days	100 mg/kg/day PO or IV in 4 divided doses for 5 days
Campylobacter jejuni	or Nalidixic acid	0.5-0.75 g PO every 6 hours for 5 days	55 mg/kg/day PO in 4 divided doses for 5 days
	Ciprofloxacin	500 mg PO every 12 hours for 5 days	Not recommended for children less than 18 years old
	or Azithromycin‡	500 mg qd PO for 3 days	
	or Erythromycin	500 mg PO every 6 hours for 5 days	50 mg/kg/day PO or IV in 4 divided doses for 5 days

Table 25-2
Treatment for Common Bacterial Pathogens Causing Acute Diarrhea Syndromes*—cont'd

Pathogen	Drug	Dosage for Adults	Dosage for Children
	or Tetracycline§	500 mg PO every 6 hours for 5 days	Not recommended for children less than 8 years old
Yersinia enterocolitica	Ciprofloxacin	500 mg PO every 12 hours for 5 days or longer	Not recommended for children less than 18 years old
	or Gentamicin	3 to 5 mg/kg/day IV in 3 divided doses for 5 days or longer	6 to 7.5 mg/kg/day IV in 3 divided doses for 5 days or longer
	or Ceftriaxone	2.0 g IV or IM once a day for 5 days or longer	50 mg/kg/day IV or IM once a day for 5 days or longer
Vibrio spp.	Tetracycline§	500 mg PO every 6 hours for 5 days	Not recommended for children less than 8 years old (Oral rehydration of greatest importance)
	Furazolidone	100 mg PO every 6 hours for 7-10 days (*V. cholerae* O139 not susceptible)	1.25 mg/kg PO every 6 hours for 7-10 days
Clostridium difficile	Vancomycin	125 PO every 6 hours for 7-10 days	12.5 mg/kg/day PO in 4 divided doses for 5 days
	or Metronidazole	500 mg PO every 6 hours for 7-10 days	15 mg/kg/day PO in 2 divided doses for 7-10 days

*Selection of antimicrobial therapy should be guided by susceptibility testing of pathogenic bacterial isolates.
†Treat only significant or life-threatening infections; no treatment recommended for simple *Salmonella* gastroenteritis; see text for treatment choices for typhoid fever.
‡See text for details of resistance to listed antibiotics.
§Doxycycline, 100 mg PO every 12 hours may be substituted (not recommended for children less than 8 years old).

ment for gastroenteritis should continue for 2 to 3 days, or until the patient becomes afebrile.

Treatment of typhoid fever or suspected extraintestinal *Salmonellosis* is mandatory. The antibiotics of choice for uncomplicated typhoid include ciprofloxacin and third-generation cephalosporins (ceftriaxone or cefoperazone); there is also some experience with ofloxacin and azithromycin. Ciprofloxacin should be given for 7 days, whereas 5 to 7 days of third-generation cephalosporin appears to be adequate. Chloramphenicol remains the choice of some clinicians, but markedly increased resistance to this and other previously effective drugs has been noted in some developing countries; treatment with chloramphenicol requires 14 days.

In severe cases of typhoid fever (fever, delirium, obtundation, stupor, coma, or shock), a clinical trial showed that *high-dose dexamethasone* (3 mg/kg IV initial dose followed by eight doses of 1 mg/kg every 6 hours) *plus chloramphenicol* reduced mortality from 55.6% to 10%. Dexamethasone therefore should be considered in critically ill patients after starting an appropriate parenteral antibiotic. See Chapter 4 for information on the typhoid vaccines.

SHIGELLA

Etiology and Transmission

Shigellosis is an acute gastrointestinal infection caused by one of four *Shigella* species: *S. dysenteriae, S. flexneri, S. boydii,* and *S. sonnei.* Each species is a distinct serogroup (A through D), and among the four serogroups, there are more than 30 serotypes. Clinical illness ranges from severe inflammatory diarrhea (blood, mucus, tenesmus) with systemic toxicity (abdominal pain, fever), commonly called bacterial dysentery, to mild nonspecific diarrhea.

Shigellosis is a strictly human infection, and outbreaks of disease have been associated with conditions favoring human fecal-oral transmission, such as poor sanitation, inadequate water supplies, contaminated food, crowded living conditions, and fly-infested environments. Thus shigellosis is commonly seen among travelers returning from developing areas of the world and among people living or working in Indian reservations, refugee camps, and institutional settings (such as daycare centers, prisons, and facilities for the mentally handicapped).

The *Shigella* bacteria are gram-negative rods that can persist in the environment on inanimate objects for weeks and can cause infections with a relatively low inoculum dose (approximately 200 bacteria).

Plesiomonas shigelloides and *Aeromonas hydrophila* are pathogenic gram-negative rods that are found worldwide in developing areas. In addition to routine diarrhea, these organisms can occasionally cause a dysenteric picture similar to *Shigella.* The approach to diagnosis and treatment is similar to that for *Shigella.*

Clinical Features

The incubation period of *Shigella* is usually 36 to 72 hours, with a presentation characterized by fever, abdominal cramps, and watery diarrhea. The illness may progress to a more serious condition with the passage of blood, mucus, and pus in diarrheal stools, accompanied by left lower quadrant pain (the distal colon and rectum), tenesmus, and some urgency. *Shigella* invade the mucosa and submucosa of the colon during this stage of the disease. The duration of symptoms is usually a week or less, although *Shigella* may persist in the stools for 1 to 3 months after cessation of clinical symptoms.

Laboratory Tests

Diagnosis is made by isolation of the causative bacteria from stool or rectal swab specimens. Portions of the specimen containing blood or mucus give the highest yield on culture. Neutrophils seen on Gram stain or methylene blue stain of a fecal smear will support the diagnosis of an inflammatory infection but are not specific for shigellosis: *Salmonella, Campylobacter, E. histolytica,* ulcerative colitis, and *C. difficile* must also be considered.

Treatment

Most strains of *Shigella* are resistant to ampicillin, trimethoprim/sulfamethoxazole, nalidixic acid, sulfonamides and tetracyclines. Five days of treatment with ciprofloxacin (or one of the other quinolones), azithromycin or ceftriaxone will shorten the duration of symptoms and terminate bacterial carriage (Table 25-2).

CAMPYLOBACTER

Campylobacter jejuni is a short, comma-shaped, gram-negative rod that has been recognized as a common cause of infectious bacterial diarrhea worldwide and that may exceed *Salmonella* and *Shigella* as an etiologic agent of acute infectious diarrhea.

Etiology and Transmission

The *Campylobacter* bacteria are worldwide in distribution. *C. jejuni* infection is commonly acquired by ingestion of contaminated food (eggs, poultry, milk) or water, although people in close contact with sick people or animals (livestock, puppies) may acquire campylobacteriosis from direct contamination. *Campylobacter fetus* subsp. *fetus* infection is less common but causes serious systemic infections in human hosts with impaired immunity.

Clinical Features

C. jejuni is a common cause of enteritis. After an incubation period of 2 to 4 days, the illness ensues with cramping abdominal pain, fever, and watery diarrhea typically lasting for less than 1 week, although recurrent attacks in untreated individuals have been noted. In some cases, colitis symptoms predominate, with lower abdominal pain and bloody stools. Rarely, colonic ulcerations and systemic infections (bacteremia) result from infection.

C. fetus subsp. *fetus* is more regularly associated with systemic infections, with diarrhea occurring in only one third of patients. Infants and immunocompromised patients appear to be more susceptible to severe complications of fulminant sepsis, endocarditis, meningitis, and thrombophlebitis caused by this organism.

Laboratory Tests

The diagnosis is made by isolation of the bacteria in stool specimens, blood specimens, and other tissues. Isolation of *Campylobacter* from stool specimens requires selective culture media. A presumptive diagnosis can be made from Gram stain of the stool, when white cells and "seagull-shaped" arrangements of gram-negative *Vibrio*-like bacteria are observed.

Treatment

Severe or prolonged gastrointestinal illness should be treated with antibiotics, especially in pregnant women or immunosuppressed patients. In general most *Campylobacter* sp. are sensitive to macrolides, quinolones, nitrofurans, and aminoglycosides. Oral therapy with erythromycin (or one of the newer macrolides such as azithromycin), a quinolone, or tetracycline is a reasonable initial option (see Table 25-2). In certain developing countries, such as Thailand where there is now significant resistance to ciprofloxacin, azithromycin should be the initial choice. For patients with suspected extraintestinal infection, gentamicin and imipenem have also been used pending the results of in vitro sensitivity testing. No *Campylobacter* vaccine is available.

YERSINIA ENTEROCOLITICA

Yersinia enterocolitica is an increasingly recognized cause of bacterial enteritis in humans. Illness caused by this microorganism can be acquired in the United States, as well as worldwide.

Etiology and Transmission

The bacteria appear to be ubiquitous in nature, with humans acquiring infections from contamination of food (milk, meat, shellfish, tofu) and ground water (contaminated by human or animal feces). Person-to-person transmission also occurs. The bacteria are able to multiply at room temperature and to survive low temperatures (4° C) for many months under a variety of environmental conditions.

Clinical Features

Infection takes place after ingestion of a relatively large inoculum (10^9 bacteria), and the infection localizes in the terminal ileum, with localized invasion and involvement of the mesenteric lymph nodes. Patients can present with cramping abdominal pain, fever, and diarrhea. Bloody diarrhea may be seen. The enterocolitis may last from 1 to 3 weeks. Occasionally, pain localized in the right lower quadrant and caused by ileitis and mesenteric lymphadenitis is severe enough to mimic appendicitis, and *Yersinia* infections have been diagnosed at the time of laparotomy for presumed appendicitis.

Postinfectious complications are seen mainly in adults and consist of autoimmune disorders. Arthritis, erythema nodosum, Reiter's syndrome, and ankylosing spondylitis are complications occurring in up to 1% to 5% of patients in the United States. Patients with the HLA-B27 histocompatibility tissue type are more likely to develop severe postinfectious arthritic complications.

Laboratory Tests

Isolation of the gram-negative *Yersinia* bacteria from stool specimens is complicated. Current laboratory techniques involve cold enrichment and selective media. The *Yersinia* bacteria may be present in the stool for weeks after symptoms resolve. Serologic tests are available at some laboratories and are useful in the evaluation of patients with postinfectious autoimmune complications.

Treatment

The course of enterocolitis and mesenteric lymphadenitis caused by *Y. enterocolitica* is a self-limited process in most cases, and the usefulness of antimicrobial therapy is uncertain. Oral antimicrobials with potential efficacy include trimethoprim/sulfamethoxazole, doxycycline, and quinolone antibiotics (norfloxacin, ciprofloxacin, ofloxacin). However, in severe clinical illness and systemic infections, appropriate antibiotics are parenteral quinolones and ceftriaxone or ceftizoxime (these are frequently combined with an aminoglycoside, such as gentamicin). Further treatment should be guided by in vitro antibiotic sensitivity testing of the causative isolate.

VIBRIO

Human infections with *Vibrio* bacteria have been associated with four species: *V. cholerae, V. parahaemolyticus, V. vulnificus,* and *V. alginolyticus.* The first two *Vibrio* species cause gastroenteritis. *V. vulnificus* can cause gastroenteritis, septicemia, or wound infections, whereas *V. alginolyticus* has been associated only with wound and ear infections.

Etiology and Transmission

The vibrios are gram-negative halophilic rods widely distributed in marine and estuarine environments and, in the case of *V. cholerae,* also found in bodies of fresh water. All three species causing gastroenteritis can be isolated from sediments, fish and shellfish, and plankton.

Cholera gastroenteritis has occurred in epidemics that have spread across continents. Although conditions of poor sanitation and contaminated water supplies have contributed to epidemic situations, the organism can be found in environments where there is no evidence of human pollution. In addition, strain-specific virulence factors probably contribute to the transmission of disease.

Tourists from Western countries rarely acquire cholera as a consequence of travel to endemic areas, owing in part to customs and dietary habits different from those of the local inhabitants, as well as to underlying good health. Relatively large inoculums (10^{10} organisms or more) are necessary to establish an infection in normal human hosts because *V. cholerae* is exquisitely sensitive to gastric acid. In patients with decreased gastric acidity as a result of disease or medication, the infectious inoculum is lower (10^{6} organisms or less).

V. parahaemolyticus is a common cause of acute gastroenteritis in countries or situations where raw, undercooked, or improperly stored and handled seafood is consumed. *V. parahaemolyticus* outbreaks have been reported in Japan, in the United States, and on cruise ships and aircraft. Sushi, precooked crabs, shrimp, lobster, and raw oysters have all been implicated in outbreak reports.

Reported cases of *V. vulnificus* gastroenteritis have been associated with eating shellfish, especially raw oysters. In addition to causing vomiting and diarrhea, *V. vulnificus* can become an invasive pathogen causing septicemia and intractable shock secondary to gram-negative sepsis. Preexisting hepatic disease was present in more than 75% of septicemic patients reported; thus patients with hepatic disease should be cautioned about eating raw oysters.

Clinical Features

The incubation period for *Vibrio*-associated diseases ranges from less than a day to several days. Cholera symptoms can vary from mild watery diarrhea to severe watery diarrhea (rice-water stools) accompanied by abdominal cramps, nausea, and vomiting. Dehydration, hypotension, and even death can ensue from severe fluid and electrolyte losses that remain uncorrected. *V. cholerae* is not invasive.

Virulence of the cholera organism is caused by attachment of the bacterium to the small bowel epithelial cells and production of an enterotoxin (cholera toxin). The toxin causes activation of the membrane-associated cyclic adenosine monophosphate system, leading to electrolyte and water loss. Up to 1 L/hr of isotonic protein-free fluid rich in sodium, potassium, chloride, and bicarbonate can be lost from the small bowel of an infected person.

V. parahaemolyticus can cause a self-limited (72 hours) cholera-like gastroenteritis owing to a heat-labile hemolysin. However, an invasive pathogenic factor that allows bacteria to penetrate into the lamina propria of the ileum has also been reported; this virulence factor associated with *V. parahaemolyticus* may present as a bacterial dysentery (*Shigella*-like) illness.

V. vulnificus can cause acute gastroenteritis with vomiting and diarrhea and can also cause septicemia in high-risk patients, as discussed previously. An alternative presentation is that of severe wound infections.

Laboratory Studies

Vibrio can be cultured from stool, tissue, or blood specimens on a variety of selective microbiologic media. The organisms appear as comma-shaped, gram-negative rods on Gram stain. They are tolerant of relatively cold temperatures (4° C) and can withstand temperatures of traditional cooking (60° C to 80° C) for 15 minutes if they are present in high concentrations in seafood. Hemolysis can be demonstrated by culture on blood agar, although enterotoxin testing involves animal tissue assays and is not routinely available. Biotyping (classic and El Tor strains), serotyping (O1 serogroup: Ogawa, Inaba, and Hikojima serotypes), and phagetyping of cholera isolates may be performed in reference laboratories for epidemiologic tracing. In 1993, a new strain of cholera identified as a non-O1 serogroup was recognized as a cause of epidemic cholera in India and Bangladesh. The new strain is called the O139 cholera strain.

Treatment

The cornerstone of treatment for severe cholera and other forms of severe gastroenteritis is the adequate replacement of fluid and electrolytes lost in the diarrheal stools. The WHO oral rehydration formula is given in Table 6-4.

Tetracycline treatment (Table 25-2) may shorten the duration of *Vibrio* infections by eradicating organisms in the stool, although symptoms may persist after institution of appropriate antimicrobial therapy because of toxins already bound to the mucosal surface. Norfloxacin, ciprofloxacin, and ofloxacin also have activity against *V. cholerae* and *V. parahaemolyticus*. The O139 cholera strain is susceptible to tetracycline, but is resistant to trimethoprim/sulfamethoxazole and furazolidone (see Chapter 6).

In cholera-endemic areas, a long-lasting immunity to cholera appears to decrease the incidence of cholera attacks in local inhabitants surviving the disease in childhood. The parenteral cholera vaccine (Chapter 4) stimulates the formation of antitoxin and vibriocidal antibodies in the serum of recipients but is only partially effective (50% protective). An oral cholera vaccine, not currently available in the United States, appears to be more effective. Thus local mucosal factors may also influence the establishment of infection. In general, travelers to endemic areas should be advised to carefully select food and water and to avoid seafood when possible.

CLOSTRIDIUM DIFFICILE

Although colitis caused by *C. difficile* (pseudomembranous colitis, antibiotic-associated colitis) is not expected to be the primary pathogenic process in travel-acquired infectious diarrhea, this microorganism should be considered in cases of diarrhea persisting after travel when the patient has been previously treated with one or more courses of antimicrobials (not an uncommon situation, since antimicrobials are available for purchase without a prescription in many countries). Clinical features include persistent and profuse watery diarrhea, sometimes containing blood and mucus. Systemic toxicity with fever and malaise may be present in severe cases. Special laboratory techniques are required to isolate the bacterium and to demonstrate the production of *C. difficile* toxin. Treatment consists of discontinuing previous antimicrobial therapy and starting oral vancomycin or metronidazole (see Table 25-2).

ROTAVIRUS AND NORWALK AGENT

Rotavirus has been recognized as a major etiologic agent in outbreaks of gastroenteritis of infants and children in many parts of the world, especially in developing countries. Epidemics of rotavirus infection also occur in adult and geriatric populations.

Norwalk virus is another enteric pathogen recognized as an important cause of nonbacterial gastroenteritis. Although rotavirus and Norwalk virus were originally termed "winter" gastroenteritis, because outbreaks of vomiting and diarrhea occurring in winter months prompted early investigation of these agents, outbreaks may occur at any time of the year.

Transmission

Rotavirus is probably acquired by ingestion of contaminated food and water and by person-to-person transmission. Human rotavirus types appear to be distinct from animal types. Infants and children from 6 months to 2 years old appear to be most susceptible. Protective antibodies in colostrum and breast milk may protect breastfed infants less than 6 months old.

Norwalk virus is a human virus that is transmitted by contaminated water supplies and foods such as salads, clams, and oysters. One large outbreak resulting from contamination of frosting on bakery products by an infected food handler has been reported.

Clinical Features

Gastroenteritis caused by rotavirus and Norwalk virus is characterized by diarrhea, abdominal cramps, and vomiting. Fever is rarely present. The disease is self-limited, and the gastrointestinal symptoms last from 1 to 4 days. In some adult patients studied, rotavirus infection was associated with upper respiratory tract symptoms without gastrointestinal symptoms.

Laboratory Studies

Development of an ELISA detection system for rotavirus antigen and antibody has facilitated detection and study of rotavirus in outbreaks of diarrhea.

The diagnosis of Norwalk virus rests on excluding bacterial pathogens in the setting of an appropriate clinical syndrome and chain of infectious transmission. A serologic test for Norwalk virus is not available commercially at this time but is used by clinical research laboratories. Virus particles can be identified in stools of individuals selected for detailed study by electron microscopy; however, this examination is not available in many routine clinical laboratories. Neither virus grows efficiently in tissue culture.

Treatment

Treatment consists of replacement of fluid and electrolytes, by oral rehydration formulas if possible (see Table 6-4). Development of a safe vaccine against rotavirus is a subject of continuing medical research on diarrheal diseases.

CHRONIC DIARRHEA

A significant number of travelers continue to experience diarrhea and ongoing gastrointestinal complaints weeks and even months after returning from their trip. It is this group of travelers, rather than those with acute episodes of TD, who are likely to seek advice from their physician. The differential diagnosis in such patients can be wide, but most are likely to be related to (1) undiagnosed infection, (2) malabsorption syndrome, or (3) previously undiagnosed gastrointestinal disease.

UNDIAGNOSED INFECTION

Presence of ongoing infection with an enteric pathogen overlooked in a previous laboratory evaluation needs to be excluded at the outset using the appropriate stool cultures and parasite diagnostics described previously. Some infections, such as those caused by *Salmonella* and *Shigella* spp., can recrudesce in patients who are carriers of these organisms, whereas others such as *Giardia* spp. can present with vague upper gastrointestinal symptoms. Colitis resulting from *C. difficile* can occur some time after a trip if antibiotics and antimalarial agents had been used.

MALABSORPTION

A state of temporary malabsorption is not uncommon following acute diarrhea and most commonly results from disaccharide intolerance resulting in a secretory or osmotic diarrhea. The damage to the intestinal mucosa and its enzymes (especially the disaccharidase lactase) possibly resulting from infection can take several weeks to recover. Patients should be advised to follow a lactose-free (or fructose-free) diet and also to avoid excessive use of dietetic chewing gum and candy, since these may contain an indigestible carbohydrate sugar substitute.

Chronic malabsorption can follow infection with *Giardia* or *Cyclopora* spp. and can also be associated with small bowel overgrowth, celiac disease, or tropical sprue. Celiac disease can often be confirmed by response to a gluten-free diet, and possibly by the presence of antigliadin tissue transglutaminase antibodies. In some cases small bowel biopsy may be required. Tropical sprue is a poorly characterized syndrome of worsening intestinal symptoms associated with continuing diarrhea and steatorrhea, which has been described in expatriates living for long periods (over 1 year) in certain geographic regions. It only occasionally occurs after an episode of TD or in short-term travelers. Although the etiology of tropical sprue is unknown, it may respond to tetracycline, 250 mg q6h, and folic acid, 5 mg/day.

Brainerd diarrhea is a recently recognized syndrome of unknown etiology characterized by acute onset of watery diarrhea (which may last for more than 36 months in some cases) and failure to respond to antimicrobial agents. In some outbreaks it has been associated with consumption of raw milk or contaminated water. Biopsies from colonic mucosa characteristically show epithelial lymphocytosis.

PREVIOUSLY UNDIAGNOSED GASTOINTESTINAL DISEASE

Physicians seeing travelers with chronic gastrointestinal complaints need to maintain a low index of suspicion for the presence of previously unrecognized gastrointestinal disease. Irritable bowel syndrome is probably the most common such illness in travelers, who may experience an abrupt onset of intermittent cramping pain, bloating and gas after a trip. Inflammatory bowel disease resulting from ulcerative colitis or Crohn's disease should be suspected in the presence of bloody diarrhea, accompanied by systemic signs such as weight loss, oral or perianal lesions, as well as extraintestinal manifestations such as arthropathies or ophthalmic symptoms. In older travelers presenting with altered bowel habits and occult blood in the stool, colonoscopy is necessary to exclude carcinoma. Finally, unrecognized human immunodeficiency virus infection may occasionally present in returning travelers with gastrointestinal complaints.

DIAGNOSTIC APPROACH

The causes of protracted diarrhea and ongoing gastrointestinal complaints will often usually reveal themselves after clinical examination and laboratory studies outlined previously; however a few cases remain unsolved and will require further diagnostic evaluation, and possibly consultation with a gastroenterologist. In such patients a complete blood count may be helpful to exclude signs of systemic infection, anemia from ongoing blood loss or malabsorption, or eosinophilia. If tropical sprue and other malabsorption syndromes are being considered in the differential diagnosis, further evaluation for malabsorption using lactose tolerance and D-xylose may be considered. The sigmoidoscopic examination is used in the next round of evaluation for protracted inflammatory diarrhea. The colonic mucosa can be inspected and biopsy material obtained from abnormal areas to rule out diseases such as Crohn's disease, ulcerative colitis, schistosomiasis, and amebiasis. Swabs of abnormal colonic mucosa and mucus may be examined as wet preparations for trophozoites of *E. histolytica.* Finally esophagogastroduodenoscopy may be useful to obtain duodenal aspirates for protozoan parasites and small bowel biopsies to exclude celiac sprue.

THERAPEUTIC APPROACH

Specific treatment for any of the underlying causes of ongoing gastrointestinal complaints discussed here should obviously be a first therapeutic step. In some cases, however, when the stools are negative for white cells and blood, and no enteric pathogens are identified, patients in whom other gastrointestinal illnesses have reasonably been excluded may benefit from empiric therapy. Commonly used antimicrobial agents in such patients include quinolones, azithromycin, metronidazole, tinidazole, or albendazole. Elimination diets can be tried excluding lactose, fructose, or gluten from the diet for a specified period. Antispasmodic medications such as hyoscyamine (Levsin) or dicyclomine (Bentyl) can be tried, especially if irritable bowel syndrome appears likely. Finally, some patients may experience improvement with dietary supplements such as digestive enzymes (such as lactase), dietary fiber bulk-forming agents such as psylium or methylcellulose, or probiotics such as lactobacillus.

REFERENCES

Alam AN, Alam NH, Ahmed T, Sack DA: Randomised double blind trial of single dose doxycycline for treating cholera in adults, *BMJ* 300:1619, 1990.

Bennish ML et al: Treatment of shigellosis. III. Comparison of one- or two-dose ciprofloxacin with standard five-day therapy, *Ann Intern Med* 117:727, 1992.

Blaser MJ, Reller LB: Campylobacter enteritis, *N Engl J Med* 305:1444, 1981.

Centers for Disease Control and Prevention: The management of acute diarrhea in children: oral rehydration, maintenance, and nutritional therapy, *MMWR* 41(RR-16):1, 1992.

Cook GC: Persisting diarrhoea and malabsorption, *Gut* 35:582, 1994.

Chinh NT et al: A randomized controlled comparison of azithromycin and ofloxacin for treatment of multidrug-resistant or nalidixic acid-resistant enteric fever, *Antimicob Agents Chemother* 44:1855, 2000.

DuPont HL et al: Five versus three days of ofloxacin therapy for traveler's diarrhea: a placebo-controlled study, *Antimicrob Agents Chemother* 36:87, 1992.

Edlitz-Marcus T et al: Comparative efficacy of two- and five-day courses of ceftriaxone for treatment of severe shigellosis in children, *J Pediatr* 123:822, 1993.

Ericsson CD, DuPont HL: Travelers' diarrhea: approaches to prevention and treatment, *Clin Infect Dis* 16:616, 1993.

Gayraud M et al: Antibiotic treatment of *Yersinia enterocolitica* septicemia: a retrospective review of 43 cases, *Clin Infect Dis* 17:405, 1993.

Hien TT et al: Short course of ofloxacin for treatment of multidrug-resistant typhoid, *Clin Infect Dis* 20:917, 1995.

Hoffman SL et al: Reduction of mortality in chloramphenicol-treated severe typhoid fever by high-dose dexamethasone, *N Engl J Med* 310:82, 1984.

Hoge CW et al: Trends in antibiotic resistance among diarrheal pathogens isolated in Thailand over 15 years, *Clin Infect Dis* 26:341, 1998.

Khan WA et al: Randomised controlled comparison of single-dose ciprofloxacin and doxycycline for cholera caused by *Vibrio cholerae* O1 or O139, *Lancet* 348:296, 1996.

Khan WA et al: Treatment of shigellosis. V. Comparison of azithromycin and ciprofloxacin. A double-blind, randomized, controlled trial, *Ann Intern Med* 126:697, 1997.

Koeleman RGM, Regensburg DF, van Katwijk F, MacLaren DM: Retrospective study to determine the diagnostic value of the Widal test in a non-endemic country, *Eur J Clin Microbiol Infect Dis* 11:167, 1992.

Kuschner RA et al: Use of azithromycin for the treatment of *Campylobacter* enteritis in travelers to Thailand, an area where ciprofloxacin resistance is prevalent, *Clin Infect Dis* 21:536, 1995.

Lindenbaum J, Kent TH, Sprinz H: Malabsorption and jejunitis in American Peace Corps volunteers in Pakistan, *Ann Intern Med* 65:1201, 1966.

Marrie TJ et al: Rotavirus infection in a geriatric population, *Arch Intern Med* 142:313, 1982.

Mintz ED et al: An outbreak of Brainerd diarrhea among travelers to the Galapagos Islands, *J Infect Dis* 177:1041, 1998.

Morse DL et al: Widespread outbreaks of clam- and oyster-associated gastroenteritis. Role of Norwalk virus, *N Engl J Med* 314:678, 1986.

Osterholm MT et al: An outbreak of a newly recognized chronic diarrhea syndrome associated with raw milk consumption, *JAMA* 256:484, 1986.

Sirinavin S, Garner P: Antibiotics for treating salmonella gut infections, *Cochrane Database Syst Rev* 2:CD001167, 2000.

Thornton SA et al: Norfloxacin compared to trimethoprim/sulfamethoxazole for the treatment of traveler's diarrhea among U.S. military personnel deployed to South America and West Africa, *Mil Med* 157:55, 1992.

Wistrom J et al: Empiric treatment of acute diarrheal disease with norfloxacin. A randomized, placebo-controlled study, *Ann Intern Med* 117:202, 1992.

CHAPTER 26

Amebiasis, Giardiasis, and Other Intestinal Protozoan Infections

Abinash Virk and Elaine C. Jong

Entamoeba histolytica and *Giardia lamblia* are the most common protozoal pathogens of the human intestinal tract. Both are cosmopolitan parasites, being found in rural and urban environments throughout the world. Current estimates place the prevalence of fecal excretion of *Giardia* or *E. histolytica* cysts or trophozoites in the United States at approximately 4% for each pathogen. Few reliable data are available, but infection rates are believed to be significantly higher in much of the developing world; migrant workers, immigrants, and refugees from these regions are frequently found to be harboring these organisms. Despite this, neither protozoan is a common cause of disease in travelers. *Giardia* accounted for only 1% to 4% of cases of traveler's diarrhea in various series, and *E. histolytica* for less than 1%. Invasive amebiasis is similarly uncommon. However, the prolonged illness and potential for serious complications in both diseases make it important that they be expeditiously diagnosed and treated.

ENTAMOEBA HISTOLYTICA

Pathogenesis

Protozoa are divided into four classes based on their method of locomotion. *E. histolytica* is the only commonly recognized human intestinal pathogen in the subphylum Sarcodina, whose members are distinguished by the use of pseudopods for locomotion. The invasive form, the *trophozoite,* is quite large, measuring between 12 and 60 μm in diameter. The major infective form is the *cyst,* which is 10 to 20 μm in size. Infection is usually acquired by transmission of cysts by direct person-to-person contact or by ingestion of cysts present in food or water. Sexual transmission (either through oral-anal-genital contact or by direct inoculation of traumatized tissue) and an outbreak related to contaminated enema equipment illustrate alternative modes of spread.

The trophozoite form is very labile, but the cysts can survive for weeks in moist surroundings and are resistant to gastric acid and the low concentrations of chlorine commonly used in commercial water purification.

Intestinal Amebiasis

The initial site of amebic infection is always the cecum and colon after *E. histolytica* excysts in the small bowel. Attachment of trophozoites to the colonic mucosa is followed by mucosal invasion, leading to both superficial and deep colonic ulcerations. Development of the ulcers is dependent on the properties of the amebae to lyse host cells, cause proteolysis of the extracellular matrix to increase invasion of tissues while evading the host immune responses. Virulent strains of *E. histolytica* have been shown to possess cytotoxins, proteolytic enzymes, and transmembrane ion channel proteins (porins). These cellular products may contribute to the cell lysis observed in host leukocytes and tissue during amebic infections. Strains from different population groups in different areas of the world have been found to vary widely in their relative virulence. Certain isoenzyme patterns that appear to serve as markers for strain virulence have been identified. A rapid assay for virulence would have great clinical significance, as it is likely that clinically avirulent strains such as *E. dispar* or *E. moshkovskii,* while morphologically indistinguishable from virulent strains, do not require treatment. For instance, the observation that the vast majority of *E. histolytica* isolates from male homosexuals in the United States and England manifest avirulent isoenzyme patterns correlates with the rarity of amebic dysentery and invasive amebiasis in this population. Presence of other bacteria in the colon, extremes of age, immunocompromised state, pregnancy, and the nutritional status of the patient influence the virulence of the amebae.

Extraintestinal Amebiasis

Once local infection and invasion are established in the colon, the amebae can gain access to the portal venous system and establish metastatic sites of infection. Symptomatic invasive amebiasis occurs in approximately 10% of patients with asymptomatic *E. histolytica* fecal carriage state. The most common location is the liver, but amebic abscesses of the lungs, brain, and, rarely, other organs do occur. These metastatic abscesses contain necrotic debris but few leukocytes or trophozoites. Trophozoites are most easily identified in the tissue at the periphery of the abscess. In addition to hematogenous dissemination, local spread of infection from the colon can result in cutaneous amebiasis or in paracolonic inflammatory masses referred to as amebomas.

Immunity

Infected individuals develop both humoral and cell-mediated immune responses to *E. histolytica.* The specific immunoglobulin response is helpful in diagnosis in nonendemic areas (see later discussions), but its importance in vivo is unknown. Cell-mediated responses are important in controlling the disease, particularly in invasive amebiasis, but only partial protection from reinfection is achieved after recovery from the primary episode. A recent study has shown that mucosal IgA anti-lectin antibody response is associated with immune protection against *E. histolytica* colonization.

Epidemiology

There is no recognized animal reservoir for *E. histolytica.* Humans serve as the principal reservoir of infection. Therefore the persistence of endemic disease in a population is dependent on crowding and poor standards of hygiene for water purification, food preparation, and waste disposal.

Amebiasis is a significant health problem in much of Africa, Latin America, Southeast Asia, and the Indian subcontinent. Within the United States, institutionalized mentally retarded individuals and promiscuous male homosexuals (secondary to sexual transmission) are known high-risk groups. The prevalence of *E. histolytica* in male homosexuals attending sexually transmitted disease clinics in New York, San Francisco, and Seattle has been in the 25% to 30% range.

Travelers to any developing country must be considered to be at risk of acquiring amebiasis, but in practice, travel to Mexico or to remote rural areas of Asia (e.g., trekking in Nepal) appears to bear the highest risk. The risk of amebiasis among travelers was 0.3% in one study.

Surprisingly, amebiasis is uncommon in Southeast Asian refugees, with eight of ten published studies reporting prevalence rates of 2% or less (compared with 2% to 4% in the U.S. population).

Clinical Features

Intestinal Amebiasis

Infection with *E. histolytica* is most often asymptomatic. Cyst excretion can be self-limited or may persist for years. When symptoms are present, they range from mild colitis to severe dysentery. Typically, there is gradual onset of colicky lower abdominal pain and diarrhea (although the volume of stool tends to be less than in other colonic infections). Mucus, tenesmus, fever, and abdominal pain usually accompany diarrhea. Stools are often bloody and may be associated with signs of hypovolemia in severe cases. Spontaneous resolution after 1 to 4 weeks, sometimes with persistent asymptomatic cyst excretion, is the usual outcome in mild, untreated cases, but persistent disease is not uncommon. Chronic disease may manifest cyclical relapses and remissions mimicking inflammatory bowel disease. Chronic amebic colitis results in anorexia, weight loss, and intermittent abdominal pain.

Several serious complications can develop in patients with amebic dysentery or extensive colonic involvement. Peritonitis may develop secondary to perforation of an amebic colonic abscess, or intestinal hemorrhage may result from erosion of an abscess into an artery. The prognosis is poor in these situations, since the colon is often diffusely necrotic, rendering surgery difficult. Fulminant amebic colitis (which may progress to a toxic megacolon) is most common in infants, pregnant women, and patients receiving corticosteroids. The incidence of these complications among patients with dysentery in endemic areas is approximately 5%. Amebomas are inflammatory mass lesions most common in the cecum, ascending colon, and descending colon; usually solitary, they can be radiologically indistinguishable from colonic neoplasms or intestinal tuberculosis. Involvement of the cecum can result in amebic appendicitis.

Extraintestinal Amebiasis

The liver is by far the most common site of extraintestinal amebic disease. Amebic liver abscesses can present coincident with the dysenteric phase of the illness or as long as several years later. They are predominantly solitary (83%) and located in the right lobe (75%) of the liver. This predilection for the right lobe results from streaming of the blood flow within the portal vein. Hepatic amebiasis develops in 3% to 9% of cases of intestinal amebiasis. However, only 14% of patients with hepatic amebiasis will have active intestinal disease at the time of diagnosis, and 67% will have neither active intestinal disease nor a history of dysentery. Age-specific incidence peaks in the 20- to 50-year-old group with a male/female case ratio of 3:1.

The duration of symptoms before presentation is less than 2 weeks in the majority of cases. Virtually 100% of patients will present with pain, usually localized to the right upper quadrant. Right lower chest pain, which may be pleuritic, is present in 25%. Other symptoms include upper abdominal swelling, weight loss, malaise, anorexia, and cough (10% to 50%). Diaphragmatic irritation can also result in referred pain to the right shoulder. High fever with chills and profuse night sweats may be present. Examination reveals tender hepatomegaly in 80%, sometimes with point tenderness. Abnormal findings at the right lung base (rales or dullness) are present in approximately half of the patients examined. Jaundice is rare.

Primary amebic abscesses of the lung or brain have few distinguishing characteristics from pyogenic abscesses of these organs. Finally, extra-intestinal disease can also result from rupture of a hepatic amebic abscess into the peritoneum, pleural cavity, or pericardium.

Diagnosis

Intestinal Amebiasis

Examination of the Stool

Traditionally, intestinal amebiasis was diagnosed by the identification of trophozoites or cysts in fresh feces. However, owing to the more prevalent nonpathogenic, morphologically identical, but genetically distinct *E. dispar* in stool, it is recommended that E. *histolytica* be diagnosed using a *E. histolytica*-specific test. E. *histolytica* trophozoites survive only 2 to 5 hours at 37° C and 6 to 16 hours at 25° C, so either prompt examination of specimens or refrigeration (survival 48 to 96 hours) is essential. In active infections, both cysts and trophozoites can be found in the stool. More often, however, the number of organisms is small and excretion is sporadic, resulting in a yield from the examination of a single specimen of only 33% to 50%. The finding of ingested red blood cells (hematophagocytosis), if present, is diagnostic of *E. histolytica* infection. Despite invasive disease, fecal leukocytes are not found because of the lytic activity of the amebae. Fecal blood (microscopic or gross) is seen in approximately 70% of patients.

Differentiation from nonpathogenic ameba species or fecal leukocytes can be difficult, and both false-positive and false-negative laboratory errors are common. Therefore in addition to clinical and epidemiologic correlation, a specific *E. histolytica* test is advised for definitive diagnosis. Tool antigen tests are available for the detection of both *E. histolytica* and/or *E. dispar* coproantigens. These tests can help differentiate *E. histolytica* from *E. dispar.* Stool *E. histolytica*-specific antigen has a sensitivity of 87% and specificity of >90% compared with culture. Molecular methods such as polymerase chain reaction are also available to differentiate *E. histolytica* from *E. dispar;* however, this method is not widely available.

Colonoscopy

Colonoscopy is preferred over sigmoidoscopy because amebic colitis lesions can be present in the ascending colon or cecum and be missed on a sigmoidoscopy. Endoscopy may be normal or reveal only nonspecific edema and inflammation of the mucosa. Characteristic ulcers are present only 25% of the time, but scrapings or brushings from the rectal mucosa or the edge of an ulcer frequently are positive for trophozoites (samples must be obtained with a glass pipette or metal implements, since the amebae adhere to cotton fibers). Endoscopic brushings or biopsy from the edge of the ulcer is more sensitive for the diagnosis of amebic colitis than fecal examination.

Radiographic Studies

No pathognomonic pattern is present on radiographic studies. Barium studies in particular should not be performed, since the barium interferes with stool examination for protozoa.

Blood Tests

Of the several serologic tests developed for amebiasis, the indirect hemagglutination test is the most widely available. Titers are elevated in about 80% of cases of invasive intestinal disease but in only 50% or less of asymptomatic cyst passers. Other immunologic tests for measurement of antiamebic antibody are gel diffusion, immunoelectrophoresis, latex agglutination, and enzyme-linked immunosorbent assay (ELISA). Of these tests, the ELISA assay may be the most sensitive in detection of low levels of anti-*E. histolytica* antibody during early stages of infection. A positive test correlates well with the development of invasive amebic disease (liver abscess and dysentery), particularly at higher serologic titers. Serologic tests need to be evaluated carefully in persons from endemic countries, since antiameba antibodies can remain elevated for years after the initial infection. Serologic tests are particularly useful in excluding amebiasis as the etiology of chronic inflammatory bowel disease before initiating steroid therapy and especially in persons from nonendemic countries.

Extraintestinal Amebiasis (Especially Liver Abscesses)

Blood Tests

Most patients with amebic liver abscesses will have a moderate degree of leukocytosis with a predominance of neutrophils. Transaminases may be slightly elevated in acute amebic liver abscess with normal alkaline phosphatase. However, in chronic amebic liver abscess, alkaline phosphatase, transaminases, and bilirubin may be elevated in approximately 20% of patients.

Radiographic Studies

Chest radiography is abnormal in the majority of cases, and elevation and hypomotility of the right hemidiaphragm and atelectasis at the right lung base are the most common abnormalities. Pleural fluid may be present, even in the absence of frank rupture of the abscess into the pleural space. Radionucleotide liver scans have a sensitivity of 80% to 95% for abscesses larger than 2 cm in diameter, but have largely been supplanted by the more sensitive modalities of ultrasonography and computed tomography. Sensitivity and specificity of these latter two procedures are similar, and the choice of which to perform initially should be based on local availability, expertise, and cost.

Special Diagnostic Considerations

None of the aforementioned tests will reliably differentiate an amebic liver abscess from a pyogenic liver abscess or from a neoplastic mass with central necrosis. Serologic tests for antiamebic antibodies are positive in 91% to 98% of patients with amebic liver abscesses, making these tests highly useful in nonendemic areas, where the background prevalence of such antibodies is low. In one study detection of circulating *E. histolytica* Gal/GalNAc lectin in the serum, the TechLab *E. histolytica* II test (TechLab, Inc., Blacksburg, VA) had a sensitivity of 96% to diagnose amebic liver abscess and was helpful in follow-up care after treatment. In endemic areas, a therapeutic trial of metronidazole or, rarely, diagnostic aspiration of the lesion may be necessary to establish the diagnosis. Fluid from an amebic abscess is characteristically thin, brownish, and odorless, but amebae may be difficult to detect without a biopsy of the wall of the abscess. In biopsy specimens, detection of the trophozoites is diagnostic for invasive *E. histolytica* infection. If possible, aspiration or surgery should be avoided because of the risk of complications, including secondary infection of the abscess cavity, and because of the excellent therapeutic outcome obtained with chemotherapy alone.

Diagnosis of amebic abscesses of other organs or of amebic peritonitis will generally require serologic evidence of amebiasis and consistent findings in aspirated fluid from the abscess or peritoneum.

Treatment

Treatment regimens for the various clinical syndromes resulting from infection with *E. histolytica* are listed in Table 26-1. Common side effects associated with these antimicrobial agents are shown in Table 26-2. All patients with active intestinal disease or with extraintestinal infection should be treated. Management of the asymptomatic individual who passes a cyst is more controversial, and differentiating between *E. dispar* and *E. histolytica* would help clarify treatment options. Patients colonized with *E. dispar* do not need to be treated. Treatment is recommended for high-risk patients with either *E. histolytica/E. dispar* complex (in situations where differentiation is not possible) or *E. histolytica* alone in the stool. Asymptomatic *E. histolytica* colonization can be treated with a luminal agent alone. However, patients with symptoms and particularly patients at high risk for severe complications (immunocompromised patients and individuals at either extreme of age) should be treated with a tissue agent followed by a luminal agent. Conversely, in areas where the risk of reinfection is high, treatment of asymptomatic individuals may not be cost effective. Test-of-cure stool examinations after completion of therapy are important, as all of the recommended regimens have significant failure rates.

Intestinal Amebiasis

Metronidazole has become the mainstay of therapy because of its availability and relatively low toxicity. Unfortunately, it fails to eradicate luminal infection in 10% to 15% of cases because of its excellent absorption from the lumen into the tissues. The following medications are primarily active against luminal disease. Diloxanide furoate is available in the United States only through the Parasitic Diseases Division of the Centers for Disease Control and Prevention (CDC). Iodoquinol, although approved by the Food and Drug Administration (FDA), may be difficult to obtain, and there is concern over the potential for optic neuritis. Paromomycin and tetracycline have activity against luminal disease, but have not been tested in rigorous controlled treatment trials with adequate follow-up monitoring. A nitroimidazole derivative, tinidazole (Fasigyn, Tinebah), is the most active single agent against *E. histolytica* (2 g PO qd × 3-5 days), and treats both luminal and tissue disease, but it is not available in the United States. Ornidazole is also effective, but it too is not available in the United States. Given these difficulties and uncertainties, a reasonable approach to treatment would be to use metronidazole as single agent primary therapy for all forms of intestinal infection and to reserve the alternative agents for documented cases of treatment failure. Others prefer to treat asymptomatic individuals who pass cysts with a luminal agent alone and to treat invasive intestinal disease with a tissue agent (usually

Table 26-1
Treatment Regimens for *Entamoeba histolytica* Infections

Drug	Adult dose	Pediatric dose
Asymptomatic Cyst Passers		
Metronidazole	750 mg tid × 10 days	35-50 mg/kg/day in 3 doses × 10 days
Iodoquinol	650 mg tid × 20 days	30-40 mg/kg/day in 3 doses × 20 days
Diloxanide furoate	500 mg tid × 10 days	20 mg/kg/day in 3 doses × 10 days
Paramomycin	25-30 mg/kg/day in 3 doses × 7 days—can be used in pregnant women	25-30 mg/kg/day in 3 doses × 7 days
Invasive Colitis		
Metronidazole	750 mg tid × 10 days 2.4 g qd × 2-3 days*	35-50 mg/kg/day in 3 doses × 10 days
Tetracycline plus chloroquine base	250 mg qid × 14 days 600 mg qd × 2 days, then 300 mg qd × 12 days	
Dehydroemetine*	1-1.5 mg/kg/day IM in 2 doses × 5 days*	
Hepatic Abscess		
Metronidazole	750 mg tid × 10 days 2.4 mg qd × 2-3 days*	35-50 mg/kg/day in 3 doses × 10 days
Dehydroemetine	1-1.5 mg/kg/day IM × 5 days*	1-1.5 mg/kg/day IM in 2 doses × 5 days*
Chloroquine base	600 mg qd × 2 days, then 300 mg qd × 14-21 days (may be added to other regimens)	

IM, Intramuscularly.
*A luminal agent (diloxanide or iodoquinol) must be used in conjunction with dehydroemetine or short-course metronidazole regimens.

metronidazole) followed by a luminal agent. Documentation of cure should be undertaken whichever course is elected. There is a 10% relapse rate if treated with a tissue agent but not followed by a luminal agent.

None of the drugs used in the treatment of amebiasis has been shown to be safe for use during pregnancy. The indications for treatment must be weighed against the potential risk to the fetus in each case.

Extraintestinal Amebiasis

Metronidazole, with or without an additional agent to eradicate luminal infection, is also the treatment of choice for all forms of extraintestinal amebiasis. Dehydroemetine (available through the CDC) is extremely toxic and is rarely indicated. Emetine is even more toxic and should be avoided. Chloroquine as a single agent is associated with a high failure rate, but it may have a role when used in combination with metronidazole.

Table 26-2
Side Effects Associated with Drugs Use in the Treatment of Intestinal Protozoal Infections

Drug	Common	Uncommon
Metronidazole	Nausea, vomiting, bloating, metallic taste	Dizziness, vertigo, ataxia, stomatitis
Diloxanide furoate	Flatulence	Nausea, vomiting, diarrhea, urticaria
Iodoquinol	Rash, acne, enlarged thyroid, nausea, diarrhea, cramps	Optic atrophy
Paramomycin	Nausea, vomiting, diarrhea	Eighth nerve damage, nephrotoxicity
Dehydroemetine	Nausea, vomiting, diarrhea, cardiac arrhythmias, precordial pain, muscle weakness (patients must be hospitalized and electrocardiographic changes monitored)	Dizziness, weakness, heart failure, hypotension
Chloroquine	Pruritus, vomiting, headache, confusion, rash, weight loss	Retinitis, nerve deafness, blood dyscrasias
Quinacrine	Vomiting, diarrhea, dizziness, headache, abdominal cramps	Toxic psychosis, hepatic necrosis, blood dyscrasias
Furazolidone	Nausea, vomiting	Allergic reactions, polyneuritis, fever, hemolytic anemia

In a series of amebic liver abscesses treated with metronidazole and followed by hepatic ultrasonography, resolution time ranged from 2 months to 20 months. After healing, the hepatic sonograph pattern was normal. However, routine follow-up ultrasounds are not recommended, since the abscess cavity is likely to remain for months to years after appropriate therapy.

Chemotherapy alone is successful in the vast majority of cases of amebic abscesses, and the prognosis is excellent unless the patient is gravely ill at the initiation of treatment. Surgery should be reserved for emergent situations, such as rupture of a hepatic abscess into the pericardium or impending rupture into the peritoneum. Needle aspiration or drainage may be useful in selected cases for symptomatic relief or for patients not responding adequately to conservative treatment. Recovery from amebiasis does not confer immunity to reinfection.

Prevention

The basic means for eradication of endemic amebiasis is to eliminate fecal contamination of food and water by improving waste disposal systems and water purification. For the traveler, avoidance of uncooked, unpeeled fruits and vegetables (particularly green leafy vegetables), and untreated drinking water is recommended, although these measures have never been proven effective. Adequate water treatment consists of boiling (at very high elevations [>14,000 ft], it may be necessary to boil water for 10 minutes), filtration, or treatment with high concentrations of iodide. Chlorine is much less effective (see Chapter 7). Prophylactic chemotherapy is not recommended. One agent available for this purpose in some countries, iodochlorhydroxyquin (Entero-Vioform), has been associated with irreversible optic neuritis. In populations at risk of sexually transmitted amebiasis, altering sexual practices to avoid fecal-oral spread may reduce the risk of transmission of amebiasis and other enteric pathogens. Additionally, efforts should be made to decrease the transmission from a cyst-passer to family members or contacts. Contacts and family members of the index case of *E. histolytica* infection should be screened.

GIARDIA LAMBLIA

Pathogenesis

G. lamblia is a flagellate protozoan first observed by Anton van Leeuwenhoek in 1681. *G. lamblia* is the human species and is also called *G. duodenalis* or *G. intestinalis.* Infection is usually acquired by ingestion of the cyst form. The free-living trophozoite is less infectious, since it is more labile in the environment and is easily killed by gastric acid. Cysts can survive up to 3 months in water at 4° C. Infection in humans can occur with ingestion of very low inoculum, as few as 10 to 100 cysts. Excystation occurs in the duodenum and proximal jejunum, which are the regions predominantly involved in the infection. The incubation period is 3 to 25 days (median 7 to 10 days) after which the cysts can be detected in the stool.

The mechanism of disease production is poorly understood. Trophozoites have a prominent "sucking disk" on their ventral surface, but it is not known whether this structure is involved in adherence to the intestinal brush border in humans. The severity of symptoms does not correlate with the extent of morphologic damage to the epithelial cells (usually limited to disruption of the brush border) or the number of organisms. Organisms have occasionally been noted to penetrate the wall of the gut to the submucosa, but this invasiveness does not appear to play a role in producing disease. No enterotoxins have been associated with *Giardia.*

The importance of the immune system in giardiasis is best illustrated by the predisposition to chronic giardiasis observed in patients with agammaglobulinemia and common variable immunodeficiency. Observations in humans suggest that the humoral immune system is the most important component of host immunity both for recovery from the initial infection and for protection from reinfection. Other studies performed in the mouse giardiasis model have established a role for cellular immunity as well. Immunity after recovery from giardiasis is only partially protective and of variable duration.

Epidemiology

Giardiasis occurs both as an endemic disease and in large, water-borne outbreaks. In developing countries, where the disease prevalence is often 7% to 10%, it is primarily a disease of children. In the United States, major outbreaks linked to contaminated drinking water obtained from surface waters have been reported from Colorado, Utah, Washington, Oregon, New Hampshire, and New York. *G. lamblia* is the most commonly diagnosed intestinal parasite in public health laboratories in the United States. Historically, each host species was believed to harbor a unique species of *Giardia,* but it is now clear that the *G. lamblia* that infects humans has cross-species pathogenicity for other mammals, and vice versa. Water-dwelling animals, such as beavers and muskrats, have been implicated as the source of the *Giardia* contamination in some of the outbreaks noted.

Direct person-to-person spread is also important in the transmission of giardiasis. The very small infectious inoculum (<100 cysts) facilitates this form of transmission. This route is undoubtedly important in developing countries and is implicated in the high attack rate of *Giardia* in day-care centers in the United States. Sexually active male homosexuals and chronically institutionalized patients are also at high risk. Food-borne transmission has been reported occasionally.

Giardia is one of the more common parasites found in refugee groups in the United States. One study detected cysts in 20% of refugee children from Central American countries. The prevalence among Southeast Asian refugees ranges from about 7% in the Vietnamese, who are of predominantly urban origin, to 12% to 15% among the more rural Lao and Hmong.

All travelers are at some risk of acquiring giardiasis, even when traveling in the United States or other industrialized countries. For instance, an outbreak in St. Petersburg in the early 1970s was associated with a high attack rate among tourist groups, and giardiasis remains a persistent problem for travelers to that city. Overall, however, it accounts for only a small percentage of cases of traveler's diarrhea. Hikers drinking untreated surface water have perhaps the greatest risk for acquisition of giardiasis.

Among the nontraveling patients in the United States, giardiasis is more common among children between 0 and 5 years old and among adults between 31 and 40 years old. Additionally, there is a seasonal variation; it occurs more during late summer and early fall—coinciding with increase water-related outdoor activities. It is estimated to cause 100,000 to 2.5 million infections each year in the United States.

Clinical Features

The acute phase of giardiasis is highly variable in severity, but typically there is sudden onset of explosive diarrhea 7 to 21 days after ingestion of the cysts. The moderate to large volume of foul-smelling, loose stools accompanied by distention, flatulence, and midepigastric cramps helps to distinguish giardiasis from other infectious diarrheas. Bacterial pathogens of the small bowel, such as enterotoxigenic *Escherichia coli* and *Vibrio cholerae,* tend to cause a more watery diarrhea with less bloating and flatulence. Infectious colitis secondary to amebiasis or *Shigella* infection typically has smaller stool volume, more severe and diffuse cramps, and less abdominal bloating than are seen with *Giardia* infection. Dysentery is highly unusual with giardiasis and should prompt an intensive search for other pathogens. Other symptoms present during acute giardiasis can include nausea, anorexia, vomiting, low-grade fever, and headache. The acute phase usually lasts 7 to 14 days but can then evolve into a chronic infection.

Chronic giardiasis symptoms may be persistent or relapsing and include loose, bulky, foul-smelling stools; distention; foul flatus; constipation; and substernal burning. Malabsorption can occur and lead to significant weight loss. Malabsorption results from trophozoites forming a physical barrier between the intestinal epithelial cells and the lumen of the intestine, thereby interrupting the absorption of nutrients from the lumen. Spontaneous resolution is the rule, but infections have been known to persist for years. Chronic infection is the usual outcome of *Giardia* infection in patients with hypogammaglobulinemia or agammaglobulinemia. Alternatively, some individuals become chronic, asymptomatic cyst-passers and become an important reservoir for spread of the parasite to others.

Diagnosis

Giardiasis should be suspected in any patient with malabsorption or with a diarrheal illness persisting longer than 1 week. Epidemiologic data may be suggestive but should never be used to exclude the diagnosis, since giardiasis is endemic in the United States and sporadic cases are not uncommon. Both the cyst and the trophozoite forms can be seen in diarrheal stool, but trophozoites are rare in formed stool. A minimum of three specimens should be examined, since cyst passage is erratic and the numbers may be small. The yield from a single specimen is 50 to 75%, but increases to 90% to 95% with three specimens collected every other day during a 5-day period. ELISA tests that can detect *Giardia* antigen in stool specimens are now available in many diagnostic laboratories and may be more sensitive than standard morphologic identification for detection of this parasite in stool specimens.

If careful examination of multiple stool specimens is negative, one has the option of performing a therapeutic trial with antimicrobial agents or of moving on to more invasive procedures and examining the duodenal fluid. This can be done either by upper endoscopy for aspiration of duodenal fluid or duodenal biopsy or by the string test (Entero-Test, Hedeco, Palo Alto, Calif). The string test consists of a gelatin capsule containing a string (Fig. 26-1). One end of the string is held outside the patient and the capsule is swallowed. The capsule is weighted with a small metal sphere and is passed through the stomach and into the duodenum, unwinding string from a hole in the proximal end. The gelatin capsule dissolves, leaving the distal end of the string free in the duodenum. After 4 hours it is withdrawn, and the material adhering to the bile-stained end is scraped off and examined for trophozoites (Fig. 26-2).

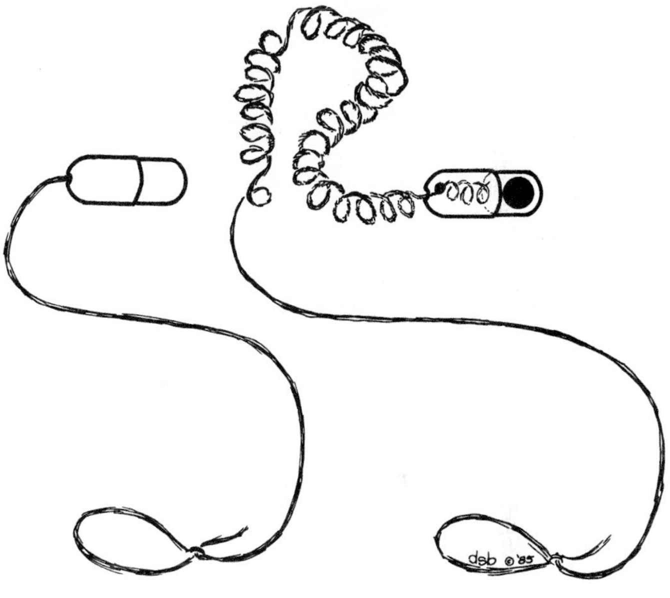

Fig. 26-1 The string test capsule.

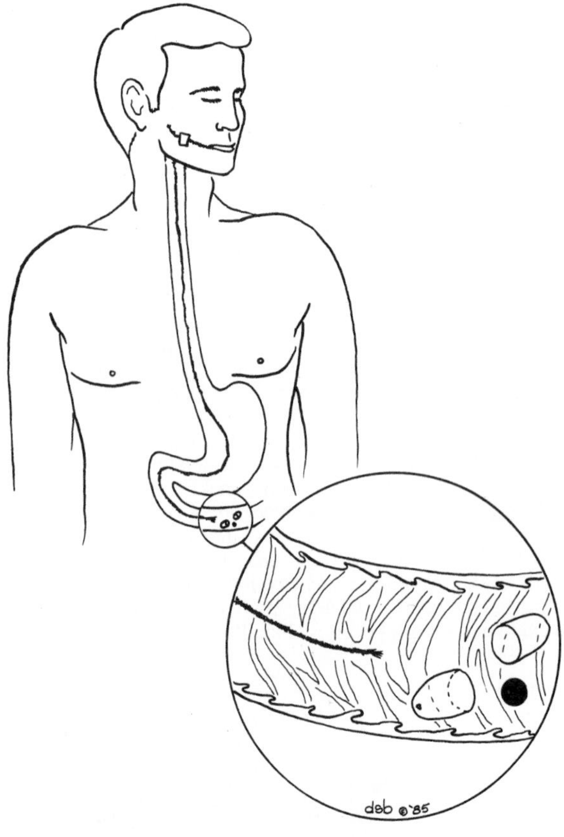

Fig. 26-2 Route of the string test in the gastrointestinal tract.

Small-bowel biopsy is most helpful in the evaluation of chronic malabsorption, one cause of which is chronic giardiasis. It has little, if any, role in the diagnosis of acute giardiasis. The histopathologic examination of the small bowel in giardiasis is usually normal but may show some nonspecific blunting of the villi. Touch preparations of the biopsy specimen are necessary to see the trophozoites, which inhabit the mucoid layer overlying the epithelial cells.

Routine blood chemistry and hematologic values are normal, and specific serodiagnostic assays for antibodies to *Giardia* are still experimental. Radiographic procedures are similarly unhelpful. Barium studies should be avoided, as they interfere with detection of cysts in the stool.

Treatment

The agents and appropriate dosage regimens used in the treatment of giardiasis are listed in Table 26-3. Common or severe side effects reported with these agents are shown in Table 26-2. Metronidazole, although not

Table 26-3
Treatment Regimens for Giardiasis

Drug	Adult dose (nonpregnant)	Pediatric dose
Metronidazole	500 mg tid × 5-10 days	5-7 mg/kg tid × 5-10 days
Quinacrine HCl	100 mg tid PC × 5 days	2 mg/kg tid PC × 5 days (max. 300 mg/day)
Furazolidone	100 mg qid × 7-10 days	1.25 mg/kg qid × 7-10 days

PC, Percutaneously.

approved for the treatment of giardiasis, has become the standard therapy in the United States because of its ready availability and its familiarity to physicians. Quinacrine, the official drug of choice, is associated with frequent severe gastrointestinal side effects that limit patient compliance. Few controlled studies have been performed comparing quinacrine with metronidazole. Although these studies had suboptimal follow-up information for late relapses, most of the data suggest that there is little difference in cure rates between these two agents, both being successful in approximately 90% of cases. Quinacrine is not easily available in the United States but can be acquired from few compounding pharmacies on a case-by-case basis.

Short-course therapy with metronidazole has been tried, but the failure rates have been high with both the 2.0-g single-dose regimen (40% to 50% treatment failure) and the two-dose (2.0 to 2.4 g qd × 2 days) regimen (20% to 25% failure rate). A regimen of 2.4 g/day for 3 days has a 91% success rate but at the cost of significant gastrointestinal toxicity; therefore it cannot be recommended over the lower-dose, longer-course regimens.

Proposed regimens for metronidazole in uncomplicated giardiasis have ranged from 250 mg three times a day for 5 days to 750 mg three times a day for 10 days. Uncontrolled studies suggest that the failure rate with the former regimen is unacceptably high; therefore a minimum dose of 500 mg three times a day for 5 to 7 days appears appropriate.

The most active agent in giardiasis is tinidazole, which produces a 92% cure rate with a single 2.0 g dose and has less gastrointestinal toxicity than is seen with metronidazole. Ornidazole has also been used, but neither it nor tinidazole is available in the United States.

Special Therapeutic Considerations

Children

Treatment of children is difficult owing to the lack of liquid preparations of quinacrine or metronidazole. The only alternative, furazolidone, is the only FDA-approved drug for giardiasis. Unfortunately, it is less active against *Giardia*. Cure rates have generally been in the 70% to 80% range.

Treatment Failures

Treatment success is generally better in acute giardiasis than in subacute or chronic cases. Drug resistance is not believed to be a major factor in treatment failures, and a second course of the same agent is as likely to be successful as switching to a second drug.

Pregnant Women

None of the drugs used in the treatment of giardiasis is approved for use in pregnancy. Unless severe or disabling symptoms are present, treatment should be deferred until after delivery. CDC recommends use of paromomycin, a nonabsorbable aminoglycoside, in the treatment of giardiasis in pregnant women.

Chronic Gastrointestinal Symptoms

Some individuals, possibly as many as 5%, develop a poorly characterized symptom complex of persistent bloating, flatulence, and upper abdominal cramps after apparently successful therapy for giardiasis. Patients with this "postgiarditic syndrome" do not have detectable persistent infections as assessed by stool examination and small-bowel aspiration and biopsy, and the giardiasis-like symptoms often persist despite repeated courses of therapy. Destruction of mucosal disaccharidases may play some role, but the symptoms have been shown to persist after recovery of the mucosal epithelium. Symptoms resolve slowly over 3 to 24 months. It is important to avoid repeated courses of antimicrobial agents in this disease if no evidence of ongoing infection is present. In refractory cases or in patients with chronic symptoms with evidence of active infection, a 14-day combination of metronidazole, 750 mg three time a day, and quinacrine, 100 mg three times a day, may be more effective.

Prevention

Contaminated water is the primary mode of transmission for *Giardia*. Boiling (30 seconds is sufficient at sea level; longer periods may be necessary at high elevations) and filtration are both adequate purification techniques (see Chapter 7). Inactivation by chlorination or by iodine treatment is less effective because these methods rely on the pH, temperature, and cloudiness of the water, thereby decreasing the reliability of the purification method. The traveler should also avoid uncooked foods that may have been washed with tap water or untreated surface water. Hikers in mountainous regions of North America should regard all surface water as potentially contaminated. No antimicrobial or other drug has been shown safe and effective for use as prophylaxis. Additionally, patients should also be advised to avoid fecal exposure and the potential of transmission during sex.

Outbreaks arising from daycare centers may be difficult to eradicate. The efficacy of epidemiologic screening or treatment of daycare staff and family members of infected children is unproven. Even the necessity for screening and treating asymptomatic children attending the daycare centers is unknown, although it would seem reasonable to screen and treat infants in diapers because of the greater potential for fecal-oral spread within and from this population.

OTHER PROTOZOA

Cryptosporidiosis

Protozoa of the genus *Cryptosporidium* are widely distributed among mammalian species, but only in the last decade has *Cryptosporidium parvum* been recognized as a significant human pathogen. Infection, acquired by ingestion of cysts, primarily involves the small intestine with highest concentration in the jejunum. Even a small inoculum as low as 30 cysts can cause an infection. In immunologically intact hosts, cryptosporidiosis is a self-limited illness that resolves spontaneously after 7 to 21 days. It is indistinguishable from giardiasis in individual cases. In the immunocompromised host (most notably in patients with acquired immunodeficiency syndrome [AIDS]), *Cryptosporidium* infection results in intractable watery diarrhea with a waxing and waning course associated with anorexia and weight loss. Among patients with human immunodeficiency virus (HIV)/AIDS, it can also cause infection of the bile duct, gallbladder, pancreas, liver, or lung. Cell-mediated and humoral immunity seems to play a role in pathogenesis.

Cryptosporidium may cause as much as 5% to 7% of pediatric diarrhea in developing countries but is implicated in only 0.3% to 1.0% of outpatient diarrhea cases in the United States. The prevalence of cryptosporidiosis among HIV/AIDS patients ranges from 14% in developed countries to 24% in developing countries. Travelers may be at slightly increased risk of acquiring this infection, and there have been outbreaks associated with daycare centers, similar to those caused by giardiasis. Veterinarians and livestock workers are also known high-risk groups.

Modified acid-fast stains of direct or concentrated stool smears are the diagnostic modality of choice, replacing small-bowel biopsies and more elaborate stool purification techniques. Patients with a clinical illness consistent with giardiasis but with multiple negative stool examinations for *Giardia* should have tests performed for *Cryptosporidium.* Commercially available stool *Cryptosporidium* antigen enzyme immunoassays are equally sensitive and specific as stool acid-fast stains. These tests are advantageous for laboratories with high stool test numbers and require less skill than microscopy.

There is no proven effective therapy, although paromomycin and high-dose azithromycin may have modest efficacy in treating chronic infections in immunocompromised patients. Subcutaneous octreotide helps ameliorate diarrhea in some people with HIV. Complete recovery is dependent on resolution of the immune defect. Initiation of immunosuppressive chemotherapy should either be delayed or the immunosuppression transiently lowered if possible in a patient with cryptosporidiosis.

Prevention of fecal-oral transmission of *Cryptosporidium* oocysts can be achieved by strict personal hygiene, eating cooked food, avoiding uncooked fruits and vegetables, and avoiding oroanal sexual exposure, and avoiding direct contact with animals, particularly calves and lambs. It is important to note that chlorination does not adequately kill the *Cryptosporidium* oocysts. Boiling water for 1 minute is perhaps the best method of decontaminating water. In addition, using filters with 1 μm or smaller pore size are effective in removing the oocysts.

Balantidiasis

Balantidium coli is the only ciliated protozoan pathogen in humans. This parasite is very large (100 μm) and is easily identified in stool specimens. It is acquired by close contact with swine or, more rarely, is transmitted within chronic care facilities for the mentally retarded. It produces invasive disease of the colon with symptoms of colitis and dysentery. Tetracycline, iodoquinol, and high-dose metronidazole are all effective in treating balantidiasis.

OTHER PROTOZOAN PATHOGENS

Isospora belli

I. belli has been reported as a rare cause of enteritis. It is distributed worldwide but is more prevalent in South America and Africa. The clinical syndrome resembles giardiasis and is acquired by contact with contaminated water or food. Persistent diarrhea associated with *Isospora* can occur in patients with AIDS. Identifying the characteristic oocysts on modified acid-fast stool smears is diagnostic. Trimethoprim-sulfamethoxazole is the agent of choice; pyrimethamine may be useful in people with HIV who are sensitive to sulfa.

Cyclospora

Cyclospora cayetanensis is a recently identified protozoan intestinal pathogen that causes diarrhea in patients in both developed and developing countries. The organism has previously been referred to as cyanobacterium-like body or as coccidian-like body (CLBs). It is presumably acquired through ingestion of contaminated water or food and not likely to be transmitted person-to-person. It has marked seasonal variation tending to occur more in the late spring and summer months. The oocysts are shed in the feces of infected patients and can be detected by modified acid-fast staining or by ultraviolet autofluorescence microscopy. The spherical cystlike organisms measure 8 to 10 μm in diameter and are larger than the oocysts of *Cryptosporidium parvum,* which are also detected by acid-fast stains.

Cyclospora infection in immunocompetent patients is associated with a prolonged but self-limited watery diarrhea lasting up to 10 weeks. During the acute phase upper abdominal symptoms, nausea, and fever accompany diarrhea. This may be followed by anorexia, weight loss, and fatigue. Symptoms may wax and wane for up to 4 to 8 weeks. *Cyclospora* infections in immunocompromised patients have been incompletely characterized, but appear to have a clinical presentation similar to that of *Cryptosporidium* infections. Cyclospora may be able to cause biliary tract disease among people with AIDS. The diagnostic differentiation between the two protozoan pathogens is significant because *Cyclospora* infections have been reported to respond to trimethoprim-sulfamethoxazole in standard therapeutic doses (adults, 160 mg trimethoprim and 800 mg sulfamethoxazole twice a day; children, 4 mg/kg trimethoprim and 20 mg/kg sulfamethoxazole twice a day) given for 3 or more days, whereas *Cryptosporidium* infections do not respond to this antibiotic. Other antimicrobials that have no or limited activity on *Cyclospora* include albendazole, trimethoprim, azithromycin, nalidixic acid, norfloxacin, tinidazole, metronidazole, quinacrine, tetracycline, and diloxanide furoate. In a patient who is allergic to sulfonamide, either desensitization to sulfonamide or perhaps treatment trial with ciprofloxacin may be an option.

Similar to *Cryptosporidium, Cyclospora* is resistant to chlorination. Therefore it is important to advise travelers regarding water precautions. Cyclosporiasis can be prevented by drinking boiled or bottled water, avoiding raw vegetables and fruits, and adhering to strict hand washing.

Dientamoeba fragilis

D. fragilis is a flagellate protozoan that has been associated with a mild, nonspecific enteritis syndrome. Iodoquinol is the treatment of choice; tetracycline and paromomycin are alternatives.

POSSIBLE PATHOGEN

Blastocystis hominis

B. hominis is a common stool commensal (up to 19% of normal controls in the United States are colonized). There is evidence that heavy infestations may be associated with cramps, vomiting, dehydration, abdominal pain, sleeplessness, nausea, weight loss, inability to work, lassitude, dizziness, flatus, anorexia, pruritus, and tenesmus.

B. hominis infections in primates have been cured with trimethoprim-sulfamethoxazole. In vitro susceptibility tests have shown that the following drugs may be effective in descending order: emetine, metronidazole, furazolidone, trimethoprim-sulfamethoxazole, iodochlorhydroxyquin (Entero-Vioform), and pentamidine. Chloroquine and iodoquinol have also been reported as effective treatments.

The role of *B. hominis* as a human pathogen is still controversial. Some published reports, based on clinical and laboratory studies, have suggested that when *B. hominis* human infections associated with diarrhea appear to respond to therapy, improvement may, in fact, be due to some other undetected organism that is actually causing the problem.

NONPATHOGENIC PROTOZOA

Numerous other species of protozoa have been detected in human feces, including *Entamoeba coli, Iodamoeba Bütschli, Endolimax nana,* and *Entamoeba hartmanni.* It is not unlikely that many of these "non-pathogens" are capable of producing disease in the proper clinical setting. At the present time, however, identification of one of these organisms in the stool is more useful as a marker of exposure to fecal-contaminated food or water. Their presence should prompt a more exhaustive search for pathogens such as *Giardia* or *E. histolytica,* which may be present in the stool in much smaller numbers.

REFERENCES

Anonymous. Giardiasis surveillance—United States, 1992-1997, *MMWR* 49/SS-7, 1, 2000.

Adams EB, MacLeod IN: Invasive amebiasis. I. Amebic dysentery and its complications. II. Amebic liver abscess and its complications, *Medicine* 56:315-323; 325-334, 1977.

Ahmed L et al: Ultrasonographic resolution time for amebic liver abscess, *Am J Trop Med Hyg* 41:406, 1989.

Black RE et al: Giardiasis in day-care centers: evidence of person-to-person transmission, *Pediatrics* 60:486, 1977.

Centers for Disease Control: Cryptosporidiosis: assessment of chemotherapy of males with acquired immmunodeficiency syndrome (AIDS), *MMWR* 31:589, 1982.

Faubert G: Immune response to *Giardia duodenalis, Clin Microbiol Rev* 13:35, 2000.

Haque R et al: Diagnosis of amebic liver abscess and intestinal infection with the TechLab *Entamoeba histolytica* II antigen detection and antibody tests, *J Clin Microbiol* 38:3235, 2000.

Herwaldt BL: *Cyclospora cayetanensis:* a review, focusing on the outbreaks of cyclosporiasis in the 1990's, *Clin Infect Dis* 31:1040, 2000.

Kean BH, William DC, Luminais SK: Epidemic of amoebiasis and giardiasis in a biased population, *Br J Vener Dis* 55:375, 1979.

Krogstad DJ, Spencer HC Jr, Healy GR: Amebiasis, *N Engl J Med* 298:262, 1978.

Ma P et al: Cryptosporidiosis in tourists returning from the Caribbean, *N Engl J Med* 312:647, 1985.

Madico G et al: Treatment of cyclospora infections with co-trimoxazole (letter), *Lancet* 342:122, 1993.

Mahmoud AAF, Warren KS: Algorithms in the diagnosis and management of exotic diseases. II. Giardiasis, *J Infect Dis* 131:621, 1975.

Markell EK et al: Intestinal protozoa in homosexual men of the San Francisco Bay area: prevalence and correlates of infection, *Am J Trop Med Hyg* 33:239, 1984.

Markell EK, Udkow MP: *Blastocystis hominis:* pathogen or fellow traveler? *Am J Trop Med Hyg* 35:1023, 1986.

Ortega YR et al: Cyclospora species—a new protozoan pathogen of humans, *N Engl J Med* 328:1308, 1993.

Petri WA Jr et al. Acquired immunity to amebiasis associated with mucosal IgA antibody against E histolytica adherence lectin in Bangladeshi children. ASTMH Annual Meeting October 2000, abstract number 1875.

Petri WA Jr, Singh U: Diagnosis and management of amebiasis, *Clin Infect Dis* 29:1117, 1999.

Pillai DR et al: *Entamoeba histolytica* and *Entamoeba dispar:* epidemiology and comparison of diagnostic methods in a setting of nonendemicity, *Clin Infect Dis* 29:1315, 1999.

Steven DP: Giardiasis: host-pathogen biology, *Rev Infect Dis* 4:851, 1982.

Zierdt CH: *Blastocystis hominis,* a long-misunderstood intestinal parasite, *Parasitol Today* 4:15, 17, 1988.

CHAPTER 27

Food Poisoning

Elaine C. Jong

Food poisoning occurs after ingestion of food improperly cooked, stored, or preserved. Bacteria present in such foods multiply and cause human illness by enterotoxins released in the food *(Staphylococcus aureus, Bacillus cereus, Clostridium botulinum)* or by elaboration of enterotoxins within the small intestine by ingested organisms *(Clostridium perfringens, B. cereus, C. botulinum).*

Onset of symptoms is usually within hours after exposure, although in a few cases of *C. botulinum,* onset has been reported to occur up to 14 days after exposure. In mild cases of food poisoning, vomiting, diarrhea, and abdominal cramping may be of short duration and be over before the afflicted person seeks medical attention.

ETIOLOGY

The bacteria commonly recognized as causes of food poisoning are *Clostridium perfringens, Staphylococcus aureus, Bacillus cereus,* and *Clostridium botulinum* (types A, B, and E). Table 27-1 presents the most common food vehicles, onset of symptoms, and major symptoms associated with each type. Web sites with excellent information on food safety are given in Table 27-2.

C. perfringens bacteria exsporulate and proliferate over 12 to 24 hours during the prolonged cooling of stews, soups, and other meat or poultry dishes at room temperature. After ingestion, the growing microorganisms multiply and sporulate in the small intestine. Sporulating *C. perfringens* produce an enterotoxin, which is then absorbed by the host. This bacterium has been identified as the causative agent in approximately 14% of food poisoning cases in the United States.

S. aureus strains producing enterotoxin are usually inoculated from hands of infected human carriers into food products (desserts, salads, baked goods, meats) served or stored at room or refrigerator temperatures. Staphylococcal enterotoxins (A, B, C, D, E) are relatively heat stable, so subsequent cooking of contaminated foods will not necessarily destroy them.

B. cereus is a ubiquitous soil bacterium present on rice, vegetables, and some meats. The illness ensuing from ingestion of *B. cereus*-contaminated food has been given the nickname "fried rice syndrome." Fried rice was associated with the first recognized outbreaks. The ingredients and the cooking technique are especially conducive to illness-producing situations

Table 27-1
Common Pathogens Causing Food Poisoning

Pathogen	Incubation	Vehicle	Major symptoms
Clostridium perfringens	6-12 hr	Meat, poultry	Cramping abdominal pain,* diarrhea
Staphylococcus aureus	2-6 hr	Creamy desserts and salads, baked goods, meats	Vomiting,* cramping abdominal pain, diarrhea
Bacillus cereus			
Toxin similar to *S. aureus* toxin	2-9 hr	Rice, vegetables, meat	Vomiting,* diarrhea
Toxin similar to ETEC LT toxin	6-14 hr	Rice, vegetables, meat	Diarrhea,* vomiting
Clostridium botulinum	12-36 hr or up to 14 days	Types A and B: Preserved (canned, pickled, cured) meats and vegetables Type E: Smoked or preserved fish	Diplopia,* blurred vision,* photophobia;* dysphonia, dysarthria, weakness of tongue; nausea and vomiting; symmetric paralysis of extremities, respiratory muscle weakness

*Major distinguishing symptoms.

Table 27-2
Web Sites for Food Safety Information

U.S. Food and Drug Administration	http://www.cfsan.fda.gov
U.S. Dept. Agriculture	http://www.fsis.usda.gov
Centers for Disease Control and Prevention	http://www.cdc.gov/foodsafety

when fried rice is improperly stored. The bacteria exsporulate during cooking and proliferate, liberating enterotoxins when the food is held for prolonged periods at room temperature. Flash cooking or brief reheating of the contaminated food before serving is not sufficient to inactivate the toxin. The short-incubation syndrome, with onset 2 to 9 hours after ingestion, is associated with preformed toxin. The long-incubation syndrome, with onset 6 to 14 hours after ingestion of contaminated food, is associated with toxin elaborated by *B. cereus* bacteria proliferating within the gastrointestinal tract.

C. botulinum bacteria proliferate in canned and preserved foods when anaerobic conditions at a relatively high pH (>4.6) exist. Cooking foods at high temperatures will inactivate the toxin (boiling 10 minutes or heating at 80° C for 30 minutes). However, the spores can survive heating at 100° C for several hours. Occasionally, ingested spores will proliferate in the human gastrointestinal tract and liberate enterotoxin that is absorbed by the host, causing symptoms. This latter mechanism is thought to account for long-incubation botulism and for infant botulism.

Because of the sometimes prolonged period before the onset of diagnostic symptoms, a careful food history should be obtained for up to the 2 weeks before the development of illness. In identified source outbreaks, contact tracing and publicity through the public health departments may help to prevent additional cases of illness and death. One reported outbreak of botulism in travelers associated with food served at a restaurant proved difficult to trace because of the widespread dispersion of the cases in two countries after the common food source was ingested.

Of the eight immunologically distinct types of *C. botulinum* toxin, types A and B are responsible for most reported cases, and type E has been associated with smoked fish. Types Cα, Cβ, and D have been isolated from animals, and types F and G are rarely isolated from humans.

DIAGNOSIS

Cramping abdominal pain is the hallmark of food poisoning caused by *C. perfringens,* and severe vomiting is the hallmark of food poisoning caused by *S. aureus. B. cereus* has two toxins, one causing a gastrointestinal illness with prominent vomiting (like *S. aureus* toxin) and one causing watery diarrhea (like the heat-labile toxin of enterotoxigenic *E. coli*). A gastrointestinal illness characterized by a relatively rapid onset of symptoms after eating, and limited to 1 or 2 days, is therefore likely to be food poisoning. The diagnosis can be best confirmed if some of the original questionable food is available for laboratory testing. Laboratory testing of patient stool specimens, vomitus, and serum is laborious but may be done by state departments of public health during large outbreaks.

In contrast, the diagnosis of botulism is extremely tricky owing to the great variation in time between ingestion of the contaminated food and onset of symptoms. In addition, ophthalmologic (diplopia and blurring of vision) rather than gastrointestinal symptoms may be seen at first presentation. Diagnosis of botulism can be confirmed if the suspected food is still available. In addition, toxin in the serum or feces of stricken patients can be detected by bioassay in laboratory animals.

TREATMENT

Antibiotics are of no known value in cases of food poisoning, since onset of symptoms is related to a certain level of the given enterotoxin being present in the gut; once formed, the toxin can exert its biologic effect independently of the continued viability of the bacterial source.

Treatment is directed toward symptomatic relief of the nausea and vomiting and replacement of fluids and electrolytes lost in watery stools and emesis. Oral rehydration is described in Chapter 6. Rarely, nausea, vomiting, and diarrhea will be so severe that parenteral rehydration is necessary. Infants, the elderly, and the debilitated are most susceptible to complications from common food poisoning.

In illness caused by *C. botulinum,* prompt therapy with polyvalent equine antitoxin against types A, B, and E may be helpful (contact the Centers for Disease Control and Prevention—see Appendix), but respiratory support for severe respiratory muscle weakness may be the most important critical intervention. The horse serum components of equine antitoxin can rarely induce an anaphylactic reaction in the recipient.

PREVENTION

Travelers are at special risk of food poisoning because of increased exposure to meals prepared outside the home under unknown conditions of preparation and storage. The handling of food by infected persons with unwashed hands is a major mode of transmission in food-borne illness (see also Chapter 6). Travelers should try to select food that is freshly prepared, thoroughly cooked, and served piping hot, or within 1 hour of preparation. For safety, chicken should be cooked to a temperature above 165° F (73.9° C), pork above 155° F (68.3° C), and ground beef above 155° F (68.3° C); and rare or pink meat or poultry should not be consumed. The new instant-read digital food thermometers may be useful for checking the internal temperature of cooked meats and casseroles. Precooked foods served at room temperature or in buffet meals, as well as baked goods with creamy fillings, should be avoided in developing areas of the world where refrigeration may be lacking. For safety, cold foods and leftovers should be refrigerated below 45° F (7.2° C) until serving. Safe selection of food is the only way to avoid food poisoning, since the contaminated food may appear, taste, and smell like normal unspoiled food.

PIGBEL

Pigbel is a form of necrotizing enterocolitis, caused by *C. perfringens* type C, that is endemic in the Papua New Guinea highlands. The *C. perfringens* bacteria are ingested in contaminated pork and other foods and appear to colonize the intestinal tract of up to 70% of normal villagers.

Rapid intestinal proliferation of *C. perfringens* with production of beta-toxin follows ingestion of meat and/or other high-protein foods. If a person has inadequate levels of proteases, the beta-toxin cannot be destroyed and causes necrotizing enterocolitis.

Children appear to be especially susceptible to pigbel owing to low levels of intestinal proteases associated with a chronic protein-deficient diet, and a low level of immunity to beta-toxin. A staple of the village diet is sweet potato, which contains trypsin inhibitors and contributes to the problem.

In most cases, cytopathic intestinal damage from beta-toxin occurs early during *C. perfringens* proliferation. Symptoms of necrotizing enterocolitis (fever, abdominal pain, intestinal obstruction) may not be manifested until several days later, too late for neutralization of beta-toxin by administration of exogenous antitoxin to ameliorate the clinical course. A pigbel vaccine employing *C. perfringens* type C beta-toxoid appears to offer protection among recipients in trials in the Papua New Guinea highlands.

REFERENCES

Case Records of the Massachusetts General Hospital: Rapidly progressive neurologic disorder following gastrointestinal symptoms (Case 48-1980), *N Engl J Med* 303:1347, 1980.

Davis MW: More on necrotizing enterocolitis: pigbel in Papua New Guinea (letter), *N Engl J Med* 311:1126, 1984.

Holmberg SD, Blake PA: Staphylococcal food poisoning in the United States: new facts and old misconceptions, *JAMA* 251:487, 1984.

Horwitz MA: Specific diagnosis of foodborne disease, *Gastroenterology* 73:375, 1977.

Hughes JM et al: Clinical features of types A and B food-borne botulism, *Ann Intern Med* 95:442, 1981.

Shandera WX, Tacket CO, Blake PA: Food poisoning due to *Clostridium perfringens* in the United States, *J Infect Dis* 147:167, 1983.

Smith LDS: *Clostridium botulinum:* characteristics and occurrence, *Rev Infect Dis* 1:637, 1979.

Terranova W, Blake PA: *Bacillus cereus* food poisoning, *N Engl J Med* 298:143, 1978.

CHAPTER 28

Fish and Shellfish Poisoning: Toxic Syndromes

Elaine C. Jong

Fish and shellfish are staples in the global diet. Today, air transport can rapidly move both passengers and fish around the world, leading to international, year-round presentation of illnesses that were previously only well recognized locally, or limited to certain seasons. The importance of seafoods as causative agents in a number of gastroenterologic and neurologic illnesses has been increasingly recognized through epidemiologic studies. Illnesses may result from bacterial, viral, or parasitic contamination of food; these are discussed in Chapters 25 through 27. The focus of this chapter is on toxic syndromes resulting from the ingestion of toxins contained in fish or shellfish.

In fish, these toxins may be concentrated in the skin, musculature, and viscera (i.e., ichthyosarcotoxic), in the reproductive organs (i.e., ichthyotoxic), or in the blood (i.e., ichthyohemotoxic). Of the nine kinds of ichthyosarcotoxism (based on types of fish), the most important are *scombroid, ciguatera,* and *puffer fish poisoning.* Likewise, a major health and economic concern in the shellfish industry are the toxic syndromes: paralytic shellfish poisoning, neurotoxic shellfish poisoning, diarrheic shellfish poisoning, and amnesic shellfish poisoning. These entities are discussed in this chapter.

A history of specific ingestion is crucial to establishing the diagnosis of fish or shellfish poisoning. There is often no uniformly reliable appearance, smell, or taste that will distinguish between safe seafood and contaminated seafood before ingestion. New pathogen-specific techniques such as polymerase chain reaction should aid in future seafood surveillance efforts.

SCOMBROID POISONING

Scrombroid poisoning is the name given to a histamine-like reaction that occasionally results from the ingestion of tuna and related species in the family Scombridae. These dark-meat fish include the skipjack tuna *(Euthynnus pelamis)*, the bonito *(Sarda sarda)*, the mackerel *(Scomber scombrus)*, and the albacore *(Thunnus alalunga)*. A nonscombroid fish, mahimahi *(Cophaena hippurus)* can also become toxic and is actually the most commonly implicated fish in scombroid outbreaks in the United States.

Fish become toxic when inadequate preservation allows for bacterial contamination. These bacteria (primarily *Morganella morganii* but also other bacteria such as *Escherichia, Proteus, Salmonella,* and *Shigella* species) degrade histidine present in the musculature to heat-stable histamine and a histamine-like substance termed *saurine.* Studies suggest that most symptoms are due to saurine, since histamine when given orally is poorly absorbed and chemically inactivated in the gastrointestinal tract. An exception may occur in patients treated with isoniazid for tuberculosis, since this medication inhibits histaminase in the gut, and may make patients more susceptible to the histamine contained in scombrotoxic fish, thus accentuating the symptoms and signs of scombroid poisoning.

Scombrotoxic fish usually appear normal, but toxicity should be suspected if the fish tastes "peppery or sharp." Within 30 minutes of ingestion of a toxic fish, a systemic histamine-like reaction occurs. Symptoms and signs include headache, flushing, abdominal cramps with nausea, vomiting, diarrhea, tachycardia, dry mouth, and occasionally urticaria, angioedema, and bronchospasm. Symptoms are transient, rarely lasting more than 8 to 12 hours, and deaths are unusual. Diagnosis is clinical but can be confirmed by measuring the histamine content of the suspected fish, which is generally 20 mg/100 g of fish muscle, or higher. (Normal histamine content is <1 mg/100 g of fish muscle.) Treatment consists of forced emesis and antihistamines. In addition to diphenhydramine (Benadryl), treatment with histamine-2 antagonists cimetidine (300 mg intravenous [IV]) or ranitidine (50 mg IV) may provide symptomatic relief. If symptoms are severe, the patient may require IV fluids, steroids, aminophylline, and epinephrine as used for anaphylaxis-like reactions.

CIGUATERA POISONING

Ciguatera poisoning consists of acute gastrointestinal and neurologic symptoms after ingestion of normally edible reef fish that contain ciguatoxin and maitotoxin. Most outbreaks occur in the Caribbean, the Indo-Pacific islands, and the Indian Ocean between 35 degrees north and 35 degrees south latitude. Although more than 425 species of fish are known to be occasionally toxic, the more commonly implicated fish include the barracuda (Sphyraenidae), red snapper (*Lutjanus bohar*), grouper, amberjack (*Seriola dumerili*), sea bass (Serranidae), surgeonfish (Acanthuridae), and moray eel (Muraenidae).

Ciguatoxin is a nonprotein toxin with water-soluble and lipid-soluble fractions (the latter with a molecular weight of 1500 to 1800 daltons). This toxin, as well as the similar maitotoxin, originates in the unicellular dinoflagellate *Gambierdiscus toxicus.* It passes through the food chain, eventually accumulating in the musculature, liver, and viscera of herbivorous and predatory reef fish. The toxin is not affected by heating, freezing, or drying; and toxic fish have normal taste, texture, and odor. Ciguatoxin induces partial membrane depolarization by enhancing sodium ion permeability in voltage-dependent sodium channels in nerve cell membranes. Maitotoxin is a calcium channel activator that increases calcium ion permeability through voltage-sensitive cells.

Symptoms develop 2 to 6 hours after ingestion of the fish and last about 1 week but occasionally can extend for months or even years. Typically, patients develop gastrointestinal symptoms such as nausea, watery diarrhea, abdominal cramps, or vomiting. Distal paresthesias are common, and the teeth may feel numb or loose. A majority of victims note an unusual hot-cold sensory reversal, in which cold objects "burn" when handled. Asthenia and arthralgias are frequent, and 10% to 45% of patients develop pruritus, usually 1 to 3 days after fish ingestion. Erythematous skin rashes that may blister or desquamate can occur in up to

20% of patients. In severe instances, ataxia, paresis, paralysis, or transient blindness occurs, often in association with sinus bradycardia and hypotension. Deaths are generally the result of respiratory depression, coma, and convulsions.

Diagnosis is made clinically but can be verified by assaying for the toxin in the implicated fish, using a bioassay (mouse, cat, mongoose, or brine shrimp), an enzyme-linked immunosorbent assay, or a radioimmunoassay.

Treatment is supportive and consists of forced emesis, IV fluids if volume is depleted and respiratory support if indicated. Intravenous mannitol (1 g/kg) has been reported to ameliorate neurologic symptoms when given acutely. Other drugs that have been reported to give symptomatic relief are amitriptyline (50 mg/day), tocainide (400 mg three times a day), and nifedipine (10 mg three times a day). A recent report described successful treatment of ciguatera poisoning symptoms with gabapentin, a drug structurally related to gamma-aminobutyric acid, and usually used as an antiepileptic. Treatment with gabapentin, 400 mg orally three times daily for up to for up to 5 weeks was reported to relieve neurologic symptoms, pruritis, and sharp, shooting pains in the legs associated with ciguatera poisoning, even though treatment was initiated 1 month after the onset of symptoms.

PUFFER FISH POISONING

Puffer fish, porcupine fish, ocean sunfishes, and related species in the order Tetraodontiformes are frequently poisonous and may produce a severe neurologic illness after ingestion. This is a particular problem in Japan, where puffer fish ("fugu") is a culinary delicacy.

The toxicity is due to the accumulation of tetrodotoxin in the ovaries, liver, intestines, and, to a lesser extent, the musculature of the fish. The toxin is believed to originate from something the puffer fish ingests; but attempts to implicate specific species of algae, jellyfish, sponges, and so forth have not been definitive. A clear correlation does exist, however, between the reproductive season of the puffer fish and its likelihood of being poisonous.

Tetrodotoxin is a nonprotein aminohydroquinazoline compound with a heterocyclic structure and a molecular weight of 319 daltons. It is water soluble and heat resistant and does not alter the taste or appearance of the fish. It appears to be similar, if not identical, to tarichatoxin, present in the California newt, and also to a toxin present in the skin of *Atelopus* frogs in Costa Rica. Physiologically, tetrodotoxin is similar to saxitoxin and (see later discussion) prevents the generation of action potentials by blocking the voltage-sensitive sodium channels in the membranes of nerves and muscle, but it has no effect on potassium conductance.

Symptoms and signs develop within hours of ingestion and include profuse sweating and salivation, hypothermia, headache, tachycardia, and hypotension. Gastrointestinal symptoms of nausea, vomiting, diarrhea, or abdominal pain may or may not be present. The hallmark of puffer fish poisoning is neurologic: paresthesias that frequently progress to numbness, ataxia, tremor, and paralysis involving both cranial and peripheral nerves. Respiratory compromise and cardiac arrhythmias may result. Occasional patients have complete flaccid paralysis with absent corneal reflexes and dilated pupils, but maintain consciousness. The mortality rate may reach 60%, but the prognosis is good with eventual full recovery if the patient survives the first 24 hours.

Diagnosis is made on clinical grounds. There is no effective antidote. If the patient is seen within 3 hours of ingestion, gastric lavage with 2 L of 2% sodium bicarbonate, followed by instillation of activated charcoal in 70% sorbitol solution may help to remove toxin from the gastrointestinal tract. Patients require supportive care with special attention to the pulmonary status. Serial vital capacity tests should be done, and early intubation is recommended if there is evidence of inadequate ventilation. There are anecdotal reports of improvement with edrophonium, pralidoxime, and atropine.

Attempts in Japan to prevent the disease have included the requirement of a special license for both restaurants and cooks wishing to serve puffer fish. Only the musculature of the puffer fish can be served and that only during the nonreproductive season (i.e., the winter months), when the fish is least likely to be toxic.

BOTULISM TOXIN E

Clostridium botulinum bacteria secreting botulism toxin type E have been reported as contaminants of improperly processed or smoked fish and fish eggs. Approximately 24 to 36 hours after ingestion of contaminated seafood, gastrointestinal symptoms may develop, followed in 3 to 7 days by cranial nerve dysfunction and symmetric descending weakness. The botulism toxin E blocks acetylcholine release at the neuromuscular junction. The diagnosis is made by clinical presentation and a history of eating preserved fish or fish eggs. Treatment consists of supportive care; trivalent ABE antitoxin should be given as soon as possible.

PARALYTIC SHELLFISH POISONING

An unusual neurologic disorder that may follow shellfish ingestion is termed *paralytic shellfish poisoning* (PSP). The disease is primarily associated with the consumption of bivalve mollusks, such as clams, mussels, and oysters; but has also been reported with gastropods, chitons, starfish, and crustaceans. Crab, abalone, and fin fish do not appear to be affected. The disease is mainly restricted to temperate climates, with most reported outbreaks in North America, Europe, and Japan, although cases have also occurred in South Africa, Papua New Guinea, and New Zealand.

The toxicity of PSP is due to the accumulation of saxitoxin and related compounds in the shellfish. Saxitoxin is a tetrahydropurine base with a molecular weight of 299 daltons. It does not affect the appearance or taste of the marine mollusks, nor is it effectively inactivated by cooking. Like tetrodotoxin, it blocks action potential generation by preventing sodium ion flow in nerve and muscle cell membranes.

Saxitoxin originates in a unicellular dinoflagellate known as *Gonyaulax*. Since bivalve mollusks are filter feeders, they concentrate the toxins from *Gonyaulax* in their digestive glands (the hepatopancreas). In the Alaska butter clam (*Saxidomus*), the saxitoxin is concentrated in the siphon as well. Toxicity of shellfish correlates with the bloom of this dinoflagellate, which is frequently associated with "red tides" and, along the Pacific Coast, usually occurs between May and October. Toxicity lessens as the dinoflagellate population decreases, but complete detoxification of shellfish may take up to a year.

Symptoms usually occur within 30 minutes after ingestion of contaminated shellfish and include distal and oral paresthesias that may progress to numbness. A sensation of "floating," gross incoordination, and paralysis with respiratory compromise may develop. The case fatality rate is 8.5%.

Diagnosis is clinical, but suspect shellfish can be analyzed in a mouse bioassay. Toxic shellfish have more than 4 MU (mouse unit)/g wet flesh (1 MU of saxitoxin is the amount that kills a 20-g mouse 15 minutes after intraperitoneal injection of a heated acid extract of the shellfish). Treatment is supportive, as with other fish poisonings.

Prevention of PSP requires public health measures, with routine surveillance using the mouse bioassay and with prompt closure of any beach to shellfish collecting when more than 4 MU/g wet flesh is detected. The Red Tide Hotline (1-800-562-5632) gives information 24 hours a day on red tide conditions in Puget Sound and the Pacific Ocean beaches.

NEUROTOXIC SHELLFISH POISONING (NONPARALYTIC)

Neurotoxic shellfish poisoning (NSP) affects people who eat mollusks from red tides off the Florida Coast. The contaminated shellfish contain brevitoxin from the dinoflagellate *Ptychodiscus brevis* in the red tides. About 1 to 6 hours after ingestion of contaminated shellfish, the affected person will experience paresthesias, reversal of hot and cold temperature sensation, ataxia, nausea, vomiting, and diarrhea. Treatment is symptomatic and supportive. When the toxin is aerosolized in rough surf, exposed people can develop a syndrome consisting of conjunctivitis, rhinorrhea, and a nonproductive cough.

DIARRHETIC SHELLFISH POISONING

Diarrhetic shellfish poisoning (DSP) can occur in people hours to days after ingesting contaminated mussels. The mussels acquire okadaic acid, a dinophysistoxin-1 from dinoflagellate algae. The syndrome is characterized by nausea, vomiting, diarrhea, and cramps. Treatment is symptomatic and supportive.

AMNESIC SHELLFISH POISONING

Amnesic shellfish poisoning (domoic acid poisoning, mussel poisoning) is a toxic encephalopathy first described among people who ate contaminated mussels from cultivated beds in Prince Edward Island, Canada in 1989. The mussels contained domoic acid, a marine toxin produced by a marine diatom *Nitzchia pungens*. Environmental factors that favor the proliferation of this algae around certain marine areas allow the toxin to be accumulated by shellfish. Since the original syndrome was described, domoic acid has been detected periodically in razor clams and dungeness crabs from the Olympic Peninsula in Washington state.

Domoic acid is related structurally to the excitatory amino acid neurotransmitter glutamate. Gastrointestinal symptoms (nausea, vomiting, abdominal cramps, and diarrhea) occur within 24 hours after the toxic ingestion, and neurologic symptoms (headache, seizures, hemiparesis, ophthalmoplegia, abnormal state of arousal ranging from agitation to coma, and antegrade memory loss) become manifest within 48 hours after ingestion. In the Canadian outbreak, gastrointestinal symptoms resolved after a day or two. However, after initial widespread neurologic dysfunction, the survivors had persistence of memory deficits and motor neuropathy. Treatment is symptomatic and supportive.

REFERENCES

Auerbach PS et al: Bacteriology of the marine environment: implication for clinical therapy, *Ann Emerg Med* 16:643, 1987.

Bagnis R, Kuberski T, Langier S: Clinical observations on 3009 cases of ciguatera fish poisoning in the South Pacific, *Am J Trop Med Hyg* 28:1067, 1979.

Blakesly ML: Scombroid poisoning: Prompt resolution of symptoms with cimetidine, *Ann Emerg Med* 12:104, 1983.

Chew S et al: Anticholinesterase drugs in the treatment of tetrodotoxin poisoning, *Lancet* 2:108, 1984.

Davis RT, Villar LA: Symptomatic improvement with amitriptyline in ciguatera poisoning, *N Engl J Med* 315:65, 1986.

Dickey RW et al: Detection of the marine toxins okadaic acid and domoic acid in shellfish and phytoplankton in the Gulf of Mexico, *Toxicon* 30:355, 1992.

Halstead BW: *Poisonous and venomous marine animals of the world,* Princeton, 1978, Darwin Press.

Halstead BW, Schantz EJ: *Paralytic shellfish poisoning,* Geneva, WHO Offset Publication No. 79, 1984.

Hughes J, Merson M: Fish and shellfish poisoning, *N Engl J Med* 295:1117, 1976.

Hughes JM, Potter ME: Scombroid-fish poisoning, from pathogenesis to prevention, *N Engl J Med* 324:766, 1991.

Johnson R, Jong EC: Ciguatera: Caribbean and Indo-Pacific fish poisoning, *West J Med* 138:872, 1983.

Laird MA, Gidal BE: Use of gabapentin in the treatment of neuropathic pain, *Ann Pharmacother* 34:802, 2000.

Lange WR, Kreider SD: Potential benefit of tocainide in the treatment of ciguatera: report of three cases, *Am J Med* 84:1087, 1988.

Lipp EK, Rose JB: The role of seafood in food borne diseases in the United States of America, *Rev Sci Tech* 16:620, 1997.

Morrow JD et al: Evidence that histamine is the causative toxin of scombroid-fish poisoning, *N Engl J Med* 324:716, 1991.

Palafox NA et al: Successful treatment of ciguatera fish poisoning with intravenous mannitol, *JAMA* 259:2740, 1988.

Perl TM et al: An outbreak of toxic encephalopathy caused by eating mussels contaminated with domoic acid, *N Engl J Med* 322:1775, 1990.

Powell CL, Doucette GJ: A receptor binding assay for paralytic shellfish poisoning toxins: recent advances and applications, *Nat Toxins* 7(6):393, 1999.

Rakita RM: Ciguatera poisoning, *J Travel Med* 2:252, 1995.

Sims JK, Ostman DC: Pufferfish poisoning: emergency diagnosis and management of mild human Tetrodotoxication, *Ann Emerg Med* 15:1094, 1986.

Teitelbaum JS et al: Neurologic sequelae of domoic acid intoxication due to ingestion of contaminated mussels, *N Engl J Med* 322:1781, 1990.

Viviani R: Eutrophication, marine biotoxins, human health, *Sci Total Environ* (suppl):631, 1992.

SECTION V

SKIN LESIONS

CHAPTER 29

Approach to Tropical Dermatology

M. Sean Strother and Roy Colven

Tropical dermatology includes those cutaneous conditions that are in some way unique to the tropics. With few exceptions, these unique skin diseases are relatively uncommon in the tropics. Many of the skin diseases common in the tropics (e.g., dermatitis, scabies, superficial fungal infections, and bacterial infections) are also common in temperate climates. Therefore the evaluation of cutaneous lesions acquired in the tropics should follow general dermatologic principles, but with appropriate consideration of tropical disease etiologies.

Diseases included in tropical dermatology may have an etiology, such as *pinta* and *Buruli ulcer* (Chapter 32), dermatophytosis (Chapter 33), leishmaniasis (Chapter 34), or Hansen's disease (Chapter 35). However, the tropics can also affect the skin through environmental factors, including increased heat and humidity as in miliaria, increased exposure to solar radiation (Chapter 30), and biting arthropods, and exposure to new contact allergens and/or irritants (Chapter 30). *Ectoparasites* and *cutaneous myiasis* are discussed in Chapter 31.

This chapter focuses on the basic approach to the patient with skin disease in, or having returned from, the tropics. A primer on topical therapy is also included.

CLINICAL APPROACH

The evaluation of the patient with a chief complaint of skin lesions or rash should include a systematic approach with physical examination, history, and appropriate diagnostic tests. In contrast to most general medical providers, dermatologists rely most on visual inspection of the skin, noting primary lesion morphology and distribution. History and laboratory tests are often used to confirm a specific diagnosis or narrow a differential diagnosis made from physical examination.

The examination of the skin should be performed in good light. Whenever possible, the entire skin surface should be examined, including the hair, scalp, nails, and mucous membranes. In certain instances it may also be important to examine the patient for lymphadenopathy and organomegaly.

A precise description of findings allows the rash to be categorized into general groups, limiting diagnostic possibilities. *Primary* changes, those directly due to the disease process, should be distinguished from *secondary* changes, which are modifications occurring over time as the result of external factors, such as rubbing, scratching, or superimposed bacterial infection, and include scale, crusts, excoriations, and lichenification. The common types of primary lesions are defined as follows:

Macules are focal alterations in skin color less than 10 mm in diameter without any change in texture or thickness.

Patches are similar nonpalpable color changes greater than 10 mm in diameter.

Papules are solid elevated lesions less than 10 mm in diameter.

Plaques are solid elevations greater than 10 mm in diameter.

Nodules are solid masses within the skin greater than 10 mm in diameter.

Vesicles are clear, fluid-filled blisters less than 10 mm in diameter.

Bullae are clear, fluid-filled blisters greater than 10 mm in diameter.

Pustules are filled with opaque purulent material.

Erosions are shallow depressions without epithelium.

Ulcers are deeper areas of epithelial loss.

Scale is visible desquamation of stratum corneum and may be a primary or secondary change.

Table 29-1 gives a partial differential diagnosis for the different types of primary lesions. This list is not complete, and some diseases are listed in several locations, since they may present in more than one way.

Important points of the history include a list of countries visited, duration of time in each location, whether urban or rural areas were visited,

Table 29-1
Differential Diagnosis of Skin Lesions

Macules	**Nodules**
Tinea versicolor	Hansen's disease
Pityriasis alba*	Furuncular myiasis
Vitiligo*	Furuncle
Hansen's disease	Chromomycosis
Onchocerciasis	Sporotrichosis
Pinta	Onchocerciasis
Tinea nigra	Mycetoma
Papules and Plaques	**Vesicles and Bullae**
Dermatitis	Dermatitis
Miliaria*	Sunburn
Scabies	Drug eruption
Insect bites	Erythema multiforme*
Bacterial infection	Insect bite
Drug eruption	Viral exanthem*
Dermatophyte infection	Pemphigus, pemphigoid*
Hansen's disease	
Tungiasis	**Ulcers**
Onchocerciasis	Leishmaniasis
Myiasis	Tropical ulcer
Cutaneous larva migrans	Buruli ulcer
Cercarial dermatitis	Sporotrichosis
Pinta	Bacterial infection
	Insect bite

*Not discussed in this book. Consult the index for the other entities.

and information about specific activities (e.g., fishing, camping). Specific details about the skin problem should include a description of the onset and evolution of the lesions, associated symptoms, and all forms of treatment used, including nonprescription treatment. A history of antecedent trauma, insect bite, suspected precipitating factors, exposure to animals, similar rash in companions, and personal or family history of similar or other skin disease should be sought.

Diagnostic tests are often needed to supplement physical diagnosis. These include Gram stain, Tzanck test, mineral oil test for scabies, potassium hydroxide (KOH) examination, and skin biopsy. The KOH examination is a quick, easy, and inexpensive test in the diagnosis of fungal infections. The technique is discussed with dermatophyte infections (Chapter 33). A Tzanck test gives a quick epithelial cell specimen to look for multinucleated giant cells, the characteristic cytopathic change seen in herpetic infections. Gram stain is invaluable for diagnosis of bacterial and some fungal (e.g., *Pityrosporum*) skin infections.

Skin biopsy may be necessary in certain cases to establish the diagnosis. A fresh lesion should be selected to minimize secondary effects, and the biopsy should be taken from an active area or edge of a lesion. The skin should be prepared with antiseptic and anesthetized with lidocaine. Most dermatologists use 3- or 4-mm biopsy punches, but an incisional biopsy is also appropriate, particularly for deep lesions. Many dermatologists elect to close the biopsy wound with nonabsorbable suture, although that is not absolutely necessary. If an unusual infectious agent is suspected, it is important to notify the pathologist so that special stains can be done on the skin biopsy specimen. A separate biopsy can be sent to the microbiology laboratory on nonbacteriostatic, saline-dampened, sterile gauze for bacterial and/or culture.

GENERAL DERMATOLOGIC TREATMENTS

Specific therapy for dermatologic diseases requires a specific diagnosis and is discussed with each disease entity in other chapters. Two aspects of dermatologic therapy, compresses and topical steroids, are discussed here.

Compresses are used to provide nonspecific relief in inflammatory dermatoses and to gently lift crust from weepy lesions. Compresses are made of several layers of cotton cloth that are soaked in a solution and partially wrung out. The active ingredient in most compress solutions used for compresses is water, although bacteriostatic or drying agents, such as aluminum acetate (Burow's solution), are frequently added. The compress is placed on the lesion and left in place for 3 to 5 minutes, then removed, soaked, wrung out, and replaced. The brief time on the lesion allows evaporative cooling and removes some exudate. The compress should be applied repeatedly for 15 to 20 minutes several times a day, more often for exudative lesions. Wet dressings should not be left on the skin for long periods, since they may macerate surrounding healthy tissue.

Topical steroids are highly effective agents for reducing the cutaneous immune response and are widely used in treating inflammatory conditions. A large number of products are available, varying greatly in potency and potential to produce side effects. In addition, different vehicles are available, including creams, ointments, lotions, solutions, gels, and sprays. It is convenient to know products of low, medium, and high potency in either cream or ointment form, since this will be adequate for effective therapy of many inflammatory dermatoses. Low-potency steroids are used in those areas most susceptible to topical steroid side effects: the face,

Table 29-2
Topical Steroids Strength Groups

Low potency	Hydrocortisone 1% cream or ointment
Medium potency	Triamcinolone acetonide 0.1% cream or ointment
	Fluocinolone 0.01% cream or solution, 0.025% ointment
	Betamethasone valerate 0.1% cream or ointment
High potency	Fluocinonide 0.05% cream or ointment
	Desoximetasone 0.25% cream

axillae, groin, and genitals. Side effects of topical steroids include atrophy, telangiectasia, striae, and steroid-induced rosacea. Medium-potency steroids are used for most other body locations, except for severe or refractory conditions, which are treated with high-potency steroids.

In general, the drier the skin condition, the more hydrophobic the topical steroid vehicle should be. In descending order of greasiness are ointments, creams, lotions, and solutions. Gels, sprays, and solutions are essentially equivalent in their low or no oil content. Solutions are useful for scalp involvement. Table 29-2 provides a simplified list of steroid preparations in each potency class.

Knowing the quantity of topical steroid to prescribe is also useful. Topical steroids should be applied sparingly and are usually dosed twice daily. A dose of 30 g of an agent is usually enough to cover an average adult's total body surface area once. Based on this amount, one can roughly estimate a desired quantity to prescribe. Container sizes typically are 15, 30, 60, 120, and 240 g; 1 lb and 1 kg sizes are available in some formulations. Prescribing large quantities with refills of high-potency topical steroids is not recommended.

REFERENCES

Freedberg IM et al: *Fitzpatrick's dermatology in general medicine,* ed 5, New York, 1999, McGraw-Hill.

CHAPTER 30

Acute Skin Reactions

Roy Colven and M. Sean Strother

Acute skin reactions are often quite symptomatic and account for the majority of skin-related complaints of travelers. Sunburn and other ultraviolet light reactions, medication-related eruptions, dermatitis, and insect bites and stings occur with brief exposure to environmental hazards or drugs, and in many cases are preventable. This chapter deals with a number of the more common acute dermatologic problems encountered by travelers.

SUNBURN AND OTHER ULTRAVIOLET LIGHT REACTIONS

The intensity of ultraviolet (UV) radiation from the sun is related to season and latitude, and the amount of UV light reaching the earth's surface is substantially greater in the tropics. This can lead to *sunburn,* but it also can unmask or aggravate *photosensitive diseases,* such as solar urticaria, polymorphous light eruption, porphyria, discoid and systemic lupus erythematosus, and dermatomyositis. A number of medications when combined with UV light in vivo can lead to *photosensitive drug eruptions.* UV light, through local immune suppressive effects, can also trigger recurrent *herpes simplex.* Over the long term, UV exposure can promote premature skin aging and skin cancer.

Etiology

Aside from heat-related conditions, the wavelengths of light responsible for clinical problems associated with sunlight are in the UV part of the spectrum. Ultraviolet B (UV-B), 290 to 320 nm, and ultraviolet A (UV-A), 320 to 400 nm, are of greatest importance. Sunburn is chiefly caused by UV-B. Individual tolerance to sun exposure is a function of constitutive skin pigmentation and genetic ability to synthesize and process melanin in the epidermis in response to UV light.

In contrast to sunburn, most photosensitive diseases and drug-induced photoeruptions are incited by UV-A, an important distinction when it comes to prevention. Also, UV-A, and not UV-B, penetrates most window glass, including the windshields of vehicles.

Prevention

Avoidance of the sun is the ultimate protection against UV-induced conditions. The highest intensity of light occurs between 10 AM and 4 PM, so limiting UV exposure during this period is helpful. Protection against sunburn and the long-term effects of sun exposure may be provided by shade and topically applied sunscreens. Brimmed hats, ideally providing shade for the face and neck, long sleeved shirts, and long pants cover the largest areas of exposed skin. Sunglasses with UV-protectant lenses will help limit sun-related effects on the eyes. Companies now market lightweight, UV-protectant clothing designed for travelers to the tropics.

Sunscreens contain chemicals that absorb or scatter ultraviolet light on the surface of the skin and reduce the amount penetrating the skin. Hundreds of products have become available with the increased awareness of the harmful effects of UV radiation. They differ in active ingredients and come in a range of efficacy. Common chemical ingredients have included *para*-aminobenzoic acid (PABA), PABA esters, salicylates, cinnamates, methyl anthralite, benzophenones, and avobenzone, also known as Parsol 1789. The last three chemicals provide protection against UV-A, as well as UV-B, though only avobenzone provides protection for near UV-A wavelengths. Mounting evidence implicates UV-A as a cause of photoaging and cutaneous carcinogenesis. Because of an unacceptable rate of fabric staining and allergic contact reactions caused by PABA, most sunscreens made now are PABA-free. So-called *sun blocks or physical sunscreens* contain zinc oxide or titanium dioxide that help to scatter UV light and to a lesser extent absorb it. Sun blocks are effective for both UV-A and B. Current formulations contain micronized zinc or titanium, making these products cosmetically acceptable.

Sun protection factor (SPF) is a ratio of the UV dose needed to develop minimal erythema to skin with sunscreen to the dose required to reach a comparable degree of erythema without sunscreen. SPF is therefore a measure of UV-B protection. The SPF is determined with artificial light sources and predetermined sunscreen dose, conditions that may vary between the laboratory and the field. Sunscreen SPFs range from 2 to 50. Clothing provides variable SPFs, depending on the weight and weave of the fabric. Typical lightweight cotton clothing provides SPFs of approximately 5 to 7. Wet clothing generally loses a third of its sun-protective ability. Dark-colored clothing generally has higher SPFs than light-colored clothing of the same fabric. Specially made sun-protective clothing can provide SPFs of greater than 30. This protection also remains stable after laundering.

A minimum recommended suncreen or sunblock SPF is 15, with higher SPF (30 or greater) for people with fairer skin. Sunscreens should be applied 20 to 30 minutes before sun exposure. Application should be liberal to all exposed skin. Many formulations are water resistant for up to 80 minutes of water immersion. Reapplication during the day is recommended, particularly after swimming or perspiring heavily, because sunscreen SPF wanes with time after application. Lip protection against UV light can be provided with specially formulated lip sunscreens.

Paint-on "tans" do not impact melanin synthesis and are not themselves sunscreens. This offers no added protection from UV exposure and should not be used as such.

Pretravel tanning to prevent tropical sunburn, whether from artificial sources or solar UV light, is controversial. Tanned skin helps prevent sunburn, but this must be weighed against the pretravel UV exposure and subsequent higher UV exposure one is likely to allow after getting a "protective" tan. Sun protection consisting of avoidance, shade, and sunscreens is the recommended prevention of both short- and long-term UV effects.

Treatment

If efforts toward sun protection fail and sunburn occurs, therapeutic options are somewhat limited. Goals of treatment are to minimize the inflammatory mediators in the skin with prostaglandin inhibitors and to provide symptomatic topical relief. *Mild sunburn* is treated with aspirin or other nonsteroidal antiinflammatory drugs (NSAIDs) and cool compresses. Topical steroids may offer limited benefit that must be weighed against cost. Emollients may be soothing, particularly when the skin begins to desquamate.

Severe sunburn often does not respond to the aforementioned measures. Though not commercially available in the United States, topical indomethacin has been reported to be highly effective in reducing erythema and tenderness when applied soon after exposure in concentrations of 0.1% to 2.5%. A single application gives relief up to 24 hours. Systemic steroids are controversial and studies have not consistently shown efficacy, but a brief course of prednisone, 40 to 60 mg/day for 3 to 4 days, may be helpful if initiated promptly.

DERMATITIS IN TRAVELERS

Dermatitis is a general term for superficial, cell-mediated inflammation of the skin. Dermatitis is classified according to etiology and clinical features. Common types include atopic dermatitis, contact dermatitis, nummular dermatitis, seborrheic dermatitis, and hand (so-called dyshidrotic) dermatitis. A tropical climate may exacerbate a preexisting dermatitis, though higher ambient humidity and UV light often help dermatitis.

Newly acquired dermatitis in travelers usually represents contact dermatitis. Contact dermatitis is further divided into irritant contact dermatitis and allergic contact dermatitis. *Irritant contact dermatitis* occurs on contact with an agent capable of causing injury and inflammation in most, if not all, persons (e.g., strong alkaline solutions). *Allergic contact dermatitis* occurs in sensitized individuals on contact with a specific antigen that does not cause dermatitis in nonsensitized individuals (e.g., poison ivy or oak).

Etiology

Irritant contact dermatitis is caused by soaps, solvents, detergents, cleansers, cutting oils, and acid or alkaline solutions. "Dishpan hands" is an example of chronic irritant contact dermatitis caused by soaps and frequent wetting of the skin. Individual susceptibility to any irritant varies greatly. Most occupational dermatitis is irritant contact dermatitis.

Allergic contact dermatitis can result from exposure to an enormous number of chemical compounds but requires specific sensitization. The most common sensitizers include nickel, chromates, rubber, formaldehyde, paraphenylenediamine, ethylenediamine, thimerosal, and neomycin. It is important to remember that many products sold for use on the skin contain sensitizers such as neomycin, benzocaine, ethylenediamine, fragrances, and lanolin.

Some topical agents can act in concert with UV light to produce *photocontact dermatitis*. Musk ambrette, a common ingredient in fragrances and cosmetics, and, ironically, sunscreen agents, such as PABA and oxybenzone, can cause photoallergic contact dermatitis. Plant-induced photodermatitis is discussed next.

Plant dermatitis (phytodermatitis) is a subset of contact dermatitis of particular importance to those traveling to rural areas. Many plants in a number of different families produce sensitizing chemicals. Poison ivy, poison oak, and poison sumac are members of the family Anacardiaceae and produce a resin containing 3-pentadecyl catechol, a potent sensitizer capable of sensitizing 70% of the population. Related plants containing cross-reacting chemicals include the Japanese lacquer tree *(Rhus verniciflua)*, the India marking nut tree, raw cashew shells *(Apacardium occidentale)*, mango rind *(Mangifera indica)*, and the fruit of the ginkgo *(Ginkgo biloba)*. Causes of plant dermatitis depend on the local flora. Mango dermatitis is the most common plant dermatitis in Hawaii. Philodendron is the most common cause in India. Primrose is a frequent sensitizer in Europe.

Phytophotodermatitis is a sun-induced plant dermatitis. Celery, limes, lemons, parsley, figs, and others contain natural psoralens that can incite a phototoxic reaction when contact with these plants is followed by sun exposure. Cases of systemic phototoxicity after ingestion of these plants followed by UV exposure are reported.

Clinical Features

The primary lesions of dermatitis are erythematous papules and vesicles. In severe cases, bullae form and papules coalesce into plaques. Chronic lesions show scale, secondary changes of lichenification, and sometimes bacterial superinfection. Pruritus is a constant feature of dermatitis. Contact dermatitis is distributed in sites of contact, often giving a bizarre or artifactual appearance. The thicker skin of the palm and soles is more resistant to irritants and is often not involved. Allergic contact may be spread with the hands to other sites of the body such as the face, eyelids, and genitals. Plant dermatitis classically shows linear vesicles or bullae where the skin brushed against the causative plant.

Diagnosis

Dermatitis is usually diagnosed clinically by the typical morphology of the rash. Biopsy may be useful in doubtful cases, but it does not identify the cause of the dermatitis. Establishing the cause of contact dermatitis requires careful questioning on exposure to plants, soaps, chemicals, topical medications, and the activities associated with the dermatitis. Patch testing is invaluable in the diagnosis of allergic contact dermatitis.

Differential diagnosis of dermatitis includes scabies, insect bites, certain drug eruptions, swimmer's itch (cercarial dermatitis), psoriasis, and onchocerciasis.

Treatment

Dermatitis of any etiology is treated in a similar manner. In the case of contact dermatitis, avoidance of the offending agent is most important. Protective clothing or gloves may be helpful when the person must continue the activities associated with the dermatitis. Excessive washing is irritating and impairs the barrier function of the skin. Similarly, mildly inflamed skin often improves with emollient alone.

Mild cases of papular or vesicular dermatitis are treated with topical steroids appropriate for the body area affected. Weeping or exudative lesions should be compressed with Burow's solution for 15 minutes, four times a day, followed by topical steroids.

Severe contact dermatitis is best treated with prednisone 40 to 60 mg/day (adult dose), tapering the dose over 2 to 3 weeks. In allergic contact dermatitis, stopping the prednisone too soon often results in recurrence of the eruption. If a sensitized person contacts an allergen, the skin should be promptly washed with soap and water to remove all possible allergen.

If secondary bacterial infection is present, it should be treated with antibiotics effective for *Staphylococcus* and *Streptococcus* sp.

DRUG ERUPTIONS

Cutaneous reactions to drugs are common and at times serious. A great variety of patterns of drug reactions occur, reflecting both the causative drug and the immune response to it. Travelers frequently take medications, either as prophylaxis or as therapy for acquired symptoms, and thus are subject to adverse reactions. In addition, new reactions from long-standing medications may occur, for example, photosensitive eruptions in the intense tropical sunlight. The frequency of reactions to different medications is quite variable.

Clinical Features

Exanthematous eruptions are the most frequently occurring pattern, accounting for almost half of all reactions. The rash begins as erythematous macules or papules over the trunk and head, which spread centrifugally and may become confluent. Petechiae may be seen in dependent areas. Symptoms may be absent, but pruritus is common. The eruptions progress over 3 to 5 days and resolve in 1 to 3 weeks after the offending agent is stopped. These eruptions are often called morbilliform, or measles-like, because of their resemblance to viral exanthems. The immunology of these eruptions is not understood. They often resolve despite continuation of the causative agent and may not recur if the drug is given again. Exanthematous eruptions may be caused by almost any drug, usually 4 to 7 days after beginning therapy, but the most common causes are ampicillin and trimethoprim/sulfamethoxazole.

Urticaria is the second most common type of drug eruption and is a manifestation of mast cell degranulation. This usually is due to immediate hypersensitivity, mediated by specific immunoglobulin E antibodies, but nonimmunologic degranulation also occurs with agents such as codeine. Onset of symptoms is rapid, generally 15 minutes to 12 hours after administration.

Urticaria is manifested by pruritic, erythematous plaques. The plaques have no scale, are often pale in the center, and have a faint peripheral white ring of vasoconstriction. Urticaria is typically transient in any one location. If a lesion is outlined with ink, it will be observed to migrate out of the ink mark over several hours. This distinguishes urticaria from the fixed lesions of urticarial vasculitis and erythema multiforme. More severe manifestations of immediate hypersensitivity include angioedema, bronchospasm, and anaphylaxis. Penicillins, blood products, and narcotics are the most common causes of urticaria. Skin testing is available for penicillin.

Drug-induced *photosensitive eruptions* include two distinct types, phototoxic and photoallergic. *Phototoxic* reactions occur 3 to 6 hours after sun exposure as an exaggerated sunburn response. Individual susceptibility is variable, but the reaction is nonimmunologic and sensitization does not occur. Erythema and a burning sensation are characteristic. *Photoallergic* eruptions occur in sensitized individuals and develop 24 to 48 hours after sun exposure. The rash is a pruritic dermatitis that may be vesicular and may involve non–sun-exposed areas. Table 30-1 lists medications used commonly in travel and tropical medicine that can produce photosensitivity.

Table 30-1
Medications Commonly Used in Travel and Tropical Medicine Associated With Photosensitivity

Phototoxic agents	Photoallergic agents
Antibiotics: Quinolones, sulfonamides, tetracyclines (doxycycline > tetracycline > minocycline), trimethoprim	Antibiotics: Sulfonamides
Antimalarials: Chloroquine, quinine	Antimalarials: Quinine, quinidine
Antifungals: Griseofulvin	Antifungals: Griseofulvin
Antiemetics: Prochlorperazine	
Diuretics: Furosemide, thiazides	Diuretics: Thiazides
NSAIDs: Naproxen, piroxicam	NSAIDs: Piroxicam

NSAIDs, Nonsteroidal antiinflammatory drugs.

Photoeruptions are recognized by their distribution. The involved areas are exposed skin with sharp outlines of clothing. Naturally, shaded areas are spared, such as the upper eyelids and under the chin and nose. The responsible wavelengths of light are usually in the UV-A spectrum.

Many other patterns of drug eruptions can occur and are not discussed here. These include fixed drug eruptions, Stevens-Johnson syndrome, toxic epidermal necrolysis, pustular eruptions, vasculitis, and drug-induced lupus.

Diagnosis

A careful history is crucial in diagnosing drug eruption. All prescribed and nonprescribed medications should be noted, as well as the date when those agents were started. Biopsy is generally nonspecific in exanthematous and urticarial rashes, but may be diagnostic in erythema multiforme and vasculitis.

Exanthematous eruptions may be difficult to distinguish from viral exanthems, although lack of constitutional symptoms and temporal relationship to the start of a new drug are helpful. Urticaria may be caused by foods, parasitic and viral infections, or physical agents, and often occurs idiopathically. The differential diagnosis of drug-induced photoeruptions includes other photosensitive rashes, such as polymorphous light eruption, lupus erythematosus, and some porphyrias.

Treatment

As a general rule, all nonessential drugs should be discontinued. This is most important in urticarial reactions, which may become more severe and result in systemic symptoms and anaphylaxis.

Antihistamines are relatively specific therapy for urticaria. Hydroxyzine, 25 to 50 mg by mouth every 4 to 6 hours, or diphenhydramine, 25 to 100 mg by mouth every 4 to 6 hours, is the usual therapy. Relatively less sedating antihistamines such as cetirizine, 10 to 20 mg/day, are useful for daytime, but this advantage must be weighed against increased cost and relatively lower potency.

In rapidly developing urticarial reactions, epinephrine 0.3 to 0.5 mg subcutaneously is helpful, together with antihistamines.

Antihistamines have no specific effect on the course of exanthematous eruptions, but in similar doses may be useful nonspecifically for pruritus. Topical steroids may provide some relief from pruritus in exanthematous eruptions and mild photoeruptions.

Prednisone has not been proven effective in drug eruptions, but is often given empirically in severe cases in doses of 40 to 60 mg/day over 1 to 2 weeks.

ARTHROPOD BITES AND STINGS

Insects are well-known vectors of disease in tropical medicine, but the symptoms and lesions they cause directly should also be emphasized. Arthropod bites and stings are the most common dermatologic complaints of tropical travelers. Although most bite reactions are self-limited, severe or fatal cases occur.

Etiology

Biting and stinging arthropods are found worldwide. Clinical disease is due to hypersensitivity to arthropod antigens, toxic effects of venoms, or both. Important venom-producing arthropods include some species of spiders, *hymenoptera* (bees and wasps), ants, centipedes, and scorpions. Non–venom-producing, biting arthropods include species of flies, mosquitoes, bedbugs, fleas, mites, and lice.

There are many biting *spiders,* but several are worth special mention. The black widow spider, *Latrodectus mactans,* and other *Lactrodectus* spp. are found worldwide. *L. mactans* is recognized by the red hourglass shape on the ventral abdomen. The bite is often painless, but a neurotoxin, alpha-lactrotoxin, is elaborated that causes systemic symptoms. *Loxosceles* spp., including the brown recluse spider, are found in North and South America, have a violin shape on the cephalothorax, and produce venom containing sphingomyelinase D, causing extensive local skin and soft tissue necrosis. The wandering spider, *Phoneutria nigriventer,* is a large South American spider measuring 3 cm in body length and producing a potent neurotoxin. Tarantulas, maligned by ages of lore, include many species of spiders and generally produce a localized bite reaction ranging from pain similar to that of a bee sting to limb edema and numbness.

Hymenoptera include bees, wasps, hornets, yellow jackets, and ants and cause painful reactions from venom injected from a posterior stinger. Depending on individual response, severe reactions to *Hymenoptera* stings also occur. Half of the fatal evenomation reactions that occur in the United States are due to *Hymenoptera.* Honey bees produce a venom containing histamine, phospholipase A, hyaluronidase, and other constituents. *Solenopsis invicta,* the imported fire ant, is common in the southern United States, Argentina, Uruguay, and Brazil.

Many species of *scorpions* are found in arid regions of the tropics and subtropics. Fatal stings are common in children in areas where species produce neurotoxic venom. Centipedes of the *Scolopendra* genus are found in Hawaii and the western United States and produce a painful local reaction to a venomous bite.

Biting *flies* have mouth parts adapted to piercing skin. The important biting flies include horseflies, black flies, sandflies, tsetse flies, midges, and mosquitoes. No venom is produced, but salivary proteins can cause hypersensitivity reactions. Black fly bites may produce a reaction that lasts for months.

Several species of *fleas* affect humans, including the human flea, *Pulex irritans,* the cat flea, and the rat flea. The burrowing flea, *Tunga penetrans,* is discussed Chapter 31.

Bedbugs include several species of bloodsucking true bugs in the family Cimicidae. Bedbugs are found worldwide. They are 3 to 4 mm oval insects that live in cracks in houses, hotels, and public places and emerge at night to feed. Bedbug infestation is uncommon in temperate climates except in older or neglected houses, but may be more common in the tropics. Bedbugs, attracted by the warmth of the host, move onto exposed skin and feed for 5 minutes before leaving the host. Bedbugs have not been established as vectors of other diseases.

Human ectoparasites, such as scabies and lice, are discussed in Chapter 31.

Clinical Features

The majority of bite reactions are mild local hypersensitivity reactions, typically one or more pruritic erythematous papules that may have a central punctum. Stings are more likely to be painful and more edematous. Most bites and stings resolve spontaneously over a few hours to several days. Exceptional reactions are discussed next.

Black widow spider bites usually have little local reaction, and systemic effects of the venom are predominant clinically. Several hours after the bite, muscle spasms, abdominal pain, nausea, and hypotension develop, which may progress to shock and death.

Brown recluse spider bites cause only a mild urticarial reaction in the majority of cases. Some bites cause severe local reactions characterized by an expanding bulla with surrounding pallor followed by cyanosis and necrosis within 48 to 72 hours after the bite. Systemic involvement with disseminated intravascular coagulation, hemolysis, and renal insufficiency is rare, but may be fatal.

Fire ant stings may cause anaphylaxis but usually produce local reactions. Stings cause an immediate wheal, which becomes a vesicle and then a sterile pustule over 12 to 24 hours.

Hymenoptera stings generally produce a painful wheal that subsides over a few hours. In sensitive individuals, systemic reactions occur owing to immediate type hypersensitivity, including urticaria, laryngeal edema, bronchospasm, and anaphylaxis. Less common systemic manifestations include toxic reactions from large numbers of simultaneous stings or a serum sickness-like syndrome that follows the sting by days to weeks.

Scorpion stings cause a painful local reaction, occasionally with some necrosis. Some species produce venom that can induce sympathomimetic, parasympathomimetic, and neurologic symptoms. Death in some cases is reported, particularly in infants and children.

Bedbug bites are usually painless; usually occur on the face, arms, ankles, or buttocks; and are often arranged in a cluster or line of two or three bites. The appearance of individual bites range from small hemorrhagic puncta to papular urticaria that last for several days.

Diagnosis

Stings usually present no problem with diagnosis because the immediate pain of the sting draws attention to the area and the arthropod is seen. With bee stings, the stinger is often left in the skin and may be visible.

Bites may be more difficult to diagnose if the injury is painless or occurs during sleep. The pruritic papules of typical bites may resemble other hypersensitivity reactions, such as urticaria or dermatitis. Bullous or necrotic reactions may mimic erythema multiforme, dermatitis herpetiformis, vasculitis, and other rashes. Definitive diagnosis is possible only if the bite is observed. Biopsy may be helpful in persistent cases.

Treatment

Most papular and mild bullous reactions are self-limited and can be treated with compresses and topical steroids or antihistamines for pruritus. As with all penetrating skin injuries, tetanus prophylaxis should be given if the patient's status is not up to date.

Black widow spider reactions may require hospitalization for analgesics, muscle relaxants, intravenous calcium, and supportive care. A specific equine antivenom is available in several countries.

Brown recluse spider bites are usually benign and can be treated symptomatically. Treatment of necrotic reactions is controversial. Ice and elevation are probably helpful to treat symptoms. Dapsone has been used with some success. Systemic corticosteroids, recommended in the past, are not helpful for skin necrosis, but may be helpful for systemic loxoscelism. Early excision of necrotic lesions is probably not warranted, although later wound excision may improve cosmesis or function. Systemic loxoscelism may be life threatening and requires hospitalization for supportive care. Antivenom is not available in the United States.

Scorpion stings are treated by local wound care, ice packs, and antihistamines. Antihypertensives or anticonvulsants may be needed in severe evenomations with sympathomimetic or neurologic effects, respectively. Antivenoms for systemic reactions are available in other countries, such as Mexico, but no FDA-approved antivenom is available in the United States. Antivenom for *Centruroides sculpturatus,* a toxic scorpion found in Arizona, is available from the Antivenom Production Laboratory at Arizona State University.

Hymenoptera stings are common, and therapy depends on the type of reaction observed. If a stinger is still in place, it should be carefully removed with forceps to avoid squeezing the venom sacs. Mild local responses are treated with compresses. Mild urticarial reactions are treated with antihistamines, more severe urticaria or angioedema with prednisone, 30 to 40 mg/day for several days. More severe generalized urticarial reactions or anaphylaxis is treated promptly with epinephrine, 0.3 mg to 0.5 mg subcutaneously repeated every 15 to 20 minutes if needed, in addition to fluid support, antihistamines, and systemic steroids. Intravenous epinephrine may be necessary if hypotension persists despite these measures.

Prevention

For persons with a history of an immediate hypersensitivity reaction to hymenoptera stings, desensitization should be considered mandatory. In addition, such persons should carry kits for therapy of stings, including antihistamines and a syringe of epinephrine. Epinephrine auto-injectors are commercially available (e.g., Ana-Kit [Hollister-Stier Laboratories, Spokane, WA] or Epipen [Meridian Medical Technologies, Columbia, MD]). Wearing protective clothing is also helpful.

For protection against biting flies, mosquitoes, ticks, and fleas, the use of protective clothing and insect repellent is useful. The most active insect repellent is diethyltoluamide (DEET). This agent protects the skin only where it is applied and should be used liberally. Because of evaporation and rubbing off of the repellent, reapplication has been necessary every 1 to 2 hours, but longer-acting formulations are now available (see Chapter 1). Insect repellents have no effect on spiders or bees. Alternative insect repellents include dimethyl phthalate, ethyl hexanediol, and dimethyl carbate butopyronoxyl.

Control of bedbugs involves treating crevices in walls and furniture with an insecticide such as 0.5% lindane or 2% malathion, or spraying bed nets with a permethrin-containing insecticide (see Chapter 1).

REFERENCES

Sun Reactions

Anonymous: Sunscreens: are they safe and effective? *Med Lett Drugs Ther* 41:43, 1999.

Gould JW, Mercurio MG, Elmets CA: Cutaneous photosensitivity diseases induced by exogenous agents, *J Am Acad Dermatol* 33:551, 1995.

Skin Cancer Foundation Internet website: www.skincancer.org

Dermatitis

Feingold S et al: Eczemas, *Curr Probl Dermatol* 10:41, 1998.

Rietschel RL, Fowler JF: *Fisher's contact dermatitis,* ed 4, Baltimore, 1997, Williams & Wilkins.

Drug Eruptions

Prussick R, Knowles S, Shear NH: Cutaneous drug reactions, *Curr Probl Dermatol* 6:81, 1994.

Bites and Stings

Carbonaro PA, Janniger CK, Schwartz RA: Scorpion sting reactions, *Cutis* 57(3):139, 1996.

Kemp ED: Bites and stings of the arthropod kind. Treating reactions that can range from annoying to menacing, *Postgrad Med* 103:88, 1998.

Wilson DC, King LE: Arthropod bites and stings. In Freedberg IM et al, editors: *Fitzpatrick's dermatology in general medicine,* ed 5, New York, 1999, McGraw-Hill.

Wright SW, Wrenn KD, Murray L, Seger D: Clinical presentation and outcome of brown recluse spider bite, *Ann Emerg Med* 30(1):28, 1997.

CHAPTER 31

Ectoparasites, Cutaneous Parasites, and Cnidarian Envenomation

M. Sean Strother and Roy Colven

This chapter describes common infestations by ectoparasites, including mites, lice, and ticks and diseases such as tungiasis, furuncular myiasis, and cutaneous larva migrans caused by less common cutaneous parasites. Swimmer's itch and cnidarian envenomation are also discussed. Travelers whose trips encompass outdoor activities, camping, or living under native conditions in developing areas of the world are more likely to return to the United States with problems of these kinds than are travelers who follow normal tourist routes.

ECTOPARASITES

Infestation of the skin with lice or scabies can cause intensely pruritic lesions of the skin. Such infestations are usually acquired from close cohabitation with affected people, including sexual contacts.

Etiology

Scabies is caused by the human "itch mite," *Sarcoptes scabiei* var. *hominis.* This microscopic mite lives on the surface of the skin. Male mites impregnate the female and subsequently die while on the skin surface. The impregnated female burrows into the stratum corneum, lays eggs along the burrow path, and then dies. The eggs hatch in 3 to 4 days, and the emerging larvae leave the burrow and travel to the skin surface. There they pass through larval and nymphal stages before maturing into adult mites. The cycle is then repeated. In most healthy people, an immune response to scabies infestation develops in 3 to 4 weeks and corresponds to the onset of symptoms. Often, few mites are found, even in cases where the skin lesions involve a large body surface area. There is no known nonhuman reservoir, and mite survival away from the host is limited.

Head lice, or pediculosis capitis, and *body lice,* pediculosis corporis, are caused by subspecies of the human louse *Pediculus humanus.* These two subspecies of lice are practically identical in appearance, but they have quite distinct patterns of infestation. *P. humanus* is a light gray insect, 2 to 4 mm long, that feeds on blood. Lice are present worldwide, but infestation is more common in conditions of poverty, crowding, and poor hygiene.

Head lice live exclusively on the scalp and deposit ova, or nits, on hairs. The total number of lice is usually less than 10, and the infestation is centered around the occiput. Nits are 0.5 mm white oval eggs that are cemented firmly to individual hairs at the point where the shaft emerges from the scalp; they grow out with the hair. Nits beyond 7 mm from the scalp have already hatched are no longer viable.

Body lice live and deposit their nits in the seams of clothing. They move onto the skin only transiently to feed. Away from their human host, lice live for only a few days.

Pubic lice, or pediculosis pubis, is caused by the crab louse *Phthirus pubis.* This 1- to 2-mm-long, brown louse is usually transmitted sexually and lives primarily in the pubic hair, although it may be found on the eyelashes, or hair of the axillae, abdomen, or other body regions.

Epidemiology

Scabies and lice are infestations are common. *Scabies* occurs worldwide, but is more common in the tropics, in areas of crowding and poverty. Scabies is epidemic in much of the developing world. In rural Central America, local prevalence may exceed 90%. Outbreaks in schools, nursing homes, prisons, and other institutions are common. Scabies is highly contagious through skin-to-skin contact. Fomites probably play a minor role, if any, in transmission. People of all ages are affected. Crusted or Norwegian scabies is an unusual clinical variant of *S. scabiei* infestation, in which thousands to millions of mites are present. It is highly contagious and is seen primarily in young children and patients with immunodeficiency, cognitive deficiency, or those who are physically unable to scratch.

Head lice is primarily a disease of children but can occur at any age. *Body lice* occur in conditions of poor hygiene, especially where clothing is not changed and washed regularly. Transmission occurs through close body contact or sharing infested articles of clothing. Lice may live for several days on clothing or bedding, but routine laundering will kill them. *Pubic lice* occur primarily in sexually active adults.

Body lice are capable of transmitting several infectious diseases including typhus, trench fever, and relapsing fever. *Staphylococcus* and group A *Streptococcus* infections have been shown to be transmitted by head lice. Although human immunodeficiency virus (HIV) has been demonstrated in lice, no epidemiologic link yet exists between lice and HIV transmission.

Clinical Features

The classic descriptions of *scabies* were written in temperate climates, and certain clinical differences may occur in the tropics. The hallmark of scabies is intense itching, generally worse at night. The primary lesions are erythematous 2 to 3 mm papules and vesicles, but the majority of lesions seen clinically are excoriated with a central crust. The distribution includes finger webs, flexor surfaces of the wrists, axillae, breasts, umbilicus, genitals, buttocks, and feet. Burrows are 3 to 5 mm, threadlike, linear lesions seen mainly in the finger webs, and on the wrists and glans penis. Secondary bacterial infection is common, and impetigo occurring in the aforementioned distribution should suggest scabies.

In temperate climates, the face and scalp are spared except in infants and elderly persons. In the tropics, the scalp and face may be involved, secondary infection is more frequent, and burrows are generally absent.

Crusted scabies may occur anywhere on the body surface, although an acral distribution is common. Hyperkeratotic plaques and crusts predominate, and burrows are often not noted because they are obscured by the overlying crusts. Pruritus is often mild or absent.

Head lice cause pruritus of the scalp and scratching leads to excoriations, frequently complicated by furunculosis or impetigo. The hair is often matted or lusterless, and regional lymph nodes may be enlarged. Lice or nits are usually readily apparent but sometimes are found only after careful scrutiny. Scalp pyoderma should always prompt an inspection for head lice.

Body lice produce generalized pruritus, with excoriations usually worse over the back, shoulders, and arms. The head, hands, and feet are spared, in contrast to head lice or scabies. Typical lesions are excoriated papules with or without secondary bacterial infection. Lice and nits are not found on the body, but may be seen in the seams of clothing.

Pubic lice cause pruritus from the umbilicus to the mid-thighs, most severely in the pubic area. Finding the tiny lice or nits may require a careful search. Often, no skin lesions are present, but excoriations or small bluish macules, called maculae caeruleae, are seen occasionally. The latter are caused by focal alteration of host blood pigment by a salivary product of the louse. Louse feces can also be seen at the base of hairs as a reddish brown material admixed with crusts or as rust-colored specks in the crotch of white underwear.

Diagnosis

A definitive diagnosis of *scabies* can be made by demonstrating the mite, eggs, or feces in skin scrapings. However, with typical lesions and exposure history, a reasonably certain clinical diagnosis is possible.

Scrapings should be made from burrows, if possible, or from lesions of the hands or genitals. With a scalpel blade coated with mineral or immersion oil, the lesions should be scraped firmly enough to cause pinpoint bleeding. The scrapings are placed on a slide with a coverslip and then examined with the low-power 4× objective of the microscope. The finding of mites or eggs is sufficient for diagnosis.

When encountering difficulty, a useful method to identify burrows involves the application of topical tetracycline or fountain pen ink to the suspected site. The area is allowed to dry, then cleansed with soap and water. Burrows treated with tetracycline will fluoresce under a Wood's lamp, whereas fountain pen ink will remain in burrows and make them more easily identifiable.

Lice are diagnosed by finding the louse or nits. *Head lice* and *crab lice* live on the skin and deposit their nits on the hair of the scalp or pubic area, respectively. The use of a hand lens may aid diagnosis. *Body lice* do not live on the skin and are found in the seams of clothing.

Treatment

Treatment for scabies includes topical use of permethrin, lindane (gamma benzene hexachloride), crotamiton, and precipitated sulfur. More recently, the use of oral ivermectin has gained popularity for its ease and effectiveness. All household members and intimate contacts, even if asymptomatic, should be treated simultaneously to avoid reinfestation. To avoid misuse, it is important to give patients careful instructions and dispense only the necessary quantity of medication. Approximately 30 to 50 ml of topical preparations should be prescribed per person for each application.

Permethrin 5% cream is the treatment of choice owing to its high cure rate and minimal toxicity. It is considered safe for infants more than 2 months old. Permethrin cream is applied from the neck down and is left in place for 8 to 12 hours before washing off.

Lindane 1% is also an effective scabicide and is applied in a manner similar to permethrin. However, systemic absorption of lindane occurs through the skin, and neurotoxicity has been reported with repeated applications. It should not be used in infants less than 6 months old. With both permethrin and lindane, retreatment in 5 to 7 days is often recommended, although a single treatment is effective in most cases.

Ivermectin, widely used in veterinary medicine, initially gained acceptance in human medicine for the treatment of the filarial disease, onchocerciasis. More recently, however, it has been used as an effective, oral alternative topical scabicides. A single oral dose of 200 μg/kg body weight is given.

Alternative treatments for scabies include 6% precipitated sulfur in petrolatum, which is applied nightly for 3 nights and washed off 24 hours after the last application. Topical sulfur is considered safe in young infants and pregnant or lactating women.

Clothing and linens should be washed in hot water at the time of treatment. Nonwashable clothing should not be worn for 3 to 5 days, which is longer than the survival time of the mites if they are without human contact. Household fumigation and other environmental management are not necessary. Secondary bacterial infection may occur and requires use of appropriate antibiotics.

Head lice are effectively treated with a 4-minute application of 1% lindane shampoo, which is repeated in 5 to 7 days. Alternative treatments include a 10-minute application of either 1% permethrin cream rinse or other pyrethrin products, according to package directions. Vinegar, used as a rinse, and a fine comb may help dislodge nits from hair. After treatment, the scalp should be examined for new nits or viable lice for several weeks. Secondary bacterial infection should be treated with antibiotics. Bed linen and hats should be laundered or dry cleaned.

Body lice are treated by destroying lice on clothing, by laundering, dry cleaning, or application of insecticide powder to the inner surface of clothing. DDT powder or 1% Malathion powder is effective. Bacterial superinfection may require antibiotics. Topical treatment of the patient is unnecessary.

Pubic lice are treated with a single 4-minute application of 1% lindane shampoo from the axillae to the thighs. An overnight application of 1% lindane lotion is an effective alternative. Pyrethrins may also be used. A second application after 1 week is rarely needed. Sexual partners should be treated simultaneously to prevent reinfestation. Crab lice infestation of the eyelashes poses a therapeutic problem. A common treatment is thick application of petrolatum to the lashes twice a day for 8 days, followed by mechanical removal of nits.

CUTANEOUS LARVA MIGRANS

Cutaneous larva migrans is a clinical syndrome caused by the larvae of various roundworms (nematodes).

Etiology

The most common cause of cutaneous larva migrans is the larva of the dog and cat hookworm, *Ancylostoma braziliense.* Eggs are passed in the stool and, under proper conditions, mature into infective larvae in the soil. These penetrate the epidermis and produce serpiginous lesions by burrowing through the skin. If untreated, the larvae usually die within 2 to 8 weeks, although chronic cases lasting as long as a year have been reported. Similar eruptions occur with the larvae of *Ancylostoma duodenale, Necator americanus, Strongyloides stercoralis,* and others. When the eruption occurs perianally, it is called larva currens and is generally due to *S. stercoralis* (see Chapter 40).

Epidemiology

The disease occurs worldwide, but is dependent on warmth and humidity for larval development. The most important risk factor is skin exposure to sandy soil contaminated with dog or cat feces. In travelers this typically occurs on beaches. Because people walk barefoot, the feet are most often involved, but skin throughout the body can be affected. Involvement of the genitalia and buttocks has been reported in travelers who have frequented nude beaches.

Clinical Features

After larval penetration, mild itching and nonspecific papules may occur and subside. After a lag period of 1 to several days, the larva begins to migrate, producing a tortuous, linear track marked by pruritus and erythema. The lesion advances a few millimeters to several centimeters each day, and there may be resolution of the older parts of the track. Excoriation and secondary infection are frequent. Multiple lesions are common. Any area of the body may be involved. In larva currens, the perianal lesions advance very rapidly, up to 10 cm/hour.

Diagnosis

The diagnosis is usually made on clinical grounds when a typical lesion occurs in a person with a history of possible exposure. Biopsy may help but often fails to demonstrate the organism, since it usually lies 1 to 2 cm away from the leading edge of the track.

Treatment

For decades the standard therapy of cutaneous larva migrans has been thiabendazole, 25 to 50 mg/kg/day, given orally in two divided doses for 2 days. Side effects of anorexia, nausea, and dizziness are common.

Because of the side effects of oral thiabendazole, there have been several studies of topical thiabendazole alone or in combination with a lower oral dose. The 10% oral suspension is applied as a lotion to lesions four times a day until the lesions have ceased to be active—usually 2 to 7 days. Side effects of local erythema and burning have occurred. Recently ivermectin, 150 (μg/kg given orally in a single dose, and albendazole, 200 mg given orally twice a day for 3 days, have been used effectively as oral alternatives to thiabendazole with fewer side effects.

MYIASIS

Myiasis refers to infestation by the larvae of flies. The three cutaneous forms are wound myiasis, dermal myiasis, and furuncular myiasis. Wound myiasis is a ubiquitous condition that occurs when flies deposit eggs into an open wound or ulcer, and larvae develop on the surface of the wound. Dermal myiasis occurs primarily in Central and South America and is a variant of cutaneous larva migrans. It is caused by larvae of the screwworm fly *(Chrysomyia macellaria)* or black blowfly *(Phormia Regina).* Furuncular myiasis occurs primarily in Central and South America and Africa and is may be found among returning travelers.

Etiology

Central and South America's furuncular myiasis is caused by the human botfly, *Dermatobia hominis.* This fly catches other biting insects in midair and attaches its eggs to their bodies. When the biting insects feed, the eggs hatch and the larvae enter through the puncture wound. The larvae develop in the dermis, breathing through an opening (pore) in the skin. After about 30 days, they leave the host.

Rare cases of North American furuncular myiasis have been associated with endemic botflies (*Cuterebra* species).

African furuncular myiasis is due to the tumbu fly, *Cordylobia anthropophaga.* This fly lays eggs on the ground and on laundry, and larvae penetrate through the skin of the mammalian host. Larvae mature and vacate the host after 6 to 7 days.

Clinical Features

Botfly myiasis may occur on any exposed surface, but commonly is found on the scalp as a single, dome-shaped, erythematous papule with a central pore. A feeling of movement in the lesion is common. Secondary bacterial infection may be present.

Tumbu fly myiasis tends to have multiple lesions of the thighs, buttocks, and scrotum. These lesions have associated erythema but fewer tendencies toward development of secondary infection.

Diagnosis

Typical lesions associated with a sense of movement are easily diagnosed. If the air hole is blocked with petrolatum, the larva may evacuate the burrow. Application of raw bacon has also been reported as effective. If the orifice is enlarged with a small incision, the larva can be extracted with forceps. A gentler method of removal consists of applying a small occlusive adhesive bandage over each lesion. The bandage is peeled off after 3 to 4 days, and the dead (asphyxiated) larva is extracted from the burrow. This technique may be recommended for patients with multiple lesions.

Treatment

Lesions are treated by extraction of the larva, as described previously. Secondary bacterial infection should be treated, if present. Prevention consists of protecting exposed body surfaces from biting insects, wearing shoes in tropical areas, and ironing all clothes in areas of tumbu fly myiasis.

TUNGIASIS

Etiology

Tungiasis is caused by *Tunga penetrans,* a 1-mm long sand flea, also known as the chigoe or jigger flea, which infests swine, human, and other mammalian hosts. The fertilized female flea burrows into the skin of the host, where she resides within the stratum corneum of the epidermis, feeds on blood, and gradually enlarges to the size of a small pea. The posterior end of the flea remains in contact with the air for respiration and discharge of ova. The eggs fall to the ground and develop into larvae, which then form a cocoon and emerge as adults after 10 days. Over the course of a few weeks, the female discharges 100 or more eggs. She then dies and is sloughed with the host's stratum corneum.

Epidemiology
Tungiasis occurs in equatorial Africa, Central and South America, and, less frequently, the southern United States. Tungiasis affects persons walking barefoot or lying in infested sand or soil.

Clinical Features
The lesions of tungiasis are pruritic, erythematous papules with a central black punctum, which is the posterior end of the female flea. The lesions are typically located on the feet and ankles, particularly the soles, toes, and under the toenails. As they develop, they become painful and may become secondarily infected. Extensive ulcerations may occur.

Diagnosis
The diagnosis is made by inspection and recovering a flea from a lesion.

Treatment
Tungiasis is treated by opening the lesions with a scalpel blade and removing the flea with forceps or a curette. Topical application of 4% formaldehyde solution, DDT, chloroform, or turpentine has also been reported as effective therapy, as has systemic niridazole. Secondary bacterial infection should be treated with appropriate antibiotics. Infection is best prevented by wearing shoes and by routine inspection of the feet; use of insecticides has also been advocated.

TICK BITES
Ticks are blood-sucking insects that are important in a number of human diseases, although humans are incidental hosts. Ticks are responsible for significant local bite reactions and systemic reactions, and are also vectors for a variety of viral, bacterial, rickettsial, and treponemal diseases.

Etiology
Ticks are members of the class Arachnida and are divided into two families: (1) Ixodidae, or hard ticks, and (2) Argasidae, or soft-bodied ticks.

Ticks are ectoparasites with larval, nymphal, and adult life stages. They are found worldwide, and more than 800 species are recognized. Ticks feed by anchoring their mouth parts in the skin and inserting a hollow proboscis to suck blood from the superficial vessels.

The different families of ticks have basic differences in host range and feeding habits. The Ixodidae live in forest and grassland areas, attach to warm-blooded hosts, and remain on the skin for days to weeks before dropping off. Ixodid ticks are vectors for Lyme disease (Chapter 21), ehrlichiosis, Rocky Mountain spotted fever, babesiosis, Colorado tick fever, tick-borne encephalitis, and many others.

The Argasidae are mainly parasites of birds and live in nesting areas. They feed at night and feed rapidly, often on several hosts in succession; this influences their role as vectors of disease. Argasid ticks are vectors for relapsing fever and others.

Clinical Features
Tick bites cause a variety of local and systemic reactions. The insertion of the mouth parts and proboscis is usually painless. Ixodid ticks often cause little tissue reaction, and the tick body may be noticed incidentally on the skin as a pea-sized tumor. Urticarial papules and pruritus may occur,

calling attention to the tick. These papules subside within a few days after removal. Argasid ticks frequently cause more inflammatory or papular reactions, which subside over several weeks.

Tick bite granuloma is a persistent pruritic reaction occurring at the site of attachment of the tick. In some cases, tick bite granuloma is associated with retention of mouth parts in the skin, but this is not a necessary condition. These granulomas are firm, slightly erythematous nodules that persist for months or years.

Tick fever is a systemic reaction with fever, headache, vomiting, and abdominal pain. This occurs after several days of attachment by the tick and subsides within 12 to 36 hours after its removal.

Tick paralysis is a rare, potentially fatal systemic reaction caused by the bite of several species of ticks endemic in the western United States, western Canada, and Australia. The paralysis appears to be due to neuromuscular blockade by a toxin elaborated by the tick. The reaction begins after 5 to 6 days of attachment, with irritability and sometimes low-grade fever. An ascending lower motor neuron paralysis develops rapidly and may result in death resulting from bulbar paralysis or aspiration. Symptoms abate rapidly after removal of the tick.

Diagnosis

If a tick is found attached to the skin, there is little doubt about the diagnosis. The bite reactions to ticks may be difficult to distinguish from those of other biting insects. Tick bite granuloma is distinguished from many other granulomatous processes by the intense pruritus that is present, but biopsy may be necessary. Tick bite fever or tick paralysis may be diagnosed only if the condition is considered and a careful inspection is made of the entire skin, including the scalp.

Treatment

When traveling in tick-infested areas, one should wear light-colored clothing, and pant cuffs should be tucked into socks. This will increase the likelihood of spotting a foraging tick before it has the chance to attach to skin. The use of insect repellent, particularly those containing DEET, and permethrin spray applied to clothing adds protection.

If a tick is found on the skin, it should be removed without leaving the mouth parts in the skin. Most ticks can be successfully removed by grasping the tick as close to the skin as possible with small forceps and applying steady, firm traction in a plane perpendicular to the skin surface. If the tick has been pulled off and mouth parts are left in the skin, they can be removed with a punch biopsy. Application of chloroform, gasoline, ethyl chloride, mineral oil, or viscous lidocaine will often cause the tick to release its hold.

Tick fever and tick paralysis are treated by removal of the tick and supportive measures. Tick bite granuloma responds to intralesional steroids. It remains controversial whether prophylactic antibiotics are of benefit following a tick bite in an area where bacterial tick-borne infections are prevalent (see Chapters 18 and 21).

CERCARIAL DERMATITIS

Cercarial dermatitis, also known as swimmer's itch, is a self-limited, common parasitic infection in which humans are an incidental host.

Etiology

Cercarial dermatitis is caused by penetration of the skin by avian or rodent schistosomal larval forms called cercariae. Snails infected with schistosome (blood fluke) species shed the infective cercariae into the water. The cercariae penetrate the wet skin of warm-blooded animals. Humans in contact with contaminated water serve as incidental and dead-end hosts. The cercariae of avian or rodent schistosomal species can penetrate the upper layers of human skin, but are unable to enter the vascular system, and soon die. In contrast, species of schistosomes pathogenic for humans travel through the skin and enter the vascular system, where maturing flukes cause systemic disease (see Chapter 43).

Epidemiology

Cercarial dermatitis occurs worldwide where either fresh or saltwater is heavily contaminated with infected rodent or avian feces. Persons become exposed by swimming or wading in contaminated water. Multiple immersions without prompt towel drying of exposed skin areas increase the risk of infection.

Clinical Features

There are two phases to cercarial dermatitis: transient symptoms, which occur soon after exposure, and delayed symptoms. Cercariae adhere to exposed areas of skin and are believed to penetrate as water evaporates. This is accompanied by a prickling sensation and transient urticarial wheals. These symptoms subside, but a number of hours later pruritic macules, papules, or vesicles develop in the same sites. These lesions reach maximal intensity in 48 to 72 hours and then subside within 1 to 2 weeks. Secondary bacterial infection can occur in excoriated lesions. Subsequent attacks tend to become more severe. Cercarial dermatitis usually spares areas covered by clothing, in contrast to seabather's eruption (see later).

Diagnosis

Diagnosis rests on the history of exposure to contaminated water, as well as the typical clinical findings. No tests are helpful in making a specific diagnosis, and biopsy rarely shows the organism. Differential diagnosis includes insect bites, contact dermatitis, and scabies.

Treatment

Prevention is the most effective therapy. If exposure occurs, immediate rubbing of the skin with a towel after leaving the water contributes to removal of adherent cercariae. Once dermatitis has developed, mild cases can be treated with compresses and topical steroids. Severe cases may require a brief course of systemic steroids. Secondary infection should be treated with appropriate antibiotics.

CNIDARIAN (COELENTERATE) ENVENOMATION

Persons swimming or wading in seawater are at risk for envenomation by cnidarians. Reactions to envenomation are usually mild, but may be serious or fatal.

Etiology

The phylum Cnidaria (formerly Coelenterata) includes more than 9000 invertebrate species that are most abundant in tropical waters. The medically significant coelenterates include (1) Portuguese man-of-war, (2) jellyfish, (3) sea anemones, and (4) stinging corals.

The injuries caused by coelenterates are due to venom-laden organelles called nematocysts. Nematocysts are microscopic spheres containing a coiled filament with a barbed end. With the proper stimulus, the filament springs out of the nematocyst and is embedded in the skin, discharging venom. Dislodged cnidarian tentacles stuck to the skin after contact often contain numerous undischarged nematocysts and are triggered by pressure and freshwater. They can be inactivated with 5% acetic acid, isopropyl alcohol, and proteolytic meat tenderizers. Nematocysts of different species contain a variety of toxins that are responsible for symptoms.

The Portuguese man-of-war, *Physalia physalis,* is perhaps the best known cnidarian to cause symptoms in humans. This large, free-floating species is found in the warmer waters of the Atlantic, has a gas-filled "sail" that may measure 30 cm, and trails nematocyst-covered tentacles that may extend for 30 meters. Stings are common and quite painful, but are usually not fatal.

A closely related species, *Physalia utriculus,* commonly called the bluebottle, is found in the Pacific and causes less painful stings than *P. physalis.* This smaller species rarely exceeds 4 to 5 cm in length.

The sea wasp or box jellyfish, *Chironex fleckeri,* is a jellyfish found mainly in the waters off of northern Australia. *Chironex fleckeri* is responsible for most deaths caused by cnidarians, with as many as 20% of stings being fatal.

Sea nettles, species of *Chrysaora* and *Cyanea,* are jellyfish causing frequent but less serious stings.

Fire corals are stinging members of the genus *Millepora.* They are not true corals, but rather sessile cnidarians.

Seabather's eruption is a form of cnidarian dermatitis thought to be caused by the larvae of the thimble jellyfish, *Linuche unguiculata,* or the sea anemone, *Edwardsiella lineata.*

Nudibranch dermatitis is a form of cnidarian dermatitis caused by contact with either of two species of nudibranch, *Glaucus atlanticus* or *G. glaucilla.* These eat the tentacles and nematocysts of the Portuguese man-of-war and deposit the undigested nematocysts on their own dorsal papillae.

Epidemiology

Persons at risk for cnidarian stings are those in contact with seawater, either through work or recreation. Nematocysts may remain active after washing ashore, so beachcombers may be at risk. All ages are affected, but most severe or fatal reactions occur in children. Sea anemone dermatitis is an occupational disease of sponge divers.

Clinical Features

Cnidarian stings present a wide range of clinical disease, including both cutaneous and systemic features. The severity of a given sting depends on the number of nematocysts discharged into the skin, the nature of the venom, and the sensitivity of the victim. The majority of the cases are mild, but reactions to the venom of certain species, such as *Chironex fleckeri,* may be fatal.

Symptoms begin immediately or soon after contact and include stinging or burning pain, which may be severe. Urticarial reactions are accompanied by pruritus. Cutaneous lesions are urticarial papules, which may become vesicular or hemorrhagic. Lesions occur on exposed skin. The distribution of lesions is often linear, in a "whiplash" pattern, when the sting is caused by *Physalia* species or jellyfish. Systemic reactions include generalized urticaria, muscle spasms, anaphylaxis, and cardiovascular collapse.

Diagnosis

The diagnosis of coelenterate envenomation should be suspected whenever pain or itching begins during contact with seawater. A specific history of activities may help to distinguish between envenomation by free-floating or sessile coelenterates. The pattern of skin lesions may also be helpful in identifying the causative organism, if it was not seen. The tentacles of the Portuguese man-of-war and jellyfish produce a characteristic whiplash appearance. Fragments of tentacles may be adherent to the skin. Different species can be identified by microscopic examination of their nematocysts.

Treatment

Treatment involves prevention of further envenomation by intact nematocysts on the skin, as well as care of the existing reaction. Undischarged nematocysts must be neutralized, and it is crucial to avoid rubbing affected areas or the application of freshwater to affected areas. Application of 5% acetic acid (vinegar) is the treatment of choice, with 40% to 70% isopropyl alcohol, ethanol, aluminum sulfate solution (Stingose), or a solution of proteolytic meat tenderizer powder as alternatives. Tentacles may then be removed by gentle shaving of the area. When these treatments are not available, rinsing affected areas with seawater and gently scraping the skin with the edge of a plastic credit card may be useful. Local reactions are treated with compresses, analgesics, and antihistamines if pruritus is prominent. Some severe cases of cutaneous pain and swelling from allergic reactions may require a short course of systemic corticosteroid therapy. Ulcerated lesions may become secondarily infected and require antibiotics. Urticarial reactions are treated with antihistamines. Anaphylaxis or shock is treated with standard supportive measures. Calcium gluconate or diazepam is sometimes used to control muscle spasms. A specific antivenin is available for stings by *Chironex fleckeri* (Commonwealth Serum Laboratory, Melbourne, Australia).

Prevention

Persons planning significant water exposure in unknown waters, such as scuba divers, should inquire about local hazardous species. Cnidarians found washed ashore should not be handled. Swimmers, divers, and others participating in water activities where risks of cnidarian envenomation exist should wear protective gloves, footwear, and other garments.

REFERENCES

Ectoparasites

Meinking TL: Infestations, *Curr Prob Dermatol* 11:73, 1999.

Cutaneous Larva Migrans

Jelinek T et al: Cutaneous larva migrans in travelers: synopsis of histories, symptoms, and treatment of 98 patients, *Clin Infect Dis* 19:1062, 1994.

Furuncular Myiasis

Arnold HL, Odom RB, James WD: Parasitic infestations, stings, and bites. In Arnold HL, Odom RB, James WD, editors: *Andrew's diseases of the skin: clinical dermatology,* ed 8, Philadelphia, 1990, WB Saunders.

Brewer TF et al: Bacon therapy and furuncular myiasis, *JAMA* 270:2087, 1993.

Elgart ML: Flies and myiasis, *Dermatol Clin* 8:237, 1990.

Kaye HDL, Higgins RP: Human botfly infestation in the United States, *JAMA* 189:64, 1964.

Tumbu Fly Larvae
Oliver PR: Tackling tumbu fly larvae (letter), *Lancet* 2:37, 1985.

Tungiasis
Reiss F: Tungiasis in New York City, *Arch Dermatol* 93:404, 1966.
Wentzell JM, Schwartz BK, Pesce JR: Tungiasis (letter), *J Am Acad Dermatol* 15:117, 1986.

Tick Bite
Sonenshine DE, Azad AF: Ticks and mites in disease transmission. In Strickland GT, editor: *Hunter's tropical medicine,* ed 7, Philadelphia, 1991, WB Saunders.

Cercarial Dermatitis
Fisher AA: *Atlas of aquatic dermatology,* New York, 1978, Grune & Stratton.
Mulvihill CA, Burnett JW: Swimmer's itch: a cercarial dermatitis, *Cutis* 46:211, 1990.

Coelenterate Envenomation
Auerbach PS, Halstead BW: Hazardous aquatic life. In Auerbach PS, Geehr EC, editors: *Management of wilderness and environmental emergencies,* ed 2, St Louis, 1989, Mosby.
Burnett JW, Calton GJ: Jellyfish envenomation syndromes updated, *Ann Emerg Med* 16:1000, 1987.
Fisher AA: *Atlas of aquatic dermatology,* New York, 1978, Grune & Stratton.
Fisher AA: Toxic and allergic reactions to jellyfish with special reference to delayed reactions, *Cutis* 40:303, 1987.

CHAPTER 32

Bacterial Skin Infections

M. Sean Strother and Roy Colven

Bacterial infections of the skin are a major problem in the tropics. Surveys of different populations have yielded estimates of prevalence of 15% to 30% in children and 11% in adults. The high prevalence is attributed to the warm, humid environment and conditions of poverty with crowding and poor hygiene. Secondary bacterial infection is common after insect bites, in traumatic lesions, and in other dermatoses such as contact dermatitis and scabies. Infection with nephritogenic strains of streptococci is more common than in temperate climates. It should be stressed that infections caused by staphylococci and streptococci are much more common in the tropics than are the exotic "tropical diseases."

PYODERMA

Pyoderma refers to a group of superficial bacterial infectious syndromes involving the skin and follicular structures. These include impetigo contagiosa, bullous impetigo, ecthyma, folliculitis, furunculosis, acute paronychia, erysipelas, and cellulitis. These infections are among the most common dermatologic diseases seen in the tropics.

Etiology

Staphylococcus aureus and group A streptococci (GAS) are the usual causative agents of pyoderma. In the past, impetigo contagiosa was thought to be the result of GAS infection; however, it is now clear that many cases result from primary *S. aureus* infection. Similarly with the other pyodermas, GAS or *S. aureus* may be the predominant pathogen for a given clinical presentation, but this is by no means a hard-and-fast rule.

Clinical Features

Impetigo contagiosa, also called impetigo vulgaris, nonbullous impetigo, or simply, impetigo, is an exceedingly common condition seen primarily in children. Invasion of the skin by pathogenic *S. aureus* or GAS often follows minor trauma. An isolated, erythematous papule or pustule accounts for the initial lesion, which often goes undetected by the patient. The primary lesion rapidly gives rise to a distinctive amber- or "honey"-crusted erosion with or without an erythematous border. Pruritus may accompany the lesions, and regional lymphadenopathy is common in protracted cases. The condition most commonly affects the central face around the nares and lips, but can occur anywhere.

Bullous impetigo is a superficial blistering condition caused by the elaboration of an exfoliatoxin produced by phage group II *S. aureus.* Children are most frequently affected and approximately 50% of patients show positive nasal and/or throat cultures for the toxin-producing *S. aureus.* Bullous impetigo presents as flaccid, well-demarcated bullae without surrounding erythema that arise rapidly from vesicles, often in intertriginous areas. The bullae rupture spontaneously in 1 or 2 days, leaving a shallow erosion covered by a light brown, varnishlike crust.

Impetiginization is a term used when *S. aureus* or GAS secondarily infects skin that has been compromised by a preexisting dermatosis. Atopic dermatitis, contact dermatitis, insect bites, dermatophyte infection, and infestations with mites or lice are frequent precursors. Lesions present as focal or widespread papules or plaques with honey-colored crusts. Close observation at the periphery may reveal the primary lesions of the underlying dermatosis.

Folliculitis is an infection of the hair follicle most often caused by *S. aureus.* Superficial folliculitis presents as follicle-based 1- to 2-mm pustules on an erythematous base, often with a central protruding hair shaft. The most frequent areas involved are the scalp, thighs, buttocks, axillae, and, in men, the beard area. Sycosis barbae is a more deeply seated folliculitis with significant perifollicular inflammation in the beard area of men.

Furunculosis refers to isolated or multiple deep-seated, cutaneous infections centered on hair follicles, which often arise by extension of a more superficial folliculitis. They occur most often in areas of friction and/or perspiration such as the axillae and buttocks. They present as painful, erythematous papules or nodules, with or without an obvious central follicular ostium. After several days, the lesion may come to a point and drain purulent material. A carbuncle refers to an indurated plaquelike mass of communicating furuncles. Both furuncles and carbuncles are often referred to by patients as “boils.”

Ecthyma is often a deeper extension of untreated impetigo or folliculitis that presents as 5- to 15-mm punched-out erosions with elevated, erythematous borders. A densely adherent, thick serum crust overlies each lesion giving a characteristic appearance. Regional lymphadenopathy is frequently observed. In untreated cases, new lesions that often start as isolated erythematous papules or vesicles may appear for months. Lesions are most common on the buttocks and legs, but can occur anywhere.

Acute paronychia is a suppurative infection of the proximal and lateral nail folds. It often follows a break in the skin resulting from minor trauma, and those exposed to recurrent hand trauma or chronic exposure to moisture are at highest risk. *S. aureus* is the most common pathogen in acute paronychia, but other organisms such as streptococci must be considered. The presentation is that of an exquisitely tender, hot, erythematous nail fold, with or without frank abscess formation.

Erysipelas is an infection of the skin and superficial lymphatic channels usually due to GAS. It classically presents as a well demarcated, brightly erythematous, hot, tender indurated plaque on the face or lower extremities. The pathogenic organisms gain entry into the skin via minor trauma or preexisting dermatitis. Cellulitis may result from untreated erysipelas, but usually arises *de novo,* and is an infection of the deeper cutaneous and subcutaneous tissues above the superficial fascial planes. Cellulitis differs from erysipelas clinically by having indistinct borders and less pronounced brawny edema. It should be noted that some authors do not differentiate between these two entities, and some cases defy clinical separation.

Diagnosis

Diagnosis of the various pyodermas is usually made primarily on clinical findings, and cultures are often unnecessary. Impetigo contagiosa may be difficult to differentiate from an exudative dermatitis, which may also have a crust. Bullous impetigo should be distinguished from other blistering disorders, such as bullous arthropod bites, pemphigus vulgaris, bullous pemphigoid, acute vesicular dermatitis, erythema multiforme, and bullous drug reactions. Folliculitis, although most often caused by gram-positive cocci, has many causes including chemical irritants, yeasts (*Candida* and *Malassezia*), gram-negative bacteria (*Pseudomonas* spp., so-called "hot tub folliculitis"), dermatophytes, herpes simplex virus, pseudofolliculitis barbae, and various drug eruptions. Hidradenitis suppurativa should be considered if furuncular lesions are localized to the axillae, groins, and intergluteal cleft. Furuncular myiasis (see Chapter 31) must be considered in anyone presenting with furunculosis after travel to an endemic area. On the lower extremities, cellulitis may be difficult to differentiate from the inflammation associated with venous stasis dermatitis, although cellulitis is rarely bilateral and symmetric.

Treatment

Systemic therapy with one of the penicillinase-resistant penicillins (cloxacillin, dicloxacillin, nafcillin, oxacillin, or amoxicillin plus clavulinate [Augmentin]) is the treatment of choice for most pyodermas. The usual course of therapy is 10 to 14 days or until signs of active infection have abated. Alternatives to penicillins include first-generation cephalosporins, clindamycin, and levofloxin. Compresses can be used if significant crusting or exudate is present. Hot compresses help to bring furuncle to a point and facilitate drainage. Any areas of localized fluctuance should be incised and drained. In cases of secondary impetiginization, the underlying disorder should be treated in conjunction with the antibiotic therapy. Mupirocin topical ointment or cream applied three times a day to infected skin areas is an effective treatment for impetigo (if not extensive), folliculitis, and infected eczema.

Prevention

Recurrent pyoderma caused by staphylococcal infection is often related to asymptomatic carriage of *S. aureus,* most commonly in the nose, but also the perineum and toe web spaces. Nasal carriage of staphylococci has a prevalence of up to 30% in the general population and should be confirmed by nasal swab sent for bacterial culture. Treatment of nasal carriage can decrease the risk of recurrent staphylococcal skin infections. Mupirocin ointment or cream applied in the anterior nares twice a day for 10 days helps to eliminate nasal staphylococcal carriage. When used regularly twice a day for 5 consecutive days each month, decreased staphylococcal skin infections have been documented.

PYOMYOSITIS

Pyomyositis, also called tropical pyomyositis, is a bacterial infection of skeletal muscle.

Etiology

Pyomyositis is caused by *S. aureus* in 85% to 90% of cases, streptococci in 10% of cases, and anaerobes and *Mycobacterium tuberculosis* in a small percentage of cases. The pathogenesis of pyomyositis is not well understood. Most cases are associated with superficial skin infection, and bacterial seeding may occur from the skin, although bacteremia or other metastatic foci of infection are not usually present. Intact, healthy skeletal muscle is quite resistant to bacterial infection; and it has been proposed that blunt trauma, ischemia, parasitic infection, or viral infection of muscles may be a contributory factor.

Epidemiology

Pyomyositis is relatively common in tropical areas of Africa, Asia, South America, and the Caribbean and Pacific islands, but is rare in temperate climates. Most patients are otherwise healthy but have a high frequency of concomitant pyoderma. In the tropics, most cases occur in young adults, but individuals of any age may be affected. In temperate climates, most reported cases are in children. Males are affected twice as frequently as females.

Clinical Features

The characteristic features of pyomyositis are pain and tenderness of the involved muscle, fever, and leukocytosis. Symptoms usually develop rapidly over a few days but may follow an indolent course over weeks. The most frequently affected muscles include those of the thigh, calf, deltoid, buttocks, iliopsoas, pectoral, and latissimus dorsi. Multiple muscle involvement occurs in a minority of tropical cases. Physical findings include fever and swelling and tenderness of the involved muscle, with a characteristic hard "woody" induration. Overlying erythema may be minimal. Later lesions may be fluctuant or may drain spontaneously through the skin.

Diagnosis

Differential diagnosis includes muscle hematoma, thrombophlebitis, neoplasm, and sickle cell crisis. Iliopsoas pyomyositis may mimic appendicitis. Diagnosis is made by recovery of pus from the affected muscle by needle aspiration (often guided by computed tomography [CT]) or surgical exploration. Various imaging modalities are useful in making the diagnosis including magnetic resonance imaging, CT, ultrasound, and tagged white blood cell scans.

Treatment

Treatment of pyomyositis involves surgical drainage and systemic antibiotics, although early cases may respond to antibiotics alone. Antibiotic therapy should be guided by cultures. Pending results, empirical therapy should be directed to cover *S. aureus.*

BURULI ULCER

Buruli ulcer, named after a district in Uganda where some of the earliest case reports occurred, is an ulcerating cutaneous infection caused by *Mycobacterium ulcerans.* It is the only extracellular mycobacterium pathogen in humans and is thought to produce one or more cytotoxic and immunosuppressive agents leading to its clinical presentation. Buruli ulcer is the third most prevalent human mycobacterial disease worldwide, behind tuberculosis and leprosy, and by some accounts its impact on human health will soon surpass that of leprosy.

Epidemiology

Buruli ulcer occurs in tropical, swampy environments near fresh and saltwater. It was initially described in Australia, with additional reports from Central and West Africa. At present, the disease is documented from most of sub-Saharan Africa, India, southern Asia, Papua New Guinea, Mexico, French Guiana, Peru, Bolivia, and Surinam. Cases acquired by travelers have been reported from the United States, Japan, Belgium, and Northern Ireland. Disease rates in some endemic populations range as high as 16% to 22%. Direct contact with contaminated soil or water appears to be the only mode of transmission, although *M. ulcerans* has never been isolated from these sources in endemic areas. No reservoir is known, but there is a single report of finding the organism in koalas. Children are most often affected; with an age span of infected persons ranging from 4 to 22 years. Evidence fails to suggest that disease prevalence or severity is different for immunodeficient patients.

Clinical Features

Early lesions of Buruli ulcer present as a firm, nontender, mobile subcutaneous nodule, usually on extremity after local trauma. Pruritus often accompanies this early lesion, as evidenced by the local term, *mputa matadi* (itching stone). In 1 or 2 months, most lesions progress to form large, indolent ulcers with indurated, undermined borders and substantial fat necrosis. Infection rarely involves soft tissues below the myofacial plane and fatalities are exceedingly rare. Ulcers heal spontaneously after months or years with significant scarring, contractures, and limb deformities. Signs of systemic illness and regional lymphadenopathy are conspicuously absent.

Diagnosis

The acid-fast bacilli may be demonstrated by Ziehl-Neelsen staining of swabs or biopsies from the undermined ulcer border. Cultures from swabbed or biopsied specimens can be grown on Löwenstein-Jensen medium kept at 33° C. Cultures may take as long as 8 weeks to turn positive.

Differential diagnosis includes, tropical ulcer (see later), tuberculous ulcers, leishmaniasis, deep fungal infections (see Chapter 33) and other noninfectious ulcerating conditions, such as pyoderma gangrenosum, venous hypertension, and arterial insufficiency.

Treatment

Early lesions may be treated by excision and grafting. Medical treatment of this condition with various drugs (rifampin, clofazimine, dapsone, and trimethoprim-sulfamethoxazole) and physical modalities (hyperbaric oxygen and hyperthermic therapy) has shown only limited success. Dramatic success in three cases treated with topical phenytoin has been recently reported, but controlled studies are not yet available. Reconstructive surgery may be required to preserve extremity function.

TROPICAL ULCER

Tropical ulcer, also called tropical phagedenic ulcer and Malabar ulcer, is a condition in which large, painful ulcers form rapidly on areas of skin prone to trauma. The etiology of this condition is unclear, but the most recent literature attributes it to polymicrobial infection with various anaerobes (*Fusobacterium* spp) and spirochetes. It is likely that several different etiologic processes give rise to clinically similar ulcerating diseases of tropical origin that have been lumped under this term.

Epidemiology

Tropical ulcer occurs commonly in most hot, humid tropical regions of the world. Previously, poor nutritional status of the host was felt to play a role in acquiring the disease, but recent evidence has failed to support this notion. Children into the teen years are most often affected. Some evidence suggests that exposure to mud or stagnant/slow-moving freshwater is a risk factor. A history of local trauma, often minor, precedes most cases.

Clinical Features

Lesions are most common on the lower extremities, but can occur anywhere. They begin as erythematous papules or hemorrhagic bullae. The initial lesion then rapidly breaks down to form a large, well-demarcated, cup-shaped ulcer, often with an indurated, undermined border. The ulcer is painful, foul smelling, and has a grayish fibrinous base. Ulcers may be deep enough to involve periosteum of underlying bone. Patients are usually febrile and systemically ill, but regional lymphadenopathy is rare. Ulcers are chronic, heal with significant scarring, and often lead to structural and functional disability of the affected site.

Diagnosis

This is a diagnosis of exclusion and other ulcerative conditions, such as tuberculous ulcer, leishmaniasis, venous stasis ulcer, pyoderma gangrenosum, Buruli ulcer, streptococcal ecthyma, and even carcinoma may need to be excluded. Biopsy of the ulcer margin may help rule out other diseases. Culture is not diagnostic, but may exclude other etiologies.

Treatment

As would be expected for a disease of uncertain etiology, many issues of therapy are unresolved. Proper nutrition has been stressed as important. Local care for the ulcer includes rest, elevations, and local wound care with appropriate bandages or compresses. Antibiotics, most frequently penicillin, metronidazole, or tetracycline, are administered until healing occurs. Reconstructive surgery may be required and early grafting may play a role.

REFERENCES

Bacterial Infections

Lee PK, Weinberg AN, Swartz MN, Johnson RA: Pyodermas: *Staphylococcus aureus, Streptococcus,* and other gram-positive bacteria. In Freedberg IM et al, editors: *Fitzpatrick's dermatology in general medicine,* ed 5, New York, 1999, McGraw-Hill.

Pyomyositis

Sissolak D, Weir WR: Tropical pyomyositis, *J Infect Dis* 29:121, 1994.

Buruli Ulcer

Adjei O, Evans MRW, Asiedu A: Phenytoin in the treatment of Buruli ulcer, *Trans R Soc Trop Med Hyg* 92(1):108, 1998.

Dobos KM et al: Emergence of a unique group of necrotizing mycobacterial diseases, *Emerg Infect Dis* 5(3):367, 1999.

Gawkrodger DJ: Mycobacterial infections. In Champion RH, Burton JL, Burns DA, Breathnach SM, editors: *Textbook of dermatology,* ed 6, vol 2, London, 1998, Blackwell Science Ltd.

Tropical Ulcer

Robinson DC et al: The clinical and epidemiologic features of tropical ulcer (tropical phagedenic ulcer), *Int J Dermatol* 27:49, 1988.

Hay RJ, Adriaans BM: Bacterial infections. In Champion RH, Burton JL, Burns DA, Breathnach SM, editors: *Textbook of dermatology,* ed 6, vol 2, London, 1998, Blackwell Science Ltd.

CHAPTER 33

Superficial and Deep Fungal Skin Infections

M. Sean Strother and Roy Colven

The often hot and humid climates of tropical areas predispose residents and travelers to a variety of superficial fungal infections of the skin. These may differ in pattern and intensity of symptoms from similar infections in temperate climates. In addition, repetitive exposure to endemic fungal pathogens through direct skin contact with soil, lumber, and plant products among agricultural workers in tropical countries can result in deep fungal infections of the skin and subcutaneous tissues. These infections occur less frequently in temperate climates, where workers are more likely to wear shoes, gloves, and protective clothing.

Fungal infections, also called mycoses, can be organized into the following groups: (1) superficial cutaneous mycoses, (2) deep cutaneous and subcutaneous mycoses, and (3) systemic mycoses. The systemic mycoses can be further subdivided into *endemic respiratory mycoses* in immunologically intact hosts (e.g., histoplasmosis, coccidiomycosis, blastomycosis, paracoccidiomycosis) and *opportunistic mycoses* in immunocompromised hosts (e.g., aspergillosis, mucormycosis, disseminated candidiasis, cryptococcosis). The systemic mycoses are beyond the scope of this chapter and are not discussed.

SUPERFICIAL CUTANEOUS MYCOSES

Superficial cutaneous mycoses result from infection by various fungi in the keratinized cutaneous structures, namely the stratum corneum, hair shaft and follicle, or nails. Immune response of the host to this invasion is variable and depends on the species of organism involved and host immune status. The following superficial mycoses are discussed in this chapter: (1) dermatophytoses, including onychomycosis, (2) conditions caused by *Malassezia furfur (Pityrosporum ovale),* (3) cutaneous candidiasis, (4) tinea nigra, and (5) piedra.

Dermatophyte Infections (Dermatophytoses)

Dermatophyte infections are due to fungal species in three genera, *Trichophyton, Microsporum,* and *Epidermophyton.* Worldwide, *T. rubrum* is the most common cause of dermatophyte infection. Each clinical syndrome described here can be caused by several fungi, except where noted. Sources of dermatophyte infection include soil and animal reservoirs, or other humans, depending on species.

Dermatophyte infections affect skin, hair, and nails. The living epidermis is not invaded. Both nonimmunologic mechanisms and cell-mediated immunity appears to be important determinants of susceptibility to infection. Delayed-type hypersensitivity, which develops after initial exposure, confers immunity in most individuals. A subset of the population, sometimes with other evidence of immune defects, is chronically infected with dermatophytes.

Epidemiology

The epidemiology of dermatophyte infection is different for each clinical syndrome and geographic area. For example, tinea pedis and nail infections are uncommon before puberty, whereas tinea capitis is primarily a disease of childhood. In temperate climates, intertriginous infections and tinea pedis predominate. In the tropics, tinea corporis and scalp infections are more common. Dermatophyte infections are enhanced by a tropical climate, and travelers typically note an exacerbation of preexisting infection. If this prior infection was asymptomatic, they may assume they acquired the infection in the tropics.

Clinical Features

Tinea capitis is mainly a disease of children, characterized by focal scaling and hair loss. Single, multiple, or generalized lesions of the scalp may occur. Occasionally, the eyelashes, eyelids, and glabrous skin may become involved. Varying degrees of inflammation may be present. When suppurative swelling of the scalp occurs, it is called a kerion, and systemic symptoms such as fever, pain, and adenopathy may develop. Kerion formation may eventually result in scarring and permanent alopecia. An "id" reaction may occur and result in widespread vesicular, papulosquamous, or pustular skin lesions. This represents a noninfective cutaneous host response to inflammatory dermatophyte infection at a separate site. Causative organisms of tinea capitis include virtually any *Trichophyton* or *Microsporum* species, but *T. tonsurans, M. audouinii,* and *M. canis* are most common. Infections caused by *M. audouinii* and *M. canis* fluoresce green under the Wood's light. Differential diagnosis includes psoriasis and seborrheic dermatitis.

Tinea corporis, or "ringworm," is a condition affecting all ages and is characterized by annular, flat plaques, with erythema and scale most prominent at the advancing border. Lesions spread centrifugally with central clearing may be multiple, and vary in size from a few millimeters to many centimeters. Pruritus is variable. The more common causative organisms include *T. rubrum, T. mentagrophytes,* and *M. canis.* Differential diagnosis includes psoriasis, nummular eczema, pityriasis rosea, and secondary syphilis. Occasionally, leprosy may resemble tinea corporis.

Favus is an uncommon variant of tinea capitis, caused by *T. schoenleinii.* It is characterized by scarring hair loss and dense, cup-shaped, yellow scales known as scutula. Wood's lamp examination induces pale green fluorescence.

Tinea cruris, or "jock itch," is mainly a disease of adult males in temperate climates and is often accompanied by tinea pedis. The rash involves the crural folds and inner thighs and may extend posteriorly to the gluteal crease. The penis and scrotum are not involved. There is mild erythema, with a well-demarcated scaly border. Causative organisms include *Epidermophyton floccosum, T. rubrum,* and *T. mentagrophytes.* Differential diagnosis includes seborrheic dermatitis, erythrasma, intertrigo, candidiasis, and psoriasis.

Tinea pedis, or "athlete's foot," is most common in temperate climates and is uncommon before puberty. Clinical variants of tinea pedis include maceration and scale of the interdigital spaces, vesicular inflammation of the plantar surface, and mild diffuse erythema and scale of the foot in a moccasin distribution. Tinea pedis typically worsens in a warm climate. Causative organisms are the same as those seen in tinea cruris. Differential diagnosis includes erythrasma, contact dermatitis, and psoriasis.

Onychomycosis, or dermatophyte infection of the nail, is less common in the tropics. Nail plate thickening, dystrophy, and subungual debris of one or several nails characterize this condition. Toenails are affected much more often than fingernails. Many organisms may cause onychomycosis, but most common are species of *Trichophyton* and *Epidermophyton.* Differential diagnosis includes psoriasis, lichen planus, candidiasis, and hereditary nail dystrophies.

A common and curious variant of tinea pedis is one hand, two foot involvement. Asymmetric scale and erythema of one hand, perhaps with nail involvement, should prompt the practitioner to inspect the feet and perform a potassium hydroxide (KOH) examination.

Diagnosis

In all forms of dermatophyte infection, diagnosis rests on demonstrating the fungus in microscopic examination of scrapings or by culture. KOH examination is a simple, rapid diagnostic tool. Scrapings should be taken from the active border of lesions, subungual debris in onychomycosis, or hair in tinea capitis. The sample should be placed on a slide, covered with a few drops of 10% to 20% KOH and a coverslip. The slide is then heated briefly to speed lysis and clearing of keratinocytes revealing the KOH-resistant fungal structures. The specimen is examined for hyphae using the 10× objective with the condenser lowered. A positive KOH examination of skin generally represents true infection by dermatophyte. In dystrophic nails, nonpathogenic molds can be present and indistinguishable from dermatophyte on KOH examination. For this reason, fungal culture is generally recommended to confirm onychomycosis. Culture of scrapings takes 2 to 6 weeks to become positive for dermatophyte.

Treatment

Topical Therapy

Topical therapy is usually adequate for tinea pedis, tinea cruris, and limited forms of tinea corporis. Topical agents include azoles (clotrimazole, miconazole, ketoconazole, and econazole), the allylamine terbinafine, and other agents (ciclopirox, naftifine, and tolnaftate). These agents are usually applied as creams twice daily until clearing occurs and 2 weeks longer to minimize recurrence.

Systemic Therapy

For tinea capitis, griseofulvin has been the drug of choice for the last 40 years. It is given in single or divided doses, 500 to 1000 mg/day of the ultramicrosized form, or 10 to 15 mg/kg/day in children. Duration of therapy is usually 6 to 12 weeks. Side effects include headache and nausea.

More recently the newer antifungals terbinafine, itraconazole, and fluconazole have been shown to be efficacious and safe alternatives to griseofulvin, with fewer side effects and shorter courses of therapy. Optimal treatment doses for these agents have yet to be determined, but the following regimens have been used effectively:

1. Terbinafine: patient weight >40 kg, 250 mg/day for 2 to 4 weeks; patient weight 20 to 40 kg, 125 mg/day and <20 kg, 62.5 mg/day, for 2 to 4 weeks
2. Itraconazole: 3-5 mg/kg/day for 4 weeks or pulse dosing of 5 mg/kg/day for 1 week followed by 1 to 3 pulses given 3 weeks apart

Duration of therapy with these agents may need to be increased if *M. canis* is involved. Adjunctive use of antifungal shampoos (selenium sulfide or ketoconazole) will help shorten the time to obtain negative cultures and may help prevent spread of infection to others.

Systemic therapy is also indicated for recalcitrant or widespread tinea corporis, cruris, and pedis. The following regimens (adult doses) have been used:

1. Terbinafine: 250 mg daily for 2 weeks
2. Fluconazole: 50 to 100 mg daily or 150 mg once a week for 2 to 3 weeks
3. Itraconazole: 100 mg daily for 2 weeks or 200 mg daily for 7 days
4. Ketoconazole: 200 mg daily for 4 weeks

Onychomycosis is treated systemically. The following regimens have been used successfully:

1. Terbinafine: patient weight >40 kg, 250 mg/day for 2 to 4 weeks; patient weight 20 to 40 kg, 125 mg/day and <20 kg, 62.5 mg/day, for 3 months for toenails (2 months fingernails)
2. Itraconazole 200 mg orally twice a day for 7 days/month for 3 months for toenails (2 pulses fingernails) or 200 mg orally daily for 3 months
3. Fluconazole 150 to 300 mg orally weekly for 6 to 12 months for toenails (3 to 6 months for fingernails)

When used systemically the azole antifungals (ketoconazole, itraconazole, and fluconazole) can have significant and drug interactions. Specific drug interaction profiles vary for each of these antifungals, and the product insert or the *Physicians Desk Reference* should be consulted before prescribing these agents to a patient who is taking other medications, including over-the-counter products.

Adjunctive Therapy

Vesicular, exudative, or very pruritic infections should be treated with compresses. Antibiotics may be indicated if evidence of secondary bacterial infection is present. Prednisone, 1 mg/kg for 2 to 3 weeks, is helpful for limiting scarring from kerion and does not affect antifungal therapy.

Conditions Caused by *Malassezia*

Malassezia furfur (*Pityrosporum ovale* or *P. orbiculare*) is a lipophilic yeast that is part of the normal human cutaneous fauna. It is believed to play a pathogenic role in several dermatologic conditions, including seborrheic dermatitis, tinea (pityriasis) versicolor, and *Malassezia* (*Pityrosporum*) folliculitis. The latter two conditions are discussed here.

Tinea Versicolor

Tinea versicolor, or pityriasis versicolor, is a common, usually asymptomatic superficial fungal infection that is most prevalent in the tropics. Under conditions of warmth, increased moisture, and complex changes in skin fatty acids, the yeast transform to the hyphal form responsible for clinical disease.

Epidemiology

It is primarily a condition of adolescents and young adults, although those of any age may be affected. Predisposing factors include hot humid conditions, pregnancy, corticosteroid therapy, and Cushing's disease. In some tropical populations, prevalence may exceed 50% among young adults. Infection is believed to reflect changes in host flora, and therefore person-to-person transmission is not thought to occur. Travelers to the tropics may experience their first episode of tinea versicolor and may assume that the condition was acquired in the tropics.

Clinical Features

The lesions of tinea versicolor are round or oval macules that coalesce into larger patches. They have a fine scale that sometimes is only evident when the lesion is scraped during the physical examination. In untanned Caucasians lesions may be subtly red-brown and go unnoticed. With ultraviolet exposure the lesions tend not to darken, giving a more striking hypopigmented spotted appearance during and after tropical travel. In more darkly pigmented patients, the lesions are slightly hypopigmented. Lesions are typically distributed over the shoulders, chest, and back, and occasionally on the neck. An inverse (intertriginous) distribution occurs uncommonly. Facial and penile involvement is rare, occurring primarily in infants or the immunocompromised. Pruritus is usually absent.

Diagnosis

In tinea versicolor, the clinical presentation is often sufficient to make the diagnosis. A KOH examination of scale scraped from lesions invariably shows the organisms and confirms the clinical suspicion. They are seen as short, curved hyphae and spherical yeast, giving a characteristic "spaghetti and meatballs" appearance. Biopsy is unnecessary but also shows organisms in the stratum corneum.

The ease of confirming the diagnosis makes differential diagnosis less important. However, the appearance of hypopigmented lesions in the tropics may raise concerns of Hansen's disease (Chapter 35), in which hypopigmented lesions are anesthetic, or vitiligo, where a Wood's lamp examination often reveals fluorescence owing to depigmentation of lesional skin.

Treatment

Topical

Many topical medications are effective in treating tinea versicolor, but recurrence is common (as high as 60% at 1 year and 80% at 2 years after treatment). Even after successful treatment, pigmentation often takes several months to return to normal. The following topical regimens have been used successfully:

1. *Zinc pyrithione shampoo:* applied to affected areas for 5 to 10 minutes, then rinsed off. Repeated daily for 1 week, then once weekly for a month, then once a month thereafter to prevent recurrences.
2. Various azole antifungal creams including *ketoconazole, miconazole, econazole, bifonazole,* and *clotrimazole:* twice daily for 2 weeks.
3. *Terbinafine:* 1% cream applied once daily for 4 weeks or as a 1% spray solution applied twice daily for 1 week.
4. *Fifty percent propylene glycol in water:* twice daily to affected areas for 2 weeks. This acts as a keratolytic agent.

Patient compliance is a common problem with these topical treatment regimens.

Systemic

Systemic therapy is indicated in recalcitrant cases or in cases with widespread involvement that makes topical therapy impractical. Three oral antifungal agents are effective against *Malassezia.*

1. Ketoconazole: single 400 mg dose
2. Itraconazole: 400 mg daily for 3 to 7 days.
3. Fluconazole: single 400 mg dose. Repeating the dose a week later may increase effectiveness.

Given the high recurrence rate with both topical and systemic therapy, continued prophylaxis is imperative. This can be achieved either with routine intermittent use of the topical agents listed above or with ketoconazole 200 mg daily for 3 consecutive days each month.

Malasseiza (Pityrosporum) Folliculitis

Malassezia folliculitis is a pruritic, follicular eruption caused by *M. furfur.* It often develops in warm, humid climates on areas of skin covered by occlusive clothing. Histopathology of this condition shows prominent follicular dilation and inflammation owing to increased colonization with the yeast forms of *M. furfur.*

Epidemiology

Malassezia folliculitis mainly affects young adults from the postpubertal teens to the mid-30s, although it has been reported in children and the elderly. In temperate climates, *Malassezia* folliculitis is reported to have a female predominance. In the tropics the patient sex ratio appears to be closer to 50:50. Predisposing factors include immunosuppression, corticosteroid therapy, diabetes, antibiotic therapy, and occlusion.

Clinical Features

In temperate climates *Malassezia* folliculitis classically presents as monomorphic, pruritic, follicular papules, and pustules distributed about the chest, upper back, and shoulders. In the tropics, the lesions may look like those of molluscum contagiosum, with a central umbilication. Facial lesions, especially in females in the tropics, are also described.

Diagnosis

Diagnosis is best made by demonstrating the yeast in the follicular plug from one of the papules by direct microscopy using either 10% KOH/Parker blue ink (50:50 mixture) or Gram stain. Serial sections of punch biopsies stained for fungi will also reveal numerous yeast forms in dilated follicles, but this is rarely necessary.

The differential diagnosis includes other folliculitides, namely bacterial (staphylococcal) and candidal, and acne vulgaris. Gram stain of an unroofed pustule helps to differentiate *Malassezia* folliculitis from other folliculitides. Acne often coexists with *Malassezia* folliculitis, but uncomplicated acne vulgaris rarely has the prominent pruritus associated the latter.

Treatment

Patients often respond dramatically to therapy, although recurrence rates are high. Many topical regimens have been used and there is no consensus on the best regimen. Adjunctive oral therapy is usually reserved for widespread cases or cases unresponsive to topical therapy. Some studies suggest that oral therapy alone is not as effective as topical therapy alone or in conjunction with oral agents. Regardless of the regimen chosen for initial treatment twice weekly prophylactic topical therapy with one of the agents listed here is usually required for sustained remission. The following regimens have been used successfully:

1. *Fifty percent propylene glycol in water:* applied to the affected areas with a gauze pad twice daily for 3 weeks.
2. *Econazole:* 1% cream applied every night for 1 week.
3. *Selenium sulfide 2.5% shampoo:* applied for 30 minutes followed by a shower for 3 consecutive days.
4. *Ketoconazole:* 2% shampoo applied to affected areas daily in combination with 200 mg orally daily for 4 weeks.

Cutaneous Candidiasis

The dimorphic fungus *Candida albicans* is a normal saprophyte of mucosal surfaces in humans. Under certain conditions and given various predisposing host factors, *C. albicans* and other less common species of *Candida* become pathogenic giving rise to several distinct clinical diseases. In addition to mucosal infections, candidiasis can occur as a cutaneous-only infection and as a systemic infection with cutaneous findings. Mucosal and cutaneous candidiasis are discussed here.

Epidemiology

The various clinical presentations of cutaneous candidiasis are quite common with the greatest prevalence in newborns and elderly persons. Numerous predisposing host factors exist and these can be broadly categorized into three groups:

1. Impaired barrier function: wounds, burns, maceration, occlusion, foreign bodies (e.g., dentures, catheters), and alterations in beneficial cutaneous flora secondary to antibiotics.
2. Altered immune states: acquired immunodeficiency syndrome, post-organ transplant immunosuppression, neutropenia/leukopenia, and various other acquired and congenital immunodeficiency disorders.
3. Others: malnutrition (including specific vitamin and mineral deficiencies), pregnancy/oral contraceptives, endocrinopathies (e.g., diabetes mellitus, hypothyroidism, hypoparathyroidism), malignancy (leukemia, lymphoma, and thymoma), and drugs (corticosteroids, antibiotics, immunosuppressive agents, cytotoxic agents, and antimetabolites).

In tropical climates increased temperature and humidity coupled with occlusive clothing predispose travelers to cutaneous candidal infections.

Clinical Features

Oral candidiasis most often presents as acute pseudomembranous candidiasis, or "thrush," with white to gray, curdlike pseudomembranes overlying a shiny, brightly erythematous painful mucosal surface on the buccal mucosa, palate, tongue or gingivae. Differential diagnosis includes leukoplakia in which the white mucosal plaques cannot be dislodged and retained food particles that lack the underlying tenderness and erythema, as well as fungal elements on KOH examination.

Less common oral presentations include the following:

- *Acute atrophic glossitis:* tender, shiny erythema of the dorsal surface of the tongue with loss of the normal papillae, seen most commonly in the setting of antibiotic or corticosteroid use.
- *Angular cheilitis (perlèche):* painful fissuring and erythema at the commissures of the lips, often associated with poorly fitted dentures.

Candidal vulvovaginitis occurs commonly in women and presents as a thick white vaginal discharge, often with associated pruritus, burning, and dysuria. The skin of the vulva often shows bright confluent erythema with scale and satellite papules and pustules. Speculum examination of the vaginal vault reveals brightly erythematous patches of vaginal mucosa with a "cottage cheese-like" vaginal discharge. Vulvovaginal involvement may extend to involve the perineum and crural folds resulting in candidal intertrigo. *Candidal balanitis* usually occurs in uncircumcised men as confluent areas of moist, bright erythema with slight scale on the glans and prepuce. Candidal balanitis may spread to involve the scrotum and crural folds.

Candidal intertrigo is a common condition occurring in closely apposed skinfolds where there is a microenvironment of increased heat, humidity, and friction. Bright red, moist erythematous patches, usually with slight peripheral scale and satellite papules and pustules, occur symmetrically in the skinfolds of the axillae, inframammary area, beneath the abdominal pannus, intergluteal fold, or crural folds. In infants the skinfolds of the anterior neck can be involved. Obesity, occlusion of the skin, and diabetes mellitus are common predisposing factors. Differential diagnosis includes psoriasis and seborrheic dermatitis, which should have findings consistent with these diagnoses in other areas. Tinea infection can involve the crural folds and would be distinguished by long, septated hyphal elements without yeast forms on KOH examination. Erythrasma, a bacterial infection caused by *Corynebacterium minutissimum,* has dull, red-brown, well demarcated patches with fine scale; lacks satellite lesions and fungal elements on KOH scrapings; and shows a characteristic coral red fluorescence on Wood's lamp examination.

Chronic paronychia is inflammation of the nail folds associated with colonization or infection by *Candida* that occurs in those whose hands are frequently immersed in water such as custodial workers, fishermen, and cooks. It presents as tender, erythematous, swollen nail folds with prominent retraction of the cuticle at the proximal nail fold. Pus or serosanguineous fluid may be expressible from the nail folds and associated nail plate changes can be seen. Concomitant bacterial infection often occurs and complicates diagnosis.

Diagnosis

Diagnosis can often be made clinically, but KOH examination of scrapings from mucosa or skin shows characteristic budding yeast cells and pseudohyphae. Culture is rarely necessary.

Treatment

All uncomplicated cutaneous candidiases respond well to most topical agents including nystatin and azole antifungals. These agents come in various forms including solutions, lotions, creams, powders, tablets, and troches. Creams and powders work well for intertrigo, and measures to reduce occlusion and friction help prevent recurrence. Tablets and troches are best suited for oral candidiasis. Although topical agents work quite well for vulvovaginal candidiasis, some physicians commonly prescribe fluconazole as a 150-mg, one-time oral dose for patient convenience. In cases of chronic paronychia, solutions and lotions probably work better than creams, and topical drying agents such as sulfacetamide or 4% thymol in chloroform are often added. In addition general measures of reduced exposure to water immersion and adequate hand drying are helpful.

It is important to search for and treat any underlying illness. The presence of oral thrush in an otherwise healthy individual should prompt an investigation of HIV risk factors and appropriate testing when indicated.

Tinea Nigra

Tinea nigra is an uncommon superficial mycosis caused most often by the melanin-producing fungus *Phaeoannellomyces werneckii* (numerous taxonomic synonyms include *Exophiala werneckii, Cladosporium werneckii, Hortae werneckii,* and many others). Some evidence suggests that other pigmented fungi may produce a similar clinical picture. The fungi live in soil, sewage, decaying vegetation, and have also been found on shower stalls in humid environments.

Epidemiology

Tinea nigra is a rare condition mainly reported in Central and South America, although cases have been identified in the Southern United States, Africa, and Southeast Asia. Inoculating the organism into the skin with minor trauma has produced experimental infections, and this is believed to be the probable mechanism for natural infection. Lesions slowly develop over years and have been observed in travelers to endemic areas.

Clinical Features

The typical lesion is an asymptomatic, nonscaly, hyperpigmented macule or patch of the palmar or plantar skin. The lesions resemble junctional nevi or melanoma, and biopsy may need to be done before the proper diagnosis is made. The pigment may be partly removed by shaving off the horny layer of the skin.

Diagnosis

KOH preparation of skin scrapings reveals hyphae. If biopsy is done, the organisms are also visible in the stratum corneum.

Treatment

Peeling away the horny layer with salicylic acid plasters or Whitfield's ointment gives good results, although recurrences are seen. Topical use of the imidazoles (econazole, ketoconazole, and miconazole) or itraconazole is also effective, although systemic griseofulvin is not. Repeatedly shaving the lesion with a scalpel may also be helpful.

Piedra

Piedra is a superficial fungal infection of the hair shaft seen most commonly in tropical climates. It presents in two distinct clinical varieties, black piedra and white piedra, caused by *Piedraia hortae* and *Trichosporon* species, respectively.

Epidemiology

Black piedra occurs in the tropical regions of the Americas and Southeast Asia. White piedra has a broader distribution including Africa, Europe, and Japan. Both types show equal age and sex distribution. Evidence suggests that some cases of white piedra may be sexually transmitted.

Clinical Features

Black piedra presents as asymptomatic, microscopic to 1 mm or larger, dark, adherent, stonelike concretions on hair shafts of the scalp or less commonly the beard. White piedra also presents as asymptomatic concretions or nodules on the hair shafts, although these are lighter in color (white to light brown) and can be easily detached unlike those of black piedra. White piedra involves facial and genital hair more often than scalp hair. In both forms, affected hair shafts may be weakened and fracture easily.

Diagnosis

Clinical inspection of the hair shafts and demonstration of fungal elements on KOH examination make the diagnosis in both forms of piedra. Culture can be performed but is usually unnecessary; *Trichosporon* species do not grow in the presence of cycloheximide, and this ingredient should be omitted from culture media when white piedra is suspected.

Differential diagnosis includes pediculosis (see Chapter 31), psoriatic and seborrheic scale, and the hair shaft abnormality, trichorrhexis nodosa. Trichomycosis axillaris and pubis, caused by *Corynebacterium* species, has yellow-tan deposits on axillary or pubic hair, and can be difficult to distinguish visually from white piedra. KOH examination of the hairs deposits will confirm the hyphae of *Trichosporon* in white piedra.

Treatment

Piedra can usually be effectively treated by cutting or shaving the affected hairs with or without the addition of an antifungal shampoo. Oral terbinafine has been reported effective in a single case. Trichomycosis axillaris responds to benzoyl peroxide wash or gel.

DEEP CUTANEOUS AND SUBCUTANEOUS MYCOSES

Deep cutaneous and subcutaneous mycoses are localized fungal infections of the subcutaneous tissues caused by several species of fungi. The infection is thought to arise after endemic fungal organisms are directly implanted into the skin and deeper tissues via trauma to unprotected skin. Chromoblastomycosis, mycetoma, and sporotrichosis are discussed next. Several rarer conditions including lobomycosis and entomophthoromycosis are not discussed.

Chromoblastomycosis

Chromoblastomycosis, or chromomycosis, is a chronic fungal infection of the skin and subcutaneous tissue. It can be caused by any of several dematiaceous (pigmented) soil and wood fungi (*Fonsecaea pedrosoi, F. compactum, F. dermatitidis, Rhinocladiella aquaspersa, Cladosporium carrionii,* and *Phialophora verrucosa*). These organisms produce an identical clinical infection and all appear in tissue sections as small (4 to 6 μm), brownish spherical forms, hence the name *chromo*blastomycosis. They are distinguished by conidiophore type in culture.

Epidemiology

Chromoblastomycosis occurs worldwide but is most common in the tropics, with 80% of reported cases occurring in tropical areas. The majority of cases occur in barefooted farm workers in rural areas. Persons of all ages may be affected, but most cases occur in adults.

Clinical Features

Lesions typically begin as a unilateral, solitary, warty nodule, most often on the lower leg or foot, which enlarges into a tumorous plaque that ulcerates. Satellite lesions occur around the primary lesion and may develop along lymphatic channels. Lesions are frequently exophytic and friable, with lobulated, keratotic surfaces. The disease progresses slowly over many years and may involve an entire extremity. Local edema of the extremity may develop, with secondary bacterial infection and lymphadenitis. Pain is uncommon in the absence of bacterial infection. Untreated infections may persist more than 20 years. In rare cases, dissemination occurs with central nervous system (CNS) or visceral involvement.

Diagnosis

The diagnosis of chromoblastomycosis rests on demonstrating the causative organism on histologic sections with confirmation of the pathogenic species by culture. Biopsy for histology and culture should be taken from the active border of a lesion. Histology shows a nonspecific granulomatous and neutrophilic response, and often the pigmented organisms ("copper pennies" known as Medlar bodies), which are diagnostic. Culture often takes 2 to 4 weeks. Serologic tests are not helpful.

Differential diagnosis includes other granulomatous processes, such as sporotrichosis, leishmaniasis, blastomycosis, and leprosy. Chromoblastomycosis can also mimic squamous cell carcinoma.

Treatment

Chromoblastomycosis is not responsive to medical therapy. For early lesions, surgical excision with skin grafting offers the best chance for cure. Extensive disease may necessitate amputation.

Among the antifungal agents, amphotericin B, flucytosine, itraconazole, and terbinafine have had reported efficacy. The most successful regimens have included flucytosine alone or in combination with amphotericin B. *Flucytosine* is usually given as 150 to 200 mg/day. Treatment continues until healing occurs, which generally takes 6 weeks. Itraconazole, 100 mg/day for 18 months, has been reported to be effective and likely has fewer side effects. Terbinafine has also had favorable results in case reports.

Surgical excision and cryotherapy have been used for very small lesions.

Mycetoma

Mycetoma, also called maduromycosis or Madura foot, refers to a chronic localized infection of the skin, subcutaneous tissue, muscle, and bone, caused by various species of saprophytic fungi (eumycetoma) or filamentous bacteria (actinomycetoma). Mycetoma has three characteristic features: tumor formation, draining fistulas, and expelled granules ("grains").

Eumycetoma may be caused by species of *Madurella, Scedosporium, Leptosphaeria, Pseudallescheria,* and *Acremonium.* Actinomycetoma may be caused by aerobic species of the Actinomycetes (e.g., *Nocardia brasiliensis, N. caviae, N. asteroides, Streptomyces somaliensis, Actinomadura madurae, A. pelletieri,* and *Actinomyces israelii*).

Epidemiology

Mycetoma is an uncommon disease caused by inoculation of the causative organism into the skin through trauma. With the exception of *A. israelii,* the causative organisms are found most abundantly in soils of tropical and subtropical climates. The disease was initially described in India, but is found in Africa, Mexico, Central and South America, and Southeast Asia. Mycetoma mainly occurs in persons working barefoot in soil or vegetation, and the vast majority of cases occur in men age 20 to 50 years old.

Clinical Features

The usual site of inoculation is the foot, but the hands or other areas may be affected. After a latent period of 1 to several months, a painless subcutaneous nodule develops and slowly enlarges. The lesion progresses to a large tumor with a nodular surface and sinus tracts draining bloody or purulent material. The lesion spreads slowly by local extension to fascia and muscle and may eventually involve bone. Pain and systemic symptoms are rare.

The sinus drainage typically contains granules, 0.1 to 5.0 mm in size, which may be white, pink, yellow, brown, or black, depending on the causative organism. Lesions are slowly progressive over many years, and later complications include amyloidosis and sepsis.

Diagnosis

The typical features of *swelling, fistula formation,* and *granules* may allow a clinical diagnosis. Specific diagnosis requires examination of the granules with culture. Granules may be obtained from drainage material or biopsy tissue. The most suitable granules for culture of fungi and actinomycetes are taken from the base of a biopsy specimen. Granules may also be crushed and examined in a KOH mount. The hyphae of eumycetoma may be distinguished from the thin filaments of actinomycetoma.

Biopsy of the lesion will also show the organisms on histologic sections and is useful in ruling out neoplasms that may be in the clinical differential diagnosis. Osteomyelitis should be looked for with radiographs of the extremity. Recently ultrasonography has been shown to be a sensitive and specific modality for diagnosing mycetoma and determining its extent. Computed tomography (CT) scans and magnetic resonance imaging (MRI) are useful in evaluating mycetomas of the head.

Treatment

Treatment varies based on the causal fungi or actinomycetes, the affected region, and the degree of invasion. Surgical excision or cauterization is often recommended for early lesions; however, this should be accompanied by chemotherapy because of the risk of recurrence even with wide-margin amputations. Actinomycetoma responds more favorably with fewer recurrences than does eumycetoma. *Nocardia* spp. can be treated with sulfonamides, minocycline, and other antibacterials. *Actinomyces* spp. are susceptible to penicillin, ampicillin, ceftriaxone, and others. Eumycetoma caused by *Pseudallescheria boydii* has been treated successfully with itraconazole and surgery. Intravenous miconazole has also been used.

Sporotrichosis

Sporotrichosis, caused by the fungus *Sporothrix schenckii,* is a common fungal infection of the skin, lymphatics, and subcutaneous tissue, which rarely becomes disseminated. *S. schenckii* is common in soil and plant debris in both temperate and tropical climates.

Epidemiology

Sporotrichosis occurs worldwide, but is more common in warm, humid climates, with the highest rates of infection occurring in Mexico, Brazil, and South Africa. Infection occurs by inoculation into sites of trauma, and most cases arise in persons whose work predisposes to injury with infected material (e.g., gardeners, florists, and farm workers). An outbreak of 3000 cases was reported in South African mine workers who were exposed by rubbing against infected timber. In the United States cases occur most often in rose gardeners and nursery workers who handle sphagnum moss.

Clinical Features

The primary lesion occurs at the site of inoculation as a painless dermal nodule that usually breaks down to form a ragged ulcer. The initial lesion may persist for weeks to months or may heal and disappear, only to be followed by further symptoms. In most cases, additional small, dusky red, painless nodules appear over weeks to months along the regional lymphatics. These may also ulcerate and form fistulae. Occasionally, the primary lesion is not followed by regional spread. These solitary lesions may become granulomatous plaques, which often develop smaller peripheral satellite lesions. Lesions may persist for years without therapy. Rarely, dissemination occurs to lungs, bone, CNS, and skin, usually in immunocompromised patients.

Diagnosis

The clinical picture of a painless, indurated ulcer on the hand, which is followed by subsequent lesions along regional lymphatics, should strongly suggest sporotrichosis. The diagnosis is established by isolating the organism, usually from a biopsy specimen. The histology of biopsied lesions shows a mixed granulomatous response but rarely reveals the organism. Fungal culture of biopsy material is the most reliable means of diagnosis, and cultures to rule out the other infections listed previously should always be performed concomitantly.

Lymphatic nodules can also be caused by atypical mycobacteria, particularly *Mycobacterium marinum,* nocardiasis, and tularemia. Solitary lesions must be distinguished from cutaneous tuberculosis, other deep fungi, anthrax, tularemia, and carcinoma.

Treatment

Spontaneous remissions occur in some patients; however, most patients are treated to ensure eradication of the infection. Itraconazole, 100 to 200 mg daily for 6 months, followed by 200 mg orally twice a day for long term, has been used successfully. Saturated solution of potassium iodide (SSKI) can be used as an alternative. Standard therapy starts with 0.5 to 1 mg/day and is increased to an effective dose of 4 to 6 mg/day. Although SSKI is inexpensive and effective, patients often do not tolerate it due to the frequently associated side effects of hypersalivation and nausea. Amphotericin B (0.5 mg/kg/d) IV and fluconazole given orally have also been used to treat sporotrichosis. Finally, hyperthermia has been used to treat the localized form of the disease. Regardless of the therapy chosen, treatment should continue for at least 4 weeks after the resolution of clinical disease.

REFERENCES

General

Elewski BE, editor: *Cutaneous fungal infections,* ed 2, Malden, Mass, 1998, Blackwell Scientific, Inc.

Dermatophyte Infections

Lesher JL: Oral therapy of common superficial fungal infections of the skin, *J Am Acad Dermatol* 40(6 Pt 2):S31, 1999.

Gupta AK, Hofstader SL, Adam P, Summerbell RC: Tinea capitis: an overview with emphasis on management, *Pediatr Dermatol* 16(3):171, 1999.

Martin AG, Kobayashi GS: Superficial fungal infection: dermatophytosis, tinea nigra, piedra. In Freedberg IM et al, editors: *Fitzpatrick's dermatology in general medicine,* ed 5, New York, 1999, McGraw-Hill.

Conditions Caused by *Malassezia*

Abdel-Razek M, Fadaly G, Abdel-Raheim M, al-Morsy F: *Pityrosporum (Malassezia)* folliculitis in Saudi Arabia: diagnosis and therapeutic trials, *Clin Exp Dermatol* 20(5):406, 1995.

Faergemann J: *Pityrosporum* infections. In Elewski BE, editor: *Cutaneous fungal infections,* ed 2, Malden, Mass, 1998, Blackwell Scientific Inc.

Gueho E et al: The role of *Malassezia* species in the ecology of human skin and as pathogens, *Med Mycol* 36(Suppl 1):220, 1998.

Jacinto-Jamora S, Tamesis J, Katigbak ML: *Pityrosporum* folliculitis in the Philippines: diagnosis, prevalence, and management, *J Am Acad Dermatol* 24(5 Pt 1):693, 1991.

Vermeer BJ, Staats CC: The efficacy of a topical application of terbinafine 1% solution in subjects with pityriasis versicolor: a placebo-controlled study, *Dermatology* 194(Suppl 1):22, 1997.

Tinea Nigra

Gupta G et al: Tinea nigra secondary to *Exophiala werneckii* responding to itraconazole, *Br J Dermatol* 137:483, 1997.

Cutaneous Candidiasis

Hay RJ: The management of superficial candidiasis, *J Am Acad Dermatol* 40(6 Part 2):S35, 1999.

Martin AG, Kobayashi GS: Yeast infections: candidiasis, pityriasis (tinea) versicolor. In Freedberg IM et al, editors: *Fitzpatrick's dermatology in general medicine,* ed 5, New York, 1999, McGraw-Hill.

Pappas AA, Ray TL: Cutaneous and disseminated skin manifestations of candidiasis. In Elewski BE, editor: *Cutaneous fungal infections,* ed 2, Malden, Mass, 1998, Blackwell Scientific Inc.

Piedra

Elewski BE: The superficial mycoses, the dermatophytoses, and select dermatomycoses. In Elewski BE (editor): *Cutaneous fungal infections,* ed 2, Malden, Mass, 1998, Blackwell Scientific Inc.

Gip L: Black piedra: the first case treated with terbinafine, *Br J Dermatol* 130:26, 1994.

Hay RJ, Moore M: Mycology. In Champion RH, Burton JL, Burns DA, Breathnach SM, editors: *Textbook of dermatology,* ed 6, vol 2, London, 1998, Blackwell Science Ltd.

Chromoblastomycosis

Elgart ML: Subcutaneous and miscellaneous mycoses. In Elewski BE (editor): *Cutaneous fungal infections,* ed 2, Malden, Mass, 1998, Blackwell Scientific Inc.

Rivitti EA, Aoki V: Deep fungal infections in tropical countries, *Clin Dermatol* 17:171, 1999.

Tagami H et al: Successful treatment of chromoblastomycosis with topical heat therapy, *J Am Acad Dermatol* 10:615, 1984.

Mycetoma

Elgart ML: Subcutaneous and miscellaneous mycoses. In Elewski BE (editor): *Cutaneous fungal infections,* ed 2, Malden, Mass, 1998, Blackwell Scientific Inc.

Fahal AH et al: Ultrasonographic imaging of mycetoma, *Br J Surg* 84(4):1120, 1997.

Sporotrichosis

Elgart ML: Subcutaneous and miscellaneous mycoses. In Elewski BE, editor: *Cutaneous fungal infections,* ed 2, Malden, Mass, 1998, Blackwell Scientific Inc.

Hull PR, Vismer HF: Treatment of cutaneous sporotrichosis with terbinafine, *Br J Dermatol* 126 (Suppl 39):51, 1992.

Rivitti EA, Aoki V: Deep fungal infections in tropical countries, *Clin Dermatol* 17:171, 1999.

CHAPTER 34

Leishmaniasis

M. Sean Strother, Roy Colven, and Russell McMullen

Several parasitic agents cause significant skin manifestations as well as systemic disease in humans. The leishmaniases are a group of chronic cutaneous, mucocutaneous, and visceral diseases caused by infection with one of several species of the protozoan parasite, *Leishmania*. Other parasitic infections that may present with significant cutaneous manifestations are presented in Chapters 31 (ectoparasites), 23 (Chagas' disease), 41 (cysticercosis), and 42 (filariasis and onchocerciasis) and 44 (trichinosis).

Members of the genus *Leishmania* are obligate intracellular parasitic protozoa in the family Trypanosomatidae. They exist as elongate, 10 to 15 μm, flagellated forms called promastigotes in their sandfly vectors. When an infected sandfly bites a mammalian host, it injects the promastigotes into the wound with its saliva. Tissue macrophages phagocytize the organisms, which then transform into round or oval, 2 to 3 μm nonflagellated forms called amastigotes. The amastigotes undergo successive asexual division until the macrophage ruptures releasing the amastigotes, which enter other macrophages to continue the cycle. When a sandfly bites an infected mammalian host, it ingests amastigote-laden macrophages along with its blood meal. The amastigotes transform into promastigotes and reproduce in the gut of the fly before migrating to the proboscis of the fly to complete the cycle with the next fly bite.

Hematophagous female sandflies in the genera *Phlebotomus* in the Old World, and *Lutzomyia* and *Psychodopygus* in the New World transmit the *Leishmania* organisms via their bite. Several nonhuman mammals serve as reservoirs for leishmaniasis including domestic and wild canines and various rodents depending on the geographic distribution and the species of *Leishmania* involved.

The taxonomy of the genus *Leishmania* remains confusing owing to the recognition of new species and subspecies by the various molecular and biochemical techniques developed over the last decade. In the past, species were recognized primarily by their clinical disease manifestations. Although certain species tend to cause relatively specific disease entities, these associations are by no means exclusive and should no longer be used as the primary means of identifying *Leishmania* species. Currently, experts recognize approximately a dozen or so species, some of which they group into complexes of closely related species, (i.e., the *L. mexicana* complex and the *L. braziliensis* complex).

CUTANEOUS LEISHMANIASIS

Cutaneous leishmaniasis is a chronic ulcerative, usually self-healing, infection caused by several species of *Leishmania,* and is divided into Old World and New World (or American) forms. Local peoples apply many common names to this disease (see following discussion). Depending on the species involved, the infecting organisms may spread by direct extension or metastasis to involve the mucosa of the upper respiratory tract (mucocutaneous leishmaniasis) resulting in painful disfigurement or even death.

Old World Cutaneous Leishmaniasis

Common names for Old World Cutaneous Leishmaniasis (OWCL) include oriental sore, Delhi boil, and Aleppo boil.

Etiology and Epidemiology

Four species, *L. major, L. tropica, L. aethiopica,* and *L. infantum,* cause OWCL.

L. major causes rural, wet, or zoonotic cutaneous leishmaniasis. The animal reservoirs are desert rodents. It is endemic in desert areas of northern Africa, Central Asia, the Sudan, and the Middle East. In certain communities, local prevalence may approach 100% and travelers may be affected.

L. tropica causes urban, dry, or anthroponotic cutaneous leishmaniasis. Experts now think that humans are the primary host and dogs may serve as a reservoir. Endemic areas include urban areas of the Mediterranean basin, Central Asia, and the Middle East.

L. aethiopica occurs mainly in Ethiopia and Kenya in rural mountain areas. Hyraxes, distant relatives of elephants, serve as the animal reservoir.

L. infantum occurs in the Mediterranean basin, China, Central Asia, and the Middle East. Adults infected with this species tend to develop a mild self-limited cutaneous disease, whereas infants tend to develop visceral disease. Animal reservoirs include domesticated and wild canines.

Clinical Features

Characteristic skin lesions generally appear within 6 week after inoculation by the sandfly, but they may be delayed for prolonged periods depending on the size of the inoculum. The lesion begins as a small, pruritic, erythematous papule that slowly enlarges and breaks down to form an ulcer up to 5 cm in diameter, with an elevated, indurated border. Lesions may be single or multiple and occur on exposed skin surfaces, but spare the palms and soles. Ulcers persist for a variable time and heal slowly with depressed scarring. Though not a universal rule, clinical features differ slightly depending on the infecting species.

L. major often causes multiple lesions with an exudative base. The infection runs a more rapid course, and the lesions may be healed in 6 months. Spread to regional lymph nodes is rare.

L. tropica usually causes a single, more indolent ulcer that may require over a year for healing. Internal organ involvement with *L. tropica* has been demonstrated in U.S. soldiers returning from prolonged deployment in the Middle East during the Gulf War (early 1990s).

L. aethiopica produces an even more indolent ulcer that may persist for several years. Diffuse cutaneous leishmaniasis, an anergic state with extensive skin infiltration by organisms resembling lepromatous leprosy, occurs in approximately 20% of endemic *L. aethiopica* infections.

Diagnosis

Diagnosis requires identification of the organism in *smears* from lesions, *biopsy,* or *culture.* Variable numbers of amastigotes, also called Leishman-Donovan bodies, are present in lesions, and they may be difficult to identify in smears or biopsies. Culture of tissue from an active lesion often grows the promastigotes. Several different culture systems are available, and cultures often take one to several weeks to provide a positive result. Promastigotes isolated from cultures can be sent to special laboratories for species identification by isoenzyme electrophoresis when warranted.

The *leishmanin skin test* gives evidence of present or past infection and is usually positive 3 months after onset of lesions except in the diffuse form. It involves a subcutaneous injection of a given inoculum of killed promastigotes and is read at 48 hours after application. A response of 5 mm or greater is positive.

Serologic tests are available in some centers, but their role in diagnosis is not well established.

Treatment

Cutaneous leishmaniasis is generally a self-limited infection, and the benefits of treatment should be weighed against potential toxicity. Indications for treatment include large, multiple, or potentially disfiguring lesions. Numerous forms of treatment have been advocated, including pentavalent antimonials, pentamidine, cryotherapy, surgery, hyperthermic therapy, amphotericin B, and many others.

The first-line therapy for uncomplicated cutaneous leishmaniasis is the pentavalent antimonial compound, sodium stibogluconate (Pentostam), 20 mg/kg/day for 28 days in two divided doses either intramuscularly or intravenous infusion. This medication is available from the Centers for Disease Control and Prevention (CDC) through their Drug Service (see Appendix). Longer treatment courses at higher doses may be required for complicated cases, lymphatic involvement, or diffuse cutaneous leishmaniasis. Some investigators believe that *L. aethiopica* responds poorly to conventional antimonial therapy and support the use of pentamidine, 2 mg/kg given intravenously every other day for seven doses.

Cryotherapy with liquid nitrogen is a locally destructive method that may be effective in early lesions. Surgical excision and grafting have been advocated for early lesions to minimize eventual scarring.

The ulcerative skin lesions of cutaneous leishmaniasis may also be secondarily infected with common skin bacterial flora. Thus treatment with appropriate antibiotics will sometimes be a valuable adjunct to the parasite-directed therapy described previously.

New World Cutaneous Leishmaniasis

Common names for New World Cutaneous Leishmaniasis (NWCL) include American cutaneous leishmaniasis, chiclero ulcer, espundia, bush yaws, uta, and picatura de pito.

Etiology and Epidemiology

NWCL is a disease of rural forest and jungle areas of most of Central and South America. Forest workers, agricultural workers, and others in rural, forested areas are primarily at risk, since the sandfly vectors do not readily bite humans. Several species belonging to the *L. braziliensis* and *L. mexi-*

cana complexes cause NWCL. Species from either complex may be principal causes of leishmaniasis in a given area. Both complexes are pathogenic throughout the range of disease in the New World, with the exceptions of southern Texas and the Dominican Republic, where *L. mexicana* is the sole identified species. Animal reservoirs include foxes, sloths, and forest rodents depending on the species.

Clinical Features

Cutaneous lesions closely resemble those of OWCL with a few specific differences. *Chiclero ulcer* refers to cutaneous disease found in the Yucatan, Belize, and Guatemala caused primarily by *L. mexicana.* Lesions tend to be solitary and occur most frequently on the ear. Ear ulcers may persist for many years before healing and may result in destruction of the ear. Lesions in other skin areas often heal within 6 months. Mucosal spread is rare.

Mucocutaneous leishmaniasis results primarily from infections caused by *L. braziliensis.* The cutaneous lesions spread along lymphatics, resembling sporotrichosis, and mucosal disease is frequent. Mucosal involvement occurs by metastatic spread of infection from the skin and presents months to years after the initial cutaneous lesions. It begins as erythema, edema, and ulceration of the nasal septum, with gradual extension to the palate, pharynx, and larynx. Occasionally, the anus and other mucosal sites may be involved. This destructive, granulomatous process of the soft tissue can involve cartilage but not bone. Perforation of the nasal septum and collapse of the nasal bridge is typical, giving the so-called tapir nose. Mucosal disease is progressive and mutilating and may be fatal. The severe form of mucosal disease is called espundia.

Diffuse cutaneous leishmaniasis occasionally occurs and is similar to this form of OWCL.

Diagnosis

Diagnosis is similar to that of OWCL.

Treatment

Systemic therapy is usually indicated for NWCL, especially when *L. braziliensis* infection is suspected or confirmed owing to the destructive nature of the lesions and the potential for metastatic spread to mucosal sites.

As with OWCL, the treatment of choice for NWCL is sodium stibogluconate or pentamidine at the dosage regimens previously described. Relapse occurs frequently if the treatment course is interrupted. Diffuse cutaneous disease may be less responsive to antimonial therapy. Patients should be reevaluated 6 weeks after the course is completed, and if lesions are not improved by at least 75%, retreatment should be considered. After completion of treatment, lesions should be monitored for relapse for 1 year.

For mucosal disease, the same regimen is recommended (20 mg/kg/day of sodium stibogluconate for 28 days) with cure rates approximating 60%. Alternatively, amphotericin B 1mg/kg IV every other day for 20 to 30 doses provides cure rates reported in the range of 75% or higher. Initial response should be assessed 3 months after completion of therapy. Because of the strong potential for relapse, it is recommended that mucosal lesions be followed for several years after completion.

VISCERAL LEISHMANIASIS*

Visceral leishmaniasis, or kala-azar, results from infection with protozoa from *L. donovani* in Africa and the India, *L. infantum* in the Mediterranean basin, and *L. chagasi* in the New World. Like the cutaneous leishmaniases, it is transmitted by the bite of phlebotomine sandflies. Reservoir animals include various rodents and domesticated or wild canines, except in India where humans are the only known reservoir.

Visceral leishmaniasis should be suspected in residents of, or recent travelers to, an endemic area who present with *intermittent fever, anemia,* and *marked hepatosplenomegaly.* Occasionally, military groups have experienced epidemics; for example, kala-azar occurred in British soldiers in India and visceral leishmaniasis has been reported in U.S. veterans of the Gulf War, although most of the latter cases appear to have been due to *L. tropica.* Infection can result from brief exposure in an endemic area.

Clinical Features

Kala-azar arising in different regions may show many variations in its clinical and epidemiologic appearance. A *cutaneous nodule* often develops at the site of the parasite inoculation in the African and Central Asian forms of the infection. Often this will have resolved before clinical illness develops. After an incubation period of 2 to 6 months, systemic manifestations develop insidiously, although the presentation may occasionally be abrupt. The earliest symptom is fever. On physical examination, the liver and spleen are large, firm, and nontender. *Lymphadenopathy* is more frequently reported in the Mediterranean countries, East Africa, and China. Brazilian and Mediterranean kala-azar occur more frequently in children. Oral and nasopharyngeal lesions may occasionally be seen in Sudan, East Africa, and India.

Clinical manifestations of kala-azar are due to invasion of the reticuloendothelial cells of the spleen, liver, bone marrow, and skin, and the subsequent multiplication of amastigotes within the cells. Untreated infections become chronic and, in addition to the physical findings already described, patients typically become markedly wasted. Patients with light-colored skin may develop a grayish cast—*kala-azar* is an Indian name meaning "black fever."

Untreated visceral leishmaniasis may be complicated by intercurrent infections such as pneumonia, pulmonary tuberculosis, and dysentery; these often prove fatal. Some patients die from gastrointestinal hemorrhage.

Immunocompromised patients, in particular those with human immunodeficiency virus infection, often follow an atypical course. They may have a short duration of symptoms, and fever and splenomegaly may be absent. They typically respond poorly to treatment and have a high mortality rate.

Long after apparently successful treatment, some patients in India and East Africa develop post-kala-azar dermal leishmaniasis, a condition that resembles leprosy and features depigmented or nodular cutaneous lesions.

Diagnosis

Diagnosis of visceral leishmaniasis should be suspected in individuals presenting with characteristic signs and symptoms, which have emigrated from or visited an area where leishmaniasis is endemic.

*This discussion of visceral leishmaniasis is based on portions of the chapter "Travel-Acquired Illnesses Associated with Fever," by the late Robert P. Aduan, MD, from the first edition of this manual.

Laboratory studies reveal anemia, leukopenia, neutropenia, and occasionally thrombocytopenia. The eosinophil count is also low. A marked hyperglobulinemia resulting from increased immunoglobulin G is usually present.

Microscopic examination and culture of bone marrow aspirates provide the best methods for reaching a definitive diagnosis of visceral leishmaniasis, although evidence suggests that splenic aspirates are probably superior. Serologic testing is available for problematic cases, but one must be certain the test used has proven sensitivity and specificity for the geographic region of origin.

Treatment

Sodium stibogluconate or meglumine antimonate are the treatments of choice for visceral leishmaniasis. The current regimen recommended by the CDC is 20 mg/kg/day for 28 days; it is better tolerated intravenously, although it can be given intramuscularly. Clinical resistance of *Leishmania* spp. to antimony compounds has been noted in some countries, India in particular. A treatment course of 40 days may be necessary in these circumstances, but should not be the routine regimen unless local resistance has been demonstrated. Patients typically feel better within a week of beginning treatment, but it may take weeks for laboratory values to normalize, and months before splenomegaly resolves. Accurate assessment for complete cure mandates follow-up at frequent intervals over a 1-year period.

Alternative regimens that can be used in the event of treatment failure with sodium stibogluconate include pentamidine given parenterally and also amphotericin B. A limited number of case reports suggest that allopurinol may be helpful in combination with antimony compounds in treating relapses.

REFERENCES

Berman JD: Human leishmaniasis: clinical, diagnostic, and chemotherapeutic developments in the last 10 years, *Clin Infect Dis* 24:684, 1997.

Bryceson ADM, Hay RJ: Parasitic worms and protozoa. In Champion RH, Burton JL, Burns DA, Breathnach SM, editors: *Textbook of dermatology,* ed 6th, vol 2, London, 1998, Blackwell Scientific Ltd.

Grimaldi G Jr, Tesh RB, McMahon-Pratt D: A review of the geographic distribution and epidemiology of leishmaniasis in the New World, *Am J Trop Med Hyg* 41:687, 1989.

Herwaldt BL: Leishmaniasis, *Lancet* 354:1191, 1999.

Herwaldt BL, Stokes SL, Juranek DD: American cutaneous leishmaniasis in U.S. travelers, *Ann Intern Med* 118:779, 1993.

Klaus SN, Frankenburg S: Leishmaniasis and other protozoan infections. In Freedberg IM et al, editors: *Fitzpatrick's dermatology in general medicine,* ed 5, New York, 1999, McGraw-Hill.

Magill AJ et al: Visceral infection caused by *Leishmania* tropica in veterans of Operation Desert Storm, *N Engl J Med* 328:1383, 1993.

CHAPTER 35

Leprosy (Hansen's Disease)

M. Patricia Joyce

Leprosy is a chronic infectious disease affecting the skin, peripheral nervous system, eyes, and testicles. Leprosy is a complex disease, with the interaction between infection and host immunity producing different clinical syndromes in different persons.

The confusing diversity of clinical forms of leprosy is best understood by using the classification system of Ridley and Jopling. This system presents leprosy as a spectrum from *localized disease* with high host immunity (tuberculoid leprosy) to *disseminated disease* with low host immunity (lepromatous leprosy). Between these two polar forms are three *midspectrum forms* (borderline leprosy). Stated another way, there is an inverse relationship between specific cellular immunity and extent of disease, or bacillary load.

Therapy, complications of disease, and prognosis are dependent on the form of disease in a given patient. The interaction between the patient's immune system and the infection is dynamic and may be influenced by many factors, including therapy, pregnancy, and certain medications. Patients with midspectrum (borderline) leprosy may move toward either tuberculoid or lepromatous forms, but the polar forms tend to be fixed.

Leprosy is almost unique among diseases for the social stigma associated with infection. For centuries, patients have been excluded from society or confined in colonies because of fear of contagion. Many persons with other skin diseases such as psoriasis probably were also mistakenly persecuted. Even today, in areas of high prevalence, visible signs of disease (e.g., skin lesions, wasting of the hand muscles, or loss of the eyebrows) may cause social rejection. Patients try to conceal their disease and may not seek medical attention for fear of exposure. These attitudes may persist when people from highly endemic areas migrate to the United States.

Today, with effective treatment, patients require no isolation, and the mutilating complications of untreated disease can mostly be prevented. Until public education removes the stigma from infection, many authorities prefer to discard the terms *leprosy* and *leper* in favor of the emotionally neutral eponyms *Hansen's disease* and *Hansen's disease patient.*

ETIOLOGY

Mycobacterium leprae, first identified by Hansen in 1873, is a weakly acid-fast, rod-shaped bacterium. *M. leprae* has never been successfully grown in artificial media, but can be propagated in the mouse footpad and the nine-banded armadillo. The organism has a long doubling time of 13 days in the mouse footpad, selectively invades peripheral nerves, and grows preferentially at temperatures of 33° to 35° C. *M. leprae* does not produce any known toxins, and tissue injury is caused by the host's immune response or by the sheer mass of infecting bacilli.

Organisms are identified using a modified acid-fast stain, the *Fite stain.* Viable organisms stain in a uniform, solid manner. With therapy, most organisms quickly lose their solid staining, appear beaded or fragmented, and are not viable in the mouse footpad.

EPIDEMIOLOGY

Leprosy is endemic in most of the world, but the majority of cases occur in the tropics. Of the estimated 10 to 15 million afflicted individuals, over half live in Africa and India, with substantial additional numbers in Southeast Asia. There are an estimated 50,000 cases in Europe and more than 6000 cases in the United States.

There has been a recent decline in the number of new cases occurring annually in the United States. From a high of 447 cases reported in 1983, there were 150 to 200 new cases reported annually in the last decade of the 20th century. Virtually all newly reported cases occur in immigrants from Mexico, the Philippines, and Southeast Asia. Low-level endemic disease in the United States is found in Texas, Louisiana, Hawaii, and Florida.

Leprosy affects males more than females, with ratios of 1.6:1 to 3:1 in different series. In children, the ratio is 1:1. All races are affected, but the predominant form of disease varies among races. In Africa, more than 90% of cases are tuberculoid, whereas in southern Asia the percentage is less than 50%. A predominance of lepromatous disease has been seen in Filipinos. Pureblooded Native American Indians are alleged to be naturally immune to leprosy. Studies of twins have shown a high degree of concordance both for developing leprosy and for the form of disease. All ages are affected, but the majority of cases occur in young adults.

The exact mode of disease transmission is unknown. Studies of disease transmission have been hampered by the lack of a culture system, the absence of serologic markers, the latent period of 2 to 15 years before disease onset, and the high degree of natural immunity in most persons. Epidemiologic studies reveal that only 3% to 5 % of people may not be able to withstand development of active infection even after prolonged exposure. In experimental animals, however, a single inoculation of small numbers of bacilli produces infection. If prolonged exposure is required, it may be related to the chance of receiving an appropriate inoculation rather than a need for multiple inoculations.

Studies of household contacts of lepromatous patients have yielded an estimated risk of infection of 2% to 4%, or attack rates of four cases per 1000 person-years. With therapy, shedding of viable organisms falls rapidly and, after several weeks, experimental infection cannot be established in the mouse footpad.

Tuberculoid leprosy patients shed no demonstrable organisms and are regarded as noncontagious, although this is unproven.

Viable-appearing organisms are shed from untreated lepromatous patients in nasal secretions, skin scales, sweat, blood, breast milk, and wound exudate. Untreated lepromatous patients have a high level of bacteremia, and viable organisms have been identified in the gut of biting insects after feeding on such patients; however, transmission through an insect vector remains unproven. The possibility of animal-to-human transmission is supported by numerous reports of cases in persons handling or consuming armadillos.

CLINICAL FEATURES

Clinical features of leprosy are a continuum between the tuberculoid and lepromatous forms of disease. There is substantial overlap in the appearance of the different forms, and careful assessment of clinical and histologic parameters is needed for accurate diagnosis. Important clinical features include (1) number of skin lesions, (2) size and morphology of skin lesions, (3) presence of neuropathy, and (4) presence of reactional states, which are caused by alterations in immune response and are described in detail in the next section.

All clinical findings must be correlated with findings on biopsies and skin smears. The disease types may be divided into paucibacillary forms (indeterminate, tuberculoid, and borderline tuberculoid) and multibacillary forms (borderline, borderline lepromatous, and lepromatous); this classification is useful to determine appropriate antibiotic therapy. Features of each type of leprosy are summarized in Table 35-1.

Tuberculoid leprosy (TT) is a localized infection in a host with a high degree of immunity. There is usually a single skin lesion or, at most, a few lesions. Lesions are large, flat plaques with well-demarcated, irregular, erythematous, raised borders and an atrophic, scaly center. Hypopigmentation is common, and there is marked anesthesia and anhidrosis of lesions. Plaques are frequently located on the face or extremities.

Neural involvement is usually confined to the area of skin lesions, with palpably enlarged peripheral nerves and motor, sensory, and autonomic deficits. Neuropathy may develop without apparent skin lesions in a subset of tuberculoid leprosy termed *pure neuritic*. Testicular and ocular infiltration does not occur, although neuropathy can cause corneal denervation, lagophthalmos, and exposure keratitis. Reactional states do not occur.

Borderline tuberculoid leprosy (BT) patients may closely resemble tuberculoid patients but have slightly lower host immunity and a higher bacillary load. There are usually several lesions that are smaller and less flat than tuberculoid lesions. Lesions are distributed asymmetrically and are moderately to markedly anesthetic. There may be more than one area of neural involvement. Biopsy shows few bacilli, rather than the rare or absent bacilli characteristic of true tuberculoid cases. Skin smears show few or no bacilli. Reversal reactions may occur.

Borderline, or *dimorphous, leprosy* (BB) is regarded as an unstable form that may move toward either polar form. Patients have moderate numbers of lesions, usually more than 10, of variable morphology. Some lesions resemble the large, irregular, flat plaques of tuberculoid leprosy, whereas others are smaller and infiltrated or raised. Annular, or ring-shaped, lesions are typical, and lesions are asymmetrically distributed. Neural involvement may occur early or late, involves multiple nerves, and may be severe. Reversal and downgrading reactions may occur with alterations of cell-mediated immunity to *M. leprae* antigens; they represent changes toward the tuberculoid and lepromatous poles, respectively. The most severe neurologic damage occurs in borderline patients because of the multiple nerves involved and the tendency for neuritis to occur with reactions. Biopsy and smears show a moderate bacillary load.

Borderline lepromatous leprosy (BL) patients resemble lepromatous patients but have fewer bacilli and higher immunity. Skin lesions are usually numerous and may be macules, papules, plaques, or nodules.

Table 35-1
Clinical Features of Leprosy

Feature	Tuberculoid	Borderline tuberculoid	Borderline	Borderline lepromatous	Lepromatous
Number of lesions	Single or few	Few	Usually >10	Many	Many
Size and morphology of lesions	Large, flat plaque, irregular border, scaly and hypopigmented	Mostly large flat plaques, scaly and hypopigmented	Variable sized, raised plaques, often annular with scaly border	Variable sized, papules and plaques, some irregular or annular, many small and regular	Small, smooth, erythematous or hyperpigmented papules and plaques; diffuse infiltration
Distribution	Asymmetric	Asymmetric	Asymmetric	Asymmetric	Symmetric
Degree of anesthesia	Marked	Moderate to marked	Variable	Minimal until late	Absent until late
Neural involvement	Occurs early; one or two nerves	Occurs early; several nerves	Variable; involves several nerves	Occurs late; several nerves	Occurs late; often diffuse sensory loss
Common reactions	None	Reversal	Reversal or downgrading	Reversal or ENL	ENL (50%), rarely Lucio's phenomenon
Other features	Corneal denervation or lagophthalmos in 10%	As in tuberculoid	Unstable form of disease		Ocular, nasal, and testicular infiltration
Number of bacilli in smears	Absent or rare	Rare	Moderate	Many	Very many

ENL, Erythema nodosum leprosum.

Some plaques may appear punched-out with a sloping outer margin and a steep inner margin. Nerve involvement occurs late and sensation is often preserved.

Lepromatous leprosy (LL) patients have unrestrained proliferation of bacilli within the skin, peripheral nerves, anterior eye, and testes. Lesions are innumerable, small, erythematous, symmetric, hyperpigmented macules, papules, and nodules. Infiltration is most prominent in cooler areas, such as the ears, upper lip, and forehead. The midline of the back is spared lesions, but all areas of skin, with or without lesions, are heavily loaded with bacilli. Diffuse infiltration of the face may occur, giving the typical leonine facies and loss of the lateral eyebrows (madarosis).

Peripheral nerves are less likely to be infiltrated and enlarged in lepromatous disease, and anesthesia occurs later or may be subtle. When anesthesia occurs, a diffuse pattern is seen, rather than focal nerve destruction; it may resemble a stocking-glove pattern. Nasal mucosal involvement causes stuffiness and epistaxis and may lead to septal perforation and collapse. Testicular involvement leads to sterility, impotence, and gynecomastia. Eye involvement includes keratitis, episcleritis, and corneal denervation. Erythema nodosum leprosum (ENL), an apparent immune-complex reaction characterized by tender cutaneous nodules and systemic symptoms, occurs in up to 50% of lepromatous patients, usually in the first several years of therapy. ENL may be a chronic complaint on diagnosis of leprosy, or may occur as late phenomena after treatment is completed. Reversal reactions rarely occur in pure lepromatous leprosy.

Indeterminate leprosy is the earliest recognizable form of the disease and may be extremely difficult to diagnose. There is typically a single hypopigmented or erythematous macule without abnormal sensation or sweating. Biopsy is nonspecific and shows rare or no organisms. The course of indeterminate leprosy is variable. Some lesions heal spontaneously with no further manifestation of disease, others are stable for months or years, and some progress into a "committed" form of persistent leprosy.

Neural involvement in leprosy is due to selective proliferation of *M. leprae* in superficial peripheral nerves. Nerve destruction occurs either from inflammation or from infiltration by masses of infecting organisms. Inflammation leads to nerve damage in conditions of high immunity, as are characteristic of tuberculoid or borderline leprosy, and also characteristic of episodes of active neuritis, such as those seen in ENL and, particularly, reversal reactions. Lepromatous and borderline lepromatous patients have massive infiltration of nerves with bacilli, which gradually destroys the nerve. The nerves most affected are those located superficially (hence cooler). They include the ulnar nerve at the elbow; the radial and median nerves at the wrist; the greater auricular nerve; and the olfactory, trigeminal, facial, peroneal, posterior tibial, and sural nerves. Sensory, motor, and autonomic neuropathy may occur together or separately. The first sensory modality lost is hot-cold discrimination, followed by light touch and pain. The central nervous system is never involved.

Ophthalmic involvement occurs in all forms of leprosy, but the type of involvement depends on the form of disease. Corneal hypesthesia and lagophthalmos from denervation are most typical of the tuberculoid end of the spectrum. Bacillary infiltration of the anterior eye occurs in borderline and lepromatous patients, causing nodular keratitis and episcleritis. ENL may cause iridocyclitis and secondary glaucoma. The sensory denervation of the eye results in the absence of symptoms despite progressive ocular injury, thus contributing to vision loss. Patients should be evaluated and followed by an ophthalmologist who is aware of the complications of leprosy. Patients with corneal anesthesia need counseling and measures to prevent exposure injury. Surgery may be useful in lagophthalmos. Inflammatory conditions associated with reactions are managed with steroids.

REACTIONAL STATES

Reactional states (also called *lepra reactions*) occur with alterations in host immune response and are important to recognize and treat because they can cause irreversible tissue damage. Several distinct types of reactions are distinguished.

Reversal reaction (or type 1 reaction) represents an increase in cellular immune response, with movement toward the tuberculoid pole of disease. This reaction is common in the borderline forms of leprosy and does not occur in the polar forms.

1. There is an increase in activated lymphocytes in areas of granulomas causes preexisting skin lesions to become erythematous and edematous. Ulceration may occur.
2. Peripheral nerves become enlarged and tender.
3. Acute neuritis may lead to rapid loss of sensory and motor function.
4. Systemic signs are usually absent, and laboratory tests are not helpful in diagnosis.

Biopsy and nerve conduction studies should be performed to confirm the diagnosis and follow the neuritis. Prompt treatment must be given to avoid permanent nerve damage. The duration of reversal reaction is often several weeks, but it may persist for many months.

Downgrading reaction refers to reactions associated with a decrease in cell-mediated immunity, that is, with movement toward the lepromatous pole. New skin lesions occur. Edema of peripheral nerves may lead to sudden functional loss.

Erythema nodosum leprosum (ENL, type 2 reaction) occurs in up to 50% of lepromatous and borderline lepromatous patients during the course of their disease and may be chronic. The immunology of ENL is not entirely understood, but the condition is believed to be mediated by immune complexes formed with *M. leprae* antigens.

1. ENL is a systematic reaction with fever, arthralgias, weight loss, neuritis, iridocyclitis, epididymoorchitis, and recurrent crops of painful skin lesions.
2. Skin lesions are erythematous papules and nodules resembling erythema nodosum or erythema multiforme.
3. Lesions usually occur on normal-appearing skin, not in plaques of leprosy, and are commonly on the thighs, forearms, and face.
4. Laboratory studies show leukocytosis, elevated sedimentation rate, and, often, increased circulating immune complexes.
5. Biopsy shows acute inflammatory panniculitis with hallmark invasion by polymorphonuclear leukocytes.
6. Chronic ENL is associated with amyloidosis and glomerulonephritis with death from renal insufficiency.

Lucio's phenomenon (erythema necroticans) is a rare reactional state seen mainly in patients from Mexico, Cuba, Brazil, or Costa Rica who have diffuse lepromatous disease of longstanding duration. Histopathologic examination reveals profound bacterial load with endovascular invasion and intravascular thrombosis. The lesions are irregular or stellate macules and papules that become purpuric and may ulcerate. Widespread cutaneous ulcers may occur, leading to secondary infection, sepsis, and death.

DIAGNOSIS

Diagnosis of leprosy requires a high index of suspicion when dealing with persons from endemic areas. There is often a delay of one or more years after medical attention is sought before the diagnosis is made. The combination of skin lesions and neuropathy should suggest the diagnosis, but neurologic findings may be subtle.

Evaluation of patients should include the following:

1. A careful inspection of the skin with diagrams of lesions should be carried out.
2. Areas of anhidrosis should be noted, because this correlates with loss of protective sensation.
3. Superficial nerves should be palpated for enlargement and tenderness.
4. Detailed sensory testing should be carried out to define deficits. Mapping of sensory deficits is helpful in following the course of neuropathy.
5. Motor testing and nerve conduction studies should be performed.
6. Examination of insensitive extremities for areas of trauma or pressure injury is important, as is assessment of the adequacy of footwear.
7. Ophthalmologic evaluation is indicated for all patients.

The differential diagnosis includes *sarcoidosis, syphilis, mycosis fungoides, vitiligo, psoriasis, miliaria profunda, pityriasis alba, tinea corporis,* and *streptocerciasis,* as well as other mycobacterial infections such as by *M. tuberculosis, M. marinum,* and *M. ulcerans.*

DIAGNOSTIC STUDIES

A definitive diagnosis requires demonstration of bacilli in tissue. Biopsy and skin smears are performed in all patients.

Biopsy should be taken from the active border of a skin lesion and stained with a Fite stain in addition to routine stains.

Skin smears aid in diagnosis, in assessment of bacillary load, and in following response to therapy. The technique involves obtaining tissue fluid and cells from the dermis and staining to analyze numbers and morphology of bacilli (Fig. 35-1):

1. A fold of skin at standard sites is pinched firmly to minimize blood flow.
2. A shallow incision is made, 5 mm long and 3 mm deep, with a scalpel or razor blade.
3. The blade is rotated 90 degrees in the wound, the sides of the wound are scraped, and material collected is smeared on a glass microscope slide for staining.
4. Numbers of organisms per high-power field are graded on a logarithmic scale called the *bacillary index.*
5. The percentage of solid-staining, hence viable, bacilli is referred to as the *morphologic index* (MI). Although bacteria persist in tissue for many years, the percentage of viable, or solid-staining, bacteria should fall to zero within 6 months of therapy. Failure of the MI to fall indicates noncompliance or drug resistance.

Nerve biopsy may be useful in tuberculoid leprosy when skin biopsy shows no organisms or when no skin lesions are present. A cutaneous sensory nerve is selected in an area of neuropathy and examined histologically for organisms and typical granulomas.

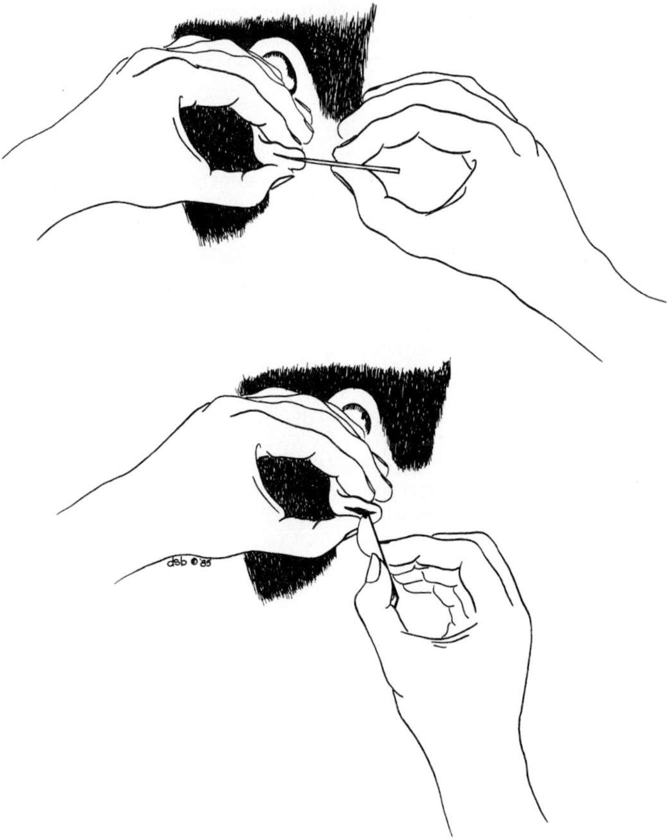

Fig. 35-1 Obtaining skin smear material for leprosy diagnosis. (Protective gloves should be worn.)

The *lepromin test* is not commonly used in the United States, but has been used to classify patients already diagnosed with leprosy. Preparations of *M. leprae* antigen from human or armadillo tissue can be injected intradermally to assess specific cellular immunity. A response resembling the tuberculin reaction occurs in 48 to 72 hours in persons with tuberculoid disease who have high cellular immunity to *M. leprae.* This is the *Fernandez reaction.* A delayed granulomatous response, called the *Mitsuda reaction,* occurs after several weeks when integral lepromin is used. Lepromatous patients who have low cellular immunity tend to be nonreactive to lepromin testing. Lepromin is too nonselective and nonspecific to be useful as a diagnostic test.

Serologic assays of antibodies against *M. leprae* cell wall components, such as phenolic glycolipid-1 or lipoarabinomannan, have been useful in epidemiologic studies but are also nonspecific or cross-reactive.

Polymerase chain reaction testing can be performed by referral laboratories on tissue biopsy samples, but has limited reliability in the setting of tuberculoid disease, where few bacteria are seen on standard microscopy.

TREATMENT

Modern and effective therapy of leprosy requires the use of several medications in combination, referred to as *multidrug therapy* (MDT). In the same way that variations in host immunity affects clinical disease, antibiotic therapy is dictated by host immunity and form of disease. Treatment recommendations are divided into *paucibacillary* or *multibacillary* therapy. Patients with paucibacillary leprosy require treatment for shorter periods, but eventually can discontinue therapy. Patients with multibacillary leprosy require longer treatment, and may be maintained on lifelong maintenance therapy if older monotherapy regimens were used. Dapsone monotherapy has been abandoned because of the emergence of dapsone resistance, but many older patients will remain on this regimen as lifelong maintenance. Treatment regimens recommended by the U.S. National Hansen's Disease Programs and the World Health Organization are summarized in Table 35-2.

The primary antibiotics used to treat leprosy are dapsone, rifampin, and clofazimine. Modern MDT regimens may involve dual therapy with dapsone and rifampin for a prescribed period of time, followed by dapsone or

Table 35-2
Current Hansen's Disease Treatment Regimens

Type of disease	World health organization study group regimen	National Hansen's disease programs (NHDP) standard regimen
Paucibacillary Forms: Indeterminate Tuberculoid Borderline tuberculoid	Dapsone 100 mg/day (unsupervised) plus rifampin 600 mg once monthly (supervised) for 6 months	Dapsone 100 mg/day plus rifampin 600 mg/day for 12 months
Single lesion Paucibacillary	Single dose of ROM therapy: Rifampin 600 mg, Ofloxacin 400 mg, and Minocycline 100 mg	Treat as Paucibacillary leprosy for 12 months
Multibacillary Forms: Borderline Borderline-lepromatous Lepromatous	Dapsone 100 mg/day plus clofazimine 50 mg/day (both unsupervised) plus rifampin 600 mg and clofazimine 300 mg once monthly in supervised setting; continue regimen for 12 months of therapy	I. Standard WHO multibacillary regimen for 2 years II. Dapsone 100 mg/day plus clofazimine 50 mg/day plus rifampin 600 mg/day for 2 years III. Dapsone 100 mg/day plus rifampin 600 mg/day for 2 years (must be proven dapsone-sensitive in mouse footpad study)

clofazimine alone. A number of other antibiotics are active against *M. leprae* and may be useful in combination as second-line therapy in the setting of drug intolerance or documented drug resistance (Table 35-3).

1. *Dapsone* is generally well tolerated but is associated with a number of potential side effects. All patients have mild degrees of methemoglobinemia and hemolysis. Persons with glucose-6-phosphate dehydrogenase deficiency will have severe hemolysis, and dapsone is contraindicated. Rare side effects include granulocytopenia and "sulfone syndrome."
2. *Rifampin* may cause liver function abnormalities, bone marrow suppression, and interstitial nephritis. Additionally rifampin will temporarily discolor urine and other body fluids.
3. *Clofazimine* is used in cases of dapsone resistance. The drug has a direct effect against ENL that is still unexplained.

Physical Therapy

Patients with insensitive extremities need counseling on the prevention of injury. The loss of digits in leprosy is the result of repetitive trauma and infection in insensitive extremities and is preventable. Common household activities such as cooking and washing pose hazards of burn or scald injuries. Knives should be used only with caution, and protective gloves should be worn. Keys, screwdrivers, and other seemingly innocuous objects can cause trauma if handled improperly. Frequent surveillance of extremities is important to detect signs of injury.

Footwear must be chosen carefully, and new shoes should be worn only for brief periods, with inspection of the feet for signs of irritation. If pressure injury of the foot occurs, special footwear may be constructed to redistribute weight.

Established areas of motor neuropathy require range-of-motion exercises or splinting to prevent contracture. Tendon transfers from unaffected muscles may restore function in selected cases. Areas of trauma or ulceration should be treated aggressively with immobilization, local dressings, and antibiotics.

Table 35-3
Chemotherapeutic Agents Against *M. leprae*

Bactericidal	Bacteriostatic
Rifampin	Dapsone*
Minocycline	Clofazimine*
Ethionamide	
Prothionamide	
Ofloxacin	
Levofloxacin	
Clarithromycin	
Amikacin	
Streptomycin	
Kanamycin	

*The combination of dapsone and clofazimine is bactericidal.

Psychosocial Therapy

All patients with leprosy need education regarding the nature of their disease. In the case of immigrants, the use of an interpreter may be invaluable. Fears of contagion and social rejection must be dealt with directly. Patients should be assured that *therapy will make them noncontagious* and that family and social relationships need not be altered. In many cases, it is best to advise patients not to tell casual contacts of their illness. An attitude of openness and reassurance is important. As in any chronic illness, it is preferable for one, or a few, health professionals to establish a relationship with the patient.

Therapy of Reactional States

The drug of choice for acute reactional states is *prednisone.* Prednisone is used, often in high doses, for limited periods of time to control the inflammatory reactions and prevent permanent sequelae, such as nerve damage. It must be remembered that rifampin alters prednisone metabolism. If patients are taking rifampin, the dose of prednisone must be doubled for comparable efficacy, or the rifampin must be temporarily discontinued or switched to a single monthly dose of 600 mg. Calcium and vitamin D should be prescribed for any patient on long-term corticosteroids.

For acute reversal reaction, prednisone should be initiated promptly in adequate dosage to control neuritis and prevent nerve damage. Doses of 30 to 100 mg/day should be continued until neuritis has resolved, and then tapered over 4 to 6 weeks. Clofazimine, 50 mg/day, may be added to paucibacillary leprosy therapy if nerve involvement is present for additional antibacterial protection in the setting of active neuropathy.

Thalidomide is the therapy of choice for acute ENL. Its use is strictly regulated because of teratogenicity and neurotoxicity. Patients may experience sedation until accustomed to thalidomide. Males and females without childbearing potential are usually controlled with thalidomide, 100 to 400 mg/day. Thalidomide should be tapered to the least dose effective in suppression of new ENL lesions. Additional treatment for acute ENL may include the use of corticosteroids and clofazimine.

In acute or chronic ENL, clofazimine, 100 to 300 mg/day, may be helpful. This medication takes approximately 6 weeks to reach full efficacy. Side effects include reversible mahogany-colored hyperpigmentation of the skin and sclera. At prolonged high doses, nausea or intestinal obstruction can occur. Chronic ENL is managed with thalidomide and clofazimine.

Therapy of Contacts

No satisfactory method has been established for managing household contacts. Trials of bacille Calmette-Guérin vaccine prophylaxis have been of minimal benefit. Dapsone prophylaxis may promote resistance and only delay, rather than prevent, onset of disease. Current practice involves initial examination of all household contacts with appropriate biopsy and periodic reexamination.

Management of Complicated Cases

Consultation in the management of leprosy can be obtained by contacting the US National Hansen's Disease Programs by telephone at (800) 642-2477 or their website at *http://bphc.hrsa.gov/nhdp/.* Additional information can be obtained through the World Health Organization website at *http://www.who.int/lep/.*

REFERENCES

Arnold HL, Odom RB, James WD: Leprosy. In *Andrew's diseases of the skin: clinical dermatology,* ed 8, Philadelphia, 1990, WB Saunders.

Bryceson A, Pfaltzgraff RE: Leprosy, ed 3, *Medicine in the Tropics Series,* Edinburgh, 1990, Churchill Livingstone.

Jacobson RR: The face of Hansen's disease in the United States. *The Star* 51:1, 1992.

Jacobson RR: Treatment. In Hastings RC, editor: *Leprosy,* ed 2, Edinburgh, 1994, Churchill Livingstone.

Jacobson RR, Krahenbuhl JL: Leprosy, *Lancet* 353:655, 1999.

Lockwood DNJ: Contributions of laboratory research to current understanding and management of leprosy, *Tropical Doctor* 22(suppl 1):22, 1992.

Lumpkin LR, Cox GF, Wolf JE: Leprosy in five armadillo handlers, *J Am Acad Dermatol* 9:899, 1983.

Meyers WM: Leprosy. In Strickland GT, editor: *Hunter's tropical medicine,* ed 8, Philadelphia, 1999, WB Saunders.

Rea TH, Levan NE: Lucio's phenomenon and diffuse non-nodular lepromatous leprosy, *Arch Dermatol* 114:1023, 1978.

Rea TH et al: Immunologic responses in patients with lepromatous leprosy, *Arch Dermatol* 112:791, 1976.

Ridley DS: Reactions in leprosy, *Lepr Rev* 40:77, 1969.

Ridley DS, Jopling WH: Classification of leprosy according to immunity. A five group system, *Int J Lepr* 34:255, 1966.

WHO Study Group on the Chemotherapy of Leprosy: *WHO Technical Report Series. No. 847: Chemotherapy of leprosy,* Geneva, 1994, World Health Organization.

SECTION VI

SEXUALLY TRANSMITTED DISEASES

CHAPTER 36

Sexually Transmitted Infections and Foreign Travel

Jeanne M. Marrazzo

Because sexually transmitted infections (STI) are defined by their transmission from one person to another during sex, travel, with its attendant opportunities for new contacts, can facilitate the transmission of STI in several ways. The number of international travelers has increased steadily in recent years, with a trend toward areas of the world endemic for STI not frequently seen in the United States. This allows for the exposure of travelers to relatively uncommon STI, such as chancroid and lymphogranuloma venereum (LGV). In addition, the prevalence of common STI, such as gonorrhea and chlamydia, is much higher in some destinations than in many parts of the United States. This may increase the likelihood of travelers' exposure to these pathogens within any given sexual encounter. Further, persons who purchase sex as part of a "travel experience" are often choosing partners who themselves have a higher likelihood of exposure to STI. Finally, certain STI, such as syphilis, are sensitive indicators of social and economic disruption; travelers to parts of the world that are experiencing wars or socioeconomic upheaval are especially vulnerable to exposure to these infections. The dynamic of STI transmission across borders has a reciprocal side: immigrants and refugees to the United States from areas with high STI prevalence may import these infections, particularly if they are clinically inapparent, as with latent syphilis.

Travelers need to be aware of the risk of STI during travel and to understand measures to protect themselves *and* their prospective sexual partners in foreign countries.

CASUAL SEXUAL ACTIVITY AND TRAVEL

Traditionally, travelers undertaking long and frequent journeys have been recognized to be at risk for STI acquisition during travel. These groups have included long-distance truckers, seafarers, and military troops. However, as more of the population travels for recreational and business purposes, the group at risk for STI acquisition has greatly increased in size and heterogeneity, and risk stratification by occupation or reason for travel becomes less precise. In considering the relationship between international travel and exposure to STI, the major determinant of risk appears to be the individual's personal behavior.

Estimates of the frequency of sex associated with travel indicate that the practice occurs rather commonly, although the magnitude of such estimates depends on the population surveyed and the gender of respondents. Among clients in Norwegian STD clinics, for example, 41% reported having had sex with a new partner abroad in the previous 5 years. Male travelers from Denmark to Greenland reported more than twice the number of lifetime partners than did nontravelers, along with more use of commercial sex and history of STI. Of 996 female travelers surveyed in Sweden, 28% described "casual" sex during travel. Surveys of short-term vacation travelers from Sweden and Australia have shown that up to 60% of travelers of both sexes may engage in casual sex (defined as sex with a previously unknown partner) during a trip. Female travelers were more likely to select partners of their own nationality, whereas male travelers were more likely to select partners from host country nationals and commercial sex workers (CSW). Factors associated with casual sex while abroad were young age, travel without a spouse or partner, and longer duration of stay.

Several studies have examined the likelihood of sexual contacts by people living or employed in foreign or developing countries for long periods, including expatriates, overseas workers, and military personnel. One survey assessed 2289 Dutch marines and naval personnel during a 6-month deployment in Cambodia. Despite an education campaign to increase awareness of STI risk and provision of freely available condoms, 45% reported sexual contact with a local CSW; however, consistent condom use was reported by 89%. Another study reported on Dutch overseas workers who had been in sub-Saharan Africa for an average of 3.7 years: 31% of males and 13% of females had engaged in sexual activity with African nationals. Factors that were highly associated with these sexual contacts included not being accompanied by a "life partner" and any history of previous STI. The length of stay in Africa was moderately to strongly associated with contact with a "non-life partner." A third study looked at Belgian men working in Central Africa: 51% reported extramarital sexual contact with a local woman, and 31% with a CSW.

Despite the known efficacy of condoms in preventing STI transmission, several studies have documented low rates of condom use in travelers. More than two thirds of 757 outpatient clinic clients surveyed in London in 1993 failed to always use condoms with new partners while abroad; exchange of sex for money was common.

SEXUAL TOURISM

Many developing countries have actively fostered development of tourism. Particularly before the recognition of the human immunodeficiency virus (HIV, HIV-1) pandemic, sexual tourism—with the lure of both homosexual and heterosexual sex—was promoted by international tourist agencies, either openly or under the guise of health or "medical treatment" tours. Some of these efforts even underplayed the magnitude of the locally emerging HIV epidemic. As fatalities resulting from AIDS have accrued, the relationship between the commercial sex implied by sexual tourism and HIV acquisition has become more difficult to ignore. However, many local tour agencies may still be reluctant to provide, or certainly to stress, relevant information (and attendant caution) regarding local prevalence of HIV and other STI for fear of discouraging potential clients.

Although specific data on sexual tourism are scarce, many studies have shown that HIV-1 infection is common among CSW: 50% to 85% of urban CSW in Africa are infected with HIV. One tragic consequence of the increased awareness of this risk has been the promotion of child prostitution because of the belief that sex with relatively young persons is safer than with older CSW. This assumption is false: one survey found that approximately 50% of Thai child sex workers were infected with HIV. Young CSW are quickly exposed to the same STI and may even be more likely to become infected with STD during sexual intercourse because of traumatic penetration.

INTERNATIONAL SPREAD OF HIV

The initial explosive spread of HIV-1 infection among residents of sub-Saharan Africa and the rapid spread of HIV through Southeast Asia and South America during the last decade were initially attributed to the high rate of CSW and genital ulcerative diseases (GUD) in these areas. Other factors have emerged as possible contributors, including chemokine receptors such as CCR-5, which confers relative protection to progression of HIV disease and is less common in blacks relative to whites. Whereas HIV transmission in North America, western Europe, Australia, and New Zealand has been predominantly among homosexual men and intravenous drug users (IDU), heterosexual transmission accounts for up to 70% of HIV infections in sub-Saharan Africa and parts of the Caribbean and Asia. In Latin America, the epidemic is shifting from the homosexual and bisexual population to a pattern of heterosexual transmission. The heterosexual transmission of HIV that is seen in developing countries has followed a consistent trend. Predominantly female CSW become infected from infected male clients (who include IDU and international travelers). Male partners of the infected CSW become infected themselves, and can then infect their female spouses at home. These infected women then transmit HIV to their children in subsequent pregnancies.

Industrialized countries are presently experiencing a rise in the proportion of HIV transmission occurring within the heterosexual population, particularly in inner cities among IDU, CSW, and immigrants from high-risk areas. Imported STI in international travelers will likely continue to contribute to this trend. Men engaging in unprotected sex with other men continue to be at risk, and some urban areas in the United States have experienced an alarming reversal of the trend toward protected sex among men who have sex with men (many of whom are infected with HIV already), which could sustain an endemic level of HIV transmission within this group.

RISKS FOR ACQUISITION OF STD AND HIV DURING TRAVEL

Travelers should be advised that unprotected casual sex with fellow travelers is most likely to expose them to infections prevalent in their home countries: predominantly genital herpes, human papillomavirus, chlamydia, and gonorrhea, and depending on the interaction, possibly HIV. Unprotected sex with host-country nationals in the developing world will also potentially expose them to syphilis, chancroid, LGV, and granuloma inguinale—diseases uncommon in Western industrialized countries.

Genital herpes, syphilis, chancroid, LGV, and granuloma inguinale are all causes of GUD. All but genital herpes are bacterial GUD and thus are curable with appropriate antibiotic treatment, and antiviral therapy can lessen the clinical symptoms and viral shedding associated with genital herpes. However, the presence of unhealed genital ulcers during intercourse increases the risk of HIV acquisition and transmission, and possibly of other viral diseases as well. In addition to HIV, sexual transmission of HIV-2 and other viruses (hepatitis B, hepatitis C, and HTLV-1) are a greater risk in parts of the developing world. Whereas GUD appears to be a major risk for increased transmission of HIV, other factors may contribute, including nonulcerative STI (notably, trichomoniasis), cervical ectopy, certain sexual practices (anal intercourse; sex during menses; use of vaginal drying agents), and frequent use of some microbicides, such as nonoxynol-9 (N-9). Among male clients of CSW in Nairobi, increased HIV acquisition appeared to be associated with lack of circumcision, as well as the presence of GUD.

Vaginal use of the spermicide N-9 without condoms reduced the risk for transmission of gonorrhea and chlamydia in one study, but there is no indication that N-9 alone prevents HIV transmission, or that it increases protection against HIV if used with condoms. Although frequent use of vaginal sponges containing high doses of N-9 increased the risk of vaginal ulceration among CSW in a study in Nairobi, not all studies have corroborated this effect. Most experts agree that any adverse effects of N-9 are likely modulated by frequency of use and dosage. The WHO recommends against relying on N-9 as a microbicide, and research into newer microbicides is proceeding.

CONDOMS

The use of condoms is strongly recommended with every act of sexual intercourse when the status of a partner with regard to HIV infection or other STI is unknown; unfortunately, even under the best of circumstances, the protection condoms provide against STI is incomplete. For one thing, the normal breakage rate during vaginal intercourse with properly applied high-quality latex condoms produced in the United States is about 2%; complete slippage occurs about 1% of the time. Similar rates probably apply for anal intercourse, although failure rates as high as 5% have been reported during anal intercourse between men. Condoms manufactured abroad may have a higher breakage rate. Improper storage conditions (heat, moisture) or oil-based lubricants (mineral oil, petroleum jelly, massage oils, body lotions, shortening, cooking oil) can weaken latex condoms and contribute to a higher breakage rate. Use beyond the expiration date also increases the likelihood of breakage.

Latex condoms offer the most reliable barrier against STI. For persons with latex allergy (estimated at 1% to 3% of the U.S. population), polyurethane (plastic) condoms offer an alternative; these are thinner than latex but reportedly stronger, and, unlike latex, are not compromised by use with oil-based lubricants. They are, however, about twice as costly as latex condoms, and may require more lubrication. Finally, natural membrane condoms (often incorrectly called "lambskin" condoms) are generally made from lamb cecum; the membranous latticework of fibers can have pores up to 1500 nm in diameter. While they will prevent the passage of sperm, the pores are more than 10 times the diameter of HIV and more than 25 times the diameter of the hepatitis B virus. Laboratory studies suggest that viral transmission can occur with natural membrane condoms; hence, although clinical data are not available, it is generally recommended that they be avoided. They are more costly than latex as well.

The relative protection that condoms afford against STI acquisition is significant, but not complete; abstinence remains the only sure method for avoiding STI. In several studies of couples who were discordant for the presence of HIV infection, use of condoms significantly reduced the risk of HIV transmission to the uninfected partner (up to a 10-fold reduction).

Table 36-1
Sources of Information Regarding Condom Usage and Effectiveness*

Source	Issues discussed
Consumer Reports: How Reliable Are Condoms? Consumer Reports, June 1999 Reprints available from: Consumer Union Bulk Reprints 101 Truman Avenue Yonkers, NY 10703-1057 (914) 378-2448	Used water test and air burst test Rates condoms by projected failure rate Includes data on features of individual brands and brand preferences of surveyed readers
Workshop summary: Scientific Evidence on Condom Effectiveness for STD Prevention (June 2000) Available at www.niaid.nih.gov	Extensive review of all available studies of condom's effectiveness in reducing STD/HIV transmission
The Latex Condom: Recent Advances, Future Directions. Family Health International Available at: www.fhi.org, or Family Health International HIV/AIDS Department 2101 Wilson Boulevard, Suite 700; Arlington, VA 22201	Monograph that describes correct placement and usage of condoms and gives an overview of efficacy of latex condoms and alternatives

*In addition to the sources cited in the table, a number of informative internet sites offer comprehensive material on ratings and availability of various condoms.

A meta-analysis of published studies on condoms and heterosexual HIV transmission concluded that although condoms correctly used were about 90% effective in preventing pregnancy, they were only about 69% (range, 46% to 82%) effective in preventing heterosexual transmission of HIV. However, this meta-analysis has been critiqued by some authors, and most experts agree that condoms afford a considerable, if not a perfect, impediment to HIV transmission.

Availability and use of the female condom have been increasing worldwide. Although its relatively high cost can present a considerable deterrent, it offers a significant advance in female-controlled methods of barrier protection. The female condom is slightly less effective for preventing pregnancy compared with male condoms; clinical studies in small numbers of women indicate protection against trichomoniasis reinfection, implying, but not yet proving, similar protection against other STI. Studies evaluating this finding are underway.

Travelers should also be advised that the use of alcohol or drugs can negatively affect their decision and ability to correctly use a condom.

ADVICE TO TRAVELERS

Limited data suggest that international travelers and expatriate workers generally purport to be aware of the risks of STI transmission and the protection afforded by condoms; furthermore, the vast majority of travelers state they would "always" use condoms during casual sex. As the studies alluded to here show, however, travelers, and especially long-term travelers, are likely to engage in casual sex, and the unfortunate reality is that condoms are used consistently by less than 25% during high-risk sex. Female travelers may be less likely than males to negotiate successful use of male condoms; availability of the female condom may offer a welcome alternative. Travelers may actually be unaware of the risks of STI, or they may be unable or unwilling to restrict themselves to safe sex practices despite recognition of the risks; regardless, compliance is low and travel medicine practitioners should make every effort to reverse this. In addition to information about risk of STI acquisition, they should ensure that the traveler is familiar with appropriate barrier protection and its proper use. Sources of condom information are given in Table 36-1.

Advice to travelers should include the following: (1) discuss the possibility of casual sex while abroad, (2) stress the importance of careful selection of partners, (3) discourage participation in exploitive sexual tourism, (4) encourage the inclusion of high-quality latex condoms in the traveler's medical kit, and (5) warn about the effects of alcohol and other mind-altering substances that can contribute to incautious behavior. Travelers should also be aware that cultural biases in sexual partners from the host country could be a strong deterrent to the use of condoms.

Finally, travelers should be strongly encouraged to overcome the understandable reluctance to talk about personal sexual matters, and to be sure to contact their personal physician or travel medicine clinic upon return from travel if any unprotected sexual exposures occurred.

REFERENCES

Artenstein AW: Multiple introductions of HIV-1 subtype E into the western hemisphere, *Lancet* 346:1197, 1995.

Arvidson M et al: Sexual risk behavior and history of sexually transmitted diseases in relation to casual travel sex during different types of journeys, *Acta Obstet Gynecol Scand* 75:490, 1996.

Centers for Disease Control: Update: barrier protection against HIV infection and other sexually transmitted diseases, *MMWR* 42:589-591, 597, 1993.

D'Oro LC et al: Barrier methods of contraception, spermicides, and sexually transmitted diseases: a review, *Genitourin Med* 70:410, 1994.

Hawkes S et al: Risk behavior and HIV prevalence in international travelers, *AIDS* 8:247, 1994.

Hawkes S et al: Risk behaviour and STD acquisition in genitourinary clinic attenders who have Traveled, *Genitourin Med* 71:351, 1995.

Hopperus Buma APCC et al: Sexual behavior and sexually transmitted diseases in Dutch marines and naval personnel on an United Nations mission to Cambodia, *Genitourin Med* 71:172, 1995.

Kreiss J et al: Efficacy of nonoxynol-9 contraceptive sponge use in preventing heterosexual acquisition of HIV in Nairobi prostitutes, *JAMA* 268:477, 1992.

Laga M et al: Non-ulcerative sexually transmitted diseases as risk factor for HIV-1 transmission in women: results from a cohort study, *AIDS* 7:95, 1993.

MacLean JD: Screening returning travelers, *Infect Dis Clin North Am* 12:431, 1998.

Melbye M, Biggar RJ: A profile of HIV-risk behaviours among travelers: a population-based study of Danes visiting Greenland, *Scand J Social Med* 22:204, 1994.

Mulhall BP: Sex and travel: studies of sexual behaviour, disease and health promotion in international travelers: a global review, *Int J STD AIDS* 7:455, 1996.
Mulhall BP: Sexual behaviour in travelers, *Lancet* 353:595, 1999.
Obbo C: HIV transmission through social and geographic networks in Uganda, *Soc Sci Med* 36:949, 1993.
Plummer FA et al: Co-factors in male-female transmission of HIV. *J Infect Dis* 163:233, 1991.
Saracco A et al: Man-to-woman sexual transmission of HIV: longitudinal study of 343 steady partners of infected men, *J Acquir Immune Defic Syndr* 6:497, 1993.
Thorpe L et al: Correlates of condom use among female prostitutes and tourist clients in Bali, Indonesia, *AIDS Care* 9:181, 1997.
Tveit KS et al: Casual sexual experience abroad in patients attending an STD clinic and at high risk for HIV infection, *Genitourin Med* 70:12, 1994.
Van den Hoek A: STDs, HIV/AIDS, ethnicity, and migrant populations. In Holmes KK et al, editors: *Sexually transmitted diseases,* ed 3, New York, 1999, McGraw Hill.
Wasserheit JN: Effect of changes in human ecology and behavior on patterns of sexually transmitted diseases, including human immunodeficiency virus infection, *Proc Natl Acad Sci USA* 91:2430, 1994.
Weller SC: A meta-analysis of condom effectiveness in reducing sexually transmitted HIV, *Soc Sci Med* 36:1635, 1993.

CHAPTER 37

Gonococcal and Chlamydial Genital Infections, and Pelvic Inflammatory Disease

Jeanne M. Marrazzo

Infections caused by *Neisseria gonorrhoeae* and *Chlamydia trachomatis* are the most common of the bacterial sexually transmitted infections (STI). In 1995 genital chlamydial infections became the most frequently reported bacterial infection in the United States. This chapter reviews the global epidemiology of these two pathogens, their associated clinical syndromes, and current guidelines for their management.

EPIDEMIOLOGY

Although the annual incidence of gonococcal infections in the United States declined from 1 million in the early 1980s to 650,000 in 1996, densely urbanized areas, particularly in the Southeast, still evidence high rates of infection. The highest rates occur in persons between the ages of 20 and 24 years, although girls aged 15 to 19 years evidence only slightly lower rates than their older counterparts. In the early 1980s, gonorrhea was a relatively common STI among men who reported sex with men (MSM). While gonorrhea rates among MSM declined markedly with the adoption of safer sex practices in response to the human immunodeficiency virus (HIV) epidemic, some areas have recently experienced an upswing in this infection, with a concomitant increase in report of unprotected anal sex between men. While gonorrhea typically infects the cervix or urethra, both rectal and pharyngeal infections occur and are an important reservoir of asymptomatic infection, which helps to promote sexual transmission.

An estimated 2 million new chlamydial infections occur annually in the United States, and 3 million occur in Europe. In 1995 the World Health Organization estimated that 89 million new cases would occur worldwide. In contrast to gonorrhea, these infections are more widely geographically distributed and peak in even younger age groups, at least in women, since the epidemiology in men has not been well defined. Biological and social factors (namely, cervical ectopy and choice of sex partners) likely play a role in placing adolescent females at highest risk for chlamydial infection. The incidence of this disease has declined dramatically in some areas, probably in response to widespread screening programs begun in the 1980s. However, the initiation of these programs was superimposed on a background of the emphasis of safer sex in response to the burgeoning HIV epidemic, which may have played some role. Chlamydia prevalence remains high in many areas of the country in which screening has not become routine, approaching or exceeding 15% to 25% in some adolescent populations.

The prevalence of gonorrhea and chlamydia infections, as well as other STI, is higher in developing countries than in the United States, although surveillance data from many areas are not comprehensive. The impact of both of these diseases goes beyond the obvious clinical and economic concerns, and beyond even that of their well-recognized sequelae for women (which include ectopic pregnancy, tubal infertility, and chronic pelvic pain). Both gonorrhea and chlamydia potentiate infectiousness for and susceptibility to HIV. Urethral infection with *N. gonorrhoeae* is associated with an eightfold increase in the amount of HIV in semen. In a prospective study of commercial sex workers (CSW) in Kenya, acquisition of cervical chlamydial infection was associated with a 2.5-fold increase in the likelihood of acquiring HIV. Thus these infections further fuel the HIV epidemic throughout Africa, Asia, and Latin America, along with other factors such as migration of refugees, population shifts from rural to urban environments, and persistence of commercial sex and illicit drug use.

URETHRITIS

Urethritis is the most common STI-related syndrome in males throughout the world, with *N. gonorrhoeae* most commonly associated with the prototypical purulent discharge characterizing this syndrome. However, in the United States, most urethritis is nongonococcal in origin (NGU); of all NGU, 30% to 40% of cases are caused by *C. trachomatis,* and the remainder by a variety of etiologic agents including *Trichomonas vaginalis,* herpes simplex virus (HSV), adenovirus, and genital mycoplasms. The role of *Ureaplasma urealyticum* in causing urethritis is still unclear (see later discussions).

The situation in many parts of the developing world is strikingly different, with *N. gonorrhoeae* accounting for up to 80% of all urethritis. The reasons for this disparity are poorly understood; inability to accurately diagnose other causes of urethritis may be partly responsible. Many studies reported from developing countries have used suboptimal methodologies for the detection of *C. trachomatis* and have probably underestimated its true contribution. The availability of nucleic acid amplified assays (NAAT) for both gonorrhea and chlamydia (discussed later) should clarify their etiologic contributions. Finally, because NGU is usually a milder disease than gonococcal urethritis, differences in the threshold for medical evaluation may exist, particularly in countries where the availability of medical care is compromised.

Most men infected with *N. gonorrhoeae* at the urethra experience purulent or mucopurulent penile discharge and dysuria, although symptomatic status is likely influenced by the duration of infection and specific strain type. Complications include epididymitis and urethral strictures; although these are rare, they are more common in developing countries. Examination of Gram-stained smears of urethral secretions reveals the gram-negative, kidney-shaped intracellular diplococci in 98% of cases and is 99% specific for the diagnosis. Gonococcal cultures are preferred in addition to Gram stain, both for confirmation of the diagnosis and for antibiotic susceptibility testing. NAAT, including ligase chain reaction (LCR), polymerase chain reaction (PCR), and transcription mediated assay (TMA), offer some increase in sensitivity (5% to 8%) over culture while maintaining specificity. Perhaps most important, NAAT can be performed on first-catch urine (not "clean-catch," or midstream urine), obviating the need for urethral swab collection.

C. trachomatis has been the traditional explanation for 40% to 60% of cases of NGU in the United States and Europe, but this percentage has recently declined, and is as low as 15% in some areas which have experienced a decline in chlamydia prevalence overall. *U. urealyticum* may be found in 30% to 40% of cases, but its role as a pathogen is debated, as it has been detected in an equal percentage of men without urethritis in some studies. Apart from gonorrhea and chlamydia, other organisms known to cause urethritis include *T. vaginalis,* HSV, (especially with primary infection), adenovirus, and genital mycoplasms (especially *Mycoplasma genitalium*). Even less is known concerning the etiology and epidemiology of NGU in developing countries.

NGU is generally a milder illness than gonococcal urethritis, presenting with less purulent discharge, but the clinical overlap is significant. Diagnostic testing is required to distinguish the etiology of urethritis, and both gonorrhea and chlamydia should be specifically sought if possible. The finding of significant numbers of polymorphonuclear leukocytes (PMN) (≥5 per high power field) *without* gram-negative intracellular diplococci is sufficient to make a presumptive diagnosis of NGU. *N. gonorrhoeae* can be easily cultured on chocolate agar; culture for *C. trachomatis,* in contrast, is not widely available due to its technical demand. A variety of antigen detection tests based on the enzyme immunoassay (EIA) and direct fluorescent antibody (DFA) are available for chlamydia, as is a nonamplified DNA probe (GenProbe). However, if available and affordable, NAAT for chlamydia (LCR, PCR, TMA) offer a marked increase in sensitivity relative to other tests and can be performed on first catch urine, without the requirement of a urethral swab. Rapid diagnostic tests for *C. trachomatis* are available, but are neither sufficiently sensitive nor specific to recommend their use.

In women, *C. trachomatis* may directly infect the urethra, inducing dysuria that may simulate bacterial cystitis. This presentation is generally characterized by the presence of PMN but no bacteria in the urine and often accompanied by a history of a new sex partner. Up to 50% of these women are also infected at the cervix, and all should undergo diagnostic cervical testing; although the urethra can be cultured, NAAT performed on urine are particularly advantageous in this situation.

CERVICITIS

Cervical gonococcal infections are usually asymptomatic. When symptoms are present, they include vaginal discharge, intermenstrual bleeding, dyspareunia, and/or abdominal pain. Similarly, only 10% of infected cervices will evidence signs, which include mucopurulent endocervical discharge, easily induced endocervical bleeding, and cervical edema. Up to 50% of women with gonococcal cervicitis may also have gonococcal urethritis with associated dysuria, but even more will have concomitant asymptomatic colonization of the urethra. Reports of disseminated gonococcal infection (DGI) to sites such as the skin and joints (causing rash and arthritis) in the United States has declined, but isolated tenosynovitis or acute arthritis is not uncommon as a manifestation of sexually acquired gonorrhea. In developing countries, the epidemiology of DGI is less well characterized. DGI occurs more commonly in women.

Gonococcal infection of the cervix may be diagnosed by culture, NAAT of the cervix or urine, or nonamplified DNA probe. Urine testing is sensitive for the detection of cervical infection because it not only detects concomitant gonococcal urethral infection, which occurs frequently, but also tests cervicovaginal secretions that have collected in the vulvar area. Obtaining rectal and pharyngeal specimens may increase the yield of case detection, particularly if receptive oral or anal intercourse is reported. Gram stain of endocervical discharge suggests the diagnosis of gonorrhea if intracellular gram-negative diplococci are seen, but this occurs in only 50% of cases, making the test too insensitive to use as the sole means of diagnosis. In cases of suspected DGI, cultures or NAAT of the genital tract should be done, as well as blood and joint aspirate cultures.

Like gonorrhea, chlamydial infections in women are usually asymptomatic (90%). Because symptoms of cervicitis are nonspecific, if at all present, chlamydial cervical infection may present exactly like gonococcal infection. Similarly, signs occur in a minority of patients (10%), and include induced endocervical bleeding, mucopurulent endocervical discharge, and edematous ectopy. Certainly, any of these should provoke diagnostic testing with the methods discussed previously. NAAT testing of cervix clearly has a higher yield than other diagnostic methods. Given the high prevalence of chlamydia in many settings, particularly in adolescent females, routine testing of young women at any presentation for STD evaluation is recommended. This is especially critical because asymptomatic untreated chlamydial infections are capable of causing tubal scarring, which can lead to infertility, ectopic pregnancy, and chronic pelvic pain.

PELVIC INFLAMMATORY DISEASE

N. gonorrhoeae and *C. trachomatis* are the causal STI implicated most often in pelvic inflammatory disease (PID), but in recent years the role of anaerobes, gram-negative rods, and genital mycoplasms has been stressed, emphasizing that PID is usually a polymicrobial process. Serious consequences of PID include infertility, ectopic pregnancy, tuboovarian abscess, chronic pelvic pain, and pelvic adhesions.

Although clinical criteria for diagnosis of PID are inexact, the diagnosis should be suspected if cervical motion, adnexal, or lower abdominal tenderness is present on bimanual pelvic examination. The finding of adnexal tenderness is the most sensitive, and a presumptive diagnosis may be made if present. Women evidencing any of these signs should be tested for gonorrhea and chlamydia, and pregnancy should be ruled out. Treatment of women with presumptive PID requires broad-spectrum coverage that includes activity against *N. gonorrhoeae* and *C. trachomatis.* A complete discussion of the diagnosis and treatment of PID is beyond the scope of this chapter; however, several up-to-date reviews have been included in the references, and recommended antibiotic treatment regimens are given in Table 37-1.

TREATMENT OF GONORRHEA AND CHLAMYDIA

Resistant strains of *N. gonorrhoeae* originally appeared in the United States as imported infections in servicemen returning from Southeast Asia in the mid 1970s. In 1994, approximately 16% of all gonococci in the United States were resistant to penicillin on the basis of either plasmid-mediated or chromosomal resistance; they are designated penicillinase-producing *N. gonorrhoeae* (PPNG). In some urban areas, the proportion of gonococcal isolates that are PPNG may approach 60% to 75%. Strains of gonococci that have also acquired plasmid-mediated tetracycline resistance are designated tetracycline-resistant *N. gonorrhoeae* (TRNG) and constituted 22% of isolates in 1994. Some multidrug-resistant strains are both PPNG and

Table 37-1
Recommendations for Treatment of Pelvic Inflammatory Disease

Outpatient Therapy
Regimen A: Ofloxacin 400 mg orally twice daily for 14 days, OR Levofloxacin 500 mg orally once daily for 14 days
WITH OR WITHOUT
Metronidazole 500 mg orally twice daily for 14 days
Regimen B: Ceftriaxone 250 mg IM once, OR Cefoxitin 2 g IM plus Probenecid 1 g orally as a single dose, OR other third-generation parenteral cephalosporin (e.g., ceftizoxime or cefotaxime)
PLUS
Doxycycline 100 mg orally twice daily for 14 days,
WITH OR WITHOUT
Metronidazole 500 mg orally twice daily for 7 days

Inpatient Therapy
Regimen A: Cefotetan 2 g IV every 12 hours OR Cefoxitin 2 g IV every 6 hours,
PLUS
Doxycycline 100 mg orally every 12 hours
Regimen B: Clindamycin 900 mg IV every 8 hours,
PLUS
Gentamicin loading dose IV or IM (2 mg/kg) then 1.5 mg/kg every 8 hours (may be given as a single daily dose instead)

From CDC: Sexually transmitted diseases treatment guidelines—2002, *MMWR* 47(RR-01):50, 2002.

TRNG. Another 10% to 15% of gonococci studied in the United States have chromosomally mediated resistance to multiple drugs (penicillin, tetracycline, second-generation cephalosporins, and erythromycin).

Most recently, gonococci have acquired resistance to fluoroquinolone (including ciprofloxacin and ofloxacin). This is particularly prevalent in Southeast Asia and the Philippines, where the percentage of resistant strains is substantial; persons being treated for gonorrhea after potential exposure in these areas should be empirically treated with a cephalosporin, and antimicrobial susceptibility of the organism assessed. Prevalence of fluoroquinolone-resistant strains in the United States is low at present (<2%) but rapidly rising in Hawaii and California. For this reason fluoroquinolones are not recommended as first line therapy in these areas.

To simplify the approach to treatment and to cover the "worst-case" scenario, the Centers for Disease Control and Prevention (CDC) recommends that all gonococcal infections be treated as if they were multidrug resistant. This is particularly applicable to gonorrhea acquired during travel abroad in developing countries. In addition, because chlamydial coinfection may be present in 10% to 30% of patients with gonorrhea, presumptive treatment for chlamydia should be provided.

Approved drug regimens are given in Tables 37-2 and 37-3. Oral regimens for gonorrhea treatment are less expensive to administer and more acceptable to patients. The single-dose treatment of azithromycin for chlamydia is preferred given its obvious advantage in compliance. Note that a cephalosporin, either ceftriaxone or cefixime, should be used for treatment of gonorrhea in pregnant women for whom fluoroquinolones are

Table 37-2
Treatment for Uncomplicated Gonococcal and Chlamydial Infections in Adults

Treatment for gonococcal infection*
Use one of the following:
- Cefixime 400 mg PO mg once
- Ceftriaxone 125 mg IM (single dose)
- Ciprofloxacin 500 mg PO once
- Ofloxacin 400 mg PO once
- Levofloxacin 250 mg PO once

Treatment for chlamydial infection
Use one of the following:
- Azithromycin 1 g PO as single dose (preferred)
- Erythromycin base 500 mg orally qid × 7 days
- Erythromycin ethylsuccinate 800 mg orally qid × 7 days
- Doxycyline 100 mg PO bid × 7 days
- Ofloxacin 300 mg PO bid × 7 days
- Levofloxacin 500 mg orally for 7 days

From CDC: Sexually transmitted diseases treatment guidelines—2002, *MMWR* 47(RR-01):33, 2002.
*Persons with documented gonococcal infection should be empirically treated for chlamydial infection as well.

Table 37-3
Treatment for Gonococcal and Chlamydial Infections in Pregnant Women

Treatment for uncomplicated gonococcal infection
Use one of the following:
- Ceftriaxone 250 mg IM (single dose)
- Cefixime 400 to 800 mg PO once
- Spectinomycin 2 g IM (single dose)

Treatment for uncomplicated chlamydial infection*
Use one of the following:
- Amoxicillin 500 mg PO TID × 7 days
- Azithromycin 1 g PO as single dose
- Erythromycin base 500 mg orally qid × 7 days
- Erythromycin base 500 mg PO qid × 7 days†
- Erythromycin ethylsuccinate 400 mg orally qid × 14 days

From CDC: Sexually transmitted diseases treatment guidelines—2002. *MMWR* 47(RR-1):35, 2002.
*Test of cure should be routine (3 weeks after initiation of therapy).
†Erythromycin estolate is contraindicated during pregnancy.

contraindicated. Amoxicillin is the recommended regimen for the treatment of chlamydia in pregnant women, but azithromycin is an alternative and has been increasingly used. Regardless of the antibiotic chosen, a test of cure at 3 weeks after completion of therapy is essential in pregnant women; no test of cure is otherwise routinely required.

Recommendations for treating rectal gonorrhea, gonorrhea in children, neonatal gonococcal infections, gonococcal ophthalmia, and complicated or disseminated gonococcal infections are covered in the CDC treatment guidelines for sexually transmitted diseases.

REFERENCES

Black CM: Current methods of laboratory diagnosis of *Chlamydia trachomatis* infections, *Clin Microbiol Rev* 10:160, 1997.

Centers for Disease Control and Prevention: Sexually transmitted diseases treatment guidelines—2002, *MMWR* 51(RR06):1, 2002

Fox KK et al: Antimicrobial resistance in *Neisseria gonorrhoeae* in the United States, 1988-1994: the emergence of decreased susceptibility to the fluoroquinolones, *J Infect Dis* 175:1396, 1997.

Marrazzo JM, Stamm WE: New approaches to the diagnosis, treatment, and prevention of Chlamydial infection. In Remington JS, Swartz MN, editors: *Current clinical topics in infectious diseases,* ed 18, Boston, 1998, Blackwell Science.

Holmes KK et al, editors: *Sexually transmitted diseases,* ed 3, New York, 1999, McGraw Hill.

World Health Organization: Sexually transmitted diseases. Press release WHO/64; 25 August 1995.

CHAPTER 38

Syphilis

Connie Celum

Syphilis is prevalent throughout much of the developing world, with 12 million cases estimated by the WHO worldwide in 1995. Reliable incidence data are rarely available. Surveys based on serologic tests are difficult to interpret because nonvenereal treponemal diseases (i.e., yaws and pinta) that were or are still endemic in many of these areas may cause reactive serologic tests for syphilis through cross-reactive antibodies. Unfortunately, the serologic assays do not differentiate between *T. pallidum* and the nonvenereal treponemes. The yaws eradication campaign of the later 1950s decreased the prevalence of these other diseases, but they have recently shown signs of resurgence in some areas.

The area of the world that currently appears to be experiencing the largest syphilis epidemic is Russia and other eastern European countries. The incidence of syphilis among women in the Russian Federation increased from 8.7 cases/100,000 to 252/100,000 between 1985 and 1996. Vertical transmission of syphilis remains a problem in Russia and countries where syphilis is prevalent in women of reproductive age, resulting in a high incidence of congenital syphilis, as well as numerous spontaneous abortions and stillbirths. In one study from Zambia, early syphilis was found in 7.6% of women attending an antenatal clinic. Control of syphilis in these countries therefore has significant public health ramifications.

In the tropics and developing countries, an increased risk of acquiring human immunodeficiency virus (HIV) has been demonstrated in the presence of genital ulcers as a result of syphilis, herpes, chancroid, and other causes. All patients with suspected or confirmed syphilis should also be tested for HIV infection. In patients with early syphilis and concurrent HIV infection, the clinical course of syphilis and the response to treatment may be altered: rapid progression to neurosyphilis (with resultant treatment failure following conventional doses of benzathine penicillin G) has been observed early in a number of HIV-infected persons. There have also been case reports of atypical and severe cutaneous manifestations of syphilis in HIV-infected persons.

ETIOLOGY

Syphilis results from infection with the spirochete *Treponema pallidum.* Numerous monographs have been written describing the protean manifestations of syphilis, and excellent recent reviews are available in the major medical and infectious disease texts. This discussion will be limited to specific aspects of syphilis relevant to understanding and treating tropical sexually transmitted infections (STIs).

CLINICAL PRESENTATION

Primary Syphilis

The classic chancre of primary syphilis is a painless ulcer with an indurated margin and a clean base that develops at the site of inoculation an average of three weeks post-infection. Unfortunately, variable clinical manifestations are sufficient to make clinical diagnosis of primary syphilis unreliable. Secondary bacterial infection of these ulcers is uncommon. Unilateral or bilateral painless, nonsuppurative inguinal adenopathy follows appearance of the chancre by several days. Spontaneous resolution of the chancre and adenopathy usually occurs within 6 weeks. Chancres may not be noticed by the patient, particularly in difficult to visualize areas such as the perianal area or labia.

Secondary Syphilis

The lesions of secondary syphilis usually appear about six weeks after the primary chancre heals. The cutaneous manifestations are extremely varied and include macular, maculopapular, nodular, pustular, or follicular skin rashes, condylomata lata (nontender, sometimes moist, wart-like papules in the genital region), mucous patches in the mouth and, less commonly, alopecia. Papular, hyperpigmented lesions appear to be particularly common in black-skinned individuals. Palmar or plantar lesions, if present, may suggest the diagnosis of secondary syphilis. The skin eruption is usually nonpruritic, but some patients complain of itching and present with excoriated lesions. Secondary syphilis must be considered in the differential diagnosis of *any* generalized skin eruption. Mild constitutional symptoms may accompany or precede the cutaneous lesions. Headache, malaise, and fatigue are the most common. Generalized nontender lymphadenopathy and hepatosplenomegaly are relatively common. If untreated, approximately 25% of patients with secondary syphilis will relapse, typically within one year.

Latent and Tertiary Syphilis

Latent syphilis as a diagnosis is often based on a positive serology in the absence of clinical disease. For the reasons noted earlier, the interpretation of positive serologies is difficult in the tropics, and hence the diagnosis of latent syphilis will often be presumptive. The major public health concern is that pregnant women with latent syphilis are capable of transmitting the infection to the fetus.

When symptomatic, late syphilis usually manifests as neurosyphilis, cardiovascular syphilis, or gummatous disease. The incidence of these manifestations seems to be declining worldwide, probably owing in part to the widespread use of antibiotics for other indications.

DIAGNOSIS

The preferred diagnostic procedure for primary and secondary syphilis is identification of spirochetes by darkfield microscopy or fluorescent monoclonal antibodies of serous exudate or scrapings obtained from lesions. Commensal spirochetes that reside in the oropharynx and intestinal tract can be difficult to differentiate from *T. pallidum* by morphologic criteria, making darkfield examination of oral and rectal lesions less reliable, unless the sample is taken from a characteristic lesion of early syphilis, for example, oral mucous patch or condylomata lata.

Serologic tests for syphilis can be classified as follows: (1) nonspecific, nontreponemal tests (i.e., Venereal Disease Research Laboratory [VDRL] or rapid plasma reagin [RPR]); and (2) specific treponemal tests (Table 38-1). The nontreponemal serologic tests are fairly sensitive and are inexpensive; the VDRL and RPR are used for screening and for quantifying the titer after to treatment. The treponemal serologic tests have a higher specificity and are used to confirm the diagnosis of syphilis following a reactive nontreponemal test. Biologic false-positive reactions are seen in both the nontreponemal and treponemal assays, but simultaneous false-positive reactions in both tests are unusual. There are a number of causes of false-positive serologic tests for syphilis, including nonvenereal treponemal diseases that induce seropositivity in either nontreponemal or treponemal tests and other diseases endemic in the tropics, such as malaria and leprosy (Table 38-2).

Approximately 80% of patients with primary syphilis will be seropositive by VDRL or RPR; the FTA typically becomes reactive earlier than the treponemal tests in primary syphilis. Virtually 100% of patients with sec-

Table 38-1
Serologic Tests for Syphilis

Nontreponemal serologic tests:	
VDRL	Venereal Disease Research Laboratory test
RPR	Rapid plasma reagin card test
Treponemal serologic tests:	
FTA-ABS	Fluorescent treponemal antibody absorption
MHA-TP	Microhemagglutination assay for antibodies to *T. pallidum*
TP-PA	Passive particle agglutination test for *T. pallidum*

Table 38-2
Causes of Biologically False-Positive Tests for Syphilis

Spirochetal diseases	Other tropical infections	Other infections	Other conditions
Yaws*	Leprosy	Varicella (chickenpox)	Connective tissue diseases
Pinta*	Malaria		
Bejel*	Chancroid	Rubeola (measles)	Illicit drug use
Leptospirosis	Lymphogranuloma venereum	Infectious mononucleosis	Advanced age
Rat-bite fever			Pregnancy
Relapsing fever	Trypanosomiasis	Other viruses	Malignancy
Lyme disease	Rickettsial infections	Immunizations	Cirrhosis
	Hepatitis	*Mycoplasma pneumoniae*	

*Nonvenereal treponematosis.

Table 38-3
Sensitivity and Specificity of Serologic

	Sensitivity by Stage for Untreated Syphilis				
	Primary	Secondary latent	Early latent	Late	Specificity*
Nontreponemal Serologic Tests:					
VDRL	78%	100%	96%	71%	98%
RPR	86%	100%	98%	73%	98%
Treponemal Serologic Tests:					
FTA-ABS	84%	100%	100%	96%	97%
MHA-TP	76%	100%	97%	94%	99%

Adapted from Larsen S, Hunter E, Kraus S (eds): *A Manual of Tests for Syphilis,* Washington, DC, 1990, American Public Health Association.
*May not apply for patients from countries with endemic nonvenereal treponematosis.

ondary syphilis will have a reactive VDRL or RPR with higher titers than other stages of syphilis (i.e., typically with VDRL or RPR ≥1:32). Antibody levels detected with the nontreponemal tests fall slowly following *treatment;* however, they also fall slowly with *time,* so that only about 70% of patients with untreated late latent syphilis will be seropositive with the nontreponemal tests (Table 38-3).

In contrast, seropositivity in the specific treponemal assays is usually present for life, particularly if the patient has not been treated. Recently, however, a study has shown that 24% of patients with primary syphilis had a nonreactive fluorescent treponemal antibody absorption (FTA-ABS) test at 36 months following treatment, and 13% had nonreactive microhemagglutination tests for *T. pallidum* (MHA-TP). Thus a nonreactive treponemal test does not rule out a past history of syphilis.

Lumbar puncture with cerebrospinal fluid (CSF) examination is used to detect central nervous system (CNS) involvement in syphilis. It should be performed on patients with latent syphilis of greater than 1 year's duration who meet specific criteria (Table 38-4). Some experts recommend performing a lumbar puncture on anyone with latent syphilis as well as HIV-infected patients regardless of syphilis stage, and it must be done for all patients with early syphilis who have evidence of meningitis or early neurologic involvement.

Patients who have lived in areas where nonvenereal treponemal diseases are prevalent are likely to have a positive syphilis serology because of exposure to these infections. It has been argued in the past that they do not routinely require lumbar puncture because of low yield from CSF examination. However, one cannot be absolutely certain that a positive serology is due to these nonvenereal infections, particularly in sexually-active persons from countries with a high prevalence of STDs and HIV. Lumbar puncture should be considered in working up a positive serology in immigrants or long-term residents of areas where treponemal diseases are endemic, factoring in their age, sexual history, clinical findings, and HIV status.

Table 38-4
Indications for Lumbar Puncture in Syphilis

Pretreatment
1. PS, SS, ELS, or LLS with meningeal, neurologic, ophthalmologic signs
2. LLS if nontreponemal serology ≥1:32
3. ELS or LLS if nonpenicillin therapy planned (If LP indicates CNS involvement, change to penicillin regimen)
4. LLS with aortitis, iritis, or gummatous disease (i.e., symptoms of tertiary disease)
5. ELS or LLS if patient is HIV antibody-positive (Some authorities would perform LP regardless of stage)

Note: LP may be considered in ELS or LLS regardless of presence of the above
If LP confirms CNS involvement, the patient must be treated with a regimen effective against neurosyphilis

Posttreatment
1. Following neurosyphilis treatment regimen (LP every 6 months until normal; retreat if not normal within 2 years)
2. Development of neurologic signs or symptoms
3. Serologic treatment failure
   a. Serologic follow-up at 3 and 6 months for PS, SS with continued follow-up quarterly if titers do not decline fourfold.
   b. Serologic follow-up at 3, 6, 12, and 24 months for ELS and LLS.
4. HIV-infected patients
   a. Requires serologic follow-up at 1, 2, 3, 6, 9, and 12 months, and some authorities would follow for life.
   b. Some authorities urge neurosyphilis treatment regimen regardless of stage of disease, and some urge follow-up LP regardless of treatment regimen used.
5. An abnormal post-treatment LP mandates retreatment with a neurosyphilis regimen

LP, Lumbar puncture, *PS,* primary syphilis; *SS,* secondary syphilis; *ELS,* early latent syphilis; *LLS,* late latent syphilis; *CNS,* central nervous system; *HIV,* human immunodeficiency virus.

TREATMENT

T. pallidum has remained exquisitely sensitive to penicillin, which remains the treatment of choice for all forms of syphilis. Treatment regimens for primary, secondary, and early latent syphilis (<1 year's duration) are well established. A recent multicenter, randomized trial of enhanced therapy (6 g of amoxicillin daily plus probenecid) demonstrated comparable clinical and serologic outcomes, compared to standard benzathine penicillin regimens (2.4 million units IM), regardless of HIV status. Thus the same treatment regimens are used for given stages of syphilis, regardless of HIV status. As mentioned previously, many experts recommend a lumbar puncture in HIV-infected persons with syphilis regardless of HIV status. The optimal management strategies for late latent syphilis, neurosyphilis, and cardiovascular syphilis (which is uncommon) are still debated; a summation of generally accepted recommendations is discussed in the following section (see also Table 38-5), but the reader is referred to the References section for sources on management, in particular the 2002 Centers for Disease Control and Prevention (CDC) guidelines. The management of congenital syphilis and syphilis during pregnancy are beyond the scope of this chapter; please consult the References section as well.

Table 38-5
Management and Treatment of Syphilis

Stage	Treatment*	Minimum follow-up testing	Special considerations for HIV disease
Primary, secondary, or if exposed to syphilis within previous 90 days (or if exposed in past year and follow-up on serology is problematic)	Benzathine penicillin G 2.4 million U IM	3 and 6 mo. Continue follow-up and consider re-treatment if < fourfold decline after six months	Follow-up at 1, 2, 3, 6, 9, 12 mo Serologic treatment failures need CSF exam; if negative, then retreat as for late latent syphilis
Latent (early) with negative CSF	Same as above	3, 6, 12, (24) mo	Pretreatment CSF exam mandatory Treat with benzathine penicillin once weekly for 3 wks
Latent (late) with negative CSF	Benzathine pencillin G 2.4 million U IM once a week for 3 wk	3, 6, 12, (24) mo	Pretreatment CSF exam mandatory Some experts treat as for neurosyphilis regardless of CSF exam results
Late latent and syphilis of unknown duration; tertiary (without neurosyphilis)	Benzathine penicillin G 2.4 million U IM once a week for 3 wk (Some authorities recommend neurosyphilis regimen for cardiovascular syphilis)	As above	Some experts treat as for neurosyphilis regardless of CSF exam results
Neurosyphilis	Aqueous penicillin G 18-24 million U IV qd × 10-14 days Procaine penicillin G 2.4 million U IM qd *and* probenecid 500 mg PO qid × 10-14 days (Some authorities follow both regimens with benzathine penicillin G 2.4 million U IM)	CSF exam every 6 mo until normal; if CSF remains positive, retreat	

Table 38-5
Management and Treatment of Syphilis—cont'd

Stage	Treatment*	Minimum follow-up testing	Special considerations for HIV disease
Penicillin allergy Primary or secondary	Doxycycline 100 mg PO bid × 14 days Tetracycline 500 mg PO qid × 14 days Azithromycin 2 g as a single oral dose Ceftriaxone 1 gm IV or IM qd × 7-10 days (inadequate data on ceftriaxone in advanced stages of disease)	As shown above for stage (see text)	Use penicillin for *all* HIV-positive patients regardless of stage; use penicillin desensitization if necessary
Latent (early) (if CSF negative)	Doxycycline 100 mg PO bid × 14 days Tetracycline 500 mg PO qid × 14 days		
Latent (late or of unknown origin) (if CSF negative)	Doxycycline 100 mg PO bid × 28 days Tetracycline 500 mg PO qid × 28 days		
Tertiary (if CSF negative)	Doxycycline or tetracycline as for late latent disease		
Neuro-syphilis and cardiovascular)	Penicillin desensitization followed by neurosyphilis penicillin regimen		

*From CDC: Sexually transmitted diseases treatment guidelines—2002, *MMWR* 51(RR-06):20, 2002.

1. Treatment regimens (adult) for primary, secondary, and early latent syphilis (<1 year's duration):
   a. Benzathine penicillin G, 2.4 million U IM one time.
   b. Doxycycline 100 mg PO bid (or tetracycline 500 mg PO qid) for 14 days. These regimens may be less effective than penicillin. They are difficult for many patients to comply with, and twice-daily doxycycline is likely easier to adhere to than the tetracycline regimen. They should be reserved for patients with *documented* penicillin allergy.
   c. Ceftriaxone. The CDC recommends regimens that provide treponemicidal serum levels for 7 to 10 days. Single-dose therapy is *not* adequate for primary or secondary syphilis; 1 g IV or IM qd for 7 to 10 days may be considered. These regimens may be considered for careful use against primary or secondary syphilis in penicillin-

allergic patients, less than 5% of whom are also allergic to cephalosporins. Compared to the other alternative oral regimens, ceftriaxone has the advantage of allowing the provider to monitor compliance.

d. Azithromycin 2 g as a single oral dose. This should only be used as an alternative for a patient who is penicillin allergic and cannot tolerate doxycycline or tetracycline, since efficacy is based on preliminary data.

The use of doxycycline, ceftriaxone, and azithromycin among HIV-infected persons has not been studied, so treatment with regimens not using benzathine penicillin among such persons must be undertaken with caution, according to current CDC guidelines.

2. Treatment regimens for syphilis of more than 1 year's duration:
   a. Benzathine penicillin G, 2.4 million U IM once a week for 3 successive weeks.
   b. There are few data that suggest that alternative regimens to penicillin are effective for syphilis of over 1 year's duration. Patients at this stage of disease should have a lumbar puncture to exclude neurosyphilis before using alternative therapy. Doxycycline, 100 mg PO bid (or tetracycline 500 mg PO qid) for 28 days, is a generally accepted alternative. Erythromycin is not recommended for late latent syphilis. At a minimum, treated patients should return at 3, 6, and 12 months after treatment to have repeat quantitative nontreponemal serologies performed (and at 24 months for latent syphilis). Indications of successful therapy are: (1) a titer that falls fourfold within 3 months of treatment for early syphilis and 12 to 24 months for latent syphilis, (2) that eventually becomes nonreactive or reactive at a very low level, and (3) that does not show a fourfold rise in titer at any time following treatment.
3. Treatment for late latent syphilis or syphilis of unknown duration:
   a. Benzathine penicillin G, 2.4 million U IM once a week for 3 successive weeks. This regimen is used for patients with latent syphilis without neurologic findings or evidence of neurosyphilis in the CSF. The alternative regimens, doxycycline or tetracycline for one month (as described earlier), should only be used for patients with a documented penicillin allergy and normal CSF examination.
   b. For patients with tertiary syphilis (e.g., cardiovascular syphilis), some people recommend treatment of cardiovascular syphilis with a neurosyphilis regimen.
4. Treatment for neurosyphilis:
   a. Aqueous penicillin G, 3 to 4 million U IV every 4 hours (18 to 24 million U/day) for 10 to 14 days.
   b. Procaine penicillin, 2.4 million U IM daily, *plus* probenecid, 500 mg PO qid, both for 10 to 14 days.
   c. To prolong treponemicidal levels of penicillin in the CSF, some experts give a single dose of benzathine penicillin, 2.4 million U IM at the conclusion of the above courses.
   d. Nonpenicillin regimens cannot be recommended. Patients with documented penicillin allergy should undergo desensitization followed by therapy with penicillin.

ASSESSING THERAPEUTIC RESPONSE

An adequate serologic response after treatment must be judged on the basis of the stage of syphilis, whether previous infection with *T. pallidum* has occurred, and on the pretreatment Venereal Disease Research Laboratory (VDRL) or rapid plasma reagin (RPR) titer. Most patients with an initial episode of primary syphilis revert to nonreactive VDRL or RPR test status within 1 year after treatment; patients in the secondary stage who are treated usually revert within 2 years.

In contrast, following treatment, many patients with latent syphilis, whether early or late, remain reactive by VDRL or RPR testing at a persistent low titer (1:1 to 1:8) for several years. These patients require careful follow-up with periodic testing: a four-fold increase in titer indicates treatment failure (or reinfection).

Lumbar puncture with CSF examination is recommended for patients with treated early syphilis whose titers do not fall adequately, or who develop signs of neurologic involvement. They should also receive testing for HIV. Lumbar puncture is recommended to follow patients after treatment for late latent syphilis if they: (1) are serologic treatment failures, (2) have signs or symptoms compatible with neurosyphilis, (3) have been treated with a nonpenicillin treatment regimen, or (4) are HIV-positive (Table 38-4). Patients treated for neurosyphilis require lumbar puncture every 6 months until the CSF no longer shows pleocytosis.

HIV AND SYPHILIS

Risk factors and behaviors that promote transmission of HIV also promote transmission of syphilis. Conversely, the presence of untreated ulcerative STDs including syphilis appears to facilitate the transmission of HIV.

Neurosyphilis has been reported to be a complication of syphilis in patients with HIV infection. *T. pallidum* invades the CNS in up to 40% of all patients with early syphilis; in 1% to 2%, it can cause acute neurosyphilis characterized by meningitis, cranial nerve abnormalities, and cerebrovascular accidents. Even if standard recommended doses of benzathine penicillin G are given, it often fails to reach treponemicidal levels in the CNS; the outcome of treatment may depend on the host's immune response, as well as antibiotic therapy. HIV patients suffer from compromised humoral, as well as cellular immunity; thus the risk of neurosyphilis may be greater in patients who are HIV-positive, and cases of relapse of neurosyphilis after standard treatment have been well-documented.

In general, standard treatment for syphilis can be given to HIV-infected patients based on the results of the randomized trial that showed comparable clinical responses in the standard and enhanced treatment arms. HIV-infected patients with syphilis should be monitored closely for clinical and serologic response after treatment. Treatment failures should be evaluated by lumbar puncture if not previously done, and should be treated with a three-dose benzathine penicillin regimen, if the CSF status shows no signs of neurosyphilis. Patients with HIV infection who have symptoms of neurosyphilis should be treated with standard neurosyphilis regimens, namely daily procaine penicillin IM with probenecid or IV penicillin G 12 to 24 million U/day for 10 to 14 days. Other therapeutic alternatives for neurosyphilis have not been well evaluated: erythromycin should not be used, and it appears that ceftriaxone is associated with a higher failure rate than parenteral penicillin G. Penicillin desensitization followed by the standard regimen is recommended for penicillin-allergic patients. A detailed discussion on the clinical management of patients coinfected with HIV and syphilis is beyond the scope of this chapter. Readers should consult the References section or call their local Public Health Department, or contact the CDC Division of HIV/AIDS in Atlanta at (404) 639-3311.

REFERENCES

Berry CD, Hooton TM, Collier AC, et al: Neurologic relapse after benzathine penicillin therapy for secondary syphilis in a patient with HIV infection, *N Engl J Med* 316: 1589, 1987.

Centers for Disease Control and Prevention: Sexually transmitted diseases treatment guidelines—2002, *MMWR* 51(RR-06):18, 2002.

Coury-Doniger PA: Syphilis: Managing patients with reactive serologic tests, *STD Bulletin* 12: 11, 1993.

Jaffe HW, Musher DM: Management of the reactive syphilis serology. In Holmes KK, Mårdh P-A, Sparling PF, Wiesner PJ, et al (eds): *Sexually Transmitted Diseases,* ed 2, New York, 1990, McGraw-Hill.

Johns DR, Tierney M, Felsenstein D: Alteration in the natural history of neurosyphilis by concurrent infection with the human immunodeficiency virus, *N Engl J Med* 316:1569, 1987.

Hook E, Marra C: Acquired syphilis in adults, *N Engl J Med* 326:1060, 1992.

Larsen S, Hunter EF, Creighton ET: Syphilis. In Holmes KK, Mårdh P-A, Sparling PF, Wiesner PJ, et al (eds): *Sexually Transmitted Diseases,* ed 2, New York, 1990, McGraw-Hill.

Larsen S, Hunter E, Kraus S (eds): *A Manual of Tests for Syphilis,* Washington, DC, 1990, American Public Health Association.

Lukehart SA, Hook EW III, Baker-Zander SA, et al: Invasion of the central nervous system by *Treponema pallidum, Ann Intern Med* 109:855, 1988.

Musher DM: Syphilis, neurosyphilis, penicillin, and AIDS, *J Infect Dis* 163:1201, 1991.

Musher DM: Early syphilis. In Holmes KK, Sparling PF, Mardh PA et al (eds). *Sexually Transmitted Diseases,* ed 3, 1999, McGraw-Hill.

Rolfs RT, Joesoef MR, Hendershoot EF, et. al. A randomized trial of enhanced therapy for early syphilis in patients with and without human immunodeficiency virus infection, *N Engl J Med* 337:307, 1997.

Romanowski B, Sutherland R, Fick GH, et al: Serologic response to treatment of infectious syphilis, *Ann Intern Med* 114:1005, 1991.

Tichinova L, Bonshenko K, Ward H et al: Epidemics of syphilis in the Russian Federation: trends, origins and priorities for control, *Lancet* 350:210, 1997.

Wasserheit J: Epidemiological synergy. Interrelationships between human immunodeficiency virus and other sexually transmitted diseases, *Sex Transm Dis* 19:61, 1992.

World Health organization Office of HIV/AIDS and Sexually Transmitted Diseases (1998). An overview of selected evaluable STDs. ASD online at http://www.who.int/asd.

CHAPTER 39

Genital Ulcer Disease

Elaine C. Jong and H. Hunter Handsfield

A genital ulcer can be defined as a discrete mucosal or cutaneous discontinuity involving the genitals, perineum, or surrounding tissues in the presence of otherwise normal skin and mucous membranes. The etiology of genital ulcer disease (GUD) varies among geographic areas and sometimes among populations characterized by demographic, behavioral, and socioeconomic markers. In industrialized countries, genital herpes has been recognized as one of the most common sexually transmitted diseases (STD) in the past two decades, and is the leading cause of GUD in sexually active young adults across all socioeconomic strata. In developing countries, syphilis and chancroid are the predominant causes of GUD, but these two infections are usually found only among poor minority populations in urban environments in developed countries. Lymphogranuloma venereum (LGV) and granuloma inguinale are relatively rare in both developing and industrialized countries.

Genital ulceration is often accompanied by inguinal lymphadenopathy and occasionally by systemic manifestations. Serious long-term sequelae are common, and GUD has emerged as a potent risk factor for sexual transmission of human immunodeficiency virus (HIV). The dominant risk factors for acquisition of GUD are those associated with all STDs—multiple sex partners, intercourse with a new partner, selection of high-risk partners, and failure to use condoms. Duration of infection also influences relative risk of transmission. The clinical course of infectious syphilis or chancroid is measured in weeks, whereas genital herpes and other viral STDs are transmissible for many years, perhaps for the life of the infected person. As a result, low rates of sexual partner change are sufficient to sustain transmission of genital herpes in a population, but syphilis and chancroid are sustained only in populations with especially high rates of partner change.

Uncircumcised men are at increased risk for chancroid, and perhaps for syphilis and herpes. It is thought that the preputial sac provides a reservoir that prolongs exposure to the partner's genital secretions, and that the skin of the glans penis is less cornified than in circumcised men and thus is more susceptible to infection. The association of an intact foreskin with HIV infection also is well documented. Infection with HIV has an adverse effect on the natural course of HSV infection and probably syphilis, and also impairs the response to therapy of herpes, chancroid, and syphilis.

SYPHILIS

Syphilis is a common cause of GUD in patients at risk for STDs in developing countries and is considered in detail in Chapter 38.

CHANCROID

Haemophilus ducreyi, the cause of chancroid, is a small gram-negative bacillus. Ribosomal MA typing suggests a closer relationship of the organism to *Actinobacillus* than to other *Haemophilus* species, although *H. ducreyi* remains the accepted name. The organism is nutritionally fastidious, slow to grow, and often difficult to isolate, even when experienced laboratories use highly enriched media.

Chancroid is the predominant cause of GUD in many developing countries, especially in tropical climates. Throughout the world, chancroid appears to be more closely linked than any other STD with prostitution, substance abuse, and economic deprivation. This may occur because asymptomatic infection is uncommon, and maintenance of a chancroid outbreak may require a population of persons who continue sexual exposure despite painful genital lesions; addiction and economic pressures may provide the necessary incentives. In industrial countries chancroid tends to occur in localized epidemics, and it persists as an occasional cause of GUD in only a few cities in the United States. Chancroid declined dramatically in the United States after 1990, and only 386 cases were reported in 1996. However, reported cases underestimate the true burden of disease, partly because bacteriologic confirmation is difficult and often not attempted.

Knowledge of the pathogenesis of chancroid is limited. Initial attachment of *H. ducreyi* to epithelial cells is followed by cell penetration and necrosis. The initial inflammatory papule rapidly evolves into a pustule and then an ulcer. Chancroid was historically called "soft chancre," reflecting the lesion's nonindurated nature compared with syphilis. Most ulcers occur on the penis, especially under the foreskin in uncircumcised men, and near the introitus in women. Typically one to three lesions are present, but there may be several, especially in women. The shape may be round, oval, or irregular. The edges are erythematous and may be undermined; the base typically is covered with purulent exudate, and the lesion usually is very tender. However, some cases are mild with nonspecific-appearing lesions.

Up to two thirds of patients with chancroid have inguinale lymphadenopathy, which may be unilateral or bilateral. Overlying cutaneous erythema and fluctuance are the rule (the "bubo"), helping to distinguish chancroid from syphilis or herpes. Untreated, and sometimes despite effective antibiotic therapy, fluctuant lymph nodes rupture and drain spontaneously. Despite the locally aggressive nature of the infection, fever and disseminated infection occur rarely, if ever. Repeated infections are common in endemic areas. Although antibodies are produced to several outer membrane proteins, their contribution to acquired immunity is unknown.

Several studies in the last decade have documented the efficacy of single-dose treatment of chancroid with ceftriaxone or azithromycin and with 3-day regimens of ciprofloxacin or other fluoroquinolones. The 2002 Centers for Disease Control and Prevention recommendations are shown in Table 39-1. Erythromycin is effective but requires compliance for 7 days. All regimens have somewhat reduced efficacy in the presence of HIV infection, an important consideration for treatment of in tropical developing countries where high transmission rates of chancroid and HIV

Table 39-1
Recommended Regimens for Treatment of Chancroid

Azithromycin 1.0 g orally in a single dose
Ceftriaxone 250 mg intramuscularly in single dose
Ciprofloxacin 500 mg orally twice a day for 3 days
Erythromycin 500 mg orally 4 times a day for 7 days

Centers for Control and Prevention: Sexually transmitted diseases treatment guidelines—2002, *MMWR* 51(RR-06):11, 2002.

infection are concomitant. Fluctuant lymph nodes should be aspirated as often as necessary to prevent spontaneous rupture.

LYMPHOGRANULOMA VENEREUM

LGV is caused by *Chlamydia trachomatis* serovars L_1, L_2, and L_3. Compared with the more prevalent oculogenital strains (Chapter 37), these serovars grow rapidly, are more cytolytic in cell culture, and are lethal to mice after intracerebral inoculation. In the United States LGV is rare, with a mean of 260 cases reported each year in the 1990s; only 75 cases were recognized in 1996.

The primary lesion of LGV is an evanescent papule or ulcer that usually resolves before the patient seeks care. Instead, it is possible that the primary infection often is manifested by urethritis or cervicitis, as for infection with other C. *trachomatis* serovars. Lymphatic spread results in regional lymphadenopathy, with central necrosis and liquefaction that typically evolves over 2 to 4 weeks. The classic presentation of LGV is bilateral inguinale lymphadenopathy. Initially the lymph nodes are moderately tender, often with overlying erythema, and may be fluctuant. Doxycycline, 100 mg orally twice a day for 3 weeks, is the recommended regimen for LGV.

Untreated, there may be repeated cycles of spontaneous rupture and drainage, and patients with chronic infection may present with indurated, matted nodes often with sinus tracts and secondary pyogenic infection. Rarely, lymphatic obstruction supervenes, with elephantiasis devolving the genitals or lower extremities; such presentations are now rare. LGV occasionally presents as acute proctocolitis, especially in homosexually active men who are the receptive partners in rectal intercourse. Fever and malaise are seen occasionally, especially in proctocolitis, and aseptic meningitis occasionally occurs.

Both humoral and cellular immune responses occur, and it is likely that delayed hypersensitivity is largely responsible for the chronic, relapsing lymphadenopathy, and lymphatic obstructions are the classic hallmarks of untreated infection.

GRANULOMA INGUINALE

Calymmatobacterium granulomatis, the cause of granuloma inguinale, is a small, pleomorphic gram-negative coccobacillus that in pathologic material typically appears intracellularly in macrophages ("Donovan bodies"). The histologic picture and course suggest that the clinical manifestations are due largely to a cell-mediated immune response. Granuloma inguinale is rare even in most developing countries; in the United States, a mean of only 11 cases were reported annually in the 1990s. The infection is most commonly recognized in the Indian subcontinent, Papua New Guinea, isolated areas of Australia, and parts of the Caribbean, and most cases in the United States probably are imported from such endemic areas.

Granuloma inguinale presents with one or more indolent, mildly tender ulcerative lesions, typically with hypertrophic granulation-like tissue in the inguinal region. Inguinal masses are due more frequently to subcutaneous extension of inflammatory tissue than to lymphadenopathy per se. Sometimes the lesions spread inexorably, rarely leading to penile autoamputation, and the appearance may be similar to that of squamous cell carcinoma. Although systemic symptoms do not occur, disseminated osteolytic lesions have been described. Doxycycline, 100 mg orally twice a day for 3 weeks, is the recommended regimen for donovanosis, as granuloma inguinale is also called. *C. granulomatis* recently has been sustained in culture for the first time, which will lead to improved characterization of the organism in the near future.

HERPES SIMPLEX VIRUSES

In contrast to industrialized countries, genital herpes has been infrequently recognized as a cause of GUD in most developing countries. However, recent studies using polymerase chain reaction (PCR) to detect herpes simplex virus (HSV) DNA have demonstrated that in some developing countries, a substantial portion of GUD is due to genital herpes. Herpes simplex virus type 2 (HSV-2) is the predominant cause of genital herpes, although the type 1 virus (HSV-1) is responsible for a substantial and apparently growing minority of cases. Seroepidemiologic studies showed that by the early 1990s an estimated 22% of the U.S. population greater than 12 years old was seropositive for antibody to HSV-2, and that the prevalence rises rapidly from age 15 to 40 years old (Table 39-2).

Most new cases of genital herpes are acquired from sex partners with subclinical viral shedding. After inoculation, HSV penetrates epithelial cells, causing ballooning degeneration and focal necrosis. There is an initial inflammatory response characterized by polymorphonuclear leukocytes followed by the production of multinucleated giant cells. The virus migrates along sensory nerve axons toward the dorsal root ganglia, where latent infection is established. Healing of the initial mucocutaneous

Table 39-2
Characteristics of Symptomatic Genital Herpes

	Type of Infection		
	Primary	**Initial nonprimary**	**Recurrent**
Lesions	Many, bilateral	Fewer	Few, unilateral
Cervicitis or urethritis	Common	Occasional	Uncommon
Neuropathic complications	Common	Uncommon	Rare
Regional lymphadenopathy	Usual	Occasional	Uncommon
Systemic manifestations	Usual	Occasional	Rare
Usual duration	2-6 wk	1-3 wk	5-10 days

lesions is associated with development of neutralizing antibody and a cellular immune response.

Primary genital herpes is defined as the patient's first infection with either HSV type. Primary genital herpes can be severe with multiple crops of extensive clustered lesions, often with urethritis, cervicitis, regional lymphadenopathy, neuropathy, or aseptic meningitis (see Table 39-2). An individual lesion evolves over 2 to 3 days from an erythematous papule to a vesicle containing clear fluid, to a pustule. The epithelial surface may be shed at any time, resulting in a discrete shallow ulcer. The ulcerations are exquisitely tender with burning pain. Early ulceration is the rule on moist surfaces, such as the vulva, partly explaining the more severe course in women compared with the usually more benign course in most men. On dry surfaces, the lesions develop crusts after several days with rapid subsequent healing. The time from papule to encrustation and healing is substantially longer in primary herpes infections than in recurrent attacks. During a symptomatic viral episode, virus is shed in the secretions from intact vesicles, and from early, moist, tender ulcers.

Prior infection with either virus type reduces susceptibility among persons reexposed to HSV and ameliorates the clinical course of infection with the opposite type. Up to 40% of symptomatic initial episodes of genital herpes is due to HSV-1, but the clinical recurrence rate is lower than for genital HSV-2. Thus, approximately 90% of clinically recognized outbreaks of recurrent genital herpes are due to HSV-2.

Initial nonprimary genital herpes is defined as the first clinically recognized herpes infection, usually with HSV-2, in a patient previous infected with HSV, usually orolabial HSV-1. Such infections usually are intermediate in severity. *Recurrent genital herpes* is the second or subsequent clinically recognized genital outbreak. Symptomatic recurrences usually are mild and brief, without mucosal involvement or systemic symptoms. Some patients with recurrent herpes experience a neuropathic prodrome, such as paresthesias that begin from a few hours to 2 days before the appearance of overt cutaneous lesions.

During the first year after symptomatic primary or initial nonprimary genital herpes caused by HSV-2, the mean frequency of symptomatic recurrences is four per year in women and five per year in men. The rate of occurrences may decline slightly thereafter, but most patients continue to have symptomatic outbreaks for several years. Persons with genital HSV-1 infection experience an average of only one symptomatic outbreak per year, and many patients have no recurrence. Among persons with recognized recurrences, HSV can be isolated from the genitals or anus up to 7% of the days between symptomatic outbreaks.

The mechanisms of reactivation, migration of HSV virions from the dorsal root ganglia along sensory nerve axons, and recurrent mucocutaneous lesions are incompletely understood. Local trauma or inflammation (e.g., sunburn) commonly results in recurrent orolabial herpes caused by HSV-1, but such triggers have not been documented for genital herpes. Anecdotal reports that menstruation, sexual intercourse, stress, fatigue, or other factors stimulate symptomatic recurrences of genital HSV-2 have not been corroborated by controlled studies.

If there are classic signs of genital herpes, such as a cluster of vesicles or tender superficial ulcers, the history and physical often will lead to a highly probably diagnosis, and initiating presumptive therapy for herpes while awaiting laboratory confirmation is reasonable. Laboratory assessment is recommended to identify virus type and to aid prognosis. HSV-1

Table 39-3
Treatment of Genital Herpes Simplex Virus Infection*

First Episode (Primary) Genital Herpes
Acyclovir 400 mg orally 3 times a day (or 200 mg orally 5 times a day) for 7-10 days; OR
Famciclovir 250 mg orally 3 times a day for 7-10 days, OR
Valacyclovir 1.0 g orally 2 times a day for 7-10 days

Severe Infection That Requires Parental Therapy
Acyclovir 5-10 mg/kg body weight intravenously every 8 hours until clinical resolution is attained, followed by oral antiviral therapy to complete 10 days total therapy

Episodic Treatment of Recurrent Herpes
Acyclovir 400 mg orally 3 times a day (OR 200 mg orally 5 times a day, OR 800 mg twice a day) for 5 days; OR,
Famciclovir 125 mg orally twice a day for 5 days, OR
Valacyclovir 500 mg orally twice a day for 3 days, OR valocyclovir 1 g orally once a day for 5 days

Suppressive Therapy†
Acyclovir 400 mg orally twice a day; OR
Famciclovir 250 mg orally twice a day; OR,
Valacyclovir 500 mg (<10 episodes/year) or 1000 mg (>10 episodes/year) orally once a day

*From specific product package inserts; standard guidelines for therapy of genital herpes in otherwise healthy adults (not pregnant); and Centers for Control and Prevention: Sexually transmitted diseases treatment guidelines—2002, *MMWR* 51(RR-06):12, 2002.
†Suppressive therapy should be interrupted at 1-year intervals to reassess the frequency of symptomatic recurrent. Treatment reduces the frequency and severity of recurrences but does not entirely prevent them, nor does it completely suppress subclinical shedding of herpes simplex virus.

and HSV-2 are double-stranded DNA viruses and have numerous genetically stable antigenic differences, notably among several outer membrane glycoproteins, the basis of type-specific antibody tests. All patients with first-episode genital herpes should be tested for other common STDs, such as syphilis, chlamydial infection, gonorrhea, and HIV infection. Table 39-3 lists the treatment regimens for genital herpes simplex virus infection.

APPROACH TO LABORATORY DIAGNOSIS OF GUD

Complete evaluation for both HSV infection and syphilis is always indicated for sexually active patients who present with GUD that does not have the classic appearance of genital herpes. Table 39-4 outlines the laboratory evaluation of sexually active patients with genital ulcer disease. At a minimum this should include a culture or other sensitive test for HSV and a serologic test for syphilis. Because herpes is the most common cause of GUD, regardless of the appearance of the lesion, failure to test for HSV often will lead to misdiagnosis. Darkfield microscopy also is indicated but is not always readily available; as an alternative, most public

Table 39-4
Laboratory Evaluation of Sexually Active Patients with Genital Ulcer Disease

Lesions Typical of Genital Herpes*
Culture or direct FA test for HSV (recommended but optional)
Screening tests for other STD (syphilis, HIV, chlamydia, and gonorrhea)

Other Genital Ulcers
Culture or direct FA test for HSV (or PCR, if available)
Darkfield microscopy or direct FA test for *Treponema pallidum*
Syphilis serology

Selected Cases
Culture for *Haemophilus ducreyi*
Culture for pyogenic bacteria
Biopsy
Type-specific HSV serology†

FA, Fluorescent antibody; *HSV,* herpes simplex virus; *STD,* sexually transmitted disease; *HIV,* human immunodeficiency virus; *PCR,* polymerase chain reaction; *GUD,* genital ulcer disease.

*For example, a cluster of superficial ulcer, or vesiculopustular lesions.
†Type-specific HSV serology may have value as a routine diagnostic test in all patients with GUD when the glycoprotein G1 (HSV-1) and glycoprotein G2 (HSV-2) assays become more widely available.

health laboratories offer the direct fluorescent antibody test for *Treponema pallidum.* If the clinical appearance or history suggests chancroid, a culture for *H. ducreyi* should be done on the lesion and, if there is fluctuant lymphadenopathy, on a needle aspirate from the lymph node. Sensitive PCR tests for *H. ducreyi* and *T. pallidum* have been developed but are not widely available.

If the diagnosis remains elusive after the initial evaluation, follow-up and repeat laboratory tests, especially syphilis serology, often are helpful. New type specific serologic tests for HSV antibody based on glycoprotein G1 (HSV-1) and glycoprotein G2 (HSV-2) have recently been approved by the FDA. These newer glycoprotein G (gG) tests are reported to have a 80% to 98% sensitivity and ≥96% specificity, and can be used to confirm a clinical diagnosis of genital herpes, or to diagnose persons with unrecognized infection. If regional lymphadenopathy is prominent, LGV should be assessed by testing the lymph node aspirate or lesion for *C. trachomatis* and performing an LGV complement fixation test; if available, type-specific chlamydia serology with the microimmunofluorecence test is recommended. If granuloma inguinale is suspected, a scraping of the lesion should be crushed between two microscope slides, stained with the Wright-Giemsa method, and examined for intracellular Donovan bodies; culture tests for *C. granulomatis* may be available soon. Some cases may require biopsy, culture of the ulcer or lymph node aspirate for pyogenic bacteria, or other special tests.

REFERENCES

Centers for Control and Prevention: Sexually transmitted diseases treatment guidelines—2002, *MMWR* 51(RR-06):11, 2002.

Fleming DT et al: Herpes simplex virus 1 and 2 in the United States, 1976 to 1994, *N Engl J Med* 337:1105, 1997.

Gordon SM et al: The response of symptomatic neurosyphilis to high-dose intravenous penicillin G in patients with human immunodeficiency virus infection, *N Engl J Med* 331:146, 1994.

Handsfield HH: *Color atlas and synopsis of sexually transmitted diseases,* New York, 1992, McGraw-Hill.

Holmes KK et al, editors: *Sexually transmitted diseases,* ed 3, New York, 1998, McGraw-Hill.

Kaplowitz LG et al: Prolonged continuous acyclovir treatment of normal adults with frequently recurring genital herpes simplex virus infection, *JAMA* 265:747, 1991.

Koutsky LA et al: Underdiagnosis of genital herpes by current clinical and viral-isolation procedures, *N Engl J Med* 326:153, 1999.

Lynch PJ, Edwards L: *Genital dermatoses,* New York, 1994, Churchill-Livingstone.

Marrazzo JM, Handsfield HH: Chancroid: new developments in an old disease, *Curr Clin Top Infect Dis* 15:129, 1995.

Morse SA et al: Comparison of clinical diagnosis and standard laboratory and molecular methods for the diagnosis of genital ulcer disease in Lesotho: association with human immunodeficiency virus infection, *J Infect Dis* 175:583, 1997.

Rothanowski B et al: Serologic response to treatment of infectious syphilis, *Ann Intern Med* 114:1005, 1991.

Wald A et al: Suppression of subclinical shedding of herpes simplex virus type 2 with Acyclovir, *Ann Intern Med* 124:8, 1996.

SECTION VII

WORMS

CHAPTER 40

Common Intestinal Roundworms

Christopher Sanford and Elaine C. Jong

The worms crawl in
The worms crawl out
The worms play pinochle on your snout.
Children's song, Anonymous

GENERAL CONSIDERATIONS

Medically important worms belonging to the phylum Nematoda (roundworms) parasitize the gastrointestinal tract of humans. The worms are commonly acquired through ingestion of contaminated food (especially raw or uncooked vegetables), through skin contact with contaminated soil, or, in some instances, from direct contact with infected persons or their fomites.

Individuals most likely to be infected with intestinal nematodes will frequently give a history of one of the following: (1) travel or residence in a developing area of the world, (2) emigration from a developing area of the world, (3) residence in a rural farming community, (4) ingestion of organically grown vegetables, (5) the use of wastewater for agriculture, or (6) pica. Developing areas of the world are areas where environmental sanitation may be a problem. In the United States, such areas may include areas of the Southeast and Southwest as well as farming communities in the temperate zone. Pica, or geophagy, is not rare; in one study in Kenya, 77% of children ate soil daily Table 40-1.

ETIOLOGY

Species of nematodes causing infections in humans include *Ascaris lumbricoides, Ascaris suum, Ancylostoma duodenale, Necator americanus, Trichuris trichiura, Strongyloides stercoralis,* and *Enterobius vermicularis.* Human intestinal infection with the marine roundworm *Anisakis* are also considered in this chapter.

CLINICAL FEATURES

1. Patients with intestinal nematodes are frequently asymptomatic.
2. Vague abdominal complaints are sometimes the only symptoms reported with light to moderate infections.
3. Chronic, heavy infections are associated with growth stunting in children.
4. Occasionally, asymptomatic patients pass a recognizable worm, which is the first sign that they have acquired an intestinal parasite.
5. At other times, the diagnosis is suspected or made on finding eosinophilia on a routine white blood cell differential analysis or on finding ova or parasites in a stool examination done for screening purposes.

Table 40-1
Prevalence of Intestinal Nematodes in Rural Regions

	A. lumbricoides	*T. trichiura*	Hookworm
Vietnam (Needham, 1998)	83%	94%	59%
China (Changhua, 1999)	63%	60%	87%
Madagascar (Kightliner, 1998)	93%	55%	27%
Venezuela (Morales, 1998)	27%	33%	6%
Ethiopia (Jemaneh, 1998)	29-38%	13%	7-24%
Brazil (Saldiva, 1999)	41%	40%	
Mali (Behnke JM, 2000)			53% (*N. americanus*)
Paraguay (Labiano Abello, 1999)			59%

Additionally, studies on Pemba Island, Tanzania, and Barru district, Sulawesi, Indonesia, showed that 58% and 17.4%, respectively, of inhabitants were infected with all three of the above parasites.
From Booth M et al: Parasitology 116(pt1):85, 1998; Toma A et al: *Southwest Asian J Trop Med Public Health* 30:68, 1999.

In general, the severity of signs and symptoms will be related to the intensity of the infection (worm burden). Young children, possibly because of unsanitary habits (a tendency to put dirty fingers and objects into their mouths, run around outdoors without shoes, and so forth) and possibly because of immature host defense mechanisms, will tend to acquire a heavier parasite load than adults living in the same area.

For salient features of infection with intestinal nematodes, see Table 40-2.

DIAGNOSIS

Hematology

The absolute eosinophil count may be normal or elevated ($>450/mm^3$).

Microbiology

Examination for ova and parasites of up to three different stool specimens collected on three different days at 2- to 3-day intervals is sufficient for diagnosis. It is not uncommon for stool examinations to be negative for diagnostic forms of *Strongyloides* or *Enterobius* (pinworm).

Serology

Both immunofluorescent assay and enzyme-linked immunosorbent assay (ELISA) serologic tests for *Strongyloides* (available through commercial laboratories or arranged through state health departments and performed by the Parasite Serology Laboratory at the Centers for Disease Control and Prevention, Atlanta, Georgia) can be helpful in making the diagnosis

Table 40-2
Intestinal Nematode Infection

Infection	Agent	Geographic distribution	Mode of infection	Clinical features	Diagnosis	Indication for treatment
Common roundworm Pig roundworm	*Ascaris lumbricoides* *Ascaris suum*	Worldwide	Raw fruits and vegetables	Pneumonitis, colicky epigastric pain, nausea and vomiting, passage of a mature pencil-sized worm*	Ova in stool or identification of mature worm	A single retained worm, multiple worms, obstruction of a viscus, or presence of other parasites requiring treatment
Hookworm (Old World) Hookworm (New World)	*Ancylostoma duodenale* *Necator americanus*	Worldwide	Percutaneous or perioral infections from contaminated soil or vegetation	"Ground itch" (rash), pneumonitis, abdominal pain, diarrhea, anemia (with large worm burdens and iron-deficient diet)†	Ova in stool	Heavy infection (>2000 eggs per gram of stool) Presence of anemia Malnutrition

Continued

Table 40-2
Intestinal Nematode Infection—cont'd

Infection	Agent	Geographic distribution	Mode of infection	Clinical features	Diagnosis	Indication for treatment
Strongyloides	*Strongyloides stercoralis*	Worldwide	Skin contact with wet, infected soil	Rash on buttocks or thighs, abdominal pain, nausea and vomiting, weight loss, eosinophilia, recurrent bacterial systemic infections with gastrointestinal flora in immunocompromised patients	Rhabditiform larvae in stool or jejunal aspirate Serology available	Documented infection
Whipworm	*Trichuris trichiura*	Worldwide	Raw fruits and vegetables, soil contact, flies on food	Mild anemia, bloody diarrhea, rectal prolapse in heavy infections	Ova in stool	Symptoms associated with heavy infection (>3000 eggs per gram of stool) Not necessary to treat patients with low egg counts
Pinworm	*Enterobius vermicularis*	Worldwide	Anus-finger-mouth cycle, or from clothing, bedding, dust	Perianal itching, irritation, restlessness, sleeplessness	Ova from perianal skin seen on Scotch tape swab	Symptomatic infection, psychosocial reasons

*Rare: bile duct obstruction, acute pancreatitis, appendicitis.
†*Ancylostoma duodenale* causes a more severe anemia than does *Necator americanus*.

in a patient with an appropriate geographic history, peripheral blood eosinophilia, and negative stool examinations for ova and parasites. ELISA sensitivity and specificity are improved if used in conjunction with the Western blot test. All serologic diagnostic tests for *Strongyloides* are complicated by cross-reactivity with filarial antigens.

The String Test

The "Enterotest" method for sampling proximal jejunal secretions may be a useful diagnostic procedure for *Strongyloides* diagnosis (see Chapter 26, diagnosis of giardiasis).

Scotch Tape Test

The diagnosis of *Enterobius* is best made from microscopic examination of Scotch tape pressed adhesive-side down on the perianal skin and then directly mounted, adhesive-side down, on a glass microscope slide. The distinctive eggs are rarely found in the stool.

Baermann Funnel Gauze Method

Strongyloides larvae do not float in hypertonic saline, which is used to concentrate other parasites. The Baermann method uses gauze, warm water, and larval sedimentation in the neck of a funnel.

TREATMENT

For treatment of common intestinal nematodes in patients without severe underlying health problems, see Table 40-3. Infection with multiple parasites is common, so Table 40-4 groups multiple parasites that may be treated with the same drug.

Table 40-3
Comparison of Spectrum of Activity of Various Antihelmintics

Organism	Albendazole*	Mebendazole	Thiabendazole	Pyrantel pamoate
Pinworm (*Enterobius*)	+	+	a	+
Ascaris	+	+	a	+
A. duodenale[†]	+[‡]	+	a	+
N. americanus	+	+	a	+
Trichuris[§]	+	+	–	–
Strongyloides[¶]	+	–	+	–
Taenia spp.	+	ni	–	–
Hymenolepis nana	+	–	–	–

+, Efficacious; –, not efficacious; *a*, when other therapy cannot be used; *ni*, not an official indication for use.
*Not available in the United States.
[†]Albendazole found to be more efficacious than mebendazole in southern region of Mali
[‡]Albendazole also efficacious for coinfection of hookworm with *Giardia lamblia.*
[§]Mebendazole superior to albendazole (85% versus 75%) in reducing Trichuris ova count in a study from Durban, South Africa.
[¶]Ivermectin is the preferred drug for *Strongyloides.*

Table 40-4
Strategy for Treatment of Intestinal Nematodes in Mixed Infections

Group	Treatment
*Ascaris** Hookworm* *Enterobius**	**Pyrantel pamoate** (Antiminth): 50-mg/ml oral suspension. *Standard dose:* 11 mg/kg in a single oral dose not to exceed a maximum dose of 1 g. Not recommended for children less than 2 years old. For *Enterobius,* repeat dose after 2 weeks.
*Ascaris** Hookworm* *Enterobius** *Trichuris**	**Mebendazole** (Vermox): 100-mg chewable tablet. *Standard dose:* 100 mg bid × 3 days for adults and children more than 2 years old. Available as chewable tablet. Infection with *Enterobius* alone requires only one 100-mg tablet for treatment, with repeat dose after 2 weeks.
*Strongyloides** *Ascaris** Hookworm* *Enterobius** *Trichuris** *Strongyloides** *Taenia** *Hymenolepis nana**	**Albendazole** (Albenza): 200-mg tablet; 100 mg/5 ml suspension. *Standard dose:* Two 200-mg tablets as single dose in adults and children at least 2 years old; 200 mg as single dose in children 1 to 2 years old (not studied in children less than 1 year old; **contraindicated in pregnancy**). Repeat dose after 2 weeks for *Enterobius.* Treatment for *Strongyloides, Taenia* spp., *Hymenolepis nana:* Two 200-mg tablets as single dose on 3 consecutive days.
Ascaris Hookworm *Strongyloides*	**Thiabendazole** (Mintezol): 500-mg chewable tablet, or 500 mg/5 ml oral suspension. *Standard dose:* 25 mg/kg bid (max 3 g/day) × 2 days. For disseminated *Strongyloides* infection, continue treatment for 5 days or more. Variable activity against *Ascaris,* and hookworm. Some consultants recommend pyrantel pamoate (as above) 1 week after thiabendazole therapy if patient is infected concurrently with *Ascaris.*

*Treatment listed for each group is appropriate for any single parasite infection marked with an asterisk within a group, or for multiple parasitism within a given group, provided that one or more asterisked parasites is present.

If *Ascaris* is present, this parasite should be covered by the first round of antiparasitic therapy, even if other drugs will be used subsequently to treat other parasites that are present. This strategy is necessary because of the propensity for mature *Ascaris* worms to migrate into unpredictable ectopic sites when they are irritated but not killed by drugs, fever, or even starvation in the host. Migrating worms may cause perforation of an abdominal viscus, appendicitis, biliary obstruction, pancreatitis, or intestinal obstruction. Antiparasitic therapy directed at ascarides may be administered concurrently with antibiotics for other infections.

If a person with an *Ascaris* infection needs anesthesia before a cure is obtained, the anesthesiologist should be informed because of the remote possibility that the anesthetic agent could cause ectopic worm migration into the trachea, causing respiratory obstruction.

Special Therapeutic Considerations

Intestinal Obstruction Caused By Ascaris

A gastrointestinal tube should be placed, retained fluids aspirated, and an appropriate dose of piperazine citrate instilled (Antepar, 75 mg/kg/day, not to exceed 3.5 g). The piperazine will paralyze the worms, allowing them to be passed out by the intestinal peristalsis of the host. If relief of the obstruction is not obtained within 1 to 2 days, a surgical procedure may be necessary, as in the other complications caused by migratory *Ascaris* worms. Approximately 20,000 people die from *Ascaris* infection each year, but given that a quarter of the world, or 1.5 billion people are infected, the case/fatality ratio is only 0.000013.

Infants

There are few data from published studies on the use of antiparasitic drugs in infants less than 2 years old. In a severely ill infant, in whom the presence of parasites is thought to contribute to the disease process (e.g., intestinal obstruction caused by ascarides, severe anemia caused by hookworm), the possible risks of antiparasitic therapy must be weighed against the effects of the untreated infection, and the dosage of the appropriate drug adjusted for weight.

Pregnant and Lactating Women

There are few data from published studies on the use of antiparasitic drugs in pregnancy and lactation. Both mebendazole and albendazole have been shown to have teratogenic potential in animal models. It would be prudent to withhold therapy during the first trimester and to delay therapy as long as possible, ideally until after delivery. There is no evidence for transplacental transmission of roundworm infections in humans.

If therapy of a lactating woman is contemplated, asking the patient to use mechanical means for milk expression during and for 48 hours after antiparasitic therapy would be prudent.

If antiparasitic therapy is inadvertently given during the first trimester of pregnancy, the patient should be cautioned that there is no consensus on the possible effects of therapy on fetal outcome. Adverse fetal outcome directly related to antiparasitic drugs given during pregnancy is thought to be a rare but possible occurrence.

In addition to teratogenic considerations, side effects—including nausea, vomiting, malaise, and Stevens-Johnson syndrome—have been associated with the use of some of the drugs mentioned in this section (see Chapter 12).

Altered Immune States

Hyperinfection syndrome (disseminated strongyloidiasis), a potentially untreatable and fatal development, has been reported in patients with chronic underlying illnesses (diabetes, alcoholism, and human T-cell lymphotrophic virus-1 infection), in patients being treated with immunosuppressive drugs (corticosteroids, cancer chemotherapeutic agents) or radiation therapy, and in patients with malignancy, particularly lymphoma and leukemia. *Strongyloides* can disseminate to all the major internal organs, including the liver, lungs, heart, and central nervous system. Along with consideration of *Pneumocystis* and *Toxoplasma* infections, disseminated *Strongyloides* infection should be considered, especially in the case of immunocompromised patients who develop bilateral pulmonary infiltrates.

It is important to consider the diagnosis in asymptomatic patients from high-risk geographic areas, and to immediately treat those who have positive stool examinations or unexplained hypereosinophilia and positive *Strongyloides* serologies. High-risk patients may be treated empirically for *Strongyloides* before corticosteroid therapy, cancer chemotherapy, or radiation therapy is instituted. If parasite dissemination in a compromised host is believed to have occurred (usually diagnosed on the basis of tissue biopsy or sputum specimens), treatment with the appropriate dosage of thiabendazole may be extended to 5 days or longer.

Another phenomenon described in immunocompromised patients and associated with disseminated *Strongyloides* infections is recurrent polymicrobial bacteremia with enteric microorganisms. The bacteria are thought to stick to the cuticle of worms and to gain access to the circulation when *Strongyloides* larvae migrate out of the gut.

Chronic Strongyloides *Infections*

Infections persisting for more than 30 years are possible because of an autoinfective cycle, in which eggs laid by mature worms in the proximal small intestine hatch in transit with the fecal stream. The resulting rhabditiform larvae undergo maturational changes, becoming infective filariform larvae by the time they reach the rectum. These are capable of exiting from the anus and perforating the skin in the perianal area, buttocks, and upper thighs, thus initiating a new cycle of infection. Local rashes (larva currens) and perianal itching may be the presenting complaints. In one study from Spain, cough was the most common symptom. Rates of infection among former Allied prisoners of war (POW) who worked on the Burma-Thailand Railroad during World War II were found 30 to 40 years later to range from 21% to 37%. Two thirds of these former POWs had episodic, recurring symptoms. Diagnosis and treatment are the same as for more acute infections with *Strongyloides.*

Pinworm

Pinworm is probably the most common worm infection in the United States, occurring mainly in school-aged children (anus-finger-mouth transmission) and their families (household environmental transmission through dust and fomites). Pinworm infections have been linked to increased risk of urinary tract infection in young girls. Rarely, pinworm infection may cause appendicitis or peritonitis. In addition to antiparasitic therapy (Table 40-3), thorough house cleaning and washing of underclothes and bedclothes in hot soapy water contribute to breaking the transmission cycle.

Other Roundworms

Ascaris suum, the roundworm of pigs, is infective for humans and is grossly indistinguishable from the roundworm of humans, *Ascaris lumbricoides.* Environmental contamination with pig excrement may account for acquisition of the common roundworm in patients who report no significant travel history.

Mixed Infections

A study in a highly endemic area in Bangladesh found that mass chemotherapy with albendazole at 18 month intervals was superior to two regimens that involved health education.

ANISAKIASIS

Anisakiasis is a gastrointestinal illness occurring when humans are infected with larval forms of marine ascarides or roundworms belonging to the family Anisakidae, most commonly *Anisakis simplex* and *Pseudoterranova decipiens.* The larvae are present in the flesh of many market fish, including salmon, chum, mackerel, cod, pollock, herring, whiting, bonito, sole, pike, and squid. Humans become infected by eating raw, pickled, or lightly salted fish. The larvae (third stage) are present in the muscles and visceral organs of the fish and can survive 51 days in vinegar, 50 days at 2° C, 6 days in 10% formalin at room temperature, and about 2 hours at 20° C. The larvae are killed in seconds at 60° C. The larvae are 18 to 36 mm long and 0.24 and 0.69 mm wide.

Epidemiology

The disease was first recognized in the 1950s in Holland among people eating raw (green) or lightly pickled herring and was called "green-herring" disease. Thousands of cases have been reported from Japan, where raw or pickled marine fish dishes are consumed (sushi, sashimi, and sunomono). Fewer cases have been reported from the United States and other countries. Gastric anisakiasis is the most common presentation in Japan, whereas in Europe and elsewhere, intestinal anisakiasis the most common form.

The parasite's definitive hosts are marine mammals: *Anisakis* spp. infect Cetacea (whales, dolphins) and *Pseudoterranova* infects Pinnipedia (seals, sea lions, walruses.) The adult parasites living in the stomach of these animals lay eggs, which exit in the feces and hatch in seawater. The larvae are eaten by squid, crustaceans, and other macroinvertebrates, which in turn are eaten by fish. Marine mammals then eat the fish, completing the life cycle. If humans eat the fish or squid, the larvae cannot reach sexual maturity and never lay eggs.

There are two forms of the disease:

1. *Gastric anisakiasis* is an acute illness occurring 1 to 12 hours after the ingestion of raw seafood, with the sudden onset of severe stomach pain, nausea, and vomiting. In more than 50% of cases, there is a peripheral blood eosinophilia of up to 40% without a marked leukocytosis; in 70% of cases, occult blood is found in gastric juices and stools. Anaphylactoid reactions are common; arthralgia and arthritis occur rarely. Untreated infections usually become chronic, with similar manifestations lasting for more than a year. Penetrating lesions, abscess formation, or granulation may occur at the site of larval attachment to the stomach.

2. *Intestinal anisakiasis* is a more chronic disease. Severe pain in the lower abdomen, nausea, vomiting, fever, diarrhea, and occult blood in the stools begin about 1 to 5 days after ingestion of raw seafood. Marked leukocytosis with no or mild eosinophilia may be present. Over months, occasionally for years, infiltrative and mass lesions of the intestinal tract occur, with continued cramping abdominal pain, diarrhea, and dysmotility. Perforation of the intestine, abscess formation, and granulation may occur at the site of the infection.

Diagnosis

The history of eating raw fish is the most important historical element. While immunologic methods of detecting specific antibodies against *Anisakis* (cutaneous skin prick with *Anisakis simplex* extract, and ELISA) may support the diagnosis of ansakiasis, usually the diagnosis is made by upper endoscopy. The histology of lesions in specimens from biopsy or resection is characterized by an eosinophilic granulomatous inflammation; the finding of characteristic larvae in cross section within the tissue confirms the diagnosis.

The gastric form is often misdiagnosed as ulcer, cancer, tumor, polyp, or food poisoning, whereas the intestinal form has been misdiagnosed as regional enteritis or appendicitis.

Treatment

Medication with antiparasitic drugs appears to be ineffective. If the larva is seen during gastroscopy, it can be removed during the procedure. In chronic disease, surgical resection of the affected part may be necessary.

Prevention

Reinfections with additional larvae can occur in acute or chronic *Anisakis* infections. The best prevention is to avoid raw, undercooked, or lightly pickled marine fish and squid. If raw fish is eaten, it should be frozen at −20° C for at least 24 hours; otherwise, it should be thoroughly cooked to a temperature of 60° C.

REFERENCES

Albonico M et al: Epidemiological evidence for a differential effect of hookworm species, *Ancyclostoma duodenale* or *Necator americanus,* on iron status of children, *Int J Epidemiol* 27:530, 1998.

Behnke JM et al: The epidemiology of human hookworm infections in the southern region of Mali, *Trop Med Int Health* 5:343, 2000.

Blumenthal DS, Schultz MG: Incidence of intestinal obstruction in children infected with *Ascaris lumbricoides, Am J Trop Med Hyg* 24:801, 1975.

Booth M et al: Associations among multiple geohelminth species infections in schoolchildren from Pemba Island, *Parasitology* 116 (Pt 1):85, 1998.

Changhua L et al: Epidemiology of human hookworm infections among adult villagers in Hejiang and Santai Counties, Sichuan Province, China, *Acta Trop* 73: 243, 1999.

Geisslet PW et al: Geophagy as a risk factor for geohelminth infections: a longitudinal study of Kenyan primary schoolchildren, *Trans R Soc Trop Med Hyg* 92:7, 1998.

Gotuzzo E et al: *Strongyloides stercoralis* hyperinfection associated with human T-cell lymphotropic virus type-a infection in Peru, *Am J Trop Med Hyg* 60:146, 1999.

Jackson TF et al: A comparison of mebendazole and albendazole in treating children with *Trichuris trichiura* infection in Durban, South Africa, *S Afr Med J* 88:880, 1998.

Jemaneh L: Comparative prevalences of some common intestinal helminth infections in different altitudinal regions in Ethiopia, *Ethiop Med J* 36:1, 1998.

Kightliner LK, Seed JR, Kightlinger MB: Ascaris lumbricoides intensity in relation to environmental, socioeconomic, and behavioral determinants of exposure to infection in children from southeast Madagascar, *J Parasitol* 84:480, 1998.

Labiano Abello N et al: Epidemiology of hookworm infection in Itagua, Paraguay: a cross sectional study, *Mem Inst Oswaldo Cruz* 94:583, 1999.

Mascie Taylor CG et al: A study of the cost effectiveness of selective health interventions for the control of intestinal parasites in rural Bangladesh, *J Parasitol* 85:6, 1999.

Morales G et al: Relationships in the prevalence of geohelminth infections in humans from Venezuela, *Bol Chil Parasitol* 53:84, 1998.

Nacher M et al: *Ascaris lumbricoides* infection is associated with protection from cerebral malaria, *Parasite Immunol* 22:107, 2000.

Needham C et al: Epidemiology of soil transmitted nematode infections in Ha Nam Province, Vietnam, *Trop Med Int Health* 3:904, 1998.

Pearson RD, Irons RP Sr, Irons RP Jr: Chronic pelvic peritonitis due to the pinworm *Entobius vermicularis, JAMA* 245:1340, 1981.
Pelletier LL Jr: Chronic strongyloidiasis in World War II Far East ex-prisoners of war, *Am J Trop Med Hyg* 33:55, 1984.
Pinkus GS, Coolidge C, Little MD: Intestinal anisakiasis. First case report from North America, *Am J Med* 59:114, 1975.
Reynoldson JA et al: Efficacy of albendazole against *Giardia* and hookworm in a remote Aboriginal community in the north of Western Australia, *Acta Trop* 71:27, 1998.
Rodriguez Calabuig D et al: 30 cases of strongyloidiasis at a primary care center: characteristics and possible complications, *Aten Primaria* 21:271, 1998.
Sacko M et al: Comparison of the efficacy of mebendazole, albendazole and pyrantel in the treatment of human hookworm infections in the southern region of Mali, West Africa, *Trans R Soc Trop Med Hyg* 93:195, 1999.
Saldiva SR et al: Ascaris-Trichuris association and malnutrition in Brazilian children, *Paediatr Perinat Epidemiol* 13:89, 1999.
Toma A et al: Questionnaire survey and prevalence of intestinal helminthic infections in Barru, Sulawesi, Indonesia, *Southwest Asian J Trop Med Public Health* 30:68, 1999.

CHAPTER 41

Cestodes: Intestinal and Extraintestinal Tapeworms, Including *Echinococcus* and *Cysticercus*

Christopher Sanford and Elaine C. Jong

Only kings, editors, and people with tapeworm have the right to use the editorial "we."

Mark Twain

Humans acquire tapeworms through ingestion of contaminated food products or dirt. Common intestinal tapeworms include *Taenia saginata* (beef), *Taenia solium* (pork), *Diphyllobothrium latum* (fish), *Hymenolepis nana* (human, rat, mice), *Hymenolepis diminuta* (rat, mice), and *Dipylidium caninum* (dog). *Echinococcus* spp. are tapeworms of carnivorous mammals whose extraintestinal larval stages cause cysts and mass lesions in humans. Cysticercosis is a disease caused by extraintestinal larval stages of *T. solium* that produce mass lesions in humans.

INTESTINAL TAPEWORMS

In the United States, tapeworm infections are uncommon in the general population but are found in certain ethnic and cultural groups owing to dietary habits and exposures. Humans accidentally become infected through ingestion of encysted larvae (plerocercoids) present in the muscles of various animals consumed as meat. Thus, *T. saginata* infections are found among people who eat raw beef dishes, such as steak tartar, and among certain immigrant groups (Ethiopians). *T. solium* is found among people exposed to undercooked pork, commonly immigrants and refugees from developing areas of the world. *D. latum* and other *Diphyllobothrium* species are found among people who eat raw, smoked, pickled, or undercooked fish. These include Eskimos, fishermen, Jewish home cooks (tasting uncooked gefilte fish), and devotees of sushi bars (raw salmon and other anadromous fish, [i.e., fish that ascend rivers to spawn], including American shad, blueback herring, shortnose sturgeon, striped bass, and steelhead trout).

H. nana and *H. diminuta* are rodent tapeworms. Humans can acquire these infections through accidental ingestion of tapeworm egg containing rodent feces *(H. nana)* or larvae-containing fleas and mealworms *(H. diminuta)* when they contaminate granola and other uncooked cereal products. Small children who indiscriminately put small objects into their mouths or who live in rodent-infested environments are also at risk. *H. nana* can be acquired through fecal-oral contamination from other infected humans and thus is common among children from areas of poor sanitation, refugees, and institutionalized populations. *D. caninum* infection usually occurs in children living in households with a dog: accidental ingestion of an infected flea can result in a human infection.

The ingested tapeworm cysts (or eggs in the case of *H. nana*) break open in the gastrointestinal (GI) tract; larvae emerge and attach to the mucosal lining of the small intestine by their head or *scolex*. The tapeworm elongates from each scolex by forming *proglottids,* which are trapezoid-shaped flat segments containing egg-filled uterine branches. The proglottids may stay attached to each other and form a "tape." Segments of proglottids break off the growing worm and are passed in the fecal stream, but the scolex remains anchored and continues to produce more proglottids. The tapeworm has no mouth or GI tract and absorbs nutrients directly through its entire surface.

Clinical Presentation

Intestinal tapeworm infections are often asymptomatic, although abdominal pain, cramps, and diarrhea have been described in heavily infected hosts. Discovery of infection often occurs when a segment or longer "tape" of tapeworm proglottids is passed from the rectum during a bowel movement or spontaneously. Infections are also detected by the presence of eggs (released from the proglottids) found in stool specimens. In the case of chronic *D. latum* infection, the clinical presentation may be that of megaloblastic anemia secondary to vitamin B_{12} deficiency, as these tapeworms compete with the human host for absorption of vitamin B_{12} in the fecal stream.

Diagnosis

Diagnosis can be made from morphologic features of gross tapeworm specimens or from microscopic identification of characteristic eggs in stool specimens. The eggs of *T. saginata* and *T. solium* are so similar in appearance that species identification usually depends on examination of proglottids. Adult *T. saginata* may be noted on GI contrast radiographs as long, translucent filling defects. Species identification of *Taenia* may be important from an epidemiologic point of view but is not necessary for treatment. When differentiating between *T. solium* and *T. saginata* infection is desired, either (1) routine embedding, sectioning, and hematoxylin-eosin (HE) staining, or (2) polymerase chain reaction (PCR) with restriction enzyme analysis, is a useful technique. In the former, the number of lateral uterine branches in the proglottids are counted, with *T. solium* having fewer than 13 lateral uterine branches per proglottid segment, and *T. saginata* having 13 or more lateral uterine branches per proglottid segment.

Treatment

Antihelminthic drugs and their dosages for treatment of tapeworm infections are listed in Table 41-1. Praziquantel and albendazole are the drugs of choice for most cestode infections. Side effects of praziquantel treatment include abdominal pain, nervousness, and weight loss. Niclosamide tablets must be taken on an empty stomach and thoroughly chewed and swallowed. The drug kills by direct contact with the tapeworms. If the scolex is covered by a layer of mucus and is thus protected from contact with the drug, the tapeworm infection will survive treatment. This problem may be avoided by drinking orange juice, lemonade, or some other acidic beverage one-half hour before taking the tablets.

Praziquantel, 25 mg/kg given as a single oral dose, is considered the treatment of choice for *H. nana* by some practitioners. Praziquantel, 5 to 10 mg/kg given as a single oral dose, is an effective treatment for *D. latum, T. saginata, T. solium,* and *D. caninum.*

Table 41-1
Treatment for Intestinal Tapeworms

Parasite	Drug	Dosage
Taenia saginata *Taenia solium* *Diphyllobothrium latum* *Dipylidium caninum*	Praziquantel	Single dose of 10 mg/kg
	or Niclosamide	*Adults:* Single dose of 1.5 g (3 tablets) chewed thoroughly *Children 11-34 kg:* Single dose of 1 g (2 tablets) chewed thoroughly *Children >34 kg:* Single dose of 1.5 g (3 tablets) chewed thoroughly
	or Albendazole	*Adults and children >2 years old:* Two 200-mg tablets as a single dose on 3 consecutive days
Hymenolepis nana	Praziquantel	*Adults and children:* Single dose of 25 mg/kg
Hymenolepis diminuta	Praziquantel	*Adults and children:* Single dose of 5-10 mg/kg

For recalcitrant infections, an alternative treatment consists of purging the adult patient with magnesium citrate and following the purge with quinacrine, 100 mg orally, every 4 to 6 hours for three doses.

Given the high prevalence of these infections in high-risk groups (21.3% of 5412 stool samples of Ethiopian immigrants to Israel were positive for *H. nana,* for example) mass treatment with praziquantel is often chosen over microscopic analysis and individualized treatment.

To test for cure of infection, stool specimens should be examined 1 month and 3 months following treatment.

Prognosis

Untreated tapeworm infections may persist for years and may be associated with mild eosinophilia in the peripheral blood of the host. Megaloblastic anemia may result from chronic *D. latum* infection owing to vitamin B_{12} deficiency. *T. solium* infections may result in a disseminated extraintestinal larval infection called cysticercosis, which is addressed later in this chapter.

EXTRAINTESTINAL TAPEWORMS

Echinococcal Infections

Hydatid disease in humans refers to pathology caused by larval stages of animal tapeworms of the genus *Echinococcus.* In humans, *E. granulosus* forms larval cysts (cystic hydatid disease) in the liver (60%), lungs (25%), and bone or brain, whereas *E. multilocularis* forms solid, tumor-like masses (alveolar hydatid disease) with local invasion of the liver and contiguous organs. *E. vogeli* causes a polycystic form of hydatid disease with lesions primarily in the liver.

Etiology and Transmission

In the United States, endemic areas for *E. granulosus* exist in sheep-raising areas of California and Utah, and in Alaska, where many dogs and wolves are infected. Immigrants from the Mediterranean region, the Middle East, and South America are also likely to have been exposed. Alveolar hydatid disease caused by *E. multilocularis* is endemic in Alaska, central North America including some regions of Canada and the United States, central Europe, Siberia, and northern Japan.

Dogs, wolves, foxes, and other carnivorous mammals harbor the adult *E. granulosus* tapeworm in their intestines. The natural hosts for the adult *E. multilocularis* tapeworm are foxes. Occasionally, dogs and cats in rural areas harbor this parasite and transmit the infection to humans.

Eggs pass with the feces and contaminate grass farmlands. The infection is then transmitted to intermediate hosts (*E. granulosus* in sheep, cattle, swine; *E. multilocularis* in rodents) by the fecal-oral route. In the duodenum, ingested eggs hatch, releasing larvae called onchospheres, which traverse the intestinal wall and enter the portal system. Space-occupying lesions develop in any organ where the onchosphere is trapped. In both infections, humans are an accidental intermediate host. *E. vogeli* is endemic to Panama, Ecuador, Colombia, Venezuela, and Brazil, where it is thought to be transmitted to humans by dogs who have had contact with feral animals.

Clinical Features

In both cystic and alveolar hydatid disease, the infection progresses over decades with minimal specific symptoms until space-occupying lesions cause signs and symptoms in the affected organs. Hepatic enlargement, right upper quadrant abdominal pain, and palpable upper abdominal masses are found in more than half the cases. Patients can present with signs and symptoms of a purulent abscess if echinococcal cysts become secondarily infected from blood-borne bacteria. Acute anaphylactic shock may occur if spontaneous rupture of a cyst occurs or if a cyst ruptures during surgical resection. Alveolar hydatid lesions may become cystic if central necrosis of the mass takes place.

Diagnosis

Eosinophilia is not a finding in the majority of cases. Serum bilirubin and other liver function tests may remain normal until advanced hepatic lesions have developed. Serologic tests performed by the Centers for Disease Control and Prevention (CDC) are the indirect microhemagglutination (IHA), enzyme-linked immunosorbent assay (ELISA), and counterimmunoelectrophoresis (CIE) tests. Specific immunoglobulin G (IgG) ELISA is the most sensitive test (83.5% sensitivity in one study). On the CIE test, the finding of *Echinococcus*-specific "arc-5" antigen is strong evidence for diagnosis, although 5% to 25% of serum samples from patients with cysticercosis may react positively on this test. The greatest number of false-positive results in all serologic tests, except immunoelectrophoresis, occurred in patients with *T. saginata* and *T. solium* cysticerci, and in patients with lymphoma and leukemia.

Radiographs, ultrasound studies, computed tomography (CT), and magnetic resonance imaging (MRI) studies all help to define the location, size, and consistency of the mass lesions. Excisional biopsy, if permitted by the location of the lesion, will yield a definitive diagnosis.

Treatment

Surgical excision of the mass lesions is the treatment of choice when the anatomy of the disease and the underlying health of the patient permit.

Oral albendazole is often efficacious in hydatid disease and is used (1) if surgical excision is not feasible or (2) presurgical and postsurgical treatment to reduce the risk of recurrence after cyst leakage during surgery. Dosage is 10 to 15 mg/kg or 400 mg twice a day in adults, in cycles of 28 days, separated by 14-day periods without treatment. The number of cycles is determined by patient response: 3 to 12 cycles have been used. The most common side effects of albendazole treatment are elevations of hepatic enzymes (aspartate aminotransferase and alanine aminotransferase) and abdominal pain. Rare complications are headache, abdominal distention, and alopecia.

Limited experience using praziquantel to treat echinococcal infections suggests that this drug will not be useful for treatment in humans.

Attempts to sterilize the contents of the cysts with injections of alcohol or dilute formalin into the cyst cavity before surgical manipulation (to prevent secondary echinococcal infections in the event of cyst rupture) may add to the risk of rupture and are not recommended. However, injection of hypertonic saline (20% to 30%), which is reaspirated after 20 minutes, has been useful in sterilizing the contents of cyst cavities.

In an experimental study in sheep, cystic echinococcus responded favorably to percutaneous albendazole sulphoxide without reaspiration.

Cysticercosis

Cysticercus cellulosae refers to the tissue lesions caused by dissemination of larval stages of *T. solium.* This disease is common in Mexico, Central and South America, Africa, India, China, Eastern Europe, and Indonesia. Cysticercosis infection of the central nervous system has been frequently diagnosed as a cause of seizures among immigrants from Latin America to the United States.

People are usually infected with *T. solium* when the eggs (passed in the stool of infected individuals) are ingested in contaminated food or water. Person-to-person transmission in household settings has been documented in nonendemic areas.

Clinical Features

When humans accidentally ingest viable eggs of *T. solium,* the pork tapeworm, the eggs hatch and liberate larvae that migrate out of the GI tract and into the soft tissues. The larvae encyst in the soft tissues; each encysted larva is called a cysticercus at this stage. This process takes place over 60 to 70 days.

If the cysts are located in muscle and subcutaneous tissue, asymptomatic space-occupying nodules may be palpated on physical examination. After excisional biopsy of such nodules, histologic examination shows a characteristic parasite larva in the center of each cyst. After approximately 5 years or more, the larva within each cyst spontaneously dies, and the cysts become calcified. Rice grain—shaped calcifications in soft tissue is seen on x-ray films; these are easily differentiated from the oval spiral calcifications associated with "burnt-out" *Trichinella spiralis* infections.

A more serious consequence of cysticercosis occurs when the larvae migrate to the central nervous system and encyst in the brain. The cysts may involve the parenchyma, the ventricles, or both. Clinical presentation is usually that of seizures and focal neurologic deficits. On CT or MRI scans, single or multiple characteristic cystic masses are seen. Viable cysts enhance with contrast, dying cysts do not enhance with contrast, and dead cysts are calcified. Cases of cysticercosis of the spinal cord have been recorded but appear to occur less frequently than disease of the brain.

Laboratory Studies

Stool specimens may or may not be positive for ova or proglottids of *T. solium* at the time the disseminated larval disease is diagnosed. Eosinophilia of the peripheral blood may be detected at the time of larval migration through the tissues but is not usually present by the time the lesions calcify. Excisional biopsy, if permitted by the location of the lesion(s), will yield a definitive diagnosis. The characteristic brain lesions on CT or MRI scans in the setting of an appropriate geographic or culinary history constitute strong evidence for the diagnosis. A serologic assay for cysticercosis is performed at the CDC (see Chapter 44) and must be requested through the local state health department. A positive result confirms the clinical diagnosis, but a negative result does not rule it out. The test is less sensitive when a solitary cyst is present.

Treatment

Cysticidal therapy for neurocysticercosis is controversial. Many apparently nonepileptic individuals have brain lesions indicative of this disease. Treatment outcome is superior in parenchymal neurocysticercosis than that observed in extraparenchymal neurocysticercosis.

Albendazole is the drug of choice for symptomatic infections when the lesions are located in areas unsuitable for surgical excision. Striking resolution of cerebral cystic lesions has been documented in the months after drug therapy. Albendazole is given at a dosage of 15 mg/kg/day orally for 28 days for the treatment of neurocysticercosis. During initial albendazole treatment, patients may manifest symptoms owing to an intense inflammatory reaction to the rapid destruction of parasites. Dexamethasone in high doses can be used to prevent intense reactions, and has the secondary benefit of increasing the plasma levels of albendazole.

The suggested dose of praziquantel is 50 mg/kg/day orally in three divided doses for 14 days. Drug treatment of cerebral lesions may precipitate cerebral edema, seizures, and acute anaphylactic reactions; for this reason, patients with neurocysticercosis are usually premedicated with corticosteroids before and during praziquantel treatment, as with albendazole. Plasma levels of praziquantel are markedly reduced when patients are treated concurrently with antiepileptics or corticosteroids, particularly carbamazepine, phenytoin, or dexamethasone. Steroids should be used to treat a severe drug-induced inflammatory reaction and may be continued for up to 3 months after drug treatment as needed. Symptomatic treatment with analgesics, antiemetics, and/or antiepileptic drugs may also be necessary.

Repeat CT scan 3 months after treatment with anticysticercal drugs can help determine if retreatment is warranted. A response to drug treatment is made on the basis of the number and diameter of cysts. CT studies performed earlier than this interval may still show residual signs of inflammation after destruction of cysticerci.

REFERENCES

Centers for Disease Control: Diphyllobothriasis associated with salmon—United States, *MMWR* 30:331, 1981.

Curtis MA, Bylund G: Diphyllobothriasis: fish tapeworm disease in the circumpolar north, *Arctic Med Res* 50(1):18, 1991.
Deger E et al: A new therapeutic approach for the treatment of cystic eichinococcis: percutaneous albendazole sulphoxide injection without reaspiration, *Am J Gastroenterol* 95:248, 2000.
Garcia-Noval J et al: An epidemiological study of epilepsy and epileptic seizures in two rural Guatemalan communities, *Ann Trop Parasitol* 95:167, 2001.
Guerrant RL, Walker DH, Weller PF: *Tropical infectious diseases,* London, 1999, Churchill Livingstone.
Kim SK et al: Outcomes of medical treatment of neurocysticercosis: a study of 65 cases in Cheju Island, Korea, *Surg Neurol* 525:563, 1999.
Matuchansky C et al: Images in clinical medicine: *Taenia saginata, N Engl J Med* 341:1737, 1999.
Mayta H et al: Differentiating *Taenia solium* and *Taenia saginata* infections by simple hematoxylin-eosin staining and PCR-restriction enzyme analysis, *J Clin Microbiol* 38(1):133, 2000.
Nahmias J et al: Mass treatment of intestinal parasites among Ethiopian immigrants, *Isr J Med Sci* 27(5):278, 1991.
Ruiz Perez A et al: [The minimum dosage of praziquantel in the treatment of *Taenia saginata,* 1986-1993]. [Article in Spanish], *Rev Cubana Med Trop* 47(3):219, 1995.
Ruttenber AJ et al: Diphyllobothriasis associated with salmon consumption in Pacific Coast States, *Am J Trop Med Hyg* 33:455, 1984.
Salinas R et al: Treating neurocysticercosis medically: a systematic review of randomized, controlled trials, *Trop Med Int Health* 4:713, 1999.
Santoyo H, Corona R, Sotelo J: Total recovery of visual function after treatment for cerebral Cysticercosis, *N Engl J Med* 324:1137, 1991.
Schantz PM et al: Neurocysticercosis in an orthodox Jewish community in New York City, *N Engl J Med* 327:692, 1992.
Sotelo J, Jung H: Pharmacokinetic optimisation of the treatment of neurocysticercosis, *Clin Pharmacokinet* 34:503, 1998.
Tanowitz HB, Weiss LM, Wittner M: Tapeworms, *Curr Infect Dis Rep* 3(1):77, 2001.
Wilson JF, Rausch RL: Alveolar hydatid disease. A review of the clinical features of 33 indigenous cases of *Echinococcus multilocularis* infection in Alaskan Eskimos, *Am J Trop Med Hyg* 29:1340, 1980.
Zarzosa MP et al: Evaluation of six serological tests in diagnosis and postoperative control of pulmonary hydatid disease patients, *Diagn Microbiol Infect Dis* 35(4):255, 1999.

CHAPTER 42

Filarial Infections

Thomas B. Nutman

Filarial worms are nematodes or roundworms that dwell in the subcutaneous tissues and the lymphatics. Although eight filarial species commonly infect humans, three are responsible for most of the pathology associated with these infections. These are (1) *Brugia malayi,* (2) *Wuchereria bancrofti,* and (3) *Onchocerca volvulus.* The distribution and vectors of all the filarial parasites of humans are given in Table 42-1.

In general, each of the parasites is transmitted by biting arthropods. Each goes through a complex life cycle that includes an infective larval stage carried by the insects and an adult worm stage *(macrofilariae)* that resides in humans, either in the lymph nodes or adjacent lymphatics, or in the subcutaneous tissue. The offspring of the adults, the *microfilariae* (200 to 250 μm long and 5 to 7 μm wide), either circulate in the blood or migrate through the skin. The microfilariae then can be ingested by the appropriate biting arthropod and develop over a 1 to 2 weeks into infective larvae, which are capable of initiating the life cycle over again. A generalized schematic is shown in Fig. 42-1.

Adult worms are long-lived, whereas the life spans of microfilariae range from 3 months to 3 years depending on the filarial species. Infection is generally not established unless exposure to infective larvae is intense and prolonged. Furthermore, clinical manifestations of these diseases develop rather slowly.

There are significant differences in the clinical manifestations of filariasis, or at least in the time course over which these infections are acquired, in patients native to the endemic areas and those who are travelers or recent arrivals in these same areas. Characteristically, the disease in previously unexposed individuals is more acute and intense than that found in natives of the endemic region; also, early removal of newly infected individuals tends to speed the end of clinical symptomatology or at least halt the progression of the disease.

LYMPHATIC FILARIASIS

There are three lymphatic-dwelling filarial parasites of humans: *B. malayi, Brugia timori,* and *W. bancrofti.* Adult worms usually reside in either the afferent lymphatic channels or the lymph nodes. These adult parasites may remain viable in the human host for decades.

Table 42-1
Filarial Parasites of Humans

Species	Distribution	Vector	Primary pathology
Brugia malayi	Southeast Asia	Mosquito	Lymphatic, pulmonary
Brugia timori	Indonesia	Mosquito	Lymphatic
Wuchereria bancrofti	Tropics	Mosquito	Lymphatic, pulmonary
Onchocerca volvulus	Africa, Central and South America	Blackfly	Dermal, ocular, lymphatic
Mansonella streptocerca	Africa	Midge	Dermal
Loa loa	Africa	Deerfly	Allergic
Mansonella perstans	Africa, South America	Midge	Probably allergic
Mansonella ozzardi	Central and South America	Midge	?

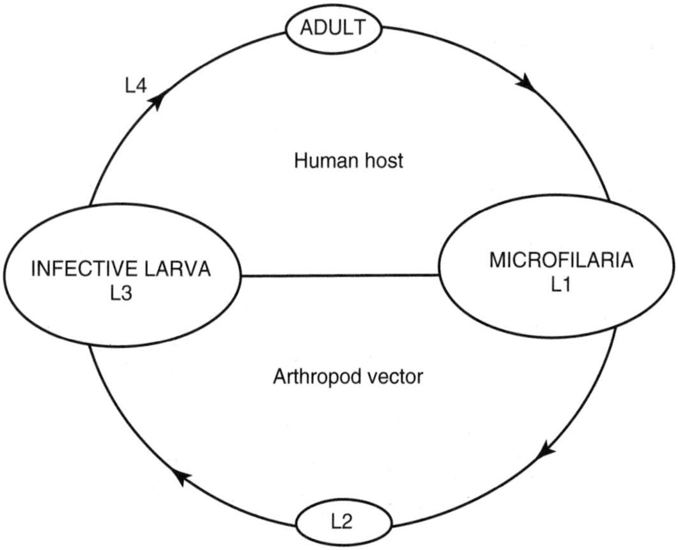

Fig. 42-1 General life cycle of the filarial parasites in humans. Microfilariae (L1) are produced by the adult worms. L2 and L3 are larval development stages in the arthropod vector. L3 larval forms are infective for humans. L4 develop from the newly arrived infective larval forms.

Epidemiology

B. malayi and B. timori

The distribution of brugian filariasis is limited primarily to China, India, Indonesia, Korea, Japan, Malaysia, and the Philippines. In both brugian species, two forms of the parasite can be distinguished by the periodicity of their microfilariae (Mf). *Nocturnally periodic forms* have Mf present in the peripheral blood primarily at night, whereas the *subperiodic forms* have Mf present in the blood at all times, but with maximal levels in the afternoon.

The nocturnal form of brugian filariasis is more common and is transmitted in areas of coastal rice fields (by mansonian and anopheline mosquitoes), whereas the subperiodic form is found in the swamp forests (mansonian vector). Although humans are the common host, *B. malayi* can be a natural infection of cats. *B. timori* has been described only on two islands in Indonesia.

W. bancrofti

Bancroftian filariasis is found throughout the tropics and subtropics, including Asia and the Pacific islands, Africa, areas of South America, and the Caribbean basin. Humans are the only definitive host for this parasite and are therefore the natural reservoir for infection. Like brugian filariasis, there is both a *periodic* and a *subperiodic* form of the parasite. Generally, the subperiodic form is found only in the Pacific Islands (including Cook and Ellis islands, Fiji, New Caledonia, the Marquesas, Samoa, and the Society Islands); elsewhere, *W. bancrofti* is nocturnally periodic. The natural vectors are *Culex fatigans* mosquitoes in urban settings and usually anopheline or aedean mosquitoes in rural areas.

Pathology

Most of the pathology of bancroftian and brugian filariasis is localized to the lymphatics. Damaged lymphatics first lead to reversible lymphedema and then to chronic obstructive changes (elephantiasis) in the limbs, breasts, or genitalia, or to chyluria. The location of the lymphatic damage determines the type and site of the pathology.

Although the underlying mechanisms of pathology in this form of the disease are not yet known with certainty, it is thought that adult worms residing in the lymph nodes or neighboring lymphatics induce local inflammatory reactions and/or changes in lymphatic function. These reactions result in dilation of the lymphatics and hypertrophy of the vessel walls, although as long as the adult worm remains viable, the vessel is said to remain patent. Death of the worm, however, leads to local necrosis and a granulomatous reaction around the parasite. Fibrosis occurs and lymphatic obstruction develops. Although some recanalization and collateralization of the lymphatics take place, lymphatic function remains compromised.

Clinical Manifestations of Those Native to the Endemic Region

The three most common presentations of the lymphatic filariases are *asymptomatic (or subclinical) microfilaremia, adentolymphangitis (ADL),* and *lymphatic obstruction.*

1. Patients with *asymptomatic microfilaremia* rarely come to the attention of medical personnel except through the incidental finding of Mf in the peripheral blood during mass surveys in endemic regions or when blood eosinophilia leads to a diagnostic evaluation for filariasis. Such asymptomatic persons are clinically unaffected by the parasites, although lym-

phoscintigraphic evaluation of these individuals suggest that lymphatic dysfunction (and tortuosity) is common.

2. Acute *filarial* ADL is characterized by high fever (and shaking chills), lymphatic inflammation (lymphangitis and lymphadenitis), and transient local edema. The lymphangitis is retrograde, extending peripherally from the lymph node draining the area where the adult parasites reside. Regional lymph nodes are often enlarged, and the entire lymphatic channel can become indurated and inflamed. Concomitant local thrombophlebitis can occur as well. In brugian filariasis, a single local abscess may form along the involved lymphatic tract and subsequently rupture to the surface. The lymphadenitis and lymphangitis occur in both the upper and the lower extremities with both bancroftian and brugian filariasis, but involvement of the genital lymphatics occurs almost exclusively with *W. bancrofti* infection. Genital involvement can be manifested by funiculitis, epididymitis, scrotal pain, and tenderness.

In endemic areas, another type of ADL secondary to bacterial or fungal infection is common. This is usually recognized as a syndrome with a clinical picture that can include high fever, chills, myalgia, and headache. Edematous inflammatory plaques clearly demarcated from normal skin are seen. Occasionally, vesicles, ulcers, and hyperpigmentation may also be noted. There is often a history of trauma, burns, radiation, insect bites, punctiform lesions, or chemical injury. Entry lesions, especially in the interdigital area, are common. This second form of ADL is usually diagnosed as cellulitis.

3. Chronic manifestations of lymphatic filariasis rarely develop before the age of 15 years, and only a small proportion of the filarial-infected population is affected. If lymphatic damage progresses, transient lymphedema can develop into *lymphatic obstruction* and the permanent changes associated with elephantiasis. Brawny edema follows the early pitting edema, and thickening of the subcutaneous tissues and hyperkeratosis occur. Fissuring of the skin develops, as do hyperplastic changes. Superinfection of these poorly vascularized tissues becomes a problem. In bancroftian filariasis, when genital involvement is evident, scrotal lymphdema or hydrocele formation occurs. Furthermore, if there is obstruction of the retroperitoneal lymphatics, renal lymphatic pressure can increase to the point at which they rupture into the renal pelvis or tubules so that chyluria is seen. The chyluria is characteristically intermittent and is often prominent in the morning just after the patient arises.

Clinical Manifestations in New Arrivals to Endemic Areas

As mentioned previously, there are significant differences in the clinical manifestations of filarial infection, or at least in the time course over which they appear, between individuals who have recently entered the endemic areas (travelers or "transmigrants") and those who are native to these areas.

Given sufficient exposure to the vector (generally 3 to 6 months), patients often present with the signs and symptoms of acute lymphatic or scrotal inflammation. Urticaria and localized angioedema are common. Lymphadenitis of the epitrochlear, axillary, femoral, or inguinal nodes is often followed by lymphangitis, which is retrograde.

Acute attacks are short-lived and, in contradistinction to filarial ADL seen in native patients, are generally not accompanied by fever. If allowed to continue (by chronic exposure to infected mosquitoes), these attacks become increasingly severe and quickly (compared with the indigenous population) lead to permanent lymphatic inflammation and obstruction. Important to note, however, is that early removal of the patients from continued reexposure seems to hasten the end of the clinical syndrome.

Diagnosis

Diagnosis of filarial diseases can be problematic, because these infections most often require parasitologic techniques to demonstrate the offending organisms. In addition, satisfactory methods for the definitive diagnosis in amicrofilaremic states can be extremely difficult. The diagnostic procedures, however, should take advantage of the periodicity of each organism as well as their characteristic morphologic appearance. Table 42-2 and Fig. 42-2 address these issues specifically. The following techniques may be used for examining blood or other fluids, such as chyle, urine, and hydrocele fluid.

Direct Examination

A small volume of fluid is spread on a clean slide. The slide is then air-dried, stained with Giemsa stain, and examined microscopically.

Nuclepore Filtration

A known volume of anticoagulated blood is passed through a polycarbonate (Nuclepore) filter with a 3-μm pore. A large volume (50 ml) of water is passed through (the water will lyse or break open the red cells, leaving the worms intact and more easily visible). The filter is then air-dried, stained with Wright's or Giemsa stain, and examined by microscopy. For studies in the field, 1 ml of anticoagulated blood can be added to 9 ml of a solution of 2% formalin/10% Teepol and stored for up to 9 months before performing filtration.

Knott's Concentration Technique

In this technique, 1 ml of anticoagulated blood is placed in 9 ml of 2% formalin. The tube is centrifuged at 1500 rpm for 1 minute. The sediment is spread on a slide and dried thoroughly. The slide is then stained with Wright's or Giemsa stain and examined microscopically.

Table 42-2
Characteristics of Microfilariae in Humans

Species	Location	Periodicity	Presence of sheath
Brugia malayi	Blood	Nocturnal, subperiodic	+
Brugia timori	Blood	Nocturnal	+
Wuchereria bancrofti	Blood, hydrocele fluid	Nocturnal, subperiodic	+
Onchocerca volvulus	Skin	None	−
Mansonella streptocerca	Skin	None	−
Loa loa	Blood	Diurnal	+
Mansonella perstans	Blood	None	−
Mansonella ozzardi	Blood	None	−

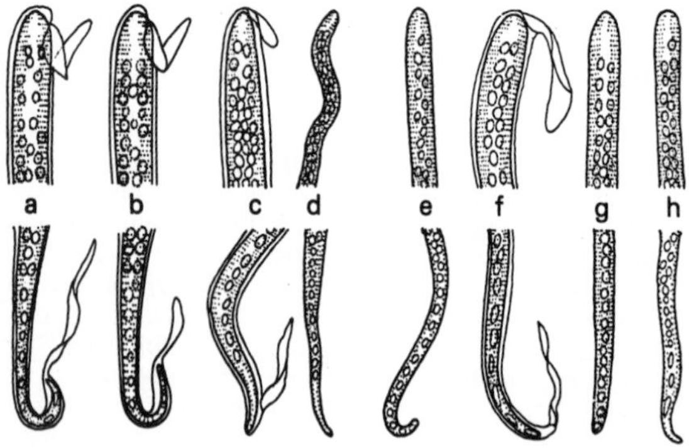

Fig. 42-2 Differential characterizations of the microfilariae: (a) *Brugia malayi,* (b) *Brugia timori,* (c) *Wuchereria bancrofti,* (d) *Onchocerca volvulus,* (e) *Mansonella streptocerca,* (f) *Loa loa,* (g) *Mansonella perstans,* (h) *Mansonella ozzardi.* (Redrawn after Faust and Russell: *Clinical parasitology,* ed 7, Philadelphia, 1964, Lea & Febiger.)

Indirect Measures

Detection of Circulating Parasite Antigen

Assays for circulating antigens of *W. bancrofti* permit the diagnosis of microfilaremic and cryptic (amicrofilaremic) infection. There are currently two commercially available tests, one in an enzyme-linked immunosorbent assay format (Trop-Ag *W. bancrofti,* manufactured by JCU Tropical Biotechnology Pty. Ltd, Townsville, Queensland, Australia), and the other a rapid-format card test (marketed by Binax, Portland, Maine). Both assays have reported sensitivities that range from 96% to 100% and specificities that approach 100%. There are currently no tests for circulating antigens in brugian filariasis.

Serodiagnosis Using Parasite Extract

Development of serodiagnostic assays of sufficient sensitivity and specificity for routine use has proven difficult, primarily because of their poor specificity. As is the case for serodiagnosis of most infectious diseases, it is difficult to differentiate previous infection or exposure to the parasite (aborted infection) from current active infection. Indeed, most residents of filariasis-endemic regions are antibody positive. Nevertheless, such serologic assays have a definite place in diagnosis, as a negative assay result effectively excludes past or present infection.

Molecular Diagnostics

Polymerase chain reaction (PCR)-based assays for DNA of *W. bancrofti* and *B. malayi* in blood have also been developed. In a number of studies evaluating PCR-based diagnosis, the method is of equivalent or greater sensitivity compared with parasitologic methods, detecting patent infection in almost all infected subjects.

Imaging Studies

In cases of suspected lymphatic filariasis, examination of the scrotum or female breast using high-frequency ultrasound in conjunction with Doppler techniques may result in the identification of motile adult worms within dilated lymphatics. Worms may be visualized in the lymphatics of the spermatic cord in up to 80% of infected men. Live adult worms have a distinctive pattern of movement within the lymphatic vessels (termed the “filaria dance sign”). This technique may be useful to monitor the success of antifilarial chemotherapy, by observing for the disappearance of the dance sign.

Radionuclide lymphoscintigraphic imaging of the limbs reliably demonstrates widespread lymphatic abnormalities both in asymptomatic microfilaremic persons and in those with clinical manifestations of lymphatic pathology. While of potential utility in the delineation of anatomic changes associated with infection, lymphoscintigraphy is unlikely to assume primacy in the diagnostic evaluation of individuals with suspected infection.

Differential Diagnosis

The diagnosis of filariasis often must be made clinically because many patients with lymphatic filariasis are not microfilaremic. In acute episodes, the differential diagnosis includes thrombophlebitis, infection, and trauma. Edema and changes associated with chronic filariasis must be distinguished from the similar changes that are seen to occur with malignancy, postsurgical scarring, trauma, and congestive heart failure, along with the less common congenital or idiopathic lymphatic system abnormalities. The many disorders associated with eosinophil and serum immunoglobulin E elevations must be considered also.

Treatment

With newer definitions of clinical syndromes in lymphatic filariasis and new tools to assess clinical status (e.g., ultrasound, lymphoscintigraphy, circulating filarial antigen assays), approaches to treatment based on infection status and pathogenesis have been proposed.

Microfilaria-Positive Individuals

A growing body of evidence indicates that although they may be asymptomatic, virtually all persons with *W. bancrofti* or *B. malayi* microfilaremia have some degree of subclinical disease (hematuria, proteinuria, abnormalities on lymphoscintigraphy). Thus early treatment of asymptomatic persons is recommended to prevent further lymphatic damage. Diethylcarbamazine (DEC), which has both macrofilaricidal and microfilaricidal properties, is the drug of choice.

Microfilaria-Negative Antigen-Positive Individuals

Because lymphatic disease is associated with the adult worm, treatment with DEC is recommended for microfilaria-negative adult worm carriers (i.e., persons who are microfilaria negative but filaria antigen or ultrasound positive).

Acute Manifestations of Lymphatic Filariasis

Filarial Adenolymphangitis (ADL)

Supportive treatment is recommended, including rest; postural drainage, particularly if the lower limb is affected; cold compresses at the site of inflammation; and antipyretics and analgesics for symptomatic relief. During the acute episode, treatment with antifilarial drugs is not recommended, because it may provoke additional adult worm death and exacerbate the inflammatory response. After the acute attack has resolved, if the patient remains microfilaria or antigen positive, DEC can be given to kill the remaining adult worms.

For patients with ADL secondary to bacterial or fungal infections, cold compresses, antipyretics, and analgesics are recommended. The patient should remain at rest, with the affected limb elevated. Antibiotic therapy must be initiated while awaiting results of cultures of blood or tissue aspirates. The bacteria isolated during these attacks are sensitive to most systemic antibiotics, including penicillin.

Chronic Manifestations of Lymphatic Filariasis

Chronic manifestations of lymphatic filariasis include lymphedema and urogenital disease. Although antifilarial drug therapy is rarely, if ever, the "definitive" treatment for these conditions, such treatment is indicated if the patient has evidence of active infection (e.g., detection of microfilaria or filarial antigen in the blood, or of the "filaria dance sign" on ultrasound examination). Not infrequently, the inflammatory response secondary to treatment-induced death of the adult worm exacerbates manifestations of chronic disease.

Lymphedema

Careful attention must be paid to the management of lymphedema once it has occurred. Elevation of the affected limb, elastic stockings, and local foot care will ameliorate some of the symptoms associated with lymphedema. Data indicate that filarial elephantiasis and lymphedema of the leg may be partially reversible with a treatment regimen that emphasizes hygiene, prevention of secondary bacterial infections, and physiotherapy. This regimen is similar to that now recommended for treatment of lymphedema of most nonfilarial causes where it is known by a variety of names including complex decongestive physiotherapy and complex lymphedema therapy. Surgical decompression using a nodovenous shunt may provide improvement in extreme cases. Hydroceles can be drained repeatedly or managed surgically.

Dosage for DEC Treatment

The currently recommended 12-day, 72 mg/kg (6 mg/kg/day in 3 doses), course of DEC treatment has remained the standard for many years; however, recent data indicate that single-dose treatment with 6 mg/kg (in 3 doses in 1 day) of DEC may have equivalent microfilaricidal efficacy. The 12-day course provides more rapid short-term microfilarial suppression.

There is some evidence that multiple courses of DEC will provide a cure: a new treatment course can be initiated 1 month after completion of the previous one. Chronic low-dose DEC may also result in cure.

Side effects of DEC treatment include fever, chills, arthralgias, headaches, nausea, and vomiting. Both the development and severity of these reactions are directly related to the number of Mf circulating in the bloodstream and may represent an acute hypersensitivity reaction to the antigens being released by dead and dying parasites. To avoid these side effects, one can either initiate treatment with a very small dose of DEC and increase the dose to the full level over a few days, or premedicate the patient with corticosteroids. DEC is not commercially available, but must be obtained from the manufacturer.*

TROPICAL EOSINOPHILIA SYNDROME

Tropical eosinophilia syndrome, or tropical pulmonary eosinophilia (TPE), was recognized as being of filarial etiology only in the late 1950s or early 1960s, when it was noted that the antifilarial drug DEC was effective in this syndrome and that patients with TPE had extraordinarily high levels of antifilarial antibodies in their blood. Although circulating microfilariae were never found, lung and lymph node biopsies occasionally revealed trapped microfilariae.

Patients with this syndrome are primarily male (4:1 predominance). Characteristically, those with this form of the disease are in their third or fourth decade of life. A majority of cases have been reported from India, Pakistan, Sri Lanka, Southeast Asia, Guyana, and Brazil.

Clinical Features

The main features of this syndrome, besides a history of residence in a filaria-endemic region, include paroxysmal cough and wheezing (usually nocturnal), occasional weight loss, low-grade fever, adenopathy, and extreme peripheral blood eosinophilia ($>3000/mm^3$). Chest radiographs may be normal but generally show increased bronchovascular markings, diffuse miliary lesions, or mottled opacities primarily involving the mid and lower lung fields. Pulmonary function testing often shows restrictive abnormalities, which may be accompanied by obstructive defects.

This syndrome is associated with marked elevations of antifilarial antibodies, as well as extremely elevated levels of total serum IgE (10,000 to 100,000 ng/ml). Furthermore, in the absence of successful treatment, permanent pulmonary damage (interstitial fibrosis) can develop.

Pathology

Tropical eosinophilia is now considered to be a form of *occult filariasis* in which rapid clearance of the microfilariae occurs, presumably on the basis of host immunologic hyperresponsiveness to the parasite. This clearance takes place in the lung, and the clinical symptoms are probably the result of allergic and inflammatory reactions elicited by the cleared parasites. In some subjects, the microfilarial trapping occurs in other organs of the reticuloendothelial system (liver, spleen, lymph nodes), in which case hepatomegaly, splenomegaly, or lymphadenopathy occurs.

Differential Diagnosis

Tropical eosinophilia must be distinguished from Löffler's syndrome, chronic eosinophilic pneumonia, allergic bronchopulmonary aspergillosis, some of the vasculitides, the idiopathic hypereosinophilic syndrome, drug allergies, and some other helminth infections. Although there is no single clinical or laboratory criterion that aids in distinguishing tropical eosinophilia from these diseases, residence in the tropics, the presence of high levels of antifilarial antibodies, and a rapid clinical response to DEC favor the diagnosis of tropical eosinophilia.

---

*In the United States, diethylcarbamazine (DEC) must be obtained directly the Centers for Disease Control and Prevention (CDC) under an IND.

Treatment

DEC is the drug of choice for treatment of TPE. Treatment for tropical eosinophilia is DEC at a dose of 6 mg/kg/day (divided into 3 doses in 1 day) for 14 days. Symptoms usually resolve between days 4 and 7 of therapy. Characteristically, respiratory symptoms rapidly resolve after treatment with DEC. Despite dramatic initial improvement after conventional treatment with DEC, symptoms recur in approximately 20% of patients 12 to 24 months after treatment, and a majority of patients continue to have subtle clinical, radiographic, and functional abnormalities. Repeat treatment may be necessary.

ONCHOCERCIASIS

Onchocerciasis, sometimes called river blindness, is caused by infection with *Onchocerca volvulus,* a subcutaneous-dwelling filarial worm. Approximately 18 million people are infected, mostly in equatorial Africa, the Sahara, Yemen, and parts of Central and South America (Guatemala, Venezuela, Mexico, Ecuador, Colombia, and Brazil). The infection is transmitted to humans through the bites of blackflies of the genus *Simulium,* which breed along fast-flowing rivers in the previously mentioned tropical areas.

Pathology

The pathology of onchocerciasis is limited primarily to the skin, lymphatic system, and eyes.

Onchocerciasis is a *cumulative* infection. Intense infections, which lead to the disease's severest complications, are believed to reflect repeated inoculation of infective larvae.

Skin

In the skin, granulomatous and fibrous reactions tend to occur in response to the adult worm. Similarly, dead microfilariae in the skin tend to produce small granulomata with eosinophilic infiltrates. Over a period of years, adult worms are encased by host tissue, thereby forming the characteristic subcutaneous nodules (onchocercomata).

Lymph Nodes

The pathology of the lymph nodes consists of scarring of the lymphoid areas (*O. volvulus* infection in Africa) or follicular hyperplasia (*O. volvulus* infection in Yemen). Histologically the lymph nodes draining areas of onchodermatitis show capsular fibrosis, atrophic follicles, and dilation of the subcapsular sinusoids and lymphatics.

Eyes

The pathologic processes that occur in the ocular tissues are not yet well elucidated. The conjunctiva can show an infiltrate with plasma cells, eosinophils, and mast cells. Punctate keratitis occurs and is believed to reflect inflammation around degenerating microfilariae. Anterior uveitis and chorioretinitis may occur and are thought to be a result of a low-grade inflammation, although autoimmune reaction may play a role.

Clinical Features

The major disease manifestations of onchocerciasis are localized to the skin, lymph nodes and lymphatics, and eyes.

Skin

Pruritus is the most frequent manifestation of onchocercal dermatitis. This pruritus may be accompanied by the appearance of localized areas of edema and erythema that is characteristically evanescent. If the infection is prolonged, lichenification and pigment changes (either hypopigmentation or hyperpigmentation) can occur; these often lead to atrophy, "lizard skin," and mottling of the skin. These skin changes can also become superinfected, particularly in the presence of excoriation or trauma.

The subcutaneous nodules contain the adult worm. In the Central American form of the disease, nodules tend to be distributed on the upper part of the body, particularly on the head, neck, and shoulders. In Africa, the onchocercomata tend to be found over bony prominences, such as the coccyx, femoral trochanter, iliac crests, lateral aspects of the knee and elbow, and head. Interestingly, it is thought that for every palpable nodule, there are probably at least five deeper nodules.

Lymph Nodes

Lymphadenopathy is frequently found, particularly in the inguinal and femoral areas. As the glands enlarge, they can come to lie within areas of loose skin (so-called hanging groins), which predisposes the affected patients to hernias. Scarring in lymph nodes may lead to regional lymphedema.

Eyes

Onchocercal eye disease can take many forms, and most can lead to severe visual loss or blindness. Usually seen in persons with moderate or heavy infections, the ocular disease spares no part of the eye. Conjunctivitis, anterior uveitis, iridocyclitis leading to secondary glaucoma, sclerosing keratitis, optic atrophy, and chorioretinal lesions can be found.

Diagnosis

Definitive diagnosis depends on finding an adult worm in an excised nodule or, more commonly, microfilariae in a skin snip.

Skin Snip

A small piece of skin is elevated by the tip of a needle or skin hook held parallel to the surface, and a razor or scalpel blade is used to shave off the skin area stretched across the top surface of the needle (Fig. 42-3). Alternatively, a sclerocorneal punch can be used to obtain a blood-free circular skin specimen.

Skin snips are generally obtained from an area of affected skin or from the scapular, gluteal, and calf areas (in the African form) and from the scapular, deltoid, and gluteal areas (in the Central American form). Once obtained, the skin snips are incubated in a physiologic solution (such as normal saline); the emergent microfilariae can be seen under a microscope after 2 to 4 hours. Occasionally, in light infections, overnight incubation is necessary.

Mazzotti Test

When no microfilariae can be detected, some have advocated the use of the Mazzotti test, which is the appearance of itching and a rash after administration of a single oral 50-mg dose of DEC. Although this test

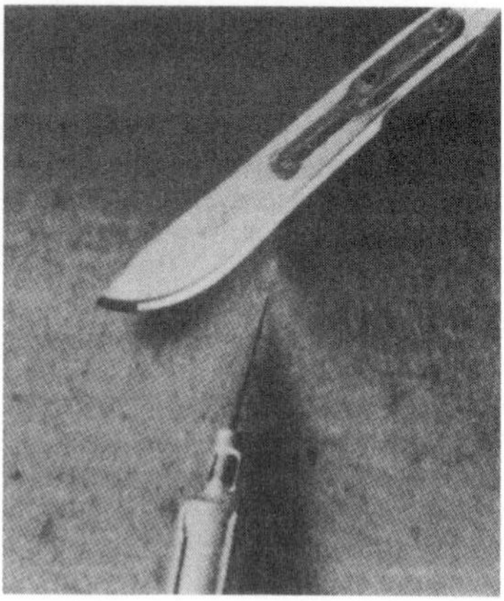

Fig. 42-3 Skin snips being removed with needle and scalpel. Note the small cone of skin that is lifted up by the needle. (From Eberhard ML, Lammie PJ: Laboratory diagnosis of filariasis, *Clin Lab Med* 11:977, 1991.)

is highly sensitive, false-negativity and serious posttreatment sequelae prevent it from being used routinely as a diagnostic modality.

A variety of serodiagnostic and antigenic skin tests have been described. Recently, recombinant onchocercal-specific antigens have been produced, a cocktail of which having been developed by the World Health Organization for diagnosis of onchocerciasis. A rapid format card test using one of these recumbinant antigens has also been developed.

Molecular Diagnosis

Highly specific and sensitive PCR-based assays have been developed for the detection of *O. volvulus* DNA in skin snips that are microscopically negative. This has proved useful in the detection of very low infection levels but requires expensive equipment and reagents, as well as rigorous training and quality control.

Differential Diagnosis

Onchocerciasis must be differentiated from scabies, contact dermatitis, and, rarely, streptocerciasis (see the following section).

Treatment

The major goals of therapy are to prevent irreversible lesions and to alleviate bothersome symptoms. Surgical excision of nodules is recommended when the nodules are located on the head because of the proximity of the microfilaria-producing adult worms to the eye, but chemotherapy is the mainstay of treatment.

Ivermectin, a semisynthetic macrocyclic lactone, is now considered first-line therapy for onchocerciasis. It is given orally in a single dose of 150 μg/kg. It is characteristically given yearly or semiannually. With treatment, most patients have a mild or no reaction. Pruritus, cutaneous edema, and/or a maculopapular rash occur in approximately 1% to 10%

of treated individuals. Significant ocular complications are extremely rare, as is hypotension (1 in 10,000). Contraindications to treatment include pregnancy, breastfeeding, age less than 5 years, and central nervous system (CNS) disorders that might increase the penetration of ivermectin into the CNS (e.g., meningitis).

Although treatment with ivermectin results in a marked drop in microfilarial density, its effect can be short-lived (much less than 6 months in some cases). Thus, it is occasionally necessary to give ivermectin more frequently for persistent symptoms.

STREPTOCERCIASIS

Mansonella streptocerca (Dipetalonema streptocerca, Tetrapetalonema streptocerca) is largely found in the tropical forest belt of Africa from Ghana to Zaire. It is transmitted to the human host by biting midges (*Culicoides* species).

The pathology of streptocerciasis is both dermal and lymphatic. In the skin, there are hypopigmented macules (and occasionally papular rashes) that are thought to be secondary to inflammatory reactions around microfilariae. The distribution of the parasite in the skin of the human host tends to be across the shoulders and upper torso. Lymph nodes of affected individuals may show chronic lymphadenitis with scarring.

The major clinical manifestations are related to the skin—pruritus, papular rashes, and pigmentation changes. Most infected individuals also show inguinal lymphadenopathy; however, many patients are completely asymptomatic.

The diagnosis is made after finding the characteristic microfilariae on skin-snip examination (see previous section on onchocerciasis diagnosis). Leprosy and granuloma multiforme are the two other diseases that must be distinguished from streptocerciasis.

DEC is particularly effective in treating infection by both the microfilarial and the adult form of the parasite. The recommended dosage is 6 mg/kg/day in divided doses for 21 days. After treatment, as in onchocerciasis, one can often see urticaria, arthralgias, myalgias, headaches, and abdominal discomfort. Ivermectin at a dose of 150 μg/kg appears to have a salutary microfilaricidal effect, although only its short-term (6 to 12 days) efficacy has thus far been assessed.

LOIASIS

The distribution of *Loa loa* is limited to the rain forests of West and Central Africa. Tabanid flies (deerflies) of the genus *Chrysops* are the intermediate hosts. The adult parasite lives in the subcutaneous tissues in humans; then microfilariae circulate in the bloodstream with a diurnal periodicity.

Pathology

The pathology associated with loiasis includes the classic "Calabar swelling" (localized areas of transient angioedema) found predominantly on the extremities; a nephropathy presumed to be immune complex mediated; encephalopathy thought to be secondary to either an acute cerebral edema or a chronic, subacute encephalitis; and cardiomyopathy presumably related to the marked hypereosinophilia that these patients have.

Clinical Manifestations

Loa loa infection may be present as asymptomatic microfilaremia, with the infection being recognized only after subconjunctival migration of an adult worm (the so-called eye worm). Other patients have episodic Calabar swellings. If associated inflammation extends to the nearby joints or peripheral nerves, corresponding symptoms develop. Nephropathy, encephalopathy, and cardiomyopathy can occur, but rarely.

There appears to be a difference between the presentation of loiasis in those native to the endemic area and those who are visitors. The latter tend to have a greater predominance of allergic symptomatology. The episodes of Calabar swellings tend to be more frequent and debilitating, and such patients rarely have microfilaremia. In addition, those who are not native to the endemic area have extreme elevation of eosinophils in the blood, as well as marked increases in antifilarial antibody titers.

Diagnosis

Definitive diagnosis is made through parasitologic examination, either by finding microfilariae in the peripheral blood, or by isolating the adult worm from the eye or in subcutaneous biopsy material following treatment. However, the diagnosis must often be made on clinical grounds, particularly in travelers (usually amicrofilaremic) to the endemic region.

Treatment

DEC, 8 to 10 mg/kg/day for 21 days, is the recommended treatment. The drug is effective against both the adult and microfilarial forms of the parasite, but multiple courses of therapy are necessary before there is complete resolution of the disease. In cases of heavy microfilaremia, allergic or other inflammatory reactions can occur; in the most severe cases, there may be CNS involvement, with coma and encephalitis. Heavy infections can be managed initially with low doses of DEC (0.5 to 1.0 mg/kg/day) and the simultaneous administration of corticosteroids. DEC (300 mg once a week) has been shown to prevent infection.

Albendazole has been shown in a double-blind, placebo-controlled study to decrease microfilarial levels in *Loa*-infected patients.

PERSTANS FILARIASIS

Mansonella perstans (formerly *Dipetalonema perstans, Acanthocheilonema perstans*) is distributed across the center of Africa and in northeastern South America. The infection is transmitted to humans through the bites of midges (*Culicoides* species). The adult worms reside in the body cavities (pericardial, pleural, peritoneal) as well as in the mesentery and the perirenal and retroperitoneal tissues. The microfilariae circulate in the blood without periodicity. As with *M. ozzardi* (see the following discussion), the pathology relating to this infection is ill defined.

Although most patients appear to be asymptomatic, clinical manifestations of this infection include transient angioedematous swellings of the arms, face, or other body parts (not unlike the Calabar swellings of *Loa loa* infection); pruritus; fever; headache; arthralgias; neurologic or psychologic symptoms; and right upper quadrant pain. Occasionally, pericarditis and hepatitis occur.

The diagnosis is made through parasitologic evaluation by finding the microfilariae in the blood or in other body fluids (serosal effusions). Perstans filariasis is often associated with peripheral blood eosinophilia and antifilarial antibody elevations. Although DEC remains the treatment of choice, there is little evidence that it is efficacious. If cure is attained, usually with multiple (8 to 10) courses of therapy, patients lose their symptoms along with their eosinophilia.

MANSONELLA OZZARDI INFECTION

The distribution of *Mansonella ozzardi* is restricted to Central and South America, as well as certain Caribbean islands. The parasite is transmitted to the human host by biting midges *(Culicoides furens)* and blackflies *(Simulium amazonicum).* Although adult worms have only twice been recovered from humans, studies on the microfilariae show that they circulate in the bloodstream with little periodicity. The pathology of *M. ozzardi* infection is poorly characterized. Furthermore, many consider this organism to be nonpathogenic. However, headache, articular pain, fever, pulmonary symptoms, adenopathy, hepatomegaly, and pruritus have been ascribed to infection with this organism. Eosinophilia accompanies *M. ozzardi* infection as well. Diagnosis is made by demonstrating the characteristic microfilariae in the peripheral blood. DEC has little or no effect on this infection, but ivermectin has been shown to be effective in reducing symptoms and circulating microfilariae.

REFERENCES

General

Eberhard ML, Lammie PJ: Laboratory diagnosis of filariasis, *Clin Lab Med* 11: 977, 1991.

Lymphatic Filariasis

Nutman TB, editor: *Lymphatic filariasis,* London, 2000, Imperial College Press.

Ottesen EA, Duke BO, Karam M, Behbehani K: Strategies and tools for the control/elimination of lymphatic filariasis, *Bull WHO* 75:491, 1997.

WHO Expert Committee on Lymphatic Filariasis: *Fifth Report. Technical Report Series No. 821,* Geneva, 1992, World Health Organization.

Tropical Eosinophilia

Ottesen EA, Nutman TB: Tropical pulmonary eosinophilia, *Annu Rev Med* 43:417, 1992.

Udwadia FE: *Pulmonary eosinophilia. Progress in respiration research,* vol, 7, Basel, 1975, S Karger.

Onchocerciasis

Ottesen EA, Campbell WC: Ivermectin in human medicine, *J Antimicrob Chemother* 34:195, 1994.

WHO Expert Committee on Onchocerciasis: *Fourth Report. Technical Report Series No. 852,* Geneva, 1995, World Health Organization.

Greene BM et al: Comparison of ivermectin and diethylcarbamazine in the treatment of Onchocerciasis, *N Engl J Med* 313:133, 1985.

McCarthy JS, Otteson EA, Nutman TB: Onchocerciasis in endemic and non-endemic populations: differences in clinical presentation and immunologic findings, *J Infect Dis* 170:736, 1994.

Taylor H, editor: Infectious causes of blindness: trachoma and onchocerciasis, *Rev Infect Dis* 7:711, 1985.

Streptocerciasis

Meyers WM et al: Human streptocerciasis: a clinicopathologic study of 40 Africans (Zairians) including identification of the adult filarial, *Am J Trop Med Hyg* 21: 528, 1972.

Loiasis

Fain A: Les problèmes actuels de la loase, *Bull WHO* 56:155, 1978.

Klion AD et al: Loiasis in endemic and non-endemic populations: immunologically mediated differences in clinical presentation, *J Infect Dis* 163:1318, 1991.

Nutman TB et al: Diethylcarbamazine prophylaxis for human loiasis: results of a double-blinded study, *N Engl J Med* 319:752, 1988.

Perstans Filariasis

Adolph PE, Kagan IG, McQuay RM: Diagnosis and treatment of *Acanthocheilonema perstans* filariasis, *Am J Trop Med Hyg* 11:76, 1962.

Clark VdeV et al: Filariasis *Dipetalonema perstans* infections in Rhodesia, *Cent Afr J Med* 17:1, 1971.

Mansonellosis

Marinkelle CJ, German E: Mansonelliasis in the Comisaría del Vaupes of Colombia, *Trop Geogr Med* 22:101, 1970.

CHAPTER 43

Schistosomiasis, Paragonimiasis, and Other Flukes

Thomas R. Hawn and Elaine C. Jong

The flukes, or trematodes, consist of long-lived parasites that can cause human disease by mechanical obstruction and by inciting local inflammatory responses in affected organs (Table 43-1). Blood flukes (*Schistosoma* spp.), hepatobiliary flukes (*Clonorchis sinensis, Opisthorchis* spp., and *Fasciola hepatica*) and lung flukes (*Paragonimus* spp.) can be associated with major systemic pathology, whereas infections with intestinal flukes (*Metagonimus yokogawai, Heterophyes heterophyes, Fasciolopsis buski,* and *Echinostoma* spp.) usually cause gastrointestinal symptoms such as diarrhea, anorexia, and abdominal pain only in heavy infections.

SCHISTOSOMIASIS

Schistosomiasis is a trematode infection caused by blood flukes. In Africa, schistosomiasis is often called Bilharzia after T. Bilharz, the German physician who first described the parasitic origin of the clinical disease. Species pathogenic for humans include *S. mansoni, S. japonicum, S. mekongi,* and *S. haematobium.* Acute infection of humans with nonpathogenic avian species of schistosomes can result in an allergic skin reaction called swimmers' itch (Chapter 30).

Schistosomiasis affects approximately 200 million people worldwide and is an important cause of morbidity and mortality in rural tropical and semitropical areas. *S. japonicum* is endemic in the Philippines and the People's Republic of China; *S. mekongi* along the Mekong River valley; *S. mansoni* in the Middle East, Africa, eastern South America, and parts of the Caribbean; and *S. haematobium* in the Middle East and Africa.

Transmission

Cercariae penetrate wet human skin during contact or immersion in freshwater inhabited by infected snails, the obligate intermediate host in the parasite life cycle. After infection, the cercariae transform into schistosomula, which develop into adult worms over 4 to 6 weeks. During maturation, the schistosomula migrate through the lungs to specific sites depending on the species. The adult male and female schistosomes couple and begin to produce hundreds to thousands of eggs per day. *S. japonicum* and *S. mekongi* worm pairs migrate to the superior mesenteric vein, *S. mansoni* to the inferior mesenteric vein, and *S. haematobium* to the venous plexus surrounding the bladder.

Table 43-1
Location, Source of Infection, and Clinical Features of Trematode Infections

Species	Location	Source of infection	Clinical features
Blood Flukes			
Schistosoma mansoni	Africa, Caribbean, S. America, Middle East	Freshwater, penetration of skin by cercaria from infected snails.	Dermatitis, abdominal pain, hematochezia, cirrhosis
S. japonicum	China, SE Asia		Same
S. mekongi	Cambodia, Laos		Same
S. haematobium	Africa, Middle East		Hematuria
Hepatobiliary Flukes			
Opisthorchis viverrini	Thailand, Laos	Freshwater fish	Asymptomatic or abdominal pain
O. felineus	Eastern Europe, Vietnam	Same	
Clonorchis sinensis	Far East	Same	
Fasciola hepatica, F. gigantica	Worldwide, sheep and cattle raising areas	Raw vegetables, especially watercress	Asymptomatic or abdominal pain, hepatomegaly, and fever
Lung Flukes			
Paragonimus westermani	Worldwide	Freshwater crustaceans such as crabs or crayfish.	Hemoptysis, cough, ± extrapulmonary involvement
P. heterotremus	Thailand, Laos, China		
P. skrjabini (*P. szechuanensis*)	China	Same	Same but also with cutaneous nodules
Intestinal Flukes			
Metagonimus yokogawai	Asia, Russia, Spain	Freshwater fish	Asymptomatic or diarrhea with abdominal pain
Heterophyes heterophyes	Middle East, Egypt	Freshwater fish	
Echinostoma spp.	Asia	Freshwater snails, fish, or vegetables	
Fasciolopsis buski	Asia	Freshwater plants	

The eggs deposited by the female worms in the blood vessels of the intestines or bladder work their way through the walls of these organs and are passed outside the body in the feces or urine. When stool or urine from infected humans is deposited into freshwater, the eggs hatch and motile miracidia emerge and infect snails of certain species, thus completing the life cycle.

The adult worms can persist in the human host for decades; thus infections acquired in endemic tropical areas can present as puzzling clinical problems years later if infected individuals emigrate to northern temperature areas, where environmental parasites are uncommon.

Clinical Features

Light infections may be completely asymptomatic.

Katayama Fever

At the time of initial parasite egg-laying (ovi-deposition), about 4 to 6 weeks after infection, the patient sometimes presents with a severe febrile illness called Katayama fever. The etiology of this systemic reaction is probably a hypersensitivity to egg-associated antigens; it has been mainly associated with *S. mansoni* and *S. japonicum* infections. This febrile syndrome presents with fevers, headache, cough, urticaria, lymphadenopathy, tender hepatosplenomegaly, and hypereosinophilia of the peripheral blood.

Bloody Diarrhea and Obstipation

Eggs deposited by the female *S. mansoni, S. japonicum,* and *S. mekongi* worms on the peritoneal side of the colon work their way through the bowel wall and cause tissue inflammation and lesions on the luminal side. This acute process can produce cramping abdominal pain and bloody diarrhea.

As the infection progresses, some eggs are retained in the bowel wall, inciting a granulomatous response with eventual fibrosis. As increasing fibrosis displaces normal bowel wall tissue, the contractile dysfunction of the colon can result in obstipation.

Hepatosplenic Disease

In chronic *S. mansoni, S. japonicum,* and *S. mekongi* infections, some eggs do not penetrate through the walls of the intestines but are carried in the direction of the portal blood flow to the liver. Egg granulomas in the portal triad area progress to extensive hepatic fibrosis (pipestem fibrosis). The result is development of portal hypertension and its sequelae of passive splenic congestion, ascites, and esophageal varices. In endemic areas, death by exsanguination from bleeding esophageal varices is not uncommon in heavily infected individuals in the second and third decades of life.

Urinary Tract Disease

The passage of eggs through the bladder wall in *S. haematobium* infections can result in microscopic or gross hematuria. Granulomatous lesions of the urinary bladder, especially in the trigone area, contribute to the development of ureteral obstruction, with subsequent reflux, hydroureter, and chronic bacterial pyelonephritis. In endemic areas, chronic *S. haematobium* infections are associated with development of carcinoma of the bladder.

Lung Disease

Eosinophilic pneumonitis results when eggs reaching the general circulation are trapped in the alveolar capillaries.

Skin Disease

Acute penetration of the skin by cercarial forms may cause a short-lived pruritic rash. In chronic infections, *S. mansoni* eggs reaching the general circulation may lodge in the skin and cause a chronic egg dermatitis.

Central Nervous System Disease

Cases of acute transverse myelitis occurring after the initial 4- to 6-week incubation period have been reported in patients infected with *S. mansoni* and *S. haematobium.* Presumably, eggs or worm pairs gain access to the spinal cord through the venous drainage system of the lower abdomen, resulting in an acute inflammatory reaction where they lodge in the spinal cord. *S. japonicum* eggs carried in the circulation to the brain are thought to be a significant cause of seizure disorders in the Far East.

Schistosomiasis in Pregnancy

Eggs lodging in the placenta may cause poor placental development and premature placental separation (Chapter 12).

Laboratory Studies

A definitive diagnosis can be made by identifying the schistosome eggs in samples of stool or urine submitted to the laboratory. The egg of each schistosome species has its own characteristic morphologic appearance and can be readily differentiated from the others. *S. mansoni* has a prominent lateral spine, *S. haematobium* has a terminal spine, and both *S. japonicum* and *S. mekongi* have a rudimentary lateral spine.

Eosinophilia of the peripheral blood may be present during the initial stages of clinical disease but is not a constant finding in late chronic infections.

Expatriates and travelers returning from schistosomiasis-endemic areas with central nervous system abnormalities should be studied by computed tomography (CT) or magnetic resonance imaging, and a diagnosis of neuroschistosomiasis considered, even in the absence of typical clinical features of acute schistosomiasis, and even if urine and stool examinations are negative.

Serologic testing with sensitive (schistosomiasis FAST-ELISA) and specific tests (immunoblot) for schistosomiasis is available from the Centers for Disease Control and Prevention (CDC). The tests may be helpful to detect low-intensity infections in travelers, expatriates, and immigrants with a history of fresh water exposure in schistosomiasis-endemic areas who have negative stool and urine examinations. The schistosomiasis tests are available through the CDC's Parasitic Diseases Branch, National Center for Infectious Diseases, at (404) 639-3311.

If the clinical picture and geographic history are strongly suggestive for schistosomiasis, but the stool or urine samples are negative for eggs, biopsies of inflamed areas of rectum or colon (via sigmoidoscopy or colonoscopy) or bladder (via cystoscopy) may reveal schistosome eggs retained in the tissues. The eggs may be seen in wet mounts of crushed tissue or histologically stained preparations of the biopsy specimens.

Treatment

Praziquantel is an oral drug and is the only drug that is efficacious against all forms of schistosomiasis. Oxamniquine is an oral drug that has efficacy against *S. mansoni* infections only. It is contraindicated in patients with a history of seizures. Metrifonate is an oral drug that has efficacy against *S. haematobium* infections. Praziquantel (Biltricide) and oxamniquine (Vansil) are both marketed in the United States. Metrifonate (Bilarcil) must be obtained from the CDC (see Appendix). Table 43-2 gives the indications and doses for each drug.

Table 43-2
Drug Treatment of Human Fluke Infections

Parasite	Drug of choice	Alternative drugs
Blood Flukes		
S. japonicum, S. mekongi	*Praziquantel:* 60 mg/kg given orally in 3 divided doses 4-6 hr apart on a single day	
S. mansoni	*Praziquantel:* 40 mg/kg given in 2 divided doses 4-6 hr apart on a single day	*Oxamniquine:* 15 mg/kg given orally once; 30 mg/kg/day given orally for 2 consecutive days for infections acquired in Egypt or South Africa or for 1 day for infections acquired in East Africa
S. haematobium	*Praziquantel:* 40 mg/kg in 2 divided doses on a single day	*Metrifonate:* 10 mg/kg given orally once every 2 weeks for 3 doses*†
Hepatobiliary Flukes		
Clonorchis sinensis, Opisthorchis spp	*Praziquantel:* 75 mg/kg given orally in 3 divided doses 4-6 hr apart on a single day	
Fasciola hepatica	*Bithionol:* 30-50 mg/kg/day given orally alternate days for 10-15 total doses*†	See text for investigational alternatives
Lung Flukes		
Paragonimus spp. (*P. westermani, P. heterotremus, P. skrjabini*)	*Praziquantel:* 75 mg/kg/day given orally in 3 divided doses 4-6 hr apart on 2 consecutive days*	
Intestinal Flukes		
Metagonimus okogawai, Heterophyes heterophyes, Echinostoma spp., *Fasciolopsis buski*	*Praziquantel:* 75 mg/kg given orally in 3 divided doses 4-6 hr apart on a single day*	

* Considered an investigational drug for this purpose. Not available in the United States.
† Not approved by U.S. Food and Drug Administration.

Treatment of acute hypersensitivity syndromes (Katayama fever, acute transverse myelitis) is directed toward general systemic support of severely ill patients. Corticosteroids may be indicated to decrease the inflammatory reaction to parasite antigens.

Prevention consists of avoiding water contact or immersion in areas known to be endemic for schistosomiasis. If accidental water contact occurs, rapid toweling to dry the skin may prevent parasite penetration.

In endemic areas where water contact is unavoidable in native populations, mass drug treatment programs combined with environmental measures to control the snails and promote sanitary disposal of human excrement must proceed concurrently to decrease the incidence and prevalence of the disease. A vaccine against schistosomiasis in humans is not available at the time of writing, although an irradiated cercarial vaccine against a bovine strain of schistosomiasis has been used in cattle in Africa with some success.

HEPATOBILIARY FLUKES: CLONORCHIS AND OPISTHORCHIS

Biliary fluke infections with *Clonorchis sinensis* or *Opisthorchis* species are common among people from Laos, Cambodia, Thailand, southern People's Republic of China, Hong Kong, Korea, Japan, and the far eastern regions of Russia.

Transmission

Humans acquire liver fluke infections from eating raw, undercooked, pickled, or smoked fish. Parasite eggs, passed in the feces, hatch in freshwater. The first intermediate hosts, snails, become infected and shed free-swimming cercariae into the water; the cercariae then infect fish and encyst in the muscles. After humans eat infected fish, the larvae (metacercariae) migrate up the bile duct and mature into adult worms. In addition to humans, dogs, cats, pigs, badgers, and ducks may be definitive hosts for the liver flukes, thus serving as a reservoir of infection in endemic areas.

Liver flukes mature in the hepatic biliary radicles, and the infection may be silent, although the parasite adults induce ductal hyperplasia and fibrosis. The eggs in the bile exit the body in the fecal stream.

Clinical Features

The majority of chronically infected individuals are asymptomatic. For patients with heavy worm burdens, right upper quadrant abdominal pain and jaundice may be present.

Acute Biliary Obstruction

This is a surgical emergency occurring in late infections characterized by heavy parasite loads. Physical obstruction by numerous flukes, as well as a narrowed bile duct lumen secondary to fibrosis, probably contribute to the condition. If acute surgical or endoscopic decompression is not necessary, treatment with praziquantel may be effective.

Acute Pancreatitis

Occasionally, the flukes migrate into the pancreatic ducts and cause obstruction and inflammation.

Recurrent Pyogenic Cholangitis

This infectious process is a clinical syndrome with fever, right upper quadrant pain, jaundice, and intrahepatic biliary gallstones. It is thought to be secondary to bacterial infection in the presence of fibrosis and foreign bodies in the biliary tree. Although recurrent pyogenic cholangitis (RPC) has not conclusively been shown to be caused by *C. sinensis* or *Opisthorchis* species, there is some epidemiologic and anatomic evidence to suggest that these flukes may be associated with this syndrome.

Cholangiocarcinoma

Primary biliary carcinoma is a relatively rare form of malignancy. However, an increased incidence has been found among people living in endemic areas for biliary fluke infection and may be related to chronic inflammation of the biliary tree.

Laboratory Studies

Infections are detected by finding the characteristic eggs in stool specimens. The eggs are among the smallest of parasite eggs and are more easily detected by stool concentration techniques.

The eggs of intestinal flukes *Metagonimus* and *Heterophyes* are relatively difficult to differentiate from the *Clonorchis* and *Opisthorchis* eggs. Fortunately, the drug of choice for biliary fluke infections is also the recommended treatment for intestinal fluke infections (Table 43-2).

In difficult cases of biliary obstruction, endoscopic retrograde cholangiopancreatography (ERCP) may be performed, with adult flukes and eggs recovered directly from the bile during the procedure.

Treatment

In light of the potentially serious consequences of long-term infection with liver flukes, even asymptomatic infections should be treated when they are detected. Praziquantel is the drug of choice and has been known to cure more than 90% of infections after a single therapeutic dose (Table 43-2).

Acute biliary obstruction caused by liver flukes requires surgical decompression and drainage. Prevention of infection consists of eating only well-cooked fish. No vaccine is available and reinfection is possible.

HEPATOBILIARY FLUKES: FASCIOLA HEPATICA

Fasciola hepatica is a large liver fluke that lives in the bile ducts of its mammalian hosts, which commonly include sheep and cattle. It is endemic in more than 40 countries including Europe, North Africa, Asia, South America, and the Western Pacific.

Transmission

Parasite eggs passed in the feces hatch into miracidia, which infect freshwater snails. Cercaria emerge from the snails after 6 to 7 weeks and attach to aquatic plants where they encyst as metacercaria. Humans become infected from ingestion of contaminated aquatic plants, such as watercress, in sheep-raising and cattle-raising areas. After ingestion, the metacercaria penetrate the intestinal wall, enter the peritoneal cavity, and then penetrate through Glisson's capsule into the liver.

Clinical Features

Acute Phase

This phase occurs during parasite migration from the duodenum to the liver via the peritoneal cavity. The classic symptoms and signs include right upper quadrant abdominal pain, fever, and hepatomegaly.

Chronic Phase

After reaching the hepatobiliary system, the chronic phase of the disease begins. Patients can develop cholangitis and cholecystitis, although it is not clear what percentage of patients progress to these complications. There is no association of *F. hepatica* with cholangiocarcinoma as there is with *Clonorchis* and *Opisthorchis.*

Laboratory Studies

Diagnosis is made by finding the characteristic eggs in stool or duodenal aspirates. The sensitivity ranges from 0% to 100% depending on the microscopy technique, intensity of infection, and phase of infection (no egg secretion during the acute migration phase). Serologic tests are also available. Ultrasound and CT scan findings include linear hepatic tracks and a subcapsular location.

Treatment

Bithionol has been the first line agent for fascioliasis at a dose of 30 to 50 mg/kg on alternate days for 10 to 15 doses (Table 43-2). It is considered an investigational drug in the United States and must be obtained from the CDC. Unfortunately, it is no longer manufactured and only limited supplies are currently available. Although praziquantel is effective for most trematode infections, treatment of fascioliasis has only been partially successful. Investigational alternatives to bithionol include emetine (cardiac toxicity), triclabendazole, niclofolan, metronidazole, and albendazole.

LUNG FLUKES

Chronic pulmonary infection with *Paragonimus westermani* and related species can mimic pulmonary tuberculosis, and the diagnosis should be considered in "atypical" cases of tuberculosis that do not seem to respond to standard chemotherapy (see Chapter 22).

Paragonimiasis is endemic in areas where freshwater crab, crayfish, or shrimp are eaten raw, pickled, or undercooked. The infection is worldwide in distribution, with cases reported from Asia, South America, and Africa. A lung fluke infection acquired in the south central United States was documented in a young man who ate a raw crayfish; however, most cases seen in the North American continent are imported infections found among immigrant and refugee populations from Asia and Southeast Asia.

Transmission

Adult flukes live in the lungs of humans and other mammals, such as cats, dogs, minks, and opossums. The worms lay eggs that are coughed up in the sputum or swallowed and passed in the feces. The eggs hatch in freshwater and develop into miracidia that infect freshwater snails. The infection in snails produces cercariae, which then infect freshwater crabs, crayfish, or prawns. The encysted parasites at this stage are called metacercariae and are in the muscle, viscera, and gills. When raw or inadequately cooked crabs, crayfish, or prawns are eaten by humans and other mammals, the parasites excyst in the small intestine, penetrate the bowel wall, and migrate through the peritoneum, diaphragm, and pleura until they reach the lung parenchyma. In the lungs, the larvae mature into adult flukes and start the life cycle over again.

Clinical Features

Pulmonary Paragonimiasis

Although hemoptysis, dyspnea, and chest pain are the classic presenting symptoms, light pulmonary infections may be completely asymptomatic. Symptoms often develop 6 months to several years after infection. On chest x-ray films, parenchymal lesions of the lung, including segmental or diffuse infiltrates, nodules, cavities, or "ring" cysts, may be seen. Less frequently, the radiographic appearance is that of a pleural effusion. Peripheral eosinophilia is commonly present.

Extrapulmonary Paragonimiasis

Approximately 30% of patients present with extrapulmonary features thought to result from ectopic migration of excysted larvae from the bowel. Involved locations include the skin, liver, kidney, peritoneum, epididymis, spinal cord, and brain. The most serious complications from lesions involving the brain include seizures, headache, motor deficits, and visual disturbances. Subcutaneous nodules are a distinct feature of *Paragonimus skrjabini* infections found in China. The nodules range in size from a few millimeters to several centimeters and are often migratory.

Laboratory Studies

The diagnosis of paragonimiasis can be made by identification of the characteristic operculated eggs in specimens of sputum or stool. Sputum concentration techniques on 24-hour sputum specimen collections may be helpful in recovering eggs when random sputum specimens are negative. Eggs present in sputum specimens may be destroyed by Gram stain or acid-fast staining techniques, so the microbiology laboratory must be alerted when specimens are being submitted for parasitologic examination.

If the sputum or stool specimen is submitted to a laboratory that does not regularly do parasitologic examinations, the eggs of *Paragonimus* species may be misinterpreted as *Diphyllobothrium latum* eggs. If *D. latum* is reported in a specimen from an immigrant or refugee patient, the clinician should ask for a review of the specimen by a consulting parasitologist. Complement fixation (CF) and immunoblot tests are available and may be helpful in establishing the diagnosis in patients from endemic areas with radiographic lesions with nondiagnostic sputum studies.

Treatment

The drug of choice in the treatment of this infection is praziquantel, a total of 150 mg/kg given orally in divided doses over 2 consecutive days (75 mg/kg/day) (Table 42-1). Adverse effects associated with drug treatment include nausea on the days of medication and urticaria during the week after treatment (presumed to be a hypersensitivity reaction to antigen released by dead and dying parasites). Bithionol was previously used for the treatment of paragonimiasis (Table 42-2) but is considered an investigational drug in the United States and can be obtained only from the CDC. In addition, bithionol treatment failures have been noted in Southeast Asians with lung fluke infections.

INTESTINAL FLUKES

Endemic areas for the intestinal flukes *M. yokogawai* and *H. heterophyes* include countries in the Far East (Japan, China, Taiwan, eastern Siberia, Korea, the Philippines, and Thailand), where humans acquire infections from eating raw or undercooked fish. *Metagonimus* infections have also been reported from Israel, Romania, and Spain, and *Heterophyes* infections from India, Egypt, and Tunisia. The life cycle of the organism is similar to that of *C. sinensis* and *Opisthorchis* species, except for the anatomic residence of the adult flukes in the intestines instead of the biliary tract.

F. buski is a relatively large intestinal fluke that is acquired in the Far East from ingestion of parasite cysts attached to aquatic plants, such as water chestnuts, contaminated by feces from infected mammals (pigs, humans). Human infection with *Echinostoma* species can be found in Indonesia, the Philippines, Taiwan, and Thailand. Transmission occurs via ingestion of infected snails, fish, or vegetables.

Clinical Features

Light infections with intestinal flukes are often asymptomatic. Persons with heavy infections may present with abdominal pain, chronic diarrhea, anorexia, nausea, and weight loss. Rarely, extraintestinal lesions may result from ectopic migration of larvae, or from eggs gaining access to the circulation and being deposited in ectopic sites.

Laboratory Studies

Diagnosis can be made by finding the characteristic parasite eggs in submitted stool samples. No diagnostic serologic tests are available.

Treatment

Treatment of choice is praziquantel (Table 42-2). Tetrachloroethylene, a drug not available for human use in the United States, is often used in developing countries because of its low cost.

REFERENCES

Arjona R et al: Fascioliasis in developed countries: a review of classic and aberrant forms of the disease, *Medicine* 74:13, 1995.

Chen MS, Mott KE: Progress in assessment of morbidity due to *Fasciola hepatica* infection: a review of the recent literature, *Trop Dis Bull* 87:R1-R38, 1990.

El Kholy A, Boutros S, Tamara F: The effects of a single dose of metrifonate on *Schistosoma haematobium* infection in Egyptian school children, *Am J Trop Med Hyg* 33:1170, 1984.

Goldsmith RS: Chronic diarrhea in returning travelers: intestinal parasite infection with the fluke *Metagonimus yokogawai, South Med J* 71:1513, 1973.

Harinasuta T, Bunnag D: Intestinal trematodiasis. In Weatherall DJ, Ledingham JGG, Warrell DA, editors: *Oxford textbook of medicine,* New York, 1987, Oxford University Press.

Harinasatu T, Pungpak S, Keystone JS: Trematode infections: opisthorchiasis, clonorchiasis, fascioliasis, and paragonimiasis, *Infect Dis Clin North Am* 7:699, 1993.

Johnson RJ et al: Paragonimiasis: diagnosis and the use of praziquantel in treatment, *Rev Infect Dis* 7:200, 1985.

Jong EC et al: Praziquantel for the treatment of *Clonorchis/Opisthorchis* infections: report of a double-blind, placebo controlled trial, *J Infect Dis* 152:637, 1985.

Kilpatrick ME et al: Treatment of *Schistosomiasis mansoni* with oxamniquine—five years' experience, *Am J Trop Med Hyg* 30:1219, 1981.

Lucey DR, Maguire JH: Schistosomiasis, *Infect Dis Clin North Am* 7:635, 1993.

Medical Letter Inc: Drugs for parasitic infections, *Med Lett* 44(1127):1, 2002.

Schwartz DA: Cholangiocarcinoma associated with liver fluke infection: a preventable source of morbidity in Asian immigrants, *Am J Gastroenterol* 81:76, 1986.

Shim Y, Cho S, Han Y: Pulmonary paragonimiasis: a Korean perspective, *Semin Respir Med* 12:35, 1991.

Upatham ES et al: Morbidity in relation to intensity of infection in *Opisthorchis viverrini:* study of a community in Khon Kaen, Thailand, *Am J Trop Med Hyg* 31:1156, 1982.

CHAPTER 44

The Eosinophilic Patient with Suspected Parasitic Infection

Christopher Sanford and Elaine C. Jong

Elevations of the peripheral blood eosinophil count (>450 eosinophils/mm^3) can occur in a wide variety of clinical situations, including parasitic infections, allergic states, collagen vascular diseases, and malignancy (Table 44-1). The eosinophilia associated with parasitic infection usually occurs when helminthic parasites are migrating or dwelling in the internal tissues of the human host.

The immune response to helminth infections is characteristically a T-cell dependent delayed type hypersensitivity (DTH) type II response associated with Th-2 type cytokines IL-4 and IL-5 leading to immunoglobulin E (Ig E) production and eosinophilia. The role of eosinophils is incompletely understood, but it appears that they are involved in the killing of infective larval stages of most helminth parasites.

The absolute eosinophil count is a more reliable indicator of the presence of eosinophilia than is the relative eosinophil count (percentage of eosinophils), which is normally 3% to 6%. For example, a person with a white blood cell count of 4000 and an absolute eosinophil count of 360 has a relative eosinophil count of 9%, which, in this situation, is not elevated.

CLINICAL FEATURES

Transient Migration of Human Intestinal Parasites

Eosinophilia occurs during the larval migration of early prepatent infections with human intestinal helminths such as *Ascaris,* hookworm, whipworm, and *Strongyloides* (see Chapter 40). A transient eosinophilic response occurs in the tissues being traversed and also is seen in the peripheral blood. The eosinophilic inflammatory tissue response is commonly manifested as a pruritic skin rash or a migratory pneumonia in this situation. After the parasites reach their appropriate life cycle location in the lumen of the gastrointestinal (GI) tract, the eosinophilia becomes less pronounced and the symptoms subside. The exceptions are *Strongyloides stercoralis* (see Chapter 40) and *Capillaria philippinensis* (see Chapter 44), whose adult forms burrow beneath the mucosal surface of the GI lumen and continue to stimulate an eosinophilic response in the host.

Prolonged Retention of Parasites in Extraintestinal Sites

Helminthic parasites whose life cycle involves prolonged retention of adult and larval stages within the tissues generally provoke a sustained

Table 44-1
Less Common Causes of Eosinophilia

Rare parasites
Eosinophilic meningoencephalitis *(Angiostrongylus cantonensis)*
Gnathostomiasis
Capillaria hepatica
Fasciolopsis buski
Skin Diseases
Eczema
Dermatitis herpetiformis
Eosinophilic cellulitis (Well's syndrome)
Malignancy
Eosinophilic leukemia
Myelogenous leukemia
Hodgkin's disease
Carcinoma of the bowel, ovary, lung, pancreas, and other solid organs
Collagen Vascular Disease
Polyarteritis nodosa
Dermatomyositis
Rheumatoid arthritis
Hypereosinophilic Syndromes
Löeffler's eosinophilic endomyocarditis
Löeffler's pulmonary syndrome
Pulmonary infiltration with eosinophilia
Eosinophilic gastroenteritis
Eosinophilic granuloma
Other
Hypersensitivity pneumonitis
Wegener's granulomatosis
Inflammatory bowel disease
Pernicious anemia
Eosinophilia-myalgia syndrome
Sarcoidosis
Hypoadrenalism

Reprinted by permission of Martin S. Wolfe MD, from Medical Clinics of North America: Travel Medicine. 83:4, Ed. by Elaine C. Jong MD, July 1999, W.B. Saunders.

tissue and peripheral blood eosinophilia. Examples of this situation are found among the filarial infections of humans (see Chapter 42). Another situation in which this occurs is when humans become accidentally infected with parasites whose *definitive host* (host in which sexual maturity and reproduction of the parasite takes place) is another animal species. The "lost" larval stage parasites wander in the tissues until they die or become encysted.

Localized eosinophilic inflammatory responses to parasites in the tissues can cause severe illness in the human host, who may present with fever, abdominal pain, altered mental status, urticaria, pruritus, painful subcutaneous swellings, pulmonary symptoms, or congestive heart failure, depending on the organ system(s) involved.

Examples of parasites transmitted from animal to humans are given in Table 44-2. Cutaneous larva migrans (see Chapter 30), "swimmers' itch"

Table 44-2
Animal Helminths Commonly Transmitted to Humans

Parasite	Common definitive host relationship	Mode of human acquisition	Disease in humans
Ancylostoma braziliense, A. caninum	Dog hookworm	Direct skin contact	Cutaneous larva migrans (creeping eruption) (see Chapter 30)
A. caninum	Dog hookworm	Direct skin contact or ingestion	Eosinophilic enteritis (see Chapter 44)
Angiostrongylus cantonensis	Rat lung worm	Ingestion of contaminated food	Cerebral angiostrongyliasis (see Chapter 44)
Angiostrongylus costaricensis	Rat abdominal worm	Ingestion of contaminated food	Abdominal angiostrongyliasis (see Chapter 44)
Anisakis spp.	Intestinal roundworm of marine mammals (seals, dolphins, whales)	Raw, preserved, or undercooked fish	Anisakiasis (see Chapter 40)
Ascaris suum	Intestinal roundworm of pigs	Ingestion of contaminated food	Gastrointestinal infection, ectopic larval migrations possible (see Chapters 40, 44)
Brugia beaveri	Systemic roundworm of raccoons and beavers	Mosquito bites	
Capillaria hepatica	Rat intestinal roundworm	Ingestion of contaminated food or drink	

Dirofilaria immitis	Dog heartworm	Mosquito bites	Subcutaneous or pulmonary nodules
Dipylidium caninum	Dog tapeworm	Ingestion of infected fleas	Tapeworms (see Chapter 41)
Gnathostoma spinigerum	Roundworm of dogs, cats, other mammals	Ingestion of raw or undercooked fish, or infected chicken or pork	Creeping eruption and visceral larva syndrome (see Chapter 44)
Multiceps multiceps	Tapeworm of dogs and wolves	Direct skin contamination by infected dirt or ingestion of contaminated food	Coenurosis (see Chapter 44)
Spirometra spp.	Tapeworm of dogs and cats	Ingestion of raw or undercooked frogs, snakes, birds, or amphibian mammals; poultices made of frogs	Sparganosis (see Chapter 44)
Taenia solium	Pork tapeworm	Ingestion of raw or undercooked pork or contaminated food	Cysticercosis (see Chapter 41)
Toxocara canis, T. cati	Intestinal roundworm of dogs and cats	Ingestion of contaminated food or dirt	Visceral larva migrans; ocular toxocariasis (see Chapter 44)
Trichinella spiralis	Rodent intestinal roundworm	Ingestion of raw or undercooked pork, bear, or walrus meat	Trichinosis (see Chapter 44)

(see Chapter 30), trichinosis, visceral larva migrans, angiostrongyliasis, and gnathostomiasis (see Chapter 44) are typical examples of illnesses caused by migratory larval forms of animal parasites in which humans are the accidental hosts.

In schistosomiasis, eosinophilic inflammatory reactions to parasite eggs retained in the body lead to fibrosis and eventual organ dysfunction (see Chapter 43).

Infection with protozoan parasites usually is not associated with eosinophilia. Exceptions are toxoplasmosis, and infection with *Isospora belli* and *Dientamoeba fragilis.*

DIAGNOSIS

The diagnosis of common intestinal helminths is usually made by finding the characteristic egg in stool specimens submitted for microscopic examination. Clinical recognition and diagnosis of extraintestinal or disseminated parasites may be more difficult.

If the stool examinations do not suggest a likely diagnosis, the following approach is suggested in the workup of the patient with suspected parasite infection.

1. The *geographic* or *travel history* of the patient with eosinophilia may indicate a past exposure to parasites. Because the patient with tissue-stage parasites can have multiple systemic or few clinical symptoms to report, and often will have negative stool examinations for ova and parasites, the geographic history is of prime importance. For instance, the history of swimming in freshwater lakes or rivers in endemic areas of Africa, South America, or Asia should suggest the possibility of schistosomiasis.
2. In the *immunocompromised patient* with fever, pneumonia, or central nervous system (CNS) signs, *Strongyloides* should be considered during the search for more common parasitic infections (e.g., *Pneumocystis, Toxoplasma*) even in the absence of eosinophilia.
3. The history of exposure to pets, livestock, and wild animals or mosquito bites in rural areas may provide valuable clues to potential parasite exposure (filariasis, *Dirofilaria, Brugia, Ancylostoma, Toxocara*).
4. The history of eating exotic or raw, smoked, pickled, or undercooked food may provide additional clues to past opportunities for parasite exposure (liver and intestinal flukes, paragonimiasis, trichinosis, cysticercosis, angiostrongyliasis, gnathostomiasis).

The diagnosis of a parasitic etiology for hypereosinophilia in a given patient is important for the following reasons:

1. Specific antiparasitic treatment may be indicated.
2. Prolonged hypereosinophilia can have uncomfortable and potentially life-threatening sequelae (pruritic skin rashes, painful subcutaneous swellings, endomyocardial fibrosis, and so forth).
3. The prompt search for other etiologies of hypereosinophilia may be indicated (allergy, occult tumor, leukemia, connective tissue disease, sarcoidosis, hypereosinophilic syndrome, hepatitis).

LABORATORY STUDIES

Biopsy of a lesion or infected organ is the most reliable way to make a definitive diagnosis of tissue parasitism. However, *serologic tests* available for some of the parasites are quite valuable in cases in which the lesion or involved organ is not easily amenable to biopsy. Tests that are currently available are listed in Table 44-3.

Table 44-3
Parasite Serologic Tests Useful in Evaluation of Eosinophilia

Disease	Test	Test laboratory*
Toxocariasis	ELISA	CDC
Strongyloidiasis	ELISA	CDC
Filariasis	ELISA	NIH
Trichinosis	BFT, CIE, ELISA	State Public Health Dept.
Cysticercosis	ELISA, Immunoblot	CDC
Schistosomiasis	ELISA, Immunoblot	CDC
Paragonimiasis	ELISA	CDC

BFT, Bentonite flocculation; *CIE,* counter immunoelectrophoresis; *ELISA,* enzyme-linked immunosorbent assay; *NIH,* National Institutes of Health.
*Serum specimens are sent to the Centers for Disease Control (CDC) via the State Public Health Dept. Before serum specimens will be accepted for testing by the CDC, the clinician must furnish sufficient clinical and epidemiologic data to justify the request for the test. Depending on the suspected diagnosis, attempts must be made to make the diagnosis by prior laboratory testing, including (1) complete blood counts, (2) stool and/or urine specimens for ova and parasite examinations (strongyloidiasis, cysticercosis, schistosomiasis, paragonimiasis), (3) skin or tissue biopsies as appropriate (filariasis, trichinosis, cysticercosis), and (4) isolation of the parasite from blood by filtration or concentration techniques (filariasis). Similar serologic tests may be offered by commercial laboratories.

Eosinophils in Cerebrospinal Fluid

The finding of eosinophilic pleocytosis in the cerebrospinal fluid (CSF) may indicate parasite invasion of the CNS (angiostrongyliasis, cysticercosis, gnathostomiasis, and so forth). However, the absence of eosinophils in the CSF does not rule out a parasite problem in the CNS. Parasite-specific antibody may be detected in the CSF and may aid in making a diagnosis. Nonparasitic diagnoses that must be considered include bacterial infection (syphilis, tuberculosis), fungal infection (coccidioidomycosis), viral infection, malignancy, drug hypersensitivity, and other CNS conditions.

Eosinophils in Pleural Effusion Fluid

Eosinophilic pleural effusions may reflect a pulmonary parasite infection (paragonimiasis) or systemic eosinophilia. Eosinophilic pleural effusions may also accompany tuberculosis, pulmonary tumors, and cirrhosis of the liver. Pleural eosinophilia is not a reliable indicator that the underlying disorder is benign.

Eosinophils, Charcot-Leyden Crystals, and Curschmann's Spirals in the Sputum

The finding of eosinophils and eosinophil-derived structures, such as Charcot-Leyden crystals or Curschmann's spirals, in the sputum, pulmonary infiltrates, and peripheral blood eosinophilia is compatible with a diagnosis of pulmonary parenchymal parasitic infection (larval migrations), although severe intrinsic asthma and other nonparasitic diagnoses must be considered.

SPECIFIC INFECTIONS

Visceral Larva Migrans

Visceral larva migrans (VLM) is a pediatric illness seen in children who have pica (geophagia) or who live in households with puppies. The disease is due to accidental human infection with *Toxocara canis,* although a similar illness may be produced by infection with *T. cati, T. leonina, Capillaria hepatica, Ancylostoma* spp., *Ascaris suum, Gnathostoma* spp., and *Dirofilaria* spp. VLM resulting from toxocariasis can be acquired in the United States, as well as all over the world, even in urban areas, owing to the widespread popularity of dogs as pets.

The patient is usually a 3- to 5-year-old child who presents with cough, wheezing, fever, convulsions, and pallor. Visual impairment and strabismus may be present or may develop. On physical examination, rales and wheezing, hepatomegaly, splenomegaly, lymphadenopathy, and skin lesions may be found. Eye ground lesions (ocular toxocariasis) may appear concurrently with VLM in very heavy infections.

Laboratory studies show a marked eosinophilia in the peripheral blood and elevation of immunoglobulins, especially IgG and IgE. The definitive diagnosis is made by biopsy of involved tissues, although a serologic test (Table 44-3) may confirm the clinical diagnosis. The most prevalent findings of abdominal ultrasound examination of children are hepatic granulomas and abdominal lymph-node enlargement.

The efficacy of treatment is controversial. The newer benzimidazole compounds albendazole and mebendazole are preferable to other antihelminthic agents including diethylcarbamazine and thiabendazole, owing to the former's better safety profile. Corticosteroids may benefit patients with severe pulmonary, myocardial, or CNS symptoms. Also, adjuvant corticosteroids blunt the inflammatory response caused by treatment with antihelmintics.

Ocular Toxocariasis

Ocular toxocariasis is thought to result from a low infectious dose with *T. canis* and is manifested by a mass lesion in the retina that often cannot be distinguished on physical examination of the fundus from a retinoblastoma. The patients with ocular toxocariasis are usually older (age range, 3 to 40 years) than the VLM patients. They present with visual defects and abnormal extraocular movements in one eye but no generalized systemic complaints.

The enzyme-linked immunosorbent assay (ELISA) serologic test for *Toxocara* diagnosis is less sensitive in ocular toxocariasis (45%) than for VLM (78%). A working diagnosis is made by correlating the history of exposure to dogs or dirt, the clinical findings, and the *Toxocara* serology test results. Definitive diagnosis is made by identification of the characteristic larva in enucleated specimens.

Treatment with antihelmintics has not been shown to be of benefit. Systemic and intraocular corticosteroids, which suppress local inflammation, have been the most effective treatment if instituted within the first 4 weeks of illness. Watchful waiting with enucleation of the infected eye for end-stage ocular disease represents the conservative approach.

Trichinosis

Human infections with *Trichinella spiralis* are worldwide in distribution wherever pork is consumed raw or undercooked. Pigs are the major reservoir of infections transmitted to humans, but other mammals can serve as definitive hosts. In livestock areas, rats probably are the reservoir of infection for pigs fed on raw garbage. In the United States, an "ethnic-related prevalence" has been noted with outbreaks among Laotian refugees (pork) and Alaskan Eskimos and hunters (bear and walrus meat). Consuming raw or undercooked horse meat is a growing cause of trichinosis, particularly in France and Italy.

The larvae encysted in infected meat excyst in the duodenum or jejunum, mature into adult males and females, and copulate; then the females produce larvae that migrate through all the internal organs (including the heart and brain) and finally settle in striated muscle. In the diaphragm; tongue; masseters; and the limb, intercostal, and extraocular muscles, and others, the larvae encyst, coiling up into spirals within the cysts. Eventually, the cysts may calcify and be recognized on x-ray study of soft tissue.

Nonspecific GI symptoms (nausea, vomiting, diarrhea, constipation, abdominal pain) may occur within 24 hours after ingestion of infected meat. Larval migrations into muscle occur beginning 1 week after initial infection and are usually accompanied by *high fever, muscle pain,* and *malaise.* A pronounced peripheral blood *eosinophilia* occurs at this time. Periorbital edema, if it occurs, is a useful sign.

The diagnosis is made by finding the characteristic larvae on muscle biopsy specimens or by serologic testing (Table 44-3).

Drug treatment with antihelmintics is only of benefit during the GI and acute severe infection phases of illness. Pyrantel, mebendazole, or albendazole are used during the GI phase, and mebendazole or albendazole in addition to prednisolone is used for acute severe infection. In moderate or mild infection, prednisolone alone may be used. In late phase illness, no treatment is advised, unless active infection is shown on biopsy; in this situation mebendazole or albendazole together with corticosteroids is recommended.

Transmission is best controlled by careful pig-raising techniques and thorough cooking of pork and other meats. The *Trichinella* larvae are killed at 62° C (144° F) after brief cooking, and at 58° C (137° F) after prolonged cooking. Irradiation of pork can be used to kill *Trichinella* larvae, but this technique is controversial and not in widespread use at this time. The encysted *Trichinella* larvae are fairly resistant to freezing, cysts in pork being killed at −15° C (5° F) after 20 days, and cysts in bear meat surviving even longer periods of freezing.

Capillariasis

Capillaria philippinensis is an intestinal infection of humans caused by a nematode with a complicated, incompletely understood life cycle. There are no known animal reservoirs. Humans acquire this parasite in Southeast Asia and the Philippines through the ingestion of raw fish.

The parasite male and female adults live in the small intestine, especially in the jejunum, but also in the upper ileum, and less frequently in the duodenum. The adults burrow into the intestinal wall to the layer of the lamina propria. Parasite eggs pass out of the body in the fecal stream. An autoinfective cycle also exists, whereby the parasites can multiply internally without an obligate life cycle stage outside the human body.

Patients with heavy infections may have features of severe malnutrition owing to malabsorption of protein, carbohydrate, and fat, as well as actual loss of protein fluid and electrolytes from the damaged intestinal lining. The diagnosis is made by the finding of characteristic eggs in stool specimens, by identification of adults or larvae in intestinal biopsies, or by serologic diagnosis (an ELISA test is available in certain research laboratories). Eosinophilia and an elevated IgE value are nonspecific findings.

Hepatic capillariasis occurs when humans ingest food or water contaminated with eggs of the rat intestinal roundworm, *Capillaria hepatica.* Additional animal reservoirs may include squirrels, muskrats, mice, hares, dogs, pigs, beavers, and monkeys. Cases have been reported from the continental United States, Hawaii, Mexico, Brazil, Turkey, South Africa, and India. The infection has clinical features of VLM, although the liver is the primary organ infected. The diagnosis is made by finding the characteristic eggs and worms in biopsy or autopsy specimens of the liver.

Gnathostomiasis

Gnathostoma spinigerum and other *Gnathostoma* species cause illnesses similar to VLM and creeping eruption. Gnathostomiasis in humans occurs in Thailand, Japan, China, Malaysia, India, Vietnam, the Philippines, Java, and Israel.

The definitive hosts for *Gnathostoma* species include dogs, cats, tigers, lions, leopards, minks, and raccoons. Humans are accidentally infected with intermediate larval forms of this animal nematode by eating infected raw or undercooked freshwater fish, eels, frogs, and snakes. If chicken and pigs have eaten infected fish, humans can acquire the infection from eating undercooked chicken and pork.

If intermediate hosts of *Gnathostoma* are eaten, encysted larvae in the muscle or connective tissue undergo excystation in the stomach of the new animal. The larvae then migrate in the internal organs or subcutaneous tissues. Symptoms of disease depend on the route of the larval migrations.

Acute larval migration is accompanied by nausea, vomiting, pruritus, urticaria, and abdominal discomfort. Peripheral blood eosinophilia may be as high as 90%. The larval migrations usually go to the subcutaneous tissues after the acute phase, causing transitory *subcutaneous swelling* accompanied by local erythema, pruritus, and discomfort. Larval migration into the CNS is a serious complication and is in the differential diagnosis of *eosinophilic myeloencephalitis.* Diagnosis is made by identification of the parasite in biopsy specimens. Enzyme immunoassay for IgG antibody against an aqueous extract of the third-stage larvae of *G. spinigerum* is a promising serodiagnostic test.

Treatment consists of surgical removal of the lesions. Albendazole, 400 mg once a day for 3 weeks, may be an effective tissue larvicidal agent for cutaneous gnathostomiasis.

Cerebral Angiostrongyliasis

In April of 2000, 10 tourists from Chicago and other U.S. cities developed symptoms and signs of meningitis a median of 10 days after leaving Jamaica. Serology indicated that *A. cantonensis* was the etiologic agent. Eight of the tourists, including five medical students from Northwestern University, required hospitalization.

In the last 50 years, *Angiostrongylus cantonensis,* the rat lungworm, which is the most common cause of eosinophilic meningitis, has spread from Southeast Asia to the South Pacific, Africa, India, the Caribbean, and recently to Australia and North America. The primary mode of spread has been via cargo ship rats. Infection in humans is acquired by eating snails or food items (prawns, crabs, planarians, vegetables) contaminated by the mucus of infected slugs, land snails, or aquatic snails. The definitive host is the rat, in which the rat lungworm, *A. cantonensis,* adult worms live in the pulmonary arteries and the right heart.

When humans become accidentally infected through contaminated food, the larvae migrate to the CNS and cause eosinophilic meningitis. The eyes may be involved also. The severe illness, lasting 2 to 4 weeks, either ends in death or becomes dormant with residual CNS findings (focal neurologic defects, mental retardation, blindness). People with light infections may spontaneously recover without neurologic residua. Diagnosis is made by identifying the parasite in the CSF or brain tissue.

There is no specific drug treatment recommended for this infection. Cautious removal of CSF at 3- to 7-day intervals, which causes marked improvement of headache, is advised until there is clinical and laboratory improvement. In severe cases, corticosteroids are used to reduce cerebral pressure. Although *A. cantonensis* is susceptible to multiple antihelmintic agents, including thiabendazole and mebendazole, these agents should not be used, since they can cause clinical deterioration or death from inflammation to dead or dying worms in the brain.

Abdominal Angiostrongyliasis

Abdominal angiostrongyliasis in humans is caused by the rat abdominal worm, *Angiostrongylus costaricensis.* This infection is found in Costa Rica and other Central American countries. Snails and slugs become infected with larvae shed in rat feces, and their mucus contaminates food or drink ingested by humans. The ingested larvae penetrate the intestinal wall and migrate to mesenteric lymph nodes or lymphatic vessels, causing an appendicitis-like picture with eosinophilia. The differential diagnosis includes mesenteric pinworm infection, *Yersinia enterocolitica* infection, abdominal tuberculosis, migratory *Ascaris* infection, and bacterial appendicitis. Diagnosis is made by finding the characteristic parasites in operative or postmortem appendiceal specimens.

Sparganosis

Human infection with dog and cat cestodes of the *Spirometra* species occurs in Asia and Southeast Asia. Humans acquire *Spirometra* infections from ingestion of undercooked infected frogs, birds, and amphibian mammals. Infection also occurs through use of raw frog flesh as a poultice. Clinical manifestations of infection include migrating subcutaneous masses and peripheral blood eosinophilia. Gnathostomiasis, sparganosis, and paragonimiasis (*Paragonimus skrjabini,* see later discussions) are among the more common parasitic etiologies of migratory subcutaneous masses, as is filariasis (*Loa loa,* see Chapter 42).

Coenurosis

Human infection with the dog and wolf cestode *Multiceps multiceps* can result in two clinical syndromes—cutaneous infections characterized by solitary, painless subcutaneous nodules, and subconjunctival lesions and CNS infections that can involve the brain, spinal cord, or eyes. Coenurosis has been reported from tropical Africa and South America, although sporadic cases have occurred in northern temperate climates. Humans acquire the infection from direct contamination of the skin or by ingestion of food contaminated with eggs from canine feces. Coenurosis should be considered in the workup of suspected cysticercosis and echinococcosis.

Paragonimus Skrjabini

This species of *Paragonimus* is acquired in Asia. The parasites migrate to subcutaneous tissues and mature; a reactive nodule forms around the adult parasites. Treatment is usually excisional biopsy, and the diagnosis is confirmed by finding the adult parasite in biopsy specimens.

Eosinophilic Enteritis

Cases of human eosinophilic enteritis caused by dog hookworm *Ancylostoma caninum* have been reported from northern Queensland, Australia. Infection is presumed to occur by direct skin contact with contaminated soil, although infection by ingestion of contaminated food is presumably possible. Patients present with severe abdominal pain, sometimes accompanied by diarrhea, weight loss, and melena. Peripheral blood eosinophilia and elevated levels of serum IgE are present. Diagnosis is made on the basis of clinical history, presentation, and the finding of *A. caninum* in intestinal biopsy specimens.

Sarcocystis

Sarcocystis organisms are coccidians that form muscle cysts in the intermediate host, or host of prey, and undergo sporogony in the intestine of a definitive or predatory host. In human muscle infection, painful muscle swellings develop, measuring 1 to 3 cm, associated with fever and myalgia. In human enteric infection, fever, vomiting, chills and diaphoresis is seen. Diagnosis of *Sarcocystis* myositis is by muscle biopsy. Diagnosis of intestinal sarcocystis is made by identifying sporocysts, each containing four sporozoites, in stool with the aid of flotation procedures. Eosinophilia is often present in both forms. Treatment consists of corticosteroids, which decreases the allergic inflammatory reactions that occur after cyst rupture.

Pulmonary Syndromes: Tropical Pulmonary Eosinophilia and Löeffler's Syndrome

Tropical pulmonary eosinophilia (TPE) results from a hypersensitivity reaction to lymphatic filarial parasites *Wuchereria bancrofti,* or, less commonly, *Brugia malayi.* It occurs in long-time residents of endemic areas, most commonly in the Indian subcontinent. Clinical features include paroxysmal cough, which is usually worse at night, wheezing, and dyspnea, together with systemic manifestations including fever and weight loss. Absolute eosinophil count is usually over $3000/mm^3$. Microfilariae are not seen in peripheral blood. A high titer of antifilarial antibody is present, and serum total IgE is elevated. Diagnosis is confirmed by a favorable response to diethylcarbamazine.

Löeffler's syndrome is caused by the migration of larvae of *Ascaris,* hookworm, or *Strongyloides,* from pulmonary capillaries to alveoli. The short-lived pulmonary symptoms include irritating, nonproductive cough, and burning substernal pain. Over half of patients have rales and wheezing. Transient infiltrates are noted on chest x-ray study, and peripheral eosinophilia is moderate. *Ascaris, Necator,* or *Ancylostoma* larvae may be present in sputum. Acute symptoms usually subside within 5 or 10 days.

CONCLUSION

Parasitic infections are an important consideration in the workup of clinical syndromes characterized by tissue and peripheral blood eosinophilia. Because the diagnosis of the extraintestinal parasites presented in this chapter may involve invasive techniques, an elaborate and aggressive workup should be pursued only if the patient has an appropriate history of geographic or exposure factors.

REFERENCES

Eosinophils

Butterworth AE: Immunological aspects of human schistosomiasis, *Br Med Bull* 54:357, 1998.

Mahmoud AAF, Austen KF, editors: *The eosinophil in health and disease,* New York, 1980, Grune & Stratton.

Martinez Garcia MA et al: Diagnostic utility of eosinophils in the pleural fluid, *Eur Respir J* 15:166, 2000.

Meeusen EN, Balic A: Do eosinophils have a role in the killing of helminth parasites? *Parasitol Today* 16:95, 2000.

Wolfe M: Eosinophilia in the returning traveler, *Med Clin North Am* 83:1019, 1999.

Visceral Larva Migrans, Ocular Toxocariasis

Baldisserotto M et al: Ultrasound findings in children with toxocariasis: report on 18 cases, *Pediatr Radiol* 29:316, 1999.

Kinceková J et al: Larval toxocariasis and its clinical manifestation in childhood in the Slovak Republic, *J Helminthol* 73:323, 1999.

Shantz PM, Meyer D, Glickman LT: Clinical, serologic, and epidemiologic characteristics of ocular toxocariasis, *Am J Trop Med Hyg* 28:24, 1979.

Other Parasite Infections

Forbes LB: The occurrence and ecology of *Trichinella* in marine mammals, *Vet Parasitol* 93(3-4):321, 2000.

Pien FD, Pien BC: *Angiostrongylus cantonensis* eosinophilic meningitis, *Int J Infect Dis* 3:161, 1999.

Treatment of Parasitic Infections

Drugs for parasitic infections, *Med Lett* April, 2002. (http://www.medicalletter.com/freedocs/parasitic.pdf)

Van den Bossche H: Chemotherapy of parasitic infections, *Nature* 273:626, 1978.

Guerrant RL, Walker DH, Weller PF: *Tropical infectious diseases,* London, 1999, Churchill Livingstone.

Pulmonary Eosinophilic Syndromes

Ong RK, Doyle RL: Tropical pulmonary eosinophilia, *Chest* 113:1673, 1998.

Zoonoses

Elliot DL et al: Pet associated illness, *N Engl J Med* 313:985, 1985.

Prociv P, Croese J: Human eosinophilic enteritis caused by dog hookworm, *Ancylostoma Caninum, Lancet* 335:1299, 1990.

APPENDIX

Selected Information Resources for Travel and Tropical Medicine

AMERICAN SOCIETY OF TROPICAL MEDICINE AND HYGIENE (ASTMH)

www.astmh.org

American Journal of Tropical Medicine and Hygiene, Annual Scientific Meeting, Directory of Travel and Tropical Medicine Clinics among Society members, list of international clinical and research opportunities for tropical medicine, The American Committee on Clinical Tropical Medicine and Travelers' Health (ACCTMTH) clinical group, ACCTMTH Internet listserv, ACCTMTH Certificate Program for clinical tropical medicine and travelers' health, Continuing Medical Education (CME) courses. (Membership fee; Registration fees for Annual Scientific Meeting, CME courses, and Certificate Program)

DIVERS ALERT NETWORK (DAN)

www.diversalertnetwork.org

Scuba diving and dive safety organization, emergency medical advice and assistance for underwater diving injuries, expert medical information for dive medicine questions, equipment updates, Instructor Trainer Workshops to teach divers oxygen first aid, training programs for automated external defibrillators (AEDs) for scuba diving, announcements of other DAN programs, and continuing medical education courses for medical personnel, dive masters and dive instructors, insurance plan for members, and more. (Nonprofit organization)

GIDEON

www.cyinfo.com

Global Infectious Disease and Epidemiology Network: Tropical medicine database providing epidemiological data on country-specific infectious diseases for over 200 countries; software program linking patient exposure history and clinical profile with epidemiological data generates list of differential diagnoses; therapeutic and microbiology modules. (Subscription)

iJET TRAVEL INTELLIGENCE

www.ijet.com

Online intelligence resource related to all aspects of travel: health, safety, and security; social, political, and economic conditions; transportation; environmental hazards; travel health insurance; custom reports; or corporate programs by request. (Subscriptions, contracts)

IMMUNIZATION ACTION COALITION (IAC) AND THE HEPATITIS B COALITION

www.immunize.org/

Publishes free e-mail newsletter on immunizations and immunization programs called the "IAC EXPRESS"; IAC's "Screening Questionnaire for Child and Teen Immunization" covering contraindications and precautions to vaccine administration is available at the website, including translations into foreign languages (e.g., Chinese, Turkish).

INTERNATIONAL ASSOCIATION OF MEDICAL ASSISTANCE FOR TRAVELERS (IAMAT)

www.iamat.org

Worldwide Directory of English-Speaking Physicians, World Climate Charts, Malaria Risk Charts, and other travel medicine information based on CDC and WHO information and expert sources. (Non-profit organization, supported by voluntary donations)

INTERNATIONAL SOCIETY OF TRAVEL MEDICINE (ISTM)

www.istm.org

Journal of Travel Medicine, International Scientific Meetings, Directory of Travel Clinics among Society members, Listserv for members, Co-sponsor with CDC of GeoSentinel Project, a worldwide surveillance network for diseases of travelers; ISTM Certificate Program covering the body of knowledge for internationl travel medicine to commence in 2003. (Membership fee; Registration fees for Scientific Meetings, and other activities)

MINNESOTA DEPARTMENT OF HEALTH

www.health.state.mn.us/divs/dpc/adps/forgnvac.htm

Website resource for information on vaccines available and used worldwide. (Public health agency)

MORBIDITY AND MORTALITY WEEKLY REPORT (MMWR)

www.cdc.gov/mmwr

Weekly epidemiology reports and public health news from the Centers for Disease Control and Prevention (CDC), including international health topics. Visit the website to obtain a free electronic subscription. (Public health agency)

PROMED-MAIL

www.healthnet.org/programs/promed.html

Free e-mail list established by the Federation of American Scientists to provide health workers with rapid information on outbreaks of emerging infectious diseases, including pathogens involving humans, animals, and plants; information is screened by volunteer moderators who are specialists in infectious diseases. (Nonprofit organization, supported by donations)

PUBLIC HEALTH FOUNDATION

http://bookstore.phf.org

Distance learning resources created by U.S. Department of Health and Social Services program projects, for public health professionals: resource materials, self-study courses, computer-based training programs, videotapes, video courses, and slide sets. The titles offered cover principles of epidemiology, communicable disease control, vaccines, environmental health, and public health topics including tropical public health, microbiology, parasitology, and vector-borne diseases. (Domestic and international orders)

THE MEDICAL LETTER, ADVICE FOR TRAVELERS

www.medicalletter.com

Tropimed software program for guiding clinical services to individual travel clinic patients based on travel medicine recommendations from international experts. United States version of software program widely used in Europe. (Subscription)

THE TRAVEL MEDICINE ADVISOR

www.ahc.com

Edited by F. Bia with contributing authors. Published by American Health Consultants, Atlanta, GA. Core information in loose-leaf binder format with chapters providing comprehensive travel medicine information, frequently updated. The subscription includes the The Travel Medicine Alert monthly newsletter, which provides updates on travel and tropical medicine topics, with CME program questions available for approved CME credit hours. (Subscription)

TRAVAX AND ENCOMPASS

www.shoreland.com

TRAVAX travel health information programs for travel clinics: clinical algorithms, country-by-country health conditions, disease risk maps, assessments of medical facilities abroad, and other reference materials organized in a looseleaf binder format with selection of weekly or monthly update service (Subscription); *Travel and Routine Immunizations,* 11th edition (updated annually) included with subscription or may be purchased separately; also, ***ENCOMPASS*** custom travel medicine programs for corporate medical departments and occupational health clinics. Published by Shoreland, Inc, Milwaukee, WI. (Contract) (Commercial)

TRAVEL HEALTHY NEWSLETTER

www.travmed.com

Monthly newsletter written for the traveling public and their health advisors. Clear journalistic style, focus on health advice of great interest to the international traveler. Edited by K. Neumann with contributing authors. Published by Travel Medicine, Inc., MA. (Subscription)

TRAVELHEALTH, ON-LINE

www.tripprep.com

Frequently updated country-by-country health conditions, recommendations for vaccines and malaria chemoprophylaxis, disease risk maps, and summary of U.S. Department of State consular information. Published by Shoreland, Milwaukee, WI. Other products include TRAVAX travel health information programs for travel clinics (Subscription), and TRAVAX Encompass custom travel medicine programs for corporations (License).

WILDERNESS MEDICAL SOCIETY

www.wms.org

Wilderness and Environmental Medicine journal; scientific meetings, continuing education courses, and wilderness workshops throughout the year;

membership composed of physicians, allied health specialists and other individuals concerned with wilderness medicine and the benefits, health, safety and medical care of the individual in the wilderness. (Membership fee; Registration fees for Scientific Meetings and other activities) (Professional society)

APPENDIX

Travel Medicine Products

CHINOOK MEDICAL GEAR
www.chinookmed.com
Medical gear, survival gear, and high tech equipment for travel, camping, sports, marine, and high altitude medical needs, including adventure travel and expeditions; pre-packed and custom medical kits, packs, water treatment devices, books and videos; website features photos and short stories from travelers, list of international travel medicine clinics, and schedule of wilderness and travel medicine meetings. (Commercial)

LIFE LINE CD
www.LifeLineCD.com
Portable copy of medical records on a mini compact disk. (Commercial)

MAGELLAN'S
www.magellans.com
Accessories, appliances, luggage, clothing, medical kits, books, videos and other travel supplies for international travelers; unique products for travel exercise, hygiene and comfort; website provides free articles and helpful travel tips. (Commercial)

MEDIC ALERT FOUNDATION
www.medicalert.org
The MedicAlert Foundation provides an emergency medical information system for its membership: the MedicAlert Service makes a member's personal medical history accessible anywhere in the world, and facilitates communication with family members and personal physician; members can obtain additional coverage for medical evacuation and repatriation through the Travel Plus program. (Nonprofit organization)

MEDIC I.D.
sales@medic-id.com
Personal medical information on stainless steel bracelets or necklaces, with sizes for children and adults; complimentary wallet medical information card. (Commercial) (Not affiliated with MedicAlert Foundation)

TRAVEL MEDICINE, INC.
www.travmed.com
Comprehensive selection of water filters, medical kits, mosquito nets, insect repellents, and other products to ensure comfort and safety while

traveling; publishes the *International Travel Health Guide—2002* by S. Rose (updated annually), and the *Traveling Healthy Newsletter* (previously mentioned), and the *Kids on the Go* newsletter; website features news from the world of travel medicine, including disease risk information from the WHO, CDC, and International Society of Travel Medicine, and travel clinic directory. (Commercial)

APPENDIX

Sources for Travel Medical Insurance and/or Medical Evacuation

ACCESS AMERICA
www.accessamerica.com
866-807-3982

DIVERS ALERT NETWORK (D.A.N.)
www.diversalertnetwork.org
800-446-2671

INTERNATIONAL SOS ASSISTANCE
www.internationalsos.com
800-523-8930

MEDEX ASSISTANCE
www.medexassist.com
888-633-3900

MEDIC ALERT FOUNDATION
www.medicalert.org
800-863-3427

MEDJET ASSISTANCE
www.medjetassistance.com
800-963-3538

TRAVELEX
www.travelex.com
800-228-9792

TRAVEL GUARD
www.travelguard.com
800-826-4919

Temperature Conversion

Temperatures are commonly expressed as Fahrenheit or Celsius temperature scale degrees.

To convert a Fahrenheit temperature into degrees Celsius:

$$Tc = (5/9) \times (Tf - 32)$$

To convert a Celsius temperature into degrees Fahrenheit:

$$Tf = (9/5) \times (Tc + 32)$$

Quick Chart—Celsius to Fahrenheit

°C	°F
0	32.0
35	95.0
36	96.8
37	98.6
38	100.4
39	102.2
40	104.0
41	105.8
100	212.0

Tc, Temperature in degrees Celsius; *Tf*, temperature in degrees Fahrenheit.
Adapted from "TexLoc Quick Reference—Celsius to Fahrenheit," TexLoc, Ltd, Mfg of Precision Fluoroplastic Tubing & Heat Shrink, Fort Worth, Texas: www.texloc.com/closet (accessed 5/18/02).

INDEX

Page numbers followed by f indicate figures; t, tables; b, boxes.

B

C

D

E

J

K

L

O

P

Q

R

S

U

V

W

X

Y

Z